PEDIATRICS

PEDIATRICS

Robert A. Wood, M.D.

*Assistant Professor of Pediatrics, Division of
Pediatric Allergy and Immunology
The Johns Hopkins Hospital
Baltimore, Maryland*

Patricia Fosarelli, M.D.

*Assistant Professor of Pediatrics
Division of General Pediatrics
The Johns Hopkins Hospital
Baltimore, Maryland*

Mark Hudak, M.D.

*Assistant Professor of Pediatrics
Division of Neonatology
The Johns Hopkins Hospital
Baltimore, Maryland*

Alan Lake, M.D.

*Assistant Professor of Pediatrics
Division of Pediatric Gastroenterology
The Johns Hopkins Hospital
Baltimore, Maryland*

John Modlin, M.D.

*Assistant Professor of Pediatrics
Division of Pediatric Infectious Diseases
The Johns Hopkins Hospital
Baltimore, Maryland*

J. B. Lippincott Company
Philadelphia
London • Mexico City • New York • St. Louis • São Paulo • Sydney

Acquisitions Editor: Charles McCormick
Editorial Assistant: Robin Levin
Manuscript Editor: Helen Ewan
Indexer: Nancy Newman
Design Coordinator: Paul Fry
Cover Design: Rita Naughton
Production Manager: Kathleen P. Dunn
Production Supervisor: Charlene Squibb
Compositor: TSI Graphics
Printer/Binder: R.R. Donnelley Sons Company

6 5 4 3 2 1

Library of Congress Cataloging-in-Publication Data

Pediatrics.

   Includes bibliographies and index.
   1. pediatrics.   I. Wood, Robert A. (Robert Alan)
[DNLM: 1. Pediatrics. WS 100 P3704]
RJ47.P44 1988   618.92   88-626
ISBN 0-397-50854-9

The authors and publisher have exerted every effort to ensure that drug selection and dosage set forth in this text are in accord with current recommendations and practice at the time of publication. However, in view of ongoing research, changes in government regulations, and the constant flow of information relating to drug therapy and drug reactions, the reader is urged to check the package insert for each drug for any change in indications and dosage and for added warnings and precautions. This is particularly important when the recommended agent is a new or infrequently employed drug.

Foreword

Too often the student of pediatrics, in an effort to learn the essentials of the subject as rapidly as possible, turns to an outline or digest. The student gains only a superficial knowledge of this rich and exciting area of medicine. Recognizing the fact that the students need to know "what they have to know," *Pediatrics* focuses, with appropriate detail, on those subjects students or house officers will most likely encounter in their first exposure to pediatrics. This first encounter may occur in either the hospital or the out-patient setting. *Pediatrics* is intended to serve as a compass, and not a compendium, a companion for that first clinical encounter. The authors, all members of a single department, share a similar approach to the principles and problems and provide a concise and coherent foundation for the student of pediatrics.

Frank Oski

Preface

As with all medical specialties, the field of pediatrics has seen an extraordinary growth in information in recent years. This rapid growth has made the task of medical education increasingly difficult, particularly for medical students and residents as they embark on their training. One must constantly strive to distinguish that information which is basic and fundamental to the practice of pediatrics from that which is more esoteric or of less practical importance. *Pediatrics* was written in response to that challenge.

In *Pediatrics*, we have sought to compose a text that will best serve medical students, residents, nurses, and other health professionals in obtaining a basic education in pediatric medicine. After initial chapters on health maintenance and the general approach to the pediatric patient, subsequent sections deal with a specific symptom or disease process. Particular emphasis is placed on pathophysiology and diagnosis in an effort to provide a better, and hopefully longer-lasting, understanding of each topic discussed.

This book is by no means intended to replace the comprehensive textbooks of pediatrics that are available. It should instead serve as a foundation upon which more detailed information can later be added. To this end, reading lists are provided for each chapter to guide the reader to more in-depth discussions of each topic.

We hope that *Pediatrics* stimulates the reader's appetite for the care of our youth, providing the background for an insight into their health and their disease.

Robert A. Wood, M.D.
Patricia Fosarelli, M.D.
Mark Hudak, M.D.

Alan Lake, M.D.
John Modlin, M.D.

Contents

VII. Gastroenterology

VIII. Renal System

IX. Cardiology

X. Pulmonology

XI. Endocrinology and Metabolism

XII. Hematology

XIII. Oncology

XIV.   Neurology

XV.   Rheumatology

Appendix

Index

Part I: Health Maintenance

1

Immunizations

At the beginning of this century, infectious illnesses killed millions of children in this country. With improved hygienic practices, better nutrition, and the development of vaccines against agents commonly causing fatal disease, infectious diseases have become less important reasons for morbidity and mortality in U.S. children. However, the same diseases against which modern immunizations protect so well are still highly prevalent and deadly in Third World countries, where poor hygiene, poverty, overcrowding, inadequate nutrition, and a lack of proper immunization practices exist. It is possible, even in this country, that some of the diseases that are preventable through adequate immunization might again become important causes of morbidity and mortality if parents, either through ignorance or fear, neglect the immunization of their children.

THE DISEASES AGAINST WHICH ROUTINE IMMUNIZATIONS PROTECT

Table 1-1 lists the vaccines commonly administered in the United States and their features.

Diphtheria

Diphtheria is caused by the gram-positive rod, *Corynebacterium diphtheriae*. After an incubation period of 1 to 6 days, the organism produces an exotoxin that causes tissue necrosis, inflammation, and exudation. A membrane consisting of necrotic tissue, blood cells, and fibrinous material frequently covers the tonsils, pharynx, and larynx. The course of the illness depends on the severity of the toxemia and its location (nasal, tonsillar, pharyngeal, laryngeal) of major involvement. Complications include myocarditis and neuritis. The mortality rate is 30% to 50%; with the administration of antitoxin, this rate drops to less than 5%. Penicillin and erythromycin are usually effective against the organism.

Pertussis

Pertussis is caused by the gram-negative rod, *Bordetella pertussis*. The organism attaches to respiratory epithelial cells, inhibiting their ciliary activity. Various toxins are also produced. After an incubation period of 7 to 10 days, the patient experiences the catarrhal phase, characterized by coryza, sneezing, cough, and fever. After 1 to 2 weeks, the par-

(Text continues on p. 6.)

3

Table 1–1. Immunizations

Name of Vaccine	Diseases (and their descriptions) Protected Against	Description of Vaccine	Route of Administration
DPT	*Diphtheria*—caused by *Corynebacterium diphtheriae,* which elaborates an exotoxin. Characterized by a membranous pharyngitis, tonsillitis, laryngitis. Cardiac and neurologic sequelae are common. Death may result in 10%.	Diphtheria toxoid (inactivated)	IM
	Pertussis—caused by *Bordetella pertussis.* Has a catarrhal phase that proceeds to paroxysmal cough with the characteristic "whoop" and post-tussive vomiting. Respiratory and CNS sequelae occur. Death may result, especially in young infants, owing to respiratory compromise.	Pertussis vaccine	
	Tetanus—caused by *Clostridium tetani,* which produces an exotoxin causing spasms and contractures of skeletal muscles. Initially, the head and neck are involved, but later all muscle groups are involved. There is a 60% fatality rate.	Tetanus toxoid (inactivated)	
TOPV, IPV	Polio—caused by poliovirus, an enterovirus. Most cases are mild viral illnesses with fever, headache, sore throat, abdominal pains, and myalgias. Some patients develop muscle weakness or paralysis due to viral destruction of anterior motor cells in the spinal cord. Case fatality is 5% to 10%.	TOPV trivalent live attenuated poliovirus vaccine (Sabin)	Orally
		IPV inactivated poliovirus vaccine (Salk)	IM
MMR	*Measles*—caused by an RNA virus. Characterized by high fever, coryza, conjunctivitis, cough, and a generalized maculopapular rash. Respiratory and CNS sequelae occur. Death is common in developing countries.	Live attenuated measles vaccine	Subcutaneously
	Mumps—caused by a paramyxovirus. Characterized by enlarged salivary glands, especially the parotids. Meningoencephalitis, orchitis, oophoritis, and pancreatitis are associated findings.	Live attenuated mumps vaccine	
	Rubella—caused by an RNA virus. Characterized by a 3-day rash with generalized lymphadenopathy; other symptoms are minimal. Disease is of importance because of its devastating effects on the developing fetus.	Live attenuated rubella vaccine	
Haemophilus influenzae	*Haemophilus influenzae,* a gram-negative rod, causes a number of serious infections, such as meningitis, epiglottitis, sepsis, pneumonia, and septic arthritis.	Capsular polysaccharide	Subcutaneously

Dose	Timetable		Common Side Effects	Contraindications
	Primary Immunization	*Boosters*		
0.5 ml	2, 4, 6 mo	18 mo and 4–5 yr; Td q 10 yr	Redness, swelling, tenderness at injection site	Pertussis is contraindicated in progressive CNS disease or when there is a history of screaming fits, high fever, or seizures after previous DPT immunizations.
0.5 ml	2 and 4 mo	18 mo and 4–5 yr	Rare (1/3 million doses) paralytic disease in recipients or their contacts	Pregnancy—if absolutely necessary, use OPV Immunodeficiency—if absolutely necessary, use IPV
0.5 ml	2, 4, 6 mo	18 mo and 4–5 yr	Local reaction at site of injection	
0.5 ml	15 mo	None	Pain, redness, swelling at injection site; evanescent generalized rash 10–14 days after injection	Pregnancy (all); febrile illness (all); tuberculosis (measles); recent reception of immune serum globulin (ISG) (all); immunodeficiency (all)
0.5 ml	2–5 yr	None	Local reaction at injection site	

oxysmal stage begins; this stage can last up to 10 weeks. The cough now consists of several short, staccato "coughs" followed by an inspiratory "whoop." During these paroxysms of cough, the child may become cyanotic. Vomiting frequently accompanies the paroyxsms. The convalescent stage marks the gradual cessation of coughing and vomiting. Complications include pneumonia and seizures. The mortality rate is 1% to 2%. Antibiotic therapy (ampicillin or erythromycin) might be indicated for children younger than 3 years.

Tetanus

Tetanus is caused by the gram-positive rod *Clostridium tetani*, which frequently is found in soil. The organism usually enters the body through a break in the patient's skin. The incubation period is 5 to 14 days. *C. tetani* produces an exotoxin which causes tonic spasms and contractions of the skeletal muscles; especially noteworthy is the contraction of the jaw ("lockjaw"). Complications include respiratory embarrassment. The mortality rate is 60%. Treatment is with antitoxin and penicillin.

Polio

Poliomyelitis is caused by the polio virus. It enters orally, multiplies in the intestine, spreads to regional lymph nodes, enters the bloodstream, and finally reaches the central nervous system (CNS). Polio infection can be inapparent, nonparalytic, or paralytic. The milder forms produce an illness similar to that produced by other enteroviruses. The onset of the parlytic form is similar to that of the milder forms, but after the patient seems to have been recuperating for several days, evidence of CNS invasion appears, accompanied by muscle pain. Complications include respiratory embarrassment and bulbar in-

volvement. The mortality rate of the paralytic form is 5% to 10%. Treatment is supportive.

Measles (Rubeola)

Measles is caused by a paramyxovirus. The incubation period is 10 to 12 days. The features of the disease are high fever, coryza, conjunctivitis, cough, Koplik's spots (red spots with blue-white elevations on the buccal and labial mucosa), and a maculopapular rash appearing on the 4th day and reaching its maximal intensity on the 6th day. Complications include pneumonia, layryngotracheitis, encephalitis, and subacute sclerosing panencephalitis. The mortality rate is high in developing countries.

Mumps

Mumps is caused by a paramyxovirus. The incubation period is 16 to 18 days. In 30% to 40% of patients, the infection is inapparent. In the other patients, fever and parotitis develop. The parotid involvement is usually bilateral (75%), reaches its peak in 3 days, and resolves by the 6th day. Orchitis and meningoencephalitis can also occur. Complications include deafness, neurologic sequelae, myocarditis, and arthritis. Fatalities are rare.

Rubella

Rubella is caused by a togavirus. The incubation period is 14 to 21 days. The disease is characterized by a generalized lymphadenopathy (especially the suboccipital, postauricular, and cervical groups), low-grade fever, and a maculopapular rash that lasts 1 to 5 days (usually 3). Most patients are only mildly ill. Complications include arthritis, encephalitis, and purpura. The real danger is to the fetus; the congenital rubella syndrome is characterized by a myriad of symptoms and signs, including growth retardation, eye defects, deafness, cardiac lesions, CNS pathology, and hepatosplenomegaly.

Haemophilus influenzae type B

Haemophilus influenzae type B is a gram-negative rod. It is a cause of many serious childhood infections, including sepsis, meningitis, epiglottitis, pneumonia, and septic arthritis.

Tuberculosis

Tuberculosis is caused by the acid-fast bacillus *Mycobacterium tuberculi*. The disease has been discussed elsewhere in this book.

Tuberculosis skin testing, while not a vaccine, is included in Table 1-1 because, like vaccines, it is an important part of disease prevention and health maintenance in the pediatric population.

BIBLIOGRAPHY

Committee on Infectious Diseases: Report of the Committee of Infectious Diseases, 12th ed. Elk Grove, IL, American Academy of Pediatrics, 1986

DeAngelis C: Immunizations. In DeAngelis C (ed): Pediatric Primary Care, 3rd ed, Boston: Little Brown and Co., 1984; pp 147, (Table 5–1), 153–159.

Krugman S, Katz S: Infectious Diseases of Children. St Louis, CV Mosby, 1981

M. 16-18
M. 10-12
R. 14-21

M 10-12   11
M 16-18   17
R 14-21   18

2

Anticipatory Guidance

Anticipatory guidance is the age-specific advice about expected developmental advances and common physical and emotional problems that the physician gives the parent (or the adolescent). Such advice helps the parent to anticipate changes or problems before they arise and to be prepared when they do occur.

The following table lists the common areas of anticipatory guidance. When the pediatric patient is very young, most anticipatory guidance deals with achievement of various motor skills; when the patient is older, most of the advice deals with psychosocial issues and sexuality.

Developmental Milestones	Related Anticipatory Guidance
Early Infancy	
1. Infant learns to roll, gains good head control.	1. Infant never should be left unattended on bed, sofa, table, or tub.
2. Infant develops different cries for different purposes.	2. Infant does not need to be fed each time he cries.
3. Infant gradually sleeps less, becomes more interested in surroundings, coos when spoken to.	3. Infant should be stimulated positively by human contact, speech, and inanimate objects in crib.
4. Infant consumes more formula/seems hungry.	4. Most infants can subsist on formula alone for the first 6 months of life. If infant consumes excessive amounts of formula (*i.e.,* >32 oz/day), rice cereal can be added to diet after 2 months of age; fruits and vegetables after 4 months of age. Do not put cereal into a bottle but feed by spoon. Do not introduce more than one new food at a time (*i.e.,* within 3 days' time) in case the infant suffers an intolerance to it.
5. Maternally derived immunoglobulins decrease as infant is building his immunoglobulin arsenal.	5. Infant may begin to become ill as he is exposed to multiple pathogens.
6. Infant becomes old enough to receive immunizations.	6. Discuss common and worrisome side effects of immunizations.

Developmental Milestones	Related Anticipatory Guidance
7. Infant may develop episodic (daily) crying spells (colic).	7. Discuss suggestions for coping with colic. These include rocking the infant, rubbing his abdomen or applying heat to it, taking the infant for a ride in the car.
8. Infant's stool pattern changes from frequent to less so.	8. Normal bowel movements may occur daily or every other day and require no intervention if the infant is not in pain. If constipation is a problem, adding 1–2 tsp Karo syrup to several bottles of formula each day usually helps.
9. Infant's presence evokes sibling rivalry and maternal stress.	9. Parents should include sibling in infant's care and should do things with the sibling alone. Parents need time together, and mother needs time to herself.
10. Infant rides in car.	10. Infant should be in car seat.

Late Infancy/Toddlerhood

1. Child learns to sit alone, walk with support, and walk alone.	1. Keep dangerous objects, household cleaning products, and medicines out of child's reach and locked up. Fence off stairway entrances. Place plastic caps in electrical sockets that are not in use. Keep child away from hot objects on the stove.
2. Child enjoys playing in tub.	2. Never leave child unattended in tub.
3. Child develops teeth.	3. Teething may be painful—teething rings may help. Parent may begin to brush teeth gently to teach child good dental hygiene. Child can begin to eat meats and table foods.
4. Child puts everything in mouth and is inattentive while eating.	4. Keep dangerous or small objects away from child. Do not feed raisins, nuts, popcorn, or hot dogs (objects most often aspirated). Cut food into small pieces. Do not permit child to walk/run while eating.
5. Child's appetite decreases.	5. This is normal at the onset of toddlerhood. Do not force child to eat.
6. Child prefers "junk" food to nutritious food.	6. Parents should be firm and should not permit child to eat "junk" if he refuses his regular meals.
7. Child's milk/formula intake decreases.	7. This is normal. Other acceptable fluids include juices of all types. Sugary or carbonated beverages are unacceptable.
8. Child develops a temper.	8. Temper tantrums are a result of the child's attempts to develop autonomy. They are best managed by ignoring them. If the child's temper outbursts are accompanied by biting, scratching, hitting, or kicking, they are best handled by parental firmness indicating that this is unacceptable behavior.
9. Child develops stranger anxiety.	9. This is normal. Have the parents remind well-meaning relatives and friends of this so that their feelings will be spared.
10. Child develops separation anxiety.	10. Child is beginning to see himself as separate from parents. Since the concept of object permanence is not fully rooted, child becomes upset when separated from parents. Parents should gently remind child that they will return.

Developmental Milestones	**Related Anticipatory Guidance**
11. Child does not want to go to bed and screams for hours.	11. Again, the child does not want to be separated from his parents, may be afraid of the dark, and may hate to give up all the fun he has during waking hours. Bedtime rituals (reading a story, playing a game) help child to have a sense of control. A nightlight may also help. If the child screams when in bed, he should be checked for a wet/soiled diaper, or evidence of pain—while still in his crib. If these are present, correct them. If they are not present, the child should be reassured. He should not be picked up, played with, or taken to the parents' bed. The parent then leaves. He/she may make another visit to the child's room if he continues to cry, but the visit should be conducted the same as the first visit. After 2 visits, the child can be allowed to cry himself to sleep.
12. Child wants to go to bed with bottle.	12. Child can have a bottle before he goes to bed but should not be put to bed with a bottle (danger of aspiration/milk bottle caries).
13. Child is learning to talk and likes to repeat words.	13. Child's receptive language is greater than expressive language; hence, the child understands more than he is given credit for. Parents need to monitor their use of profanity. Parents should not laugh (in child's presence) if he uses undesirable words but gently explain that those are not nice words. Parents should monitor the television programs the child is exposed to and should encourage educational programs such as *Sesame Street,* which teaches by repetition. Parents should read to child, talk to him, and encourage him to name the object he wants.
14. Child has nightmares.	14. Limit exciting activities, including television programs and videos.
15. Child masturbates.	15. This is probably a universal phenomenon. If the child does not masturbate in public or excessively, ignore it.
16. Child will not be toilet trained.	16. Child is not neurologically ready for toilet training until the end of the second year of life. Pressuring the child to perform to parental expectations before he is ready will only lead to mutual frustration.

Early–Middle Childhood

1. Child can ride tricycle/bicycle, run, jump rope, climb stairs, and get around on his own; wants to use household instruments (knife, scissors) that parents use.	1. Teach child vehicular and pedestrian safety rules. When the child is younger, he should always be supervised when climbing, swinging, and riding. Forbid young child to use knife or sharp scissors.
2. Child is friendly and talkative.	2. Teach child not to talk to strangers.
3. Child enjoys riding in car.	3. Make sure child buckles seat belt.
4. Child does not want to go to school/day-care center.	4. Separation anxiety is frightening at any age. The child may feel that his parent is never coming back (abandonment) or that something evil is going to happen to his parent if is not there to stop it.

Developmental Milestones	Related Anticipatory Guidance
	Sometimes, a child does not want to go to school/day-care center because he dislikes his teacher, classmates, or the bus, or is afraid of failing. Find out the cause of child's reluctance and deal with it. Be firm and gentle: the child should go to school/day-care center and not be permitted to stay home.
5. The boy has become "Mama's little man"; the girl has become "Daddy's little girl".	5. In the preschool years, attraction to the parent of the opposite sex (Oedipus complex) is a normal developmental stage. Parents should not become jealous or angry, should not make a big issue of it (it *will* pass), and should not strongly encourage the behavior when the "scorned" parent is not present. The child needs, loves, and wants *both* parents.
6. Child spends most of his free time watching television.	6. Watch television with the child to provide guidance. Limit the amount and type of programs that the child can watch.
7. School-age child wants money.	7. Provide household chores so that child can earn money for things that he wants.
8. Child is a "picky eater" and loves "junk" food.	8. Insist that child eat what is provided at mealtime. If he refuses the family dinner, he should not be allowed to eat "junk" food to avoid "going to bed hungry."
9. Child masturbates.	9. This is probably universal. If he masturbates in public or constantly (an indication of anxiety), tell him that such behavior is private and inappropriate in public; try to determine why he is so anxious.
10. School-age child is frustrated with his abilities in school, sports, and socially.	10. Accentuate his positive qualities and reassure him that everyone has limitations. Tell him pertinent experiences from your own life. Do not harass him about his grades or compare him to his siblings.
11. Child is afraid of being abducted or sexually abused.	11. When younger, children should always be supervised. Parents should know where their children are or are going and their estimated time of arrival. Child should know his name, address, phone number and parent's names. He should be taught how to answer the telephone and not to answer the door if the parents are out. Child should not wear or carry items with his name on them. Child should be at home before dark. Parents should know child's friend and should screen babysitters carefully. If a child says he has been abused, he should be believed.
12. Child is constipated.	12. Frequently, merely limiting his intake of junk foods (high carbohydrate) and encouraging ingestion of fruits and fiber will relieve the child's constipation.
13. Child likes to be with other children, likes to play sports.	13. When he is old enough, encourage child to join a service/school organization (Scouts) or to join a team. However, do not push him into sports or criticize his performance.
14. Siblings fight.	14. Most of this is normal if the action does not get violent. Parents should ensure they are not contribut-

Developmental Milestones

Related Anticipatory Guidance

ing to this behavior by always taking one child's side or comparing one child with another.

15. Child wants to know where he came from, how babies are made, what sex is, etc.

15. The parent should keep calm and not become flustered. Information should be geared to the child's developmental level and need not be a treatise on the history of human sexuality. Find out what the child already knows and what he specifically wants to know. Ideally, this topic has been one of open communication in the past.

Preadolescence and Adolescence

1. Embarrassed about body.

1. Pubertal changes are beginning to occur, and child is uncomfortable with his or her body. Be patient.

2. Wears wild/unusual clothes.

2. Peer pressure and peer-group identity are very strong pulls on the teenager. Set dress standards that are reasonable but not restrictive.

3. Enjoys rock music, music videos, and portable audio cassette players.

3. Part of being a teenager. Limits *may* be set on how loud the stereo can be played and how long music videos can be watched, and when these activities can be indulged in (*e.g.,* only on weekends, only for 1 hour per day or when homework is done, etc).

4. Wants a later curfew, wants to go places parent does not approve of, etc. ("Everyone else is doing it.")

4. Set limits that both parents can agree on and live with, but be flexible and discuss the situation with the teenager. Always listen to his ideas. Contrary to popular opinion, teenagers need and want appropriate limit-setting by parents.

5. Shows interest in opposite sex.

5. This is quite normal. Younger teenagers should date in a group before pairing off.

6. Wants to "go steady."

6. Encourage the teenager to grow through relationships with many individuals. Discuss the pros and cons of partner exclusivity in adolescence.

7. Parent discovers child is sexually active (or pregnant).

7. Avoid initial inclination to vent anger. Discuss reasons that people are physically intimate and let teenagers present their views on this. Reassure teenagers that they should not be pressured into sexual relations if they are not ready. Discuss need to safeguard against pregnancy and venereal diseases. If girl is pregnant, seek medical consultation.

8. Teenager suddenly loses interest in school, friends, and home, has behavior problems, or is losing weight.

8. Teenager may be depressed, suicidal, or using ilicit drugs. Discuss problem calmly with teenager; may need professional help.

9. Parent discovers teenager is using drugs or alcohol regularly.

9. As above.

10. Teenager is argumentative, questions authority, refuses to accept criticisms, suggestions, or compliments.

10. Developmental task of adolescence is to establish one's identity separate from one's parents. Some of this behavior is expected, but rudeness need not be tolerated.

11. Teenager wants to quit school, get a job, or live on his own.

11. Provide teenager with hard financial facts. Encourage completion of school with, perhaps, after school, weekend, or summer employment.

Developmental Milestones	Related Anticipatory Guidance
12. Teenager says he is gay.	12. Be open and understanding; seek professional help.
13. Teenager vacillates between acting like an adult and acting like a child.	13. Autonomy permits one to do what one wants, but it can be hard and lonely. Being a child who is taken care of is sometimes attractive to the developing adult.

3

Nutrition

The process of physiologic growth in childhood involves the complex interaction of nutritional, genetic, and environmental factors. Nutritional requirements obviously vary with age, and diet must therefore be adjusted accordingly to achieve optimal growth. Although this process is successfully completed in the majority of children in developed countries, the incidence of nutritional disorders remains unacceptably high, often in spite of abundant resources. In this chapter, we will discuss three common nutritional disorders encountered in pediatrics—failure to thrive, obesity, and anorexia nervosa.

FAILURE TO THRIVE

There are four major growth tasks of childhood. The first is physiologic growth, in which the child achieves a rate or velocity of growth consistent with that of other children his age and the genetic potential of his family. The second is psychological growth, or the child's recognition of the significance of increasing age and maturity on his own behavior. The third is cognitive growth, or the intellectual achievement of the child. The last is social growth, or the growth in interactive skills. The major emphasis of this chapter will be on physiologic growth, but the failure to achieve the other growth tasks are often of equal or greater long-term concern. It is also important to recognize that short stature alone does not equate with failure to thrive, and that significant reduction in growth velocity may occur without the child's falling below the "magic third percentile" in cumulative growth.

Figure 3-1 summarizes the factors necessary for the achievement of normal growth in childhood. The interaction of a large number of variables is clearly apparent. The significance of each factor will vary as a function of age, being maximal in infancy and adolescence, the times of peak growth velocity.

Worldwide, the major factor is the first, suboptimal nutrient intake, attributed to economic and nutrient deprivation. Sociocultural factors, usually due to lack of awareness of optimal intake, are, regrettably as prevalent in advanced societies as in the Third World. For example, in this category would fall inappropriate parental restriction in dietary intake, as

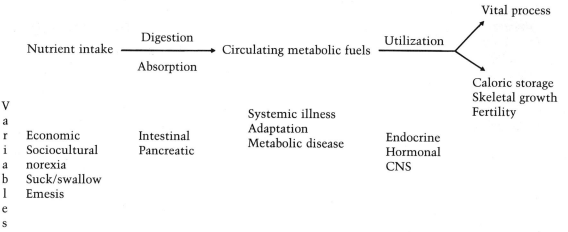

FIGURE 3–1. *Factors in normal growth.*

occurs in fear of childhood obesity, an increasingly recognized cause of suboptimal growth.

In the same category of reduced intake are the organic and psychological causes of anorexia. Table 3-1 summarizes the organic components to anorexia and includes examples of clinical syndromes in which they are prevalent.

The next phase in the pathway to normal growth is restricted by any condition in which maldigestion and/or malabsorption limits the uptake of nutrient delivered. In this category are children with cystic fibrosis, celiac disease, and short bowel syndrome.

The uptake of nutrient creates metabolic fuels. In some conditions, the demand for this fuel is increased, as in systemic illness, chronic cardiopulmonary disease, or hyperthyroidism. In other situations, the utilization of the nutrient is inefficient, as in malnutrition or metabolic disorders such as renal tubular acidosis, chronic alkalosis, or diabetes.

Fuel utilization is thus controlled primarily by hormonal factors, under the direct influence of the central nervous system (CNS).

Both primary and secondary alterations in hormonal levels may be seen. With restriction in fuel availability, vital processes are maintained at the expense of "luxury" functions such as caloric storage, skeletal growth, and fertility. The associated secondary hormonal adaptations to suboptimal intake include reduction in somatomedin-C and the sex steroids. End-organ unresponsiveness, as in chondrodystrophy, also limits growth in this phase.

One specific condition that combines many factors is the syndrome of deprivation dwarfism, in which psychosocial factors are combined with CNS defects in growth hormone secretion. These children present with severe growth failure in the absence of systemic disease. They often have bizarre eating habits, including pica, drinking from toilet bowls, or ingesting garbage. They may alternate polyphagia to the point of emesis with self-starvation. Behavioral features also include temper tantrums, sleep disturbance, enuresis, encopresis, and self-inflicted injury. Both motor and intellectual developmental delays are prominent. The diagnostic (and therapeutic)

Table 3–1. Organic Factors in Anorexia

Factors	Example
Oro-Motor function	Pierre-Robin, cleft palate
Esophageal dysfunction	TEF, achalasia, stricture
Delayed gastric emptying	Pylorospasm, stenosis
Small bowel dysfunction	Malrotation, obstipation
Inflammatory enteritis	Celiac, allergic, IBD
Cardiopulmonary	BPD, congestive failure
Metabolic	Adrenal insufficiency, hypothyroidism
Systemic	Lead poisoning, UTI
Neurologic	Hydrocephalus, degenerative

endeavor mandated is "parentectomy," or the removal of the child to a more nurturing environment. This must be combined with psychological and educational support of the parents. Dramatic acceleration of growth and development and improved behavior will be noted, and the secretion of growth hormone will return to normal.

Recognizing that nonorganic factors account for most cases of growth failure in childhood, the physician must initiate the evaluation by assessing the parent–child interaction, the appropriateness of the nutrient offered, and the response to increased caloric intake. The response to increased caloric intake may take 2 weeks to achieve steady weight gain and several months to achieve acceleration of height velocity. To achieve "catch-up" growth, the caloric demands approach 150% of that expected for age, in the absence of metabolic or chronic respiratory disease. Obviously, catch-up will only occur with organic disorders with the recognition and treatment of the underlying disease.

If increasing the caloric intake does not achieve the desired increase in growth or if the history suggests possible organic factors, the initial tests for organic failure to thrive are administered. These consist of screening studies as outlined in Table 3-2. Further studies, such as pyelograms, cardiograms, chest x-rays, malabsorption studies, or barium con-

Table 3–2. Screening Tests for Organic Factors in Growth Failure

Complete blood count with sedimentation rate
Urinalysis and culture
Stool examination for polys and blood
Serum electrolytes, urea nitrogen, and pH
Bone films for bone age and skeletal changes
Sweat test
Thyroid function tests
Buccal smear (females)

trast studies are individualized according to the results of these preliminary studies or unique features of the child's history or examination. It is critical that the physician maintain close communication with the family, explaining in a nonthreatening manner the indication for and desired result of each investigation. A team approach, incorporating the input of a nutritionist, social worker, and psychologist, is ideal. Hospitalization may be mandated to limit parental interference and allow close nursing observation of the child's feeding, bowel pattern, and behavior. Management of growth failure accounts for 3% to 5% of pediatric hospital admissions, although growth failure complicating the primary cause of admission is far more common.

While discussions of "failure to thrive" are usually limited to review of reductions in growth, it applies equally to those with excessive growth. When faced with the child with excessive growth rates, increased caloric intake is addressed first. One must also consider a number of endocrinologic and neurologic disorders, including familial or constitutional gigantism, Marfan's syndrome, neurofibromatosis, hyperthyroidism, adrenogenital virilization, Albright's syndrome, lipodystrophy, or acidophilic adenomas.

In all conditions of altered growth, it is essential to document carefully the responses to intervention. Weight, height, head circumference, midarm circumference, and triceps skin fold are considered the minimal anthropometric determinations. When possible, height should be plotted on a velocity curve rather than just the cumulative curve commonly employed. The early recognition of growth failure not only allows for early treatment of organic disease, but also minimizes the developmental and emotional sequelae of impaired growth.

OBESITY

Obesity is defined as a weight that is 20% greater than the child's ideal weight for age and sex. Not all large children are obese; some have large skeletons, and some have increased muscle mass. Therefore, all growth parameters must be taken into account before a diagnosis of obesity is entertained.

A child who has been obese since infancy probably has both hyperplasia and hypertrophy of adipose cells; a child whose obesity dates from childhood or adolescence has predominantly hypertrophy of adipose tissue. Because genetics plays a major role in obesity, a child has a 40% or 80% chance of obesity if one or both parents, respectively, are obese. A dysfunction of the hypothalamic satiety center may be operant in obese individuals so that they are not aware of normal satiety cues.

By adolescence, 12% of individuals are obese; most of these (>95%) were obese as children, and most (>80%) will become obese adults. Obese individuals tend to be rather sedentary, consume high-carbohydrate and high-fat diets, eat rapidly, eat a large amount at any given meal, eat when anxious or bored, and indulge in night eating or binge eating.

The obese child or adolescent may be ridiculed by peers and subsequently isolate himself as a response to his feelings of inferiority. In adolescence, obesity may be associated with fear of rejection by the opposite sex. Some older children and adolescents, feeling emotionally deprived, consume food as a substitute for love (parental or peer).

Eating habits may be firmly established early in infancy. Some parents feed their infants whenever they cry; others insist that children "clean their plates," or regularly provide multiple helpings of high-calorie food. Other families regularly ingest high-carbohydrate desserts or high-calorie "fast foods" (french fries, hamburgers, soda, milkshakes).

The obese child warrants a thorough history and physical examination. Important historical information includes complete daily diet history (*i.e.*, type and amount of foods/fluids ingested), amount and type of daily activity, mealtime behaviors, the child's birth weight and serial weights, the parents' and siblings' heights and weights, and the prevalence of obesity (and short stature) in other family members. The obese child's height and weight should be plotted against age. Triceps skin fold thickness may be measured in children and adolescents. The distribution of fat is noted. Despite the popular opinion that obesity is due to a "gland" problem, endocrine causes of obesity are uncommon and are rare if the child does not also have short stature. Unless there is some striking historical or physical finding suggesting an endocrine etiology, the obese child may require only a determination of serum cholesterol and lipoproteins.

The parents of infants can be urged not to feed the child every time he cries, to limit his intake of formula, and to limit his intake of sweetened fluids or other sugary foods. The parents of toddlers can be urged to limit his intake of "junk foods," to insist that he eat what the family eats during meals (in reasonable amounts), and to avoid the temptation of allowing the child to eat his favorite foods when he rejects the family's meal so that he "doesn't starve" or "doesn't go to bed hungry." These restrictions are extremely difficult to enforce if the parents themselves are obese.

The older child or adolescent who is obese will lose weight only if he is motivated to do so. No amount of coercion or scare tactics about the morbidity and mortality of obesity can make an unwilling child lose weight. His family must be supportive in attitude and in action; the amount of high-calorie food in the house should be limited, and the family should not consume sweets in front of the child if he is not permitted to eat them. The child's physician also should be supportive and be willing to see him for weight checks every week or two.

The obese individual may benefit from an organized peer group (such as Weight Watchers). He should be encouraged to be physically active and may require the company of family members to achieve this increased activity.

A realistic diet is important. If the caloric intake of a rapidly growing child can be stabilized and if he increases his exercise, he will lose weight. For children who are in a slow stage of growth or adolescents who have completed their growth, decreasing caloric intake by 300 calories/day is a reasonable goal. Eventually, the child should lose 1 to 2 pounds/week. He should be involved actively in this process by keeping his own diet record and by selecting foods (within dietary bounds) that he prefers. The parents can provide nutritious meals and low-calorie snacks. Small, frequent meals are preferable to large, infrequent ones. Finally, caloric intake should be reduced by first eliminating high-fat or high-carbohydrate foods.

Behavior modification techniques may be useful. The most successful of these is a personalized reward system for reasonable weight loss. The child must remain patient, since the process of weight loss is a slow one, with both successes and failures.

ANOREXIA NERVOSA

Anorexia nervosa is characterized by marked weight loss due to self-induced food restriction. Within several months, the patient (usually a female preadolescent or adolescent) loses 25% to 40% of her weight in the absence of obvious organic pathology. The female to male ratio is 10:1. As many as 4 to 5/1000 adolescent girls may be affected. There is a 5% mortality rate.

The typical patient is intelligent and motivated, a "perfect" child who wants to please her strict parents. Although she was of normal size, she decides that she is too heavy and begins to diet (frequently in response to a casual or teasing comment about her weight). Dieting becomes a morbid obsession. She may experience hunger but denies it. She claims to have no appetite or to become nauseous or bloated after eating minuscule amounts. She may become fanatical about adopting a strenuous exercise program. She cannot or refuses to see her own emaciated body and continues to believe she is fat. She denies that she has any problems other than that of obesity.

The girl may have occasional binges of eating (bulimia), after which she induces herself to vomit manually or by use of ipecac. She may also abuse laxatives. Paradoxically, she becomes interested in planning meals or buying food for her family or friends. As starvation and weight loss progress, she may become withdrawn and refuse to talk even to close friends.

If she has reached puberty, the anorexic is probably amenorrheic; most of these patients have low serum concentrations of luteinizing hormone, possibly due to an unexplained interruption of the pathway from the hypothalamus to the anterior pituitary. Other physical findings include hypotension, bradycardia, bradypnea, hypothermia, fine hair, and scaly skin. The patient has a normal bone age, thyroid-stimulating hormone (TSH), serum gonadotropin and growth hormone (GH) levels.

The differential diagnosis of anorexia nervosa includes malignancies, chronic infections, malabsorption (usually accompanied by steatorrhea and hypoproteinemia), adrenal insufficiency, hyperthyroidism, primary ovarian dysfunction (lack of secondary sex characteristics and menarche, increased [FSH]), and hypothalamic injury due to chronic encephalitis (presents with signs of panhypopituitarism). Evaluation is tailored to the history and physical findings.

Treatment of the anorexic patient is twofold. First, the girl's malnutrition must be corrected, and her normal physiologic state must be restored. Although some patients can be managed as outpatients, others require hospitalization and even tube-feedings. To encourage weight gain, the girl is deprived of all privileges; they are reinstituted one-by-one as she gains weight. Enumeration of the details of privilege reinstitution by weight gained is best formalized by a contract between physician and patient. Patient and parents should understand that the patient controls what she eats, whether she gains weight, and, hence, whether she regains her privileges or whether intravenous or nasogastric feeding is needed.

The second goal of therapy is to improve the patient's sense of autonomy and self-esteem. The girl with anorexia is a compliant, eager-to-please person whose parents have controlled her behavior through their overinvolvement with and overprotection of her. Food becomes an issue because the girl can control her own intake (or purge herself if she eats too much). Refusal of food is a rejection of the parents who provide it, since food is often equated with love. Malnutrition also prevents growth and, more importantly, the attainment of adult sexuality, autonomy, and responsibility.

The family must relinquish its control of the patient and allow the physicians (pediatrician and psychiatrist) to help her in their own way. Family counseling is a necessary adjunct to the girl's therapy, since anorexia nervosa is a manifestation of intrafamily dysfunction.

BIBLIOGRAPHY

Failure to Thrive

Barbero GJ, Shaheen E: Environmental failure to thrive: Clinical view. J Pediatr 71:639–644, 1967

Gardner LI: The endocrinology of abuse dwarfism. Am J Dis Child 131:505–507, 1977

Gordon M, Craithamel C, Post EM et al: Psychosocial aspects of constitutional short stature: Social competence, behavior problems, self-esteem, and family functioning. J. Pediatrics 101:477–480, 1982

Hannaway PJ: Failure to thrive—A study of 100 infants and children. Clin Pediatr 9:96–99, 1970

Powell GF, Brasel JA, Blizzard RM: Emotional deprivation and growth retardation simulating idiopathic hypopituitarism N Engl J Med 276:1271–1283, 1967

Pugliese MT, Lifshitz F, Grad G et al: Fear of obesity: A cause of short stature and delayed puberty. N Engl J Med 309:573–578, 1983

Rosenn DW, Loeb LS, Jura MB: Differentiation of organic and nonorganic failure to thrive. Pediatrics 66:698–704, 1980

Sills RH: Failure to thrive: The role of clinical and laboratory evaluation. Am J Dis Child 132:967–969, 1978

Obesity

Brownell K, Wadden T: Confronting obesity in children–Behavioral and psychological factors. Pediatr Ann 13:473–480, 1984

Cusack R: Dietary management of obese children and adolescents. Pediatr Ann 13:455–464, 1984

Dietz WH: Childhood obesity: Suscseptibility, cause, and management. J. Pediatr 103:676–686, 1983

Hervey GR: The physiological background of obesity. Pediatr Ann 13:543–555, 1984

Hofmann A (ed): Adolescent Medicine, pp 319–322. Reading, MA, Addison-Wesley, 1983

Shen JTY: The Clinical Practice of Adolescent Medicine, pp 192–195. New York, Appleton-Century-Crofts, 1980

Suskind R, Varma R: Assessment of nutritional status of children. Pediatr Rev 5:195–202, 1984

Weil W: Obesity in children. Pediatr Rev 3:180–189, 1981

Anorexia Nervosa

Harper G: Anorexia nervosa: What kind of disorder? Pediatr Ann 13:811–828, 1984

Herzog D: Pharmacotherapy of anorexia nervosa and bulimia. Pediatr Ann 13:915–923, 1984

Hofmann A (ed): Adolescent Medicine, pp 322–324. Reading, MA, Addison-Wesley, 1983

Shen JTY: The Clinical Practice of Adolescent Medicine, pp 196–204. New York, Appleton-Century-Crofts, 1980

Part II: Development

4

Normal Growth and Development

The pediatrician must constantly consider his patient's stage of growth and development. Strictly speaking, growth is the process of becoming larger. The growing child becomes taller and heavier, and his internal organs also become larger and heavier. Development, on the other hand, is the child's gradual progression toward his potential as a mature individual. Development occurs on many levels: motoric, neurological, cognitive, verbal, social, emotional, and spiritual. These personal features do not develop at the same rate, do not begin or complete development simultaneously, and may not be developed to the same degree in the mature individual.

The child's weight, height, and head circumference are three important growth parameters, which can be plotted by age on growth curves. In this way, a child's growth can be compared with that of other children of the same age. Growth curves were developed using serial measurements of weight, height, and head circumference of many children. Individuals normally tend to follow their own growth curves; that is, if a child's weight is at the 95th percentile (he is larger than 95% of other children) at 9 months, his weight is likely to be at the 95th percentile at 5 years. For ease of plotting parameters, growth curves are outlined at the following percentiles: 5th, 10th, 25th, 50th, 75th, 90th, and 95th. The curves are demonstrated in Figures 4-1 to 4-4. When the child is younger, the rate of growth is accelerated; as the child ages, the rate of growth slows. This property of human growth explains the shape of the curves: steep slopes in infancy and early childhood and flattened slopes in childhood.

The features of growth and development will be discussed by age.

NEWBORN

Growth

The average full-term newborn weighs 3.5 kg, is 50 cm long, and has a head circumference of 35 cm. He has a head that is relatively large and limbs that are relatively small for his size. His face is round, and his abdomen is protuberant. Because of his intrauterine position, he prefers to be in partial flexion at rest. The newborn's respiratory rate is approximately 30 to 40 breaths per minute, and his heart rate is 120 to 150 beats per minutes.

(Text continues on p. 28.)

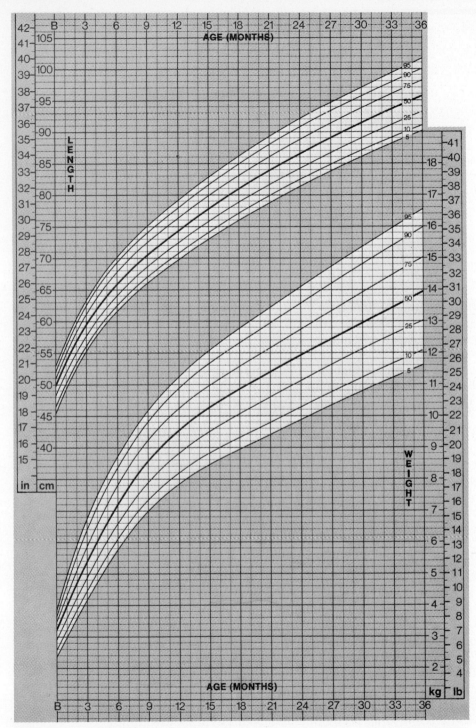

FIGURE 4–1. Girls: birth to 36 months—physical growth NCHS percentiles. (Adapted from: National Center for Health Statistics: NCHS Growth Charts, 1976. Monthly Vital Statistics Report. Vol. 25, No. 3, Supp. (HRA) 76–1120. Health Resources Administration, Rockville, Maryland, June, 1976. Data from The Fels Research Institute, Yellow Springs, Ohio. ©1976 ROSS LABORATORIES)

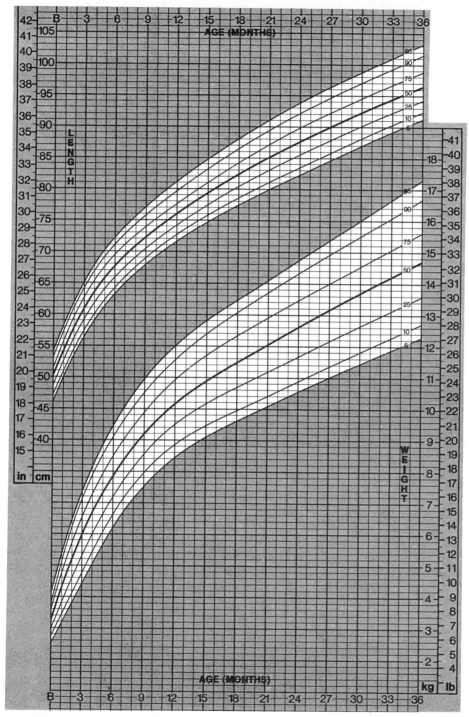

FIGURE 4–2. Boys: birth to 36 months—physical growth NCHS percentiles. (Adapted from: National Center for Health Statistics: NCHS Growth Charts, 1976. Monthly Vital Statistics Report. Vol. 25, No. 3, Supp. (HRA) 76–1120. Health Resources Administration, Rockville, Maryland, June, 1976. Data from The Fels Research Institute, Yellow Springs, Ohio. ©1976 ROSS LABORATORIES)

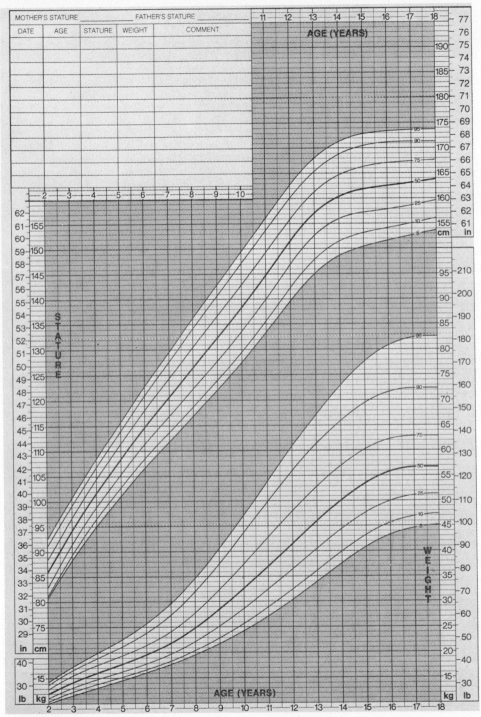

FIGURE 4–3. Girls: 2 to 18 years—physical growth NCHS percentiles. (Adapted from: Hamill PVV, Drizd TA, Johnson CL, Reed RB, Roche AF, Moore WM: Physical growth: National Center for Health Statistics percentiles. Am J Clin Nutr 32:607–629, 1979. Data from the National Center for Health Statistics [NCHS] Hyattsville, Maryland. © 1982 ROSS LABORATORIES)

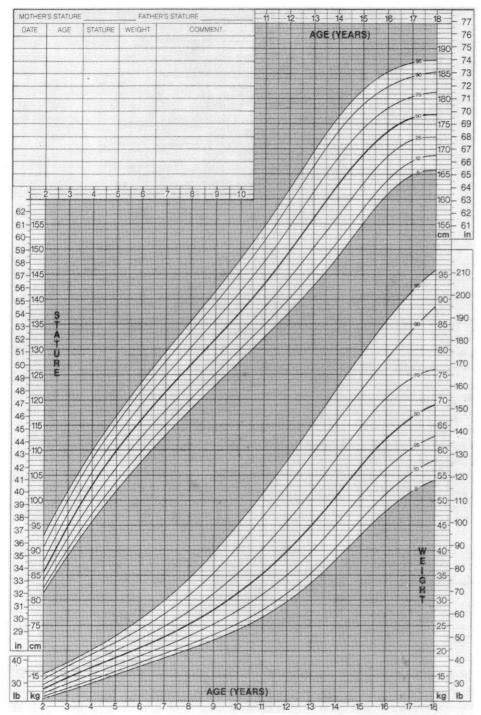

FIGURE 4–4. Boys: 2 to 18 years—physical growth NCHS percentiles. (Adapted from: Hamill PVV, Drizd TA, Johnson CL, Reed RB, Roche AF, Moore WM: Physical growth: National Center for Health Statistics percentiles. Am J Clin Nutr 32:607–629, 1979. Data from the National Center for Health Statistics [NCHS] Hyattsville, Maryland. © 1982 ROSS LABORATORIES)

Development

The neonate can turn his head toward the nipple or other stimulus ("rooting"), suck, gag, and swallow. He uses these skills to satisfy his hunger and feeds every 2 to 4 hours. Feeding may be followed closely by stooling. Because the neonate's weight has a large component of water, in the first few days of life he may lose up to 6% of his birth weight. This is usually regained by the 10th to 14th day of life.

The infant's kidneys have only a limited ability to concentrate and to clear urea. Certain enzymes of the digestive tract are not fully developed. The neonate's hemoglobin averages 17 to 19 g/dl, and the white blood cell count averages 10,000 to 14,000. His serum glucose and calcium levels may be relatively low. Maternal hormones and IgG cross the placenta, and so the neonate has a high level of IgG and may show the effects of estrogen (enlarged breasts, milk from the breasts, vaginal bleeding).

The neonate can discern light from dark, can hear, startles in response to loud noises (the Moro reflex), and cries when hungry, cold, or in pain, or when experiencing other discomfort. He cannot raise his head or roll.

THE FIRST MONTH OF LIFE

Growth

The infant should gain 20 to 30 g/day and requires 110 calories/kg/day for this growth. His birth weight is usually regained by the 10th to 14th day of life.

Development

The infant still prefers to lie in flexion, although by the end of the 4th week, he demonstrates more extension of his legs. When prone, the infant moves his head from side to side; by the 4th week, he will be able to hold up his chin. When supine, he is stiff, but by the 4th week, he is more relaxed. The Moro, stepping, placing, and grasp reflexes are present. (See Chapter 7 for their description.)

The infant will fixate visually on objects; by the end of the 4th week, he follows objects a few degrees and stares at people. The infant continues to cry to make his needs known. He usually sleeps 18 to 20 hours of the day.

MONTHS 2 TO 3

Growth

The infant continues to gain 20 to 30 g/day.

Development

When prone, the infant can raise his head higher; at 12 weeks, with arms extended, he will be able to lift his head and chest off the surface. When the infant is supine, a tonic neck posture predominates. If pulled to a sitting position, his head lags, although at 3 months, he will gain head control (albeit with some bobbing). After 3 months, his Moro reflex will disappear. He follows objects visually in a 180° arc.

The infant considers himself one with his environment, especially his mother. He has developed different cries for different purposes (hunger, cold, anger, etc.). He smiles and is attentive to voices and music. He will coo (vowel sounds), especially saying "oooh" and "aaah." He sleeps less than when a neonate but probably does not sleep through the night.

MONTHS 4 TO 6

Growth

Still continuing to gain 20 to 30 g/day, the infant will double his birth weight and will add 12 to 15 cm to his length. His head circumference at 6 months of age will be 9 to 10 cm greater than at birth. His posterior fontanelle closes by 4 months, and his patent anterior fontanelle slowly decreases in size.

Development

The infant's head control is good, and when prone, he can lift his head and chest up using his extended arms for support. After 6 months, he can roll, first from prone to supine and later from supine to prone. When lying on his back, he can maintain his head in midline comfortably and can bring his hands together in the midline. He may reach for objects of interest and attempt to put them into his mouth.

When he is pulled to a sitting position, his head no longer lags or bobs. By the 6th month, his head will be held erect and steady consistently. He can sit with support (perhaps only briefly) at 4 months, but by 6 months, he may be able to sit alone without truncal support. When pulled from sitting to standing, he bears weight on his legs and may bounce. He enjoys being upright.

At 4 months, the infant can grasp medium-sized objects; by 6 months, he can transfer large objects from hand to hand. Also at 6 months, he *begins* to attempt to pick up small objects with a raking motion.

The infant laughs out loud and coos. He shows excitement at the sight of loved ones, favorite toys, and food. By 6 months he prefers contact with those he knows. He cries, screams, or whimpers if his wishes are thwarted. He sleeps about 10 to 14 hours/day (12 hours during the night plus daytime naps) and has 1 to 2 bowel movements/day.

MONTHS 6 TO 12

Growth

The infant gains 15 g/day and typically triples his birth weight by the end of the first year; thereafter, his appetite decreases. His length increases by 50% over his birth length, and his head circumference is 33% larger than at birth. At 12 months, his brain is two-thirds its adult size. His head is becoming relatively small in relation to his body as his trunk and limbs elongate. The anterior fontanelle continues to decrease in size. The first tooth appears at 6 to 7 months of age, and it is usually a lower central incisor. In order of appearance, the erupting teeth are the lower central incisors, upper central incisors, upper lateral incisors, and lower lateral incisors. By 12 months of age, the infant has 6 to 8 teeth. A handy rule of thumb for the number of teeth an infant should have is "a tooth a month after 6 months of age."

Development

The infant can sit alone. When lying on his back, he can lift his legs and put his feet in his mouth. When on his stomach, he can, at 6 to 8 months, pivot in pursuit of an object and reach for it. By 8 to 10 months, he can creep or crawl, and he can stand and walk if his hands are held. By the end of the first year, he can "cruise" (i.e., walk holding onto objects) and may be able to walk alone.

By 9 or 10 months, the infant picks up small objects using his thumb and forefinger. By 12 months of age, he can release an object if asked, especially if the requestor touches the object or holds out his hand. When the infant is 9 to 10 months old, the infant will look for a dropped object and reach for it. In addition, if a toy is covered, he will try to uncover it, and if a cloth covers his face, he will pull it off with a giggle.

The infant babbles (consonant and vowel sounds) and by the end of the first year, he will be able to say a couple of words in addition to "dada" and "mama" ("dada" generally precedes "mama") and will recognize his own name. He enjoys imitating the actions of others (coughing, waving bye-bye, etc.). He enjoys his family, especially his mother. By 9 months, stranger anxiety usually becomes manifest as the infant cries at the presence of individuals other than his family. About the same time, he may develop separation anxiety, crying lustily when loved ones leave the room or give him to others for holding. This is because the infant recognizes he is separate from his mother. The infant likes to watch his image in the mirror.

When thwarted, the infant cries angrily and may toss things on the floor in frustration. He is becoming more autonomous and wants to feed himself and learn to drink from a cup; if his parent is reluctant to let him do this, the infant will object loudly. The infant generally sleeps 10 to 12 hours/night and several hours during the day. He has one bowel movement every day or every other day.

MONTHS 12 TO 18

Growth

By 18 months, the child's weight increases by 1.0 to 1.5 kg, his height by 6 cm, and his head circumference by 1 cm over his measurements at 12 months. He continues to erupt a tooth per month.

Development

By 12 to 15 months, the infant walks alone; by 15 months, he can crawl up steps; and by 18 months, he can run awkwardly and walk up stairs (one step at a time) if his hand is held. The child likes to empty drawers, cabinets, and trash cans and put objects into his mouth.

The child's fine motor skills are developing. He can put a small object into a container and try to remove it, first by using his fingers and later by dumping the object from the container. The 15 month old can stack two cubes, whereas the 18 month old can stack three cubes. He can scribble with a crayon early in his second year and, by 18 months, can imitate a vertical line. He enjoys feeding himself.

The child has a 10-word vocabulary by 18 months. He can name familiar objects and people and can follow simple commands. The 18 month old also uses jargon with appropriate voice inflections. He points to desired objects and seeks help when needed. He imitates others but also enjoys solitary play.

Because the child recognizes his own helplessness, his desires, and his need for parental love, he becomes frustrated. He likes to explore his environment but when exploration is met with a parental "no," the child may scream, cry, hold his breath, kick, or hit. He is ambivalent—both sunny and negative, independent and dependent, lovable and aggressive. He sleeps 8 to 12 hours/night and may or may not take daytime naps. He has a bowel movement every day or every other day.

MONTHS 18 TO 24

Growth

The same rate of growth that occurred during months 12 to 18 occurs during months 19 to 24. The anterior fontanelle closes around 18 months. The child's body continues to elongate, causing his head to appear smaller relative to the rest of his body. His abdomen protrudes because of his lordatic posture. By 24 months, he will have 14 to 16 teeth, including the first molars and cuspids.

Development

The 18 month old who ran awkwardly and could only walk up the stairs develops into the 24 month old who runs well and can walk down the stairs with his hand held. He can climb onto furniture. He continues to open drawers, cabinets, and doors in his ever-present quest to conquer his environment.

At 24 months, his fine motor skills include the ability to stack six cubes, copy horizontal lines, and draw circular shapes.

By 24 months, the child can compose three-word sentences (pronoun, verb, object). He enjoys listening to stories and may tell family members his own stories (albeit limited by his vocabulary). He imitates words, so that parents must watch their use of expletives.

He helps undress himself and feeds himself using a spoon well. The myelination of the pyramidal tracts occurs at 18 months of age; such neurological development permits the child to begin to control his bowel and bladder. Toilet-training is easier if the child is older than 24 months of age at its onset.

The same emotional developmental tasks and patterns of sleep and elimination described for months 12 to 18 are operant during months 18 to 24.

YEARS 2 TO 5

Growth

The child gains 2 kg in weight and 6 to 8 cm in height each year. The lordosis and "pot-belly" disappear by year 4. By 30 months of age, the preschooler has his 20 primary teeth.

Development

By 30 months, the child can jump, alternate feet when climbing steps, and ride a tricycle or "Big-Wheel." By 48 months, he can alternate feet when descending stairs, hop on one foot, climb, and throw a ball; within a year, he will learn to skip.

The child's fine motor skills also continue their progression. By 30 months, he can stack eight cubes and draw a crude closed circle. By 36 months, he can stack nine cubes, make a three-cube bridge, and copy a cross. By 48 months, he can build a five-cube bridge, copy a cross and square, draw a man with two to four body parts in addition to the head, and indicate the longer of two lines. By 60 months, he can copy an object with slanting lines (a triangle).

The 30 month old knows his name and can use the pronoun "I" appropriately. The 36 month old knows his age and sex and can count to three. At 4 years, the child can count to four and can tell a story; by 5 years, he knows four colors and can count to ten.

The younger preschooler helps with simple household tasks and plays simple games. By 36 months, he assists in dressing himself and washing his hands. At 49 months, he toilets himself alone and enjoys playing with other children. Finally, the 60 month old dresses and undresses himself, asks "why?" and "what's that?" and enjoys playing "mommy" or "daddy" and "doctor."

The younger preschooler develops a conscience (superego) about right and wrong, good and evil, and desirable character traits based on the values that his parents instill in him. His play is imaginative, with inanimate objects taking on the qualities of people.

Because the child knows his gender, he identifies with the same-sex parent, imagining what it would be like to be a father (or mother, if the child is female). The child then develops a "crush" on the opposite-sex parent; this may be complicated by genital feelings, since he has already learned to obtain pleasure through stimulation of his genitalia. Thus, the young preschooler shifts between allegiance to the same-sex parent and the "crush" on the opposite-sex parent (Oedipus complex). He fears the loss of love if he takes one side or the other and may demonstrate aggression. Also operant is the child's magical thinking in which he believes that his thoughts control the environment (a method for him to ease anxieties). Since he periodically wishes that the same-sex parent would disappear, he fears that this will happen and that he will be punished; a boy especially fears injury to his penis. Ultimately, the child's ego strength increases, and his superego intervenes. He gives up romantic attachment to the opposite-sex parent and replaces it with filial love. At the same time, he identifies more closely with the same-sex parent. However, the child assimilates desirable qualities of both parents. The child's pattern of sleep and elimination is established.

MIDCHILDHOOD YEARS

Growth

The child gains 3.0 to 3.5 kg in weight and 5 to 6 cm in height per year. Head circumference growth is much slower, on the order of 0.3 to 0.5 cm per year. By age 12, the brain is of adult size.

The first molars erupt in the seventh year of life. Shedding of primary teeth follows the same order of their acquisition. Primary teeth are replaced at a rate of four teeth per year over the next 7 years.

Development

As his central nervous system matures, the child develops his gross motor skills in response to the games in which he participates. He enjoys interactive games with same-sex children, while professing an aversion to opposite-sex children.

Fine motor skills and cognitive skills develop in response to the demands of school and peer pressure. If the child's (or parent's) expectations of his school performance do not match reality, the child experiences failure.

His frustration may lead to conflicts in the family or acting-out behavior. He may demonstrate school phobia and attempt to escape school attendance when he experiences psychosomatic complaints (stomachaches, headaches, etc.).

The child's sexuality is expressed in his affiliation with same-sex friends and clubs. In addition, masturbatory activity continues, usually in private.

Parents are no longer viewed by the child as omnipotent, since he now has the opportunity to judge his parents by comparing them with other adults. Other adult role-models (teachers, coaches) are sought. Fascination with rock musicians, media stars, or sports personalities begins in this age-group.

Girls of this age are generally 1 to 2 years ahead of boys in cognitive skills and emotional maturity.

ADOLESCENCE

Growth

During adolescence, the child attains his adult height, gains weight with a redistribution of subcutaneous tissues, erupts his second and, occasionally, his third molars, and develops into an adult sexually.

Adolescence has its onset at about age 10 in girls and age 12 in boys. Up to age 8 to 10, boys are somewhat larger than girls. However, at age 10 or so, girls experience a growth spurt so that they are taller than similarly aged boys. Girls begin to accumulate subcutaneous fat tissue 1 to 2 years before their growth spurts and retain most of this tissue into their adulthood. Boys also accumulate fat tissue before their growth spurts but tend to lose most of it during adolescence, replacing it with muscle mass. Adolescent boys tend to have more muscle mass than girls.

As the growth spurt begins, secondary sex changes occur. These changes have been preceded first in midchildhood, by increased production of adrenal steroids and, later, of estrogen and androgen.

In girls, estrogen production increases greatly at age 9 to 11. Hips widen, and breasts begin to enlarge. Breast development is followed first by the appearance of pubic hair and, later, of axillary hair. About 1½ to 2½ years after these secondary sex changes occur, a girl begins to menstruate. The establishment of menstruation, or menarche, is the onset of puberty in females. It is preceded by a recurrent, clear, vaginal discharge with an acidic pH (vaginal secretions had been alkaline in childhood). The first few menstrual periods may be anovulatory, irregular in occurrence, and irregular in amount of blood lost. Some girls experience very heavy periods, whereas others merely spot. These characteristics may be present for the first year of the girl's puberty. Although most of the girl's growth has occurred before her first period, she may gain several inches in height after its occurrence.

In boys, increased androgen production increases between 12 and 14 years of age. Initially, the boy's testes and scrotum enlarge; later, his penis also enlarges, with a few pubic hairs at its base. Some unilateral or bilateral breast enlargement may occur; the tissue usually regresses with time. As the testes, scrotum, and penis continue to enlarge, the latter two become darker. Pubic hair becomes coarser and thicker. The boy's voice begins to change (deepen) as the larynx grows. Nocturnal emissions are common. Finally, the adolescent's testes and penis achieve adult size, and his pubic hair extends toward his umbilicus. The boy's maximum growth spurt occurs about 2 years after secondary sex characteristics appear.

It is mid to late adolescence before fully adult distributions of pubic hair and, in the male, axillary, chest, and facial hair appear and before the adult configuration of the female breast occurs. Both boys and girls experience acne in their teens because of increased sebaceous gland activity. Adolescent boys have slightly higher blood pressures, higher respiratory rates, and greater hemoglobulin concentrations than girls. Adolescent girls, on the other hand, have higher basal body temperatures and pulse rates than boys.

The progression of an individual's sexual development occurs in stages. The Tanner stages assist in characterizing the adolescent's stage of physical development. Hence, the physical examination of all adolescents should include the Tanner staging of their genitalia and, if female, breasts.

Development

Because of his rapid growth, the adolescent is frequently ill at ease with his new body. He may now be physically awkward, whereas he was agile previously. This occurs in early adolescence; by mid- to late adolescence, the person has come to terms with his body. With their increase in muscle mass, boys frequently participate in sports; girls may participate in team sports, gymnastics, or dance. Adolescents of both sexes enjoy dancing to popular music. Adolescent girls are very weight conscious and may diet constantly.

Because of their newly developing secondary sex characteristics, adolescents of both sexes are somewhat embarrassed initially. A boy may worry if he has acne, feels he is too short (or too tall), feels he is too fat (or too thin), has facial hair, lacks facial hair, has a voice that is changing, or feels that he is otherwise unattractive to girls. He may worry about the size of his testes and penis, believing that the larger they are, the more manly he is. A girl may also worry about her complexion, her weight (in particular), her height, whether her breasts are too small (or too large), whether she has begun to develop too early, or whether she develops too late. She may also have free-floating anxiety about her attractiveness to boys. In early adolescence, these anxieties manifest themselves as shyness or frank silliness around members of the opposite sex. Boys are frequently loud and impulsive around girls, who are giggly and flirtatious around them. Group-dating and dances are popular. The young adolescent rapidly falls in (and out) of love and has numerous "crushes." the mature ability to form an intimate relationship with a member of the opposite sex is achieved in later adolescence.

Despite this relative immaturity, the adolescent may be under peer pressure to be active sexually without fully understanding the ramifications of such activity. The possibility of pregnancy may not even be considered; hence, birth control methods are not used. If the adolescent contracts a venereal disease or is involved in a pregnancy, the sense of shame and guilt can be overwhelming. In addition, most adolescents are reluctant to inform their parents of their sexual activity. In many cases, unfortunately, the sexual activity comes to the parent's attention when the adolescent contracts a venereal disease or becomes pregnant. The adolescent girl is ill-prepared to make a decision about the pregnancy's outcome (keeping the baby, giving the baby up for adoption, terminating the pregnancy); the decision is all the more painful and difficult if she chooses to make it alone, if her family has rejected her, or if her family is pressuring her to make a decision contrary to her wishes.

The adolescent is very conscious of his appearance. He is narcissistic, feels that everyone is looking at him, and may spend hours in front of a mirror in an attempt to make himself look "perfect." He is clothes conscious, but wants to dress like his peers because of the unbelievably strong influence of peer pressure. If his group is attired in ragged jeans and leather jackets, his clothes-consciousness will reflect this style of dress. If a girl's group is attired in short, baggy, mismatched clothes, she will prefer these (much to the consternation of her parents!). The adolescent's anxiety about himself makes him susceptible to peer pressure (i.e., safety in numbers) and it is only in later adolescence that he develops his own style of dress and behavior.

The adolescent attempts to develop his own identity by questioning authority and reassessing family values. Hence, the parent of an adolescent frequently finds himself at odds with his formerly compliant child. The teenager may be argumentative, rude, and rebellious and may constantly test his parent's limits (and sanity!). In the adolescent's mind, everyone—from similarly aged friends to rock stars—knows more than his parents. Every other adolescent has "better" parents than he does. Part of this behavior is normal and resolves as the child grows older and develops adult values and concerns. However, if the child did not have a satisfying relationship with his parents before adolescence, the relationship can only worsen in his teen years. If such a child is miserable, falls in with the wrong crowd, and is overly susceptible to peer suggestions, he may easily become involved with drug use, alcohol abuse, self-destructive behavior, school failure, truancy, or antisocial acts such as stealing.

Another task of adolescence is to decide about one's ultimate plans, especially for schooling or employment. Although some adolescents reject school and have no plans for adulthood, most teenagers do have vocational plans. A highly academically oriented adolescent takes the necessary courses to ensure his acceptance by a college of his choice, which will prepare him for his adult occupation. A less academically oriented teenager decides what training he requires to succeed in his chosen vocation.

Adolescence does not last forever (although many parents think it does!). If the adolescent has had a satisfying relationship with his parents, and if both he and they have approached each other with mutual love, respect, and humor, he has an excellent chance of develop-ing into a mature adult, one who is much more like his parents than he ever dreamed possible.

BIBLIOGRAPHY

Litt I, Vaughan V: Developmental pediatrics. In Behrman R, Vaughan V: Nelson Textbook of Pediatrics, 13th ed, pp 6–35. Philadelphia, WB Saunders, 1987

5

Abnormal Development

DEVELOPMENTAL DELAY

When a child does not meet the age-specific developmental milestones, he is said to be developmentally delayed. The child can be globally delayed or can be delayed in only one facet of development.

Delay may result from intrauterine or extrauterine causes. Intrauterine causes include chromosomal abnormalities; maternal infections (such as rubella, syphilis, toxoplasmosis, cytomegaloviral disease); maternal medication, drug, or alcohol exposure, irradiation; trauma; central nervous system hemorrhages, malformations, and anoxia; maternal malnutrition, and severe immunologic diseases. Extrauterine causes include prematurity; birth asphyxia/anoxia; central nervous system hemorrhages and anoxia, infections; severe malnutrition; isolated system defects (such as orthopedic abnormalities, deafness, blindness); severe chronic illnesses; metabolic disturbances; chronic poisoning (i.e., lead); seizure disorders; trauma; and maternal deprivation.

All developmental milestones have a range of time for their expected appearance. Children whose development does not meet the

age-specific standards by parental report deserve a comprehensive history and physical examination (Chapters 6 and 7) to detect any of the possible causes of delay as enumerated above. The physician should perform a complete neurological examination (see Chapter 7), with special emphasis on detecting hypertonicity, hypotonicity, or abnormal reflexes, which might be indicative of cerebral palsy (see Chapter 90). A developmental screening test such as the Denver Developmental Test should be performed to determine the levels on which the child is delayed. Note should also be made of whether the delay is accompanied by abnormal growth deceleration or cessation (i.e., "failure-to-thrive"; see Chapter 3) or by abnormal growth acceleration (such as accelerated head growth in hydrocephalus).

The work-up of failure to thrive has been discussed in Chapter 3. Evaluation of developmental delay depends on the history and physical findings. For example, the infant with a disproportionally large head merits a cranial ultrasound; the infant with abnormal facies or organomegaly deserves investigation of the possibility of congenital infection. No single laboratory test is an absolute test of developmental delay. Formal developmental testing by a team of neurologists, developmentalists, and psychologists may be required. A social worker may help to evaluate family functioning.

The treatment of developmental delay depends on its cause. A child with new-onset delay due to hydrocephalus may benefit from the placement of a ventriculoperitoneal shunt, whereas a child with delay due to inborn errors of metabolism or an endocrine disorder (such as hypothyroidism) may benefit from dietary manipulations or hormonal replacement, respectively. Chelation therapy may benefit a child with delay due to chronic lead poisoning; a child with a seizure disorder benefits from appropriate control of the seizures. A child with an orthopedic defect with isolated motoric delay may benefit from surgical correction of the defect. A child whose delay has stemmed from severe malnutrition or deprivation benefits from an adequate diet or removal from his usual environment. Finally, most children with developmental delay benefit from the services of infant-stimulation programs or developmental centers, whose staffs work with both children and parents at the center and in the home. Staff members develop an individualized teaching/management plan for each child so that parents can help them reach their potential. Staff members also serve as support resources for the parents, who are under a great deal of stress and feeling guilty about their child's condition.

DEVELOPMENTAL ACCELERATION

The child who reaches developmental milestones prematurely usually does not elicit the concern that a child with delay does. One exception would be the child with precocious sexual development (see Chapter 65).

The child who is cognitively gifted is often considered a "problem." Such a child demonstrates verbal, reading, or problem-solving skills far beyond those of his cohorts. He may be pushed by parents to excel and may be advanced in school too rapidly. Despite his gifts, he may continue to function emotionally at his true age level; this causes conflicts because he may be expected to behave as an older child would. Such children, under a great deal of pressure to do well, may be ill-prepared to handle this stress. The physician of a gifted child should counsel the parent about the age-appropriate emotional needs of the child and solicit the child's feelings about the stresses in his life.

Finally, some children have accelerated heights and weights for their ages. However, they possess only age-appropriate cognitive and emotional skills. They, too, may be expected to act as an older child would because they look older. This leads to the child feeling frustration because he cannot meet these demands. Again, parental counseling is indicated.

BIBLIOGRAPHY

Committee on Children with Disabilities: Screening for developmental disabilities. *Pediatrics:* 78:526–528, 1986

Fagan J, Singer L, Montie J et al: Selective screening device for the early detection of normal or delayed cognitive development in infants at risk for later mental retardation. *Pediatrics* 78:1021–1026, 1986

Keele D: The developmentally disabled child— Spotting the problem in infancy. *Contemp Pediatr* 1:63–79, 1984

Keele D: The developmentally disabled child— Step by step through the workup. *Contemp Pediatr* 1:77–96, 1984

Keele D: The developmentally disabled child— Pursuing the etiologic workup. *Contemp Pediatr* 2:51–62, 1985

Part III: The Diagnostic Process

6

The Interview

The collection of historical data through conversing with the patient, known as the *interview*, is a crucial part of the medical encounter. Through the information the patient gives and, more importantly, the manner in which he presents or emphasizes certain data, the physician can learn a great deal about the patient's personality and the importance of the presenting illness (or health maintenance).

Pediatrics is unique in that the historian is frequently not the patient, but his parent, who may or may not correctly interpret the child's cues or behaviors. Obviously, dependence on the parent to provide a history is unavoidable when treating the preverbal child. However, once a child is verbal, the physician should attempt to solicit the child's perspective on his health, illness, or emotional problems. The child may not wish to talk to the physician because of shyness, fear, or anger; that is his perogative. Nevertheless, the physician should always extend the courtesy of communication to the child.

Initially, a young child may be quite shy and may respond to "Hello. How are you?" by averting his eyes and refusing to speak. If the child is not prodded to speak and the physi-

cian periodically addresses him in a friendly, nonthreatening manner, the child may begin to speak when he feels more at ease. Sometimes, the child can be persuaded to talk if the physician engages in play with him.

The normal older preschooler is only too willing to talk to the physician, and, if encouraged, he will readily give his perspectives (often quite insightful) on his health, illness, and anything else about which he is questioned. The preschooler's response to "Hello. How are you?" is frequently a furtive glance at his parent, giggles, and a "Hi. Fine." Unlike the toddler and younger preschooler, who may view direct eye contact with the physician as extremely threatening, the older preschooler enjoys being addressed and being the center of attention. He may initiate conversation with the physician if he thinks he is not receiving enough attention.

Although historical information elicited from a preschooler may be somewhat diffuse, it is imperative to include him in the interview process so that his importance as an individual is appreciated.

The younger school-aged child also usually is eager to talk with the physician and can provide valuable insights into his health, illness, or other problems. To the greeting, "Hello. How are you?", this child is likely to respond "I'm OK. How are you?" if he is healthy, or "I don't feel good. My head (stomach, chest, etc.) hurts" if he is ill. Both he and his parent should be addressed in the interview. If their answers are at variance, try to clarify the issue without causing an argument.

Preadolescents and adolescents may present to medical attention willingly and unwillingly. Hence, such patients may respond to "Hello. How are you?" with a smile and a "Hi. I'm fine. How are you doing?" if willing to be present, or a scowl and a "Hmmm" (or no answer at all) if unwilling to be present. These patients can offer extremely valuable perspectives on themselves and should be the primary historians. They can be questioned in their parent's absence if they so desire. If the parent remains but constantly interrupts the child or answers for him, the physician must gently, but firmly, inform the parent that, although his or her perspectives are important and will be discussed, the child is the patient, and thus his perspectives are paramount.

Whenever sensitive material is being discussed with the child, the parent should be asked to leave the room. Most parents will readily do so. However, if the child strongly objects to the parent's exclusion, the parent should be permitted to stay (or stand right outside the door). Sensitive material includes the possibility of and circumstances surrounding abuse (physical, sexual, emotional), sexual activity, venereal diseases, pregnancy, and behavior problems at home, at school, or in social situations.

The interview should always begin with the physician greeting the parent and patient and introducing himself, if he is not already known to them. The interviewer should face the family, be friendly and courteous, speak in nontechnical terms, and make eye contact.

Although, as mentioned earlier, young patients might be threatened by eye contact, older children and adults usually view this behavior as indicative of honesty. To make them more comfortable, young children should be looked at occasionally and always in a friendly manner.

Since the content of the interview varies according to the patient's reason for seeking medical attention, the following discussion will highlight separately the historical data to be elicited during health-maintenance visits and illness visits.

HISTORY DURING A HEALTH-MAINTENANCE VISIT

The interview should always begin with an assessment by the parent (and by the patient, if possible) of the patient's overall state of health. Ask, "How's he (or how have you) been doing since the last checkup?" If the response reveals that the child has been doing well, you may proceed with your agenda. If the response reveals that the parent (or patient) believes that there was (or is) a problem, you should explore this problem completely before proceeding. If possible, both the parent's and child's perspectives should be sought and the issues elucidated to the mutual satisfaction of all present. (See the "Illness" section for important data to elicit by presenting complaint.)

If this is the child's first visit, such as is the case with a young infant, gather information about the child's birth history. Was the mother's pregnancy complicated by illness, medication, drug or alcohol use, trauma, vaginal bleeding, or premature labor? If "yes," obtain details. Was her labor spontaneous or induced? How long did labor last? Where was the baby born? Was the infant's birth accomplished vaginally or by Cesarean section? Was the mother under the effect of medications at the time of the birth? Which ones? Was she awake at the time of the birth, and did she hear the neonate cry? Did the baby require resuscitation, suctioning, or oxygen administration? How much did the baby weigh, and how long was he at birth? Did the nursery personnel report that he had respiratory, cardiovascular, or gastrointestinal problems in the nursery? Was the infant breast-fed or bottle-fed in the hospital? How well did he feed? Did he vomit his feedings or seem to tire after them? When did the infant pass his first stool? How many days did he stay in the hospital before going home? How much did he weigh at discharge? If the patient is several weeks old at this first visit, inquire about the time of the umbilical stump's separation.

Nutrition

1. If the patient is an infant. Is the infant breast-fed or bottle-fed? How frequently? If breast-fed, does he empty one or both breasts at a feeding? If bottle-fed, how many ounces does he take at a feeding? What kind of formula does he ingest? How does the parent prepare the formula? What other fluids does the infant ingest and in what quantities? What other foods does he ingest and in what quantities? Specifically, has he been introduced to cereals, fruits, vegetables, or meats? If "yes," which ones and how frequently does he ingest them? How much does he ingest at a feeding? Has he ever had an adverse reaction to any food? If "yes," which food and what reaction?

2. If the patient is a toddler or preschooler. Is the child drinking formula or whole milk? How much milk or formula does he drink each day? What other fluids does he regularly drink each day? Does he require a nighttime bottle? Does the child eat from each of the

basic food groups each day? What is a typical breakfast, lunch, and dinner for him? What does he eat for snacks? What "junk foods" does the child prefer, and how often does he get them? Does he have any food intolerances? If so, which ones?

3. If the child is 5 years or older. Use the same question as in (2), eliminating the questions about bottles and formula. Do ask, however, how much milk he drinks each day.

If the child, regardless of age, is extremely thin or obese, the physician should obtain a detailed daily dietary history, including types and amounts of foods ingested at meals and for snacks.

Elimination

How many stools does the child have each day? What do they look like (*i.e.*, color, consistency, and volume)? (This question is more pertinent to infants and to children of any age with recurrent or chronic stooling disorders or possible dietary intolerances.) If constipation is reported, define what the interviewee means by "constipation." What methods are used to relieve the constipation (laxatives, suppositories, enemas)? How frequently does the child require these aids? If diarrhea is reported, define what is meant by "diarrhea," how frequently it occurs, its appearance, and which home remedies or dietary alterations are used to resolve the episodes.

How many times does the child urinate each day? If the child is already toilet-trained, determine the age at which bowel and bladder training was achieved. Do accidents occur? When? Does he urinate at night? Does he wet or soil the bed? Does he drink a lot of fluids during the day? If "yes," how much? Does the urine have an unusual odor or color? Does he have symptoms of urgency, hesistancy, polyuria, or dysuria?

Sleep

How many hours of sleep does the child need each night? When does he go to bed, and when does he awaken? Does he take regular naps during the day? If "yes," how many and for how long? Does he ever fall asleep at inopportune times (such as in school)? Does the child snore loudly or seem to have gaps in his breathing? Does he have nightmares or sleepwalk? Where does he sleep and with whom?

Sexuality

1. Younger child. Has the parent noticed the child masturbating at any time? Reassure the parent that masturbation is normal behavior. How has the parent handled the situation?

2. Older child or adolescent. *Note:* It is preferable to question the patient, not the parent. *Males:* Have his penis and testes enlarged? Has he developed pubic, axillary, chest, or facial hair? Is his voice changing? Has he had a wet dream? Is he sexually active? Has he ever had a venereal disease? *Females:* Has she developed pubic or axillary hair? Have her breasts started to develop? Has she begun to menstruate? When? When was her last period? What is her usual period like? Is she sexually active? Has she ever had a venereal disease? Has she ever been pregnant or had an abortion? Is she using any method of contraception? If "yes," which one(s)?

Developmental Milestones

This series of question obviously varies according to the child's age. Chapter 4 describes the developmental milestones by anticipated age of attainment. One should ask the parent of an infant or young child about developmental milestones achieved since the last visit.

1. If the patient is a young infant. Does the baby appear to see and hear? Does he coo? Startle? Smile? Comfort easily or with difficulty? Lift his head off the bed when he is prone? Move all extremities?

2. If the patient is an older infant. Does the baby smile, coo, laugh audibly, and babble? At what age could he first sit without support? Crawl? Walk with support? Walk alone? Feed himself finger foods? Drink from a cup? Say an understandable word? Transfer objects from one hand to another? Develop stranger or separation anxiety? When did he develop his first tooth?

3. If the patient is a toddler. At what age did he walk? Use a spoon independently? Give up his bottle? String words together to compose short phrases? How many words (and which ones) can he say? Can he run? Climb steps? Jump? Can he manipulate blocks and other toys? Is he bowel toilet-trained? Is he bladder toilet-trained?

4. If the patient is a preschooler. Is he toilet-trained? Can he speak in sentences? Can he tell short stories? Can he feed himself? To what extent can he dress himself? Can he brush his teeth? Wash his hands and face? Can he run? Skip? Jump? Walk up and down steps? Ride a tricycle or a Big-Wheel? Draw? Color? Manipulate blocks or clay?

5. If the child is of school age or older. Has he continued to increase his gross motor, fine motor, language, cognitive, and social skills? Does the parent have any concerns about any developmental stage?

Temperament

1. If the patient is an infant. Is he an "easy" baby or "difficult" one? Does he experience recurrent daily crying spells in which he is difficult to console? Does he cuddle or hold himself stiffly when held? How does he interact with his parents and siblings?

2. If the patient is a toddler. Is he generally happy? How does he handle frustrations? Does he have temper tantrums? What does he do? Does he bite? Kick? Scratch? Throw objects? How do the parents handle such actions? Do the parents discipline the toddler? How? Does he attend a day-care center? How has he adjusted to this? How has he adjusted to stranger and separation anxiety? How much television is he exposed to? How does he interact with his parents and siblings?

3. If the patient is a preschooler. Is he generally a happy child? How does he handle frustrations? How do the parents discipline him? How does he interact with his parents? Sibling? Peers? Does he attend a day-care center? If so, how has he adjusted to such care? Does he have problems with school phobia? Interaction with his teacher or classmates? Can he share? Is he easily angered? Easily frightened? Anxious? How much television does he watch? What are his favorite programs?

4. If the patient is a younger school-aged child. Is he generally a happy child? How does he handle frustrations? How is he disciplined? How does he get along with his parents? Siblings? Peers? Teachers? How does he do in school? Does he like school? Is he school phobic? If "yes," how does he manifest his phobia? Is he overly fearful, anxious, or angry? Why? Has he begun to demonstrate any antisocial behaviors? If so, which one(s)? Is he involved in sports? Which one(s)? How does he do? How does he handle defeat? How much television does he watch? What are his favorite programs?

5. If the patient is an adolescent. Same questions as in (4), eliminating questions about school phobias and antisocial behaviors. Replace those with the following questions: Does he attend school? Does he like it? How well does he do? Does he smoke? Drink alcohol? Use drugs? Which one(s)? How often? Has he been in trouble with the law? Do he and his parents have a lot of fights? Do his parents like his friends? How much television does he watch? What are his favorite programs?

Miscellaneous

Has he ever been hospitalized? If "yes," for what and at what age? Has he ever had an operation? If "yes," for what and at what age? Has he ever injured himself so that he required stitches? Fractured a bone? Burned himself? Does he have any recurrent or chronic physical, psychosomatic, or emotional problems? If so, which ones and how have they been managed? Does he have any chronic medical conditions? If "yes," which ones(s)? Does he take medication(s) on a constant basis? If "yes," which one(s)? Does he have any allergies? If "yes," to which substances? Has he received the appropriate number and type of immunizations for his age? Has he experienced any adverse reactions to any immunization? If "yes," which reaction to which vaccine?

Review of Systems

General. Has he experienced weight loss or weight gain? How many pounds? Does he have a good appetite? Is he a quiet or noisy child, sedentary or active, shy or friendly, happy or sad (or angry)?

Head. Does he have headaches? How often and how long do they last? When do they occur (day and time of day)? Where is the pain located? What precipitates the headaches? What relieves them? Are they associated with abdominal pain, nausea, vomiting, or auras? Do other family members have headaches? Who? Has he experienced head trauma? When and under what circumstances?

Eyes. Does he have difficulty seeing? Does he walk into objects? Does he wear eyeglasses? Does he experience chronic tearing, itching, or redness of his eyes? Do his eyes appear disconjugate? Has he ever had an eye infection? If "yes," when and how was it treated? Has he ever sustained eye trauma?

Ears. Can the child hear loud noises? Soft voices? Has he had ear infections? If "yes," how many and when did they occur? How were they treated? Has he ever sustained trauma to his ears? Has he ever had tubes placed in his ears?

Nose. Can the child smell? Does he have chronic rhinorrhea or nasal congestion? Does he frequently rub his nose? What medications has he taken for this? How many acute upper respiratory infections has he had in the last year? Has he ever sustained serious nasal trauma? Does he experience recurrent nosebleeds?

Mouth. How many teeth does he have? Are they brushed daily? If an infant, is he routinely put to bed with a bottle? Has he ever seen a dentist? Has he ever had a toothache? Has he lost any teeth through trauma? When? If an infant, does he have difficulty sucking? Does the child have difficulty speaking clearly? Has the infant or young child experienced severe oral candidiasis? Has the patient ever sustained a "cold sore" on his lips, gums, or tongue? Does his tongue seem too large, and does he protrude it frequently?

Throat. Does he get recurrent sore throats? Has a streptococcal infection ever been documented? Have his tonsils or adenoids been removed? If "yes," why? Does he ever experience dysphagia or feel as if there is a "lump" in his throat?

Neck. Does he have enlarging masses or adenopathy in his neck? Has he sustained any neck trauma?

Respiratory. Does he have a chronic respiratory illness? Has he ever had pneumonia? If "yes," when? How was it treated? Has he ever wheezed? If "yes," when and how was it treated? Is wheezing precipitated by exercise? Noxious stimuli? Has he ever been cyanotic or short of breath? When?

Cardiac. Does the child have a known cardiac condition or heart murmur? (If "yes," clarification is needed.) Does he tire easily during feeding? Crying? Playing? Walking? Climbing stairs? Has he ever experienced chest pain? When? What precipitated it, and what relieved it? What is the character (location, radiation, quality, severity, duration) of the pain? Has it ever been associated with syncope? A sensation of rapid or irregular heartbeats? Cyanosis? Pallor? Does any family member have cardiac disease? If so, who? Do they experience pain?

Gastrointestinal. Does the child eat rapidly? Belch frequently? Regurgitate? Complain of abdominal pain immediately before or after eating? Does he have recurrent abdominal pain? When (day and time of day) does it occur? What are the characteristics (location, duration, radiation, quality, severity) of the pain? What precipitates the pain, and what relieves it? Is the pain associated with nausea, vomiting, diarrhea, or constipation? Does the child have recurrent episodes of vomiting? What precipitates them, and what relieves them? Has the vomitus ever contained blood or bile? Does the child have recurrent diarrhea? What foods or emotional factors precipitate the episodes? How are the episodes resolved (*i.e.*, what dietary managements, if any, are used)? Does the diarrhea ever contain blood? Does the child have chronic constipation? (See "Elimination" section for pertinent questions.) Is the child encopretic? Has the child ever had hepatitis or sustained significant abdominal trauma? If yes, when?

Genitourinary. Does the child experience chronic urinary symptoms (dysuria, urgency, hesistancy, nocturia, polyuria)? Has he ever had a urinary tract infection? If "yes," when? How was it treated? Did he have a radiographic work-up of his GU tract? If "yes," what was found? Is the child enuretic—during the day, at night, or both? Was he ever dry (*i.e.*, is the enuresis of new onset)? Have attempts been made to control the enuresis? Elaborate. Has the child ever been treated for a venereal disease? When and which one? How did he acquire the infection?

Back. Does the child seem to have a curved spine or walk "stoop-shouldered"? Has he sustained trauma to his spine?

Muscular. Does the child have muscle weakness, fasciculations, atrophy, asymmetry, or pain? When do (did) these occur?

Extremities. Does he walk with a limp or have weakness of a particular extremity? Are there asymmetries of appearance or function between left and right extremities? Does he have joint swelling, redness, heat, or limitation of motion? If yes, which joints and how often do joint symptoms occur? Does he have limb pain? Which limb? Has he ever fractured a bone? Which one?

Neurological. Has the child ever had a seizure? If "yes," was it associated with a fever? How old was he at the first seizure? What medication, if any, does he take for seizures?

Has he experienced any weakness, paresthesias, paresis, or loss of function of a limb? Has he ever experienced syncope, vertigo, or "light-headedness"? If "yes," when and under what circumstances? What made the symptoms better? Are these symptoms associated with GI or cardiovascular symptoms? If "yes," which ones?

Dermatological. Does the child have a chronic skin eruption? Where is it located? What does it look like (type, size, and quality of lesions)? What precipitates the eruption and what improves it? Is the eruption pruritic? Has the child had scalp infections? If so, which ones? Is the child's skin exposed to over-the-counter skin preparations? If so, which ones?

Family History. What are the ages of the parents, siblings, and grandparents? How are their states of health? Has any relative died in infancy, as a child or adolescent, or as a young adult? Of what cause? Are there any chronic illnesses that run in the families? Specifically, does anyone (identify affected person) have a disease of the cardiovascular system? Respiratory system? Gastrointestinal system? Genitourinary system? Muscular system? Neurological system? Does any family member have a malignancy? A mental disorder? Allergies or hay fever?

Social History. How many siblings does the child have? With how many people does he live? (If there are more people than his parents and his siblings, determine the identity of these other individuals.) Does he live in a house or apartment? Does he have a pet? What kind? Are his parents married, unmarried but living together, divorced, or separated? Is he in a single-parent family? Because of divorce? Death? Disappearance of one parent? Is there a stepparent or boy-/girlfriend in the family? Who cares for the child when the parent cannot? What support systems does the family have? Where do they live? Are there friends in the neighborhood? Does the family receive medical assistance? Do the parents work outside the home?

HISTORY DURING AN ILLNESS VISIT

The history obtained during an illness visit must be pertinent to the presenting complaint. Hence, the history may be brief if the child presents with a broken arm, may be moderately long if he presents with a vague complaint ("tired all the time," "no appetite"), or may be extended if he presents with failure-to-thrive.

Certain questions are applicable to all illnesses. The physician must know the onset, duration, and severity of the presenting complaint and whether it is worsening over time. Does the presenting symptom interfere with the child's usual levels of activity and mood,

sleep, or appetite? In what way? What other associated symptoms accompany the principal one? When was the child last well? Did any physical or emotional event seem to trigger this illness? What therapies, medication, dietary managements, or home remedies have been tried to alleviate the child's distress? Has the child ever had a similar illness in the past? When? How did the illness resolve? Does the child have a chronic condition that might complicate the presenting illness?

BIBLIOGRAPHY

Chun M, DeAngelis C: Problem oriented health record system. In DeAngelis C: Pediatric Primary Care, 3rd ed, pp 3–53. Boston, Little, Brown & Co, 1984

DeAngelis C, Fosarelli P: Interviewing to obtain a health history. In DeAngelis C: Pediatric Primary Care, 3rd ed, pp 55–70. Boston, Little, Brown & Co, 1984

7

The Pediatric Physical Examination

The pediatric physical examination provides an opportunity to verify historical information and to discover new clues to the child's state of health. Unless the child's life is immediately at risk, the physical examination should be conducted in a relaxed manner. Success in achieving this atmosphere depends on knowledge of the child's developmental level and the examiner's ability to act on this knowledge by tailoring his examination to the age of the patient and to the circumstances of the visit.

Until he develops stranger anxiety, the infant generally enjoys the physical examination and interaction with the examiner. Once stranger anxiety and separation anxiety become firmly established (usually near the end of the first year), not only does the toddler dislike the physical examination and fear the stranger who is performing it, but he may also cry incessantly during the entire visit. Unfortunately, this stage may last for 1 or 2 years; fortunately, there *are* ways to work around these fears.

By the time he is a verbal 3 year old, the preschooler usually is a little shy when initially approached; however, with minimal friendly encouragement, he becomes a coop-

erative, talkative, sometimes giggly patient, and the visit is a real joy. This easy relationship between child and examiner continues until age 10 or 11 years, when the child may again become somewhat reticent. This reticence may be more pronounced if the child and examiner are not of the same sex. This shyness has its basis in the child's embarrassment about his newly developing body. Finally, the adolescent patient is usually friendly and cooperative, but may also be quiet and shy or frankly distrustful. The latter attitude is related to the developmental task in adolescence of establishing oneself as an independent person by questioning authority.

Within each age-group, there are techniques to facilitate the physical examination. However, regardless of age, the examination is generally more successful if conducted in a gentle, friendly fashion. It is not just a body that is being examined; it is a person with fears and insecurities, but also with strengths and positive qualities. Attempting to reach that person, regardless of age, is part of the art of medicine. Appreciation of the child will also be welcomed by the parent and will strengthen the physician–parent bond.

The very young infant should be handled

gently and spoken to softly, with occasional rises in voice inflection to detect his responses to changes in voice. He should be held by the examiner to assess his "holdability." Most infants enjoy cuddling close to those who hold them. Occasionally, infants do not enjoy being held and actually stiffen their bodies when held. This could, of course, have deleterious effects on the mother–child bond. If the young infant cries, he should be held by the examiner and spoken to. This allows the examiner to assess how easily he can be comforted.

Most young infants do not object to the physical examination, with the possible exception of the ear and throat examination, which are somewhat invasive. Many infants cry when these parts are examined. Thus, these examinations should be done after the rest of the physical is completed.

As the infant becomes older, but before stranger/separation anxiety sets in, other maneuvers are useful to get to know the child. Infants between 2 and 7 to 8 months of age are incredibly friendly; they coo or babble, laugh, and generally enjoy interacting with other human beings. The examiner can capitalize on this friendliness by performing the examination while talking to, making noises at, or tickling the infant. Again, since the ear and throat examinations are the most invasive, they are done at the end.

The fearful toddler should be spoken to gently but firmly. In general, his fear prevents him from being attracted by the examiner's charm, so his protestations should not be taken personally. If his mother is cooperative and able to hold him, the toddler is best examined on her lap so that her physical nearness can reassure him. If he is kicking his legs, his mother can restrain them between her knees so that no one is hurt. The toddler usually fears all the medical instruments and might benefit from touching them himself before they are used on his body. He should not,

however, be forced to touch instruments if he strongly objects. Sometimes, the toddler will permit the stethoscope to be placed on his chest if he can help to hold it or if he has seen that the stethoscope on his teddy bear, his mother, his shoe, or his hand did not hurt. If an older sibling is present, he can also assist in showing the toddler that the instruments do not hurt. As mentioned earlier, the ear and throat examinations should be held until the end. During the entire physical examination, tell the child what you are going to do before you do it ("Jeremy, now I'm going to look at your ears with my light"). The examination of a toddler can be very difficult in spite of these maneuvers. Because of previous hospitalizations, chronic or recurrent medical problems, previous unpleasant experiences with health professionals, or overwhelming stranger anxiety, the child may be inconsolable and hysterical during the entire procedure. When this occurs, remain even tempered but gently firm and perform the examination as completely and as quickly as possible.

Most preschoolers and younger school-aged children enjoy talking to the examiner, answering his questions, or playing with his medical instruments. These children should also be informed of what the examiner is going to do during the visit. The examiner should be prepared to explain the reasons for different parts of the physical examination, since children of these ages are quite inquisitive. Knowing what is going to occur during the visit gives the child a sense of control over the situation and renders it less threatening. The conversation that the examiner has with the child should reflect the child's age and interests.

The older school-aged child or adolescent may initiate little spontaneous conversation and may respond to queries ("Does this hurt?" or "Can I check that rash on your back?") monosyllabically. The examiner should not take this reluctance to speak personally.

Sometimes, the adolescent will respond to serious questions ("Does this hurt?") with flippant comments ("What do you think—that it tickles?"). An even-tempered demeanor will assist the examiner with this type of patient. Preadolescents and adolescents usually appreciate knowing what the examiner is going to do and what he will expect the patient to do. Making small talk with the preadolescent or adolescent patient is not impossible, but the examiner should avoid assuming teenage jargon ("How ya doin', my main man?"); it is usually forced, and the patient knows it. Similarly, when an examiner makes small talk by feigning interest in an unlikely subject ("Punk rock? I listen to it all the time"), this strategy is likely to be transparent and unsuccessful.

The specifics of the health-maintenance examination, with age-appropriate comments, are given below. As a general rule, younger patients want their parents to be present, whereas older children and adolescents may or may not want their parents in the room. These older pediatric patients should be allowed to decide for themselves, and all concerned should abide by their wishes.

General Description. Note the patient's appearance. Is he happy or sad? Talkative or quiet? Crying or placid? Clean or unkempt? Well nourished or poorly nourished? At ease, disinterested, or fearful? Alert or dull? If the patient is an infant, how does the mother hold the baby?

Head. Measure the infant's head circumference. This is done by placing a tape measure around the head at the levels of the occipital prominence and the glabellae. The percentiles of the head circumference should match those of the child's weight and length.

Palpate the skull for asymmetries, areas of swelling, or areas of tenderness. Palpate the infant's skull for the posterior fontanelle (usually closed by 2 months of age), the anterior fontanelle (usually closed between 18 to 24 months of age), widened or overriding sutures, or resolving hematomas. The infant's head should be inspected for congenital skin markings (nevi, hemangiomas), unusual blood vessel patterns, rashes, or unusual hair loss or distribution. Many infants are bald so that these findings are easy to note. A particularly common pattern of hair loss is a band of loss in the occipital area. This occurs when an infant is left on his back for long periods. This may be a sign of neglect, but some normal infants who enjoy the self-stimulation of shaking their heads also present with this pattern of hair loss. In the older patient, hair loss may occur because of trauma (tight braiding, rough brushing, trichotillomania), local disease (tinea capitis), a systemic disease (certain endocrine disorders, malignancies), or may be idiopathic.

Rashes on the scalp vary by age. Infants frequently have "cradle cap" or seborrheic dermatitis. It can appear as dry flakes of desquamated skin in the scalp or hair or greasy adherent plaques on the scalp, on the eyebrows, behind the ears, or along the hairline. The scalps of older children should be checked for the integrity of the hair, dandruff, and the presence of rashes or lice infestation. Small pustules (folliculitis) may be present on the scalp at the sites of tight hair braiding; the hair breaks at the scalp line causing a microscopic break in the skin which becomes very superficially infected. Tinea capitis may present as areas of hair loss, areas of desquamation, areas of papular eruption, or areas of boggy inflammation (kerion).

Eyes. Inspect the patient's eyes for asymmetry, disconjugate gaze, esotropia/exotropia, unilateral or bilateral lid ptosis or proptosis, scleral injection and icterus, and conjunctival erythema and discharge. The degree of conjugate gaze can be assessed grossly by the patch test. Standing directly in front of the child, place a patch over one eye while shining a light at him. When the child fixes on the light, remove the patch and the position of the covered eye; note it should be in the same direction as the uncovered eye with the light reflex in the same position bilaterally. Repeat the procedure with the other eye. The patient must be cooperative during this procedure for the results to be meaningful. Note any deviation of the eye outward (exotropia) or inward (esotropia). Infants and children with these conditions should be referred to an ophthalmologist.

Note the pupil's size, equality at rest, and equality of reaction to light. Shining a light at the infant or child will permit you to determine if there is a photophobia (aversion to light) and whether the child sees. Very young infants may not be able to follow a light fully but may squint at a light or follow it briefly. Older infants and children will follow the light in all directions because of their curiosity about it. Thus, the examiner should move the light in a wide circle and observe the child's ability to follow and the presence of disconjugate gaze in certain directions. Determination of visual field cuts on the boundaries of peripheral vision may be possible in older children and adolescents. Such determinations are usually unsuccessful in infants because they are preverbal and in young children because they do not understand what they are supposed to do or are uncooperative.

The presence of purulent discharge, from one or both eyes, in the presence of an erythematous conjunctiva usually denotes an infection. The responsible organisms are usually respiratory pathogens and occasionally staphylococci, but in neonates and young infants, conjunctivitis due to *Neisseria gonorrhoeae* or *Chlamydia* must be considered (see Chapter 34, Sexually Transmitted Diseases). A watery discharge with conjunctival stippling is associated with allergic diseases, whereas a watery discharge with the sensation that the eye is scratchy or has a foreign body in it is associated with a corneal abrasion. Applying fluorescein to the cornea with subsequent examination with ultra violet light will reveal a green-fluorescing abrasion. Ocassionally, young infants will present with (a) chronically draining eye(s). This is usually due to nasolacrimal duct obstruction, which usually responds to massage of the area overlying the duct and rarely requires surgical probing.

The fundoscopic examination is easily performed in cooperative patients. Note the quality of the optic disc and vessels, and the presence of hemorrhages. Although it is sometimes imperative to see the fundus in infants, visualization of a red reflex bilaterally is usually sufficient. The red reflex is produced by shining the light of the ophthalmoscope into the pupils; the vascular fundus reflects the light. Failure to elicit this reflex occurs in cataracts and certain ocular tumors.

Ears. Examine the external ears for position, deformities, areas of dimpling, redness, tenderness, or discharge, and rashes. With the pneumatic otoscope, examine the canals for evidence of discharge, skin eruptions, and foreign bodies, and examine the tympanic membrane for its color (usually translucent or pearly gray), visibility of bony landmarks, its ability to reflect the otoscope's light, and its mobility (usually very mobile both on positive and negative pressures). Discharge from the ear canal can be due to external otitis or otitis media. Unlike otitis media, external otitis is associated with pain on manipulation of the external ear. Otitis media is an infection of the middle ear. If the pressure in the middle ear is too great, the tympanic membrane may perforate, and purulent material from the middle ear may drain from the ear. In nonperforated otitis media, the mobility of the tympanic membrane is the most sensitive indicator of disease. Hence, the pediatric ear examination is incomplete unless tympanic membrane mobility is assessed.

Finally, perform the Weber's and Rinne tests in verbal children. In the Weber's test, a vibrating tuning fork is placed on the top of the patient's head; the sound should be heard equally in both ears. In the Rinne test, the handle of a vibrating tuning fork is placed on each mastoid process. When the patient can no longer hear the sound (bone conduction) the fork is brought to the ear to determine air conduction. Air conduction normally lasts twice as long (in seconds) as bone conduction.

Nose. Examine the nose for deformities externally or internally, such as a deviated septum. Note the color of the mucosa, the size of the turbinates, and the presence of discharge (and its color and odor). A child with an allergy frequently has swollen blue turbinates with a thin, watery nasal discharge; a child with an upper respiratory infection usually has reddened mucosa and turbinates with a mucoid discharge. Children with nasal streptococcal infections or foreign bodies frequently present with a highly malodorous nasal discharge.

Mouth. Examine the lips and oral mucosa for color, dryness, fissuring, lesions, or swelling. Assess the tongue for appearance and presence of rashes or lesions. An enlarged tongue is commonly seen in hypothyroidism. Thrush is a common oral infection caused by *Candida albicans*; it occurs in infants, in persons with extremely poor oral hygiene, and in immunosuppressed patients. It appears as adherent white plaques on the tongue and oral mucosa. Irregular darkening of the tongue may be attributable to geographic tongue, a benign condition of unknown etiology. Vesicles and

ulcers anywhere in the mouth may be due to local trauma (biting, burns) or to viral infections, especially herpes and coxsackie.

Note the number of teeth, their color, shape, and approximation with each other, and their state of repair. Beginning at about 6 months of age, the child "cuts" a tooth per month, on the average, until 24 teeth are present. These primary teeth begin to be replaced, one by one, at age 6 to 7 years by the secondary (adult) teeth; replacement takes several years for completion. With eruption of primary teeth, there is a range of time in which the process can begin. For that reason, a 9 month old without teeth is not abnormal, whereas an 18 month old without teeth is abnormal. Teeth color can be affected by genetic factors, *in utero* exposure to certain drugs (especially tetracycline), malnutrition, systemic diseases, and exposure to certain drugs (tetracycline in a child younger than age 8 or 9) or substances (nicotine, coffee, etc.). Chronic phenytoin therapy may cause so much gum hypertrophy that the teeth are barely visible. The shape of teeth can be genetically determined or can be due to congenital infections (such as syphilis) or early systemic illnesses. The proper alignment of the teeth is known as the "bite." An overbite occurs when the upper teeth overhang the lower ones, whereas underbite occurs when the lower teeth jut out beyond the upper teeth. The child should be asked to bite down on his back teeth while the teeth alignment is noted. If severe malalignments are present, referral to a dentist is indicated.

Note the state of repair of the teeth and gums, especially the presence of hard, cream-colored plaques (tartar) on the teeth, areas of inflamed gums (gingivitis), and dental caries (appearing as variable-sized dark depressions on the dental surfaces). The patient with poor dental hygiene usually has halitosis despite brushing his teeth. A peculiarly pediatric pattern of caries is "milk-bottle caries," in which a young child presents with rotting of the upper and lower front teeth with spacing of teeth in the back. The history is that the child has been (and still is) put to bed each night with a bottle containing milk or other sweet fluid, with chronic exposure to sugar causing tooth destruction. Any child with caries of either primary or secondary teeth should be referred to a dentist.

Throat. Examine the throat for evidence of inflammation, exudate, and lesions. Note the positions of the uvula and tonsillar pillars. Also note the appearance and size of the tonsils. Tonsillar size is graded on a 4-point scale, with "1" representing tonsils that do not protrude from the planes of the pillars, and "4" representing tonsils that touch in the midline. With their multiple respiratory illnesses, children frequently have tonsils in the "2" to "3" range.

Neck. Inspect the neck for asymmetry. Note lesions and areas of dimpling (possibly representing fistulous tracts). Palpate the sternocleidomastoid muscles for their mass and any areas of tenderness or shortening (torticollis). Palpate the carotid pulses for equality of impluse. Attempt to palpate the thyroid, although it may not be palpable in infants and normal children of all ages. A thyroid that is easily palpable is an unusual finding in pediatrics and merits further consideration. When a thyroid is palpable, note its size, shape, symmetry and tenderness.

Palpate to detect adenopathy in submandibular, submental, preauricular, supraclavicular, axillary, and cervical chains (anterior and posterior). Because of their multiple respiratory illnesses, pediatric patients frequently have "shotty" adenopathy in their anterior cervical chains. If a previous or current scalp infection exists, posterior cervical nodes may also be present. When adenopathy is present, describe the number, size, consistency, mobility, and tenderness to palpation (along with overlying skin warmth and erythema). Suppurative nodes are very tender, warm, and red, and have enlarged very quickly. They may be fluctuant. Adenopathy due to chronic illnesses or malignancies is usually nontender, firm or hard, and poorly mobile.

The neck should also be examined for meningeal signs: nuchal rigidity on forward bending of the neck, a positive Kernig's sign (with the thigh flexed on the abdomen, knee extension is resisted), and a positive Brudzinski's sign (neck flexion causes reflex flexion of the knees and hips).

Chest. Inspect the chest for areas of asymmetry, inflammation, vascular patterns, other lesions of the skin, and bony deformities of the ribs, sternum, or clavicles. Palpate the bony structures for areas of tenderness. Tenderness may be associated with new or old trauma, neoplasms, or inflammation. One type of inflammation that is common in pediatrics is costochondritis, an inflammation of the costochondral junction presenting clinically as chest pain and rib tenderness.

Note the size, contour, Tanner staging (see Growth and Development), and symmetry of breast tissue, as well as the presence of accessory nipples. Young infants, especially those who are breast-fed, may have enlarged breasts due to the effect of maternal hormones. Young children may have small amounts (<1 cm) of unilateral or bilateral breast tissue. In preadolescence, one breast may enlarge before the other in girls, and one or both breasts may become a little larger in boys. Finally, many adolescent females may have breast asymmetry. When breast tissue is present, evidence of redness, tenderness, masses, skin changes, and discharge from the nipple should be sought. Masses due to breast malignancies are rare in adolescents, but those due to fibroadenomas or fibrocystic disease are not. The consistency, size, and change of mass should be reassessed 2 weeks after its initial discovery, since masses due to fibrocystic disease change in size, consistency, and tenderness in different stages of the menstrual cycle, whereas other masses do not.

Lungs. After inspection of the chest, auscultate the lungs. This and the cardiac examination are easily performed in older children, but in struggling or crying infants and toddlers, lung sounds may be difficult to appreciate. To calm such a child, the parent can quietly reassure or distract the child with a toy or bottle. Many toddlers are less threatened if the examiner averts or closes his eyes so that the child is not being stared at.

Note the presence, quality, and equality of normal breath sounds, as well as the presence and location of other sounds (rales, wheezes, rhonchi) that are not usually present. Estimate the respiratory rate and the inspiration:expiration duration ratio (usually 1:1 or 1:1.5). The respiratory rate normally varies with age. Rates in the 40s are normal in early infancy, whereas rates in the 20s are normal in older preschoolers and rates in the low teens or 20s are normal in older children and adolescents.

Rales are inspiratory sounds that are "wet" or crackling. They are due to fluid in the airways. Wheezes are high-pitched whistling sounds due to small airway compromise. Rhonchi are harsh, "snoring" sounds due to larger airway involvement. Finally, a pleural friction rub is a grating sound due to pleural inflammation.

Whenever respiratory disease is suspected, the child should be observed for flaring of his nostrils as he breathes, cyanosis, and retractions of his supraclavicular, substernal, and intercostal muscles.

Heart. Palpate the point of maximum cardiac impulse. Normally, the impulse is best palpated in the fifth intercostal space medial to the midclavicular line. In children with cardiomegaly, the impulse may be located in a different position. In children with dextrocardia, the impulse is best appreciated on the right side of the chest. Also inspect the chest for visual evidence of the cardiac impulse.

Auscultate the heart with the warm stethoscope. Determine the rate and regularity of rhythm. Sometimes children have slightly irregular rhythms, especially with respiration. The heart sounds are then auscultated. The first heart sound (S_1) is usually heard best at the cardiac apex; the second sound (S_2) is louder at the base of the heart. S_2 splits during inspiration under normal conditions. A third heart sound (S_3) is indicative of a ventricular gallop and is not normal. It is caused by the vibrations of rapidly filling ventricles. A fourth heart sound (S_4) is indicative of atrial gallop and is caused by ventricular vibrations as the atria contract at the end of diastole. Whenever an S_3 or S_4 is heard, note the location of loudest sound and the variation in sound by position (supine, sitting, standing).

While listening to the heart sounds, note whether a pericardial friction rub is present. This sound is grating and synchronous with the heart rate. If the child holds his breath, the sound will be heard clearly. It is caused by a lack of lubrication when inflamed pericardial layers rub together. Also note the loudness of the heart sounds. Muted sounds may be indicative of fluid in the pericardial sac, although obese individuals may have soft sounds transmitted through their subcutaneous tissues.

Determine if any cardiac murmurs are present. Murmurs are the result of vibrations caused by turbulent blood flow through the heart or great vessels. Murmurs are characterized by their location in the cardiac cycle (systolic—early, mid-, late, or holo; diastolic—early, mid-, late), their quality (high-pitched, blowing, low-pitched, rumbling), their response to changes in position (since standing decreases blood pooled in the cardiopulmonary bed, standing is associated with murmur decrease), radiation, and loudness. Murmurs are graded on a 6-point scale: I/VI—barely audible; II/VI—quiet but easily heard; III/VI—quickly heard; IV/VI—loud and accompanied by a thrill (a palpable vibration like the purring of a cat); V/VI—very loud; and VI/VI—audible without a stethoscope. Murmurs should be auscultated with both the bell and diaphragm of the stethoscope.

Holosystolic murmurs represent the blood flow from high ventricular pressure to low atrial pressure and are associated with mitral/tricuspid regurgitation or ventricular septal defect. Systolic ejection murmurs represent the blood flow from the ventricles to the pulmonary artery or aorta and may be innocent (rapid blood flow across normal valves produces an early systolic ejection murmur) or associated with aortic or pulmonic stenosis. Diastolic insufficiency murmurs represent the failure of the aortic or pulmonic valves to close completely and are associated with insufficiency of these valves. Diastolic filling murmurs represent ventricular filling *via* diseased mitral/tricuspid valves and are associated with stenosis of these valves.

Measure blood pressure in all patients older than 3 years and in anyone with a murmur. The blood pressure need only be measured in one arm at heart level with the child in a sitting position if no murmur was heard. If a murmur was heard, measure the blood pressure in both arms and a leg.

The cuff width should be two-thirds the upper arm length, and the cuff bladder should encircle the arm. This is crucial because ill-fitting cuffs give inaccurate readings. Blood pressure may rise as much as 20 to 40 mm Hg in response to pain, fear, crying, or excitement, and so the child should be as calm as possible during the determination. The final reading also depends on the observer's hearing acuity, the patient's movement, and the accuracy of the instrument used.

Apply the cuff to the arm and inflate it to 20 mm Hg above the point of radial pulse disappearance. Then release the pressure at 2 to 3 mm Hg/second. The first Korotkoff sound indicates the systolic pressure, the pressure exerted against the aortic wall during stroke volume. The first sound is measured at the beginning of faint sound. As pressure is further released, the second sound is heard. This is a swishing sound caused by turbulent flow through a narrowed vessel. The third sound is loud and crisp and is followed by the fourth sound, which is muffled. The fifth Korotkoff sound is the point of sound cessation. Blood pressures should be recorded by the first, fourth, and fifth sounds, even if the fourth and fifth sounds are identical.

Abdomen. Inspect the abdomen for asymmetries, protuberances, vascular patterns, skin markings, and defects in the muscular wall (diastasis recti abdominis, umbilical hernia). The normal toddler and preschooler have "potbellies" because of their lordotic spinal curvatures and muscle laxity. Infants and toddlers frequently have "fat bellies" due to their superabundance of subcutaneous fat. Asymmetries may indicate masses or organomegaly. Skin markings may provide evidence for systemic illnesses; examples include café-au-lait spots (neurofibromatosis) and ash-leaf spots (tuberous sclerosis). Defects in the abdominal wall are common. Diastasis recti is the midline separation of the rectus muscle; it is accentuated during crying or contracting of abdominal muscles. Umbilical hernias are very common in infants, with spontaneous resolution in most patients. There is a bulge at the umbilicus, accentuated by crying, laughing, coughing, or sneezing. The bulge is much larger than the defect itself, which is measured by palpating the muscles around the umbilicus and estimating its size. Such hernias rarely become incarcerated.

Palpate the abdomen gently to detect the presence of organomegaly, masses, feces, and areas of tenderness, guarding, or rigidity. The young child may cry throughout the examination, tensing his muscles, and rendering the examination difficult to perform. The child should be calmed as much as possible, and you should palpate (with warm hands) gently. The child may be more cooperative if he is permitted to "control" the examiner's hand by placing his hand atop that of the examiner. The presence of tenderness is detected by the patient's affirmation or by such involuntary indicators such as a change in cry, eye blinking or tearing, or facial grimacing. Verification of the pain elicited by manual palpation can be elicited by palpation through the stethoscope. Patients with real organic pain will respond in the same manner to palpation with either method, whereas patients with a strong psychogenic component to their pain will frequently respond more intensely to palpation by hand by than by stethoscope.

Areas of guarding (tensing of the muscles) and rigidity of the muscles (associated with intra-abdominal pathology) can be appreciated by palpation. The presence of rebound tenderness (increased pain when the examiner suddenly releases his hand from the abdominal wall compared to the pain of direct palpation), radiation of pain, and fluid waves are also elicited through palpation.

Organomegaly may be due to congenital disorders (e.g., glycogen storage diseases), acquired systemic diseases (e.g., malignancies), or infectious diseases (e.g., mononucleosis). The kidneys may be palpated in the neonate, but after early infancy, the kidneys are not usually palpable and easy detection denotes abnormal enlargement. The spleen tip may be palpated in normal children or in those who have recently experienced minor viral illness.

Splenic enlargement may be present in states of infectious illnesses, malignancies, and certain hematological disorders (such as early sickle cell disease). The spleen may also be palpable if it has been traumatized and if a splenic hematoma is present. Hepatomegaly may also be present in certain infectious illnesses, malignancies, hematological disorders, and hereditary metabolic diseases. The liver may be easily palpable in congestive heart failure and in respiratory disorders. When the liver is palpable, its edge (smooth or rough), degree of tenderness, and size should be noted. Size may be estimated by measuring how far the liver descends below the right costal margin or by measuring its span through percussion. Tenderness in the upper abdominal quadrants is not always hepatic and splenic in origin; it may be gastrointestinal, respiratory (as occurs with basilar pneumonia), or musculoskeletal. One way to evaluate abdominal tenderness is to ask the patient to rapidly jump down from the examining table; a child in moderate pain will do so slowly, and a child in severe pain will usually refuse to do the manuever.

Any masses detected by palpation are also characterized by location, size, contour, mobility, tenderness to palpation, and changes in the overlying skin.

Auscultate the abdomen to discern the presence and quality of bowel sounds, other bowel sounds such as rushes and high-pitched "tinkles," and vascular sounds such as bruits. Bowel sounds are classified as hypo-, normo-, and hyperactive. Hyperactive sounds occur in states of high gastric motility (as in gastroenteritis); hypoactive sounds may occur in severe, systemic illnesses and in ileus. Evaluate all quadrants for bowel sounds; their absence should not be concluded until you have listened in each area for several minutes. Lack of bowel sounds is indicative of obstruction.

Genitals

Male. Inspect the patient's genitalia. Note the patient's circumcision status, his penile size, and his Tanner stage. Note the size and location of the urethral meatus; a meatus on the ventral penis is hypospadias and one on the dorsal penis is epispadias. If the patient has complained of difficulty in urinating, observe his stream of voiding.

Inspect the penis for areas of trauma, inflammation, lesions, and urethral discharge. A discharge in the male is almost always secondary to infection with a venereal agent. Inspect and palpate the scrotum. The testes and their appendages should be descended bilaterally. If the room or the examiner's hands are cold, the testes may retract. Gentle pressure at the inguinal ring with one hand and palpation of the scrotum's contents with the other helps to limit the movement of the contents. Assess the size of the testes and their epididymis and cords. Testicular size varies by age, with a range of 1 to 2 cm in young infants to 3 to 4 cm in adults.

Other scrotal contents include hernias and hydroceles. Because of a defect in the inguinal wall, a loop of bowel enters the scrotum. The patient (or his parent, if he is quite young) will report that the scrotal bulge increases with exertion (crying, sneezing, coughing, laughing, Valsalva's maneuver) and decreases at rest. The older patient may recall an injury that predated the bulge. As long as the scrotal bulge is reducible (i.e., the bowel can move from the scrotum back to the abdominal cavity), there is no acute problem, although the hernia should be repaired at some point. If the hernia is "stuck" in the scrotum (or incarcerated), the patient will be in pain, and a medical emergency exists.

The diagnosis of an uncomplicated hernia is easy: the sausage-shaped scrotal mass bulges with exertion, and the mass contains bowel sounds. However, an incarcerated hernia may contain a dying loop of bowel without bowel sounds. Hernias are frequently confused with hydroceles, which are round or oval masses that are cystic. They are devoid of bowel sounds, are present at rest, and transilluminate light, which hernias fail to do. Transillu-

mination is performed by shining a bright light directly against the scrotal wall. A large hydrocele will cause the involved side of the scrotum to "light up" when transilluminated, whereas the uninvolved side does not. Hydroceles in childhood usually regress spontaneously and rarely require surgery.

Exquisite tenderness, swelling, and redness of the scrotum are associated with epididymitis, testicular torsion, and, uncommonly in pediatrics, testicular cancer. Epididymitis is an infection, usually by one of the venereal organisms, which is readily treated with antibiotics. Torsion is mechanical and constitutes a medical emergency. If the torsion is not repaired surgically, the testis will die. Prehn's sign helps to differentiate the two: when the affected side is supported in the examiner's hand, the pain improves with epididymitis but not with torsion.

Finally, the perineal skin is examined for rashes. Male and female infants frequently develop diaper rashes because of ever-present moisture and episodic maceration of the skin. The most common cause of diaper rash is an infection by *Candida albicans*. This is a highly erythematous maculopapular rash. Areas of rash may coalesce to involve the entire perineum, and small erythematous masculopapules (satellite lesions) may be present a few centimeters from the principal rash. Monilial rashes may also include pustular areas. Another common rash is that caused by *Staphylococcus aureus* in which vesicles and intact bullae, which proceed to become denuded bullae, occur.

Perineal rashes are uncommon between infancy and adolescence. In adolescence, fungal infections and infestations by lice and mites may occur in the pubic area.

Female. Inspected the female genitalia and perineum, noting any lesions, signs of trauma, rashes, or discharge, and the Tanner stage. Examine the labia, clitoris, urethral orifice, and vaginal introitus. The hymenal ring may or may not be intact, since the tissue may have been lacking from birth or may have been disrupted by any vigorous activity or fall. The vaginal orifice should be proportionally small in infancy and increases in size as the girl grows older; a woman who has had several children may have an introitus several centimeters in diameter. A large vaginal orifice in infancy and childhood is not a normal finding, and its discovery raises the issue of sexual abuse.

The presence of a discharge may be due to a sexually transmitted disease (see Chapter 34 for the characteristics of discharges caused by different agents), another infectious disease, a yeast infection, irritation, or a foreign body. Streptococcal or *Salmonella* infections may cause a purulent, sometimes bloody vaginal discharge. *Candida albicans* causes a discharge that is pruritic, thick, whitish, and cheesy. Irritation due to chemical agents such as soaps, shampoos, or bubble bath may cause a thin, clear, white or yellow discharge that is pruritic. Foreign bodies in the vagina (most commonly, bits of toilet paper) cause a highly malodorous yellow-green discharge that may be bloody. Regardless of the cause, vaginal irritation, inflammation, and infection may be accompanied by symptoms of dysuria, frequency, hesitancy, and enuresis.

Another cause of bloody discharge from the perineum is urethral prolapse. The inner surface of the urethra prolapses through its orifice, revealing a raw, bleeding surface. This condition is sometimes confused with the rare but malignant tumor, sarcoma botyroides, a purplish red tumor at the vaginal orifice. Although position alone can distinguish the two, massive swelling of the perineum sometimes makes this impossible. The child can be observed while voiding to see if urine emanates from the involved area; if it does, the condition is in the urethra. Treatment of urethral prolapse is through sitz baths; rarely,

surgery is indicated for recalcitrant cases. Treatment for botyroides is surgical.

Labial adhesions may involve sections of the entire length of the labia. Frequently, there has been an antecedent rash or irritation along the labia, which subsequently healed together. As long as the child can urinate well, can maintain good hygiene, and does not develop a urinary tract infection, no treatment is necessary. The adhesions will break apart when estrogenization occurs near puberty. If the child cannot void, cannot maintain good hygiene, or develops a urinary tract infection, the adhesions can be treated with an estrogen cream. Mechanical separation of the labia is contraindicated because it promulgates the process that originally led to the adhesions.

If a pelvic examination is to be performed after inspection and palpation of the perineum, it should be done as gently as possible. Generally, it is indicated only in sexually active girls. If such an examination is needed in a young child because of sexual assault or to remove a solid foreign body, it is best done under anesthesia.

The first pelvic examination is very frightening to the girl. If she desires, her mother or other supportive person should be allowed to stay with her. Explain what is going to occur and permit the girl to see and touch the instruments if she desires. The speculum used should be of an appropriate size and warmth.

The cervix must be visualized. The easiest way to do this is to insert your finger in the vagina prior to speculum insertion to locate the cervix and its orientation. The cervix feels like the end of a nose and is easily palpated. When the cervix's orientation is determined, insert the speculum slowly in that direction. Sometimes, insertion is easier if the girl breathes through her mouth. Once the cervix is visualized, the make note of its color, its os (closed or open), its surface (erosions, lesions), presence of a discharge, and the location of the string of an intrauterine device, if present. Sample the discharge for cultures and examination for yeast and *Trichomonas*. If a Papanicolaou's smear is to be done, take the sample from the endocervical area.

Remove the speculum after surveying the vaginal cavity for abnormalities. Then perform the bimanual examination. With one hand on the surface of the lower abdomen and two fingers of the other hand inserted into the vagina, approximate the hands. Cervical motion tenderness, present with pelvic inflammatory disease, is appreciated through this method, as are the size and tenderness of the adnexae, the size of the ovaries, and the size and tenderness of the uterus.

With two fingers of one hand in the vagina and one finger in the rectum, approximate the fingers along the area to detect pathology in the uterine ligaments.

Anus/Rectum. The anus should be inspected in all patients to detect its patency and associated findings such as skin tags, hemorrhoids, lesions attributable to venereal diseases, and evidence of trauma. Skin tags are normal growths of skin tissue connected to the body by a stalk. Hemorrhoids are engorged, tortuous, painful blood vessels that occur in severe constipation/straining and pregnancy. Lesions attributable to venereal diseases may be chancres (syphilis), vesicles (herpes), or warts (condyloma acuminata). These lesions are discussed in detail in Chapter 34. Finally, areas of trauma may be due to abuse, foreign body insertion, and straining with bowel movements. Infants and toddlers sometimes develop anal fissures in which the skin breaks open and bleeding occurs. The position of the fissure is described according to its position on a clock, with "12 o'clock" ventrally oriented and "6 o'clock" dorsally oriented. Treatment of a fissure is by sitz baths, lubrication of the area, and elimination of the constipation through dietary management.

If a rectal examination must be performed, it is done gently. In small infants, anal tone may admit only the little finger; in older children, the index finger is usually admitted. Young children are frightened by this examination, and older ones are embarrassed by it. Therefore, it is best to do this examination as quickly (but completely) as possible. Anal tone should admit a finger and not be too lax or too tight. Evaluate the rectal vault for size, content (stool, masses), and areas of tenderness. The stool present should be described as hard, soft, or watery. Areas of tenderness will be difficult to assess in young children who are crying. Consequently, a rectal exam should be done only when indicated by presenting complaint, history, or other physical findings.

Extremities and Back. Examine the extremities for symmetry of length and appearance and for equality of radial and brachial pulses in the arms and femoral and dorsalis pedis pulses in the legs. Palpate the limbs to detect any areas of masses, tenderness, or tightening of the muscles. Also estimate muscle mass. Assess the patient's muscular strength by asking him to oppose your attempts to move the body part passively; even a child should be able to limit your attempts. Areas of muscle rigidity, laxity, fasciculations, weakness, tenderness, and vacillating strength (clasp-knife response) are important.

Examine joints for their appearance, range of motion, and presence of crepitus, catches, or pain on passive and active motion. An acutely swollen, red, painful joint is considered infected until proven otherwise; a joint with chronic exacerbations and remissions of swelling with variable amounts of limitation and pain suggests a collagen-vascular disease.

Assess the child's gait. He should walk

evenly without listing and bear weight on both extremities. He should not sway, demonstrate a pelvic tilt, or walk on only certain parts of his feet.

Disturbances in walking may result from pathology at any point in the leg, abdomen, or spine. Inspect the spine visually and palpate with the child erect to detect areas of curvature. Then, with the child bent forward at the waist with arms dangling downward, stand behind the child and observe whether the pelvis tilts or the scapulae are unsymmetrical. Such findings suggest scoliosis, which may worsen during the adolescent growth spurt.

Palpate the muscles of the back and scapulae. Percuss the costovertebral angle to detect tenderness over the kidneys.

Several orthopedic problems commonly seen during infancy and early childhood deserve mention. Normal infants are bowlegged and have supple inturning of their forefeet due to their intrauterine positions. As the infant ages, he initially walks with a bowlegged gait; by the time he is 2 or 3 years of age, his normal gait will be somewhat knockkneed.

Evidence of congenital hip dislocation should be sought in infants younger than 12 months of age. Place the child on his back with his hips and knees flexed. Slowly abduct the upper legs to a 90° arc. If a hip is dislocated, the head of the femur will ride back into the acetabulum during this maneuver, with a palpable click (Ortolani's sign). If an infant has a hip click, he warrants immediate referral to an orthopedist.

Metatarsus adductus is the inturning of the forefoot. Take the infant's foot in your hand and gently attempt to move the forefoot to a neutral position. If the adductus is supple, this is easily done, and the parent can be reassured. If the adductus is rigid, the maneuver will be difficult, if not impossible, to perform. If this is the case, the child warrants orthopedic evaluation.

Tibial torsion (i.e., inward bowing of the tibia) also occurs frequently in infancy and toddlerhood. To estimate the degree of torsion, flex the knee at 90° and determine position of the medial malleolus relative to the lateral malleolus. A neonate's malleoli are parallel, whereas an adult's medial malleolus is anterior to the lateral one. The orientation of the infant's malleoli should be between these two. Imagine a horizontal line between the two malleoli and then imagine a second line connecting the patella and the medial malleolus. The intersection of these lines forms an angle that should be $-5°$ to $-20°$ in the infant. Although many cases of tibial torsion resolve spontaneously by 18 months of age, referral to an orthopedist is indicated for (1) severe gait abnormality, (2) persistence past 18 months, and (c) extreme angular torsion.

Skin. Survey the skin for evidence of rashes, inflammation, congenital lesions, growths, bruises, petechiae, and signs of abuse (especially bruises in unusual areas, bruises with a specific appearance such as linear bruises associated with belt beatings or perfectly circular bruises on the trunk, eight on the back and two on the front—finger marks—associated with shaking the child). A number of skin findings commonly found during health-maintenance visits have been described in this section by body part.

Neurological System. First observe the child to detect any tics or twitching. Then test the cranial nerves. Usually, this is easier to accomplish if the child is verbal and cooperative. Assess the olfactory nerve (I) by the patient's ability to identify a familiar odor. The optic nerve (II) has already been assessed by the measurement of visual acuity and the fundoscopic examination of the (flat) optic disc. The oculomotor nerve (III) is intact if the child can look in all directions without moving his head. The trochlear nerve (IV) is intact if the child can look downward. Assess the trigeminal nerve (V) by noting the equality of masseter muscle tension when the child clenches his teeth. The abducent nerve (VI) is intact if the child can gaze laterally. The facial nerve (VII) is intact if the smiling or crying face is symmetrical. The auditory nerve (VIII) is intact if the child hears normally. The glossopharyngeal nerve (IX) is intact if the child gags when his posterior pharynx is stimulated. The vagus nerve (X) is intact if the uvula is midline. The spinoaccessory nerve (XI) is intact if the child can hunch his shoulders against a downward force. The hypoglossal nerve (XII) is assessed by having the child protrude his tongue and determining if it is positioned in the midline.

The sensory examination can be accomplished by asking the child to close his eyes and tell you where you are touching him. The motor examination can be accomplished by asking the child how strong he is and to prove his strength by (1) squeezing your finger, (2) keeping his eyes closed while you try to open them, (3) keeping his mouth open while you try to close it, and (4) opposing your attempts to extend his flexed limb and to flex his extended limb.

Assess the strength (on a 4-point scale, with 4 being the strongest) and equality of deep tendon reflexes at the elbow, knee, and ankle by tapping the tendons with a reflex hammer. Reflexes may be asymmetric, absent, or hyperreflexive if the child is "trying to help." If this occurs, distract him with another activity.

Assess cerebellar function by determining the child's equilibrium when tandem-walking (i.e., tightrope walking), observing the child for tremors when he holds his arms straight out in front of him with his hands open, and observing whether the child can accurately touch his finger to his nose when his eyes are closed.

A young infant's neurologic status is assessed by noting whether he is alert, has a good suck, had good head control by 3 to 4 months (tested by gently pulling him to a sitting position), has a startle (Moro's) reflex (tested by presenting the supine infant with a loud noise; the infant startles, extends all extremities and then flexes them, perhaps with a cry), and whether palmar and plantar grasps are present. The Moro's reflex and the grasp reflex disappear by 3 to 4 months of age. Other reflexes characteristic of the young infant are the stepping reflex (standing infant "walks" by moving feet alternately), the placing reflex (standing infant "climbs" by lifting feet when the dorsi are stimulated), and the asymmetric tonic neck reflex (infant whose head is held to one side extends the limbs on the side he is facing and flexes the contralateral limbs).

Finally, elicit Babinski's reflex. When the lateral part of the sole is stimulated in a noxious fashion, the foot should dorsiflex and the toes should fan out. Up to 1 year of age, an abnormal Babinski's (i.e., extension of toes) is a normal finding.

Psychological. If you have been interacting with the patient throughout the examination, you will have a good idea of the child's state. Extensive psychological evaluation should be obtained when indicated.

BIBLIOGRAPHY

Carcio H: Manual of Health Assessment. Boston, Little, Brown & Co, 1985
DeAngelis C: The physical examination. In DeAngelis C: Pediatric Primary Care, 3rd ed, pp 71–104. Boston, Little, Brown & Co, 1984

Part IV: The Emergency Room

8

Respiratory Disorders

Alterations in respiration are common presenting complaints in the pediatric emergency room. In this chapter, several abnormal patterns of respiration will be described, and a general classification of the causes of respiratory distress will be given. Finally, two specific physical signs, stridor and wheezing, will be discussed in some detail.

Dyspnea is the general term used to describe labored or difficult breathing; it is a symptom, not a specific diagnosis, as are the other terms defined below. It implies a degree of discomfort or distress perceived by the patient, something that may not necessarily be present in pediatric patients, in which case the term *respiratory distress* might be more appropriate.

Apnea refers to the absence of breathing, *bradypnea* to slow breathing, *tachypnea* to rapid breathing, and *hyperpnea* to respirations of increased depth. *Hyperventilation* describes breathing in excess of the body's needs and might more accurately be termed *over-ventilation*.

The causes of dyspnea may be catagorized as follows:

1. Mechanical, such as with airway obstruction (*e.g.*, congenital anomaly or foreign body), bony defects of the thorax, pleural effusion, or abdominal distention.
2. Pulmonary insufficiency, as seen with pneumonia, bronchiolitis, pulmonary edema, atelectasis, or interstitial fibrosis.
3. Hypoxic drive, not due to pulmonary insufficiency but rather to other conditions limiting oxygen delivery to the tissues, as may be seen in cases of severe anemia or cyanotic congenital heart disease.
4. Neuromuscular, as with muscular dystrophy or Guillain-Barré syndrome.
5. Central nervous system, as with acidosis, salicylate poisoning, and meningitis.
6. Psychological/emotional.

STRIDOR

Stridor, a sign of upper airway obstruction, is a harsh sound that occurs predominately on inspiration. It may be the result of a congenital abnormality (*e.g.*, laryngeal web, hemangioma, or tracheal malacia), compression of the airway (*e.g.*, tumor or retropharyngeal abscess), angioneurotic edema, foreign body aspiration, or an acute inflammatory process. It is a significant symptom that should never be taken lightly, particularly since it is the primary manifestation of two serious pediatric diseases, croup and epiglottitis.

Croup (Acute Laryngotracheobronchitis)

Acute laryngotracheobronchitis refers to an acute inflammatory process involving primarily the large airways. It must be differentiated from epiglottitis and from two other less common forms of croup, bacterial tracheitis and spasmodic croup. It is almost always of viral etiology, with the parainfluenza viruses implicated as the cause of almost three quarters of all cases. Outbreaks typically occur in the autumn and early winter. The disease is characterized by edema and inflammation of the subglottic area.

The clinical picture of acute laryngotracheobronchitis is very familiar to all pediatricians. The illness is most common in children younger than 3 years of age. It is usually preceded by mild upper respiratory tract symptoms for a few days. Then, the disease commonly declares itself with the sudden onset of a harsh, barking cough with varying degrees of inspiratory stridor. Symptoms may then wax and wane over several days and typically will be worse at night. Most patients recover fully without any treatment, although some do require hospitalization and a few will even progress to respiratory failure.

Bacterial tracheitis is much less common than viral croup. It also frequently is preceded by a viral upper respiratory infection. Bacteria that have been implicated as causes include *Staphylococcus aureus*, *Corynebacterium diphtheriae*, and *Haemophilus influenzae*. In addition to edema and inflammation, a purulent exudate is usually present. Bacterial tracheitis may progress rapidly and require aggressive management.

Spasmodic croup is a third distinct entity. There usually is no prodrome, and stridor may develop almost instantaneously. Interestingly, it may resolve nearly as quickly as it began. Spasmodic croup may recur and has been associated with atopic disease; some cases actually appear to be a variant of asthma and may respond to treatment with bronchodilators.

The diagnosis of croup is generally made based on the historical points noted above and the classic physical signs of stridor and barking cough. There frequently will be intercostal or suprasternal retractions. Significant fever may or may not be present. The most critical steps in the evaluation of a patient with croup are (1) to gauge the severity of the obstructive process and the possibility of respiratory failure and (2) to rule out other possible causes of stridor, especially epiglottitis, an illness that may, without prompt intervention, rapidly progress to complete airway obstruction. If the diagnosis is unclear and the patient is stable, lateral and anteroposterior x-rays of the neck may be used to help clarify the diagnosis. If, however, the patient appears at all unstable or if there is any concern about airway maintenance, the patient should be taken quickly to the operating room for endoscopic evaluation and intubation under highly controlled circumstances, with physicians trained in pediatric airway management and tracheostomy working in an organized team.

Once the diagnosis of croup has been established, management is largely supportive for most patients. Arterial blood gases should be obtained if there is any indication of impending respiratory failure. Nebulized racemic epinephrine may be highly effective in aborting an acute attack, probably acting locally as a vasoconstrictor to decrease edema. Its effect may be quite short-lived, however, and a rebound phenomenon has been described, making observation for several hours after administration imperative. Mist therapy has become a standard component in the management of croup, although its real benefit appears minimal in controlled studies. Even more confusing is the role of steroids in croup, since several studies have given conflicting results; it is probably most accurate at this time to say that steroids may have some beneficial effect and should be used in severe cases, particularly those requiring intensive care. While no standard dose has been established, most protocols recommend the use of intramuscularly injected dexamethasone (0.5 to 1.5 mg/kg), given in one or two doses early in the course of illness.

Croup is thus a term used to describe several clinical entities. It is a common disease, with a highly variable course, although most children recover over several days with no untoward effects. Keep in mind that although croup is the most common cause of stridor in children, its differential diagnosis is broad and includes one of the truly life-threatening diseases in pediatrics—epiglottitis.

Epiglottitis

Epiglottitis is an acute inflammatory condition involving not only the epiglottis but also adjacent supraglottic structures, including the arytenoid cartilage and arytenoepiglottic folds. The clinical course is fulminant and requires immediate intervention. The illness is almost always caused by *Haemophilus influenzae* type b.

Although stridor and respiratory distress are common presenting complaints, epiglottitis has many distinct features that usually set it apart from croup. Patients appear toxic, and positive blood cultures are, in fact, common. There is usually rapid development of high fever, complaints of a sore throat, and intense dysphagia. Children with epiglottitis tend to be a bit older than those having croup, with most cases occurring in the 2-to-6-year age-group. The classic picture of a patient with epiglottitis is a child who looks ill and who is sitting upright with his head forward and his neck hyperextended, usually drooling because of dysphagia.

Any child suspected of having epiglottitis deserves prompt attention. A skilled team should be assembled, including a pediatrician, an otolaryngologist, and an anesthesiologist skilled in pediatric airway management. While these preparations are being made, the child should be disturbed as little as possible, and no attempts at visualizing the pharynx or epiglottis should be made. X-rays of the neck may be indicated in a child in whom the diagnosis is in question and who appears very stable. Unnecessary manipulation of the child, however, may precipitate complete airway obstruction and must be avoided. If at all possible, the parents should be allowed to remain with the child to provide reassurance. Blow-by oxygen may also be administered by a parent.

Airway stabilization is the most critical aspect of management in epiglottitis. Once the appropriate team members are present, along with ancillary personnel, the child is taken to the operating room and electively intubated. If intubation is impossible, a tracheostomy should be performed immediately. The patient must then be monitored in an intensive care unit, usually under heavy sedation, until the inflammation has subsided sufficiently to allow for safe extubation.

Once an airway has been established, antibiotic drugs and intravenous fluids may be administered. The antibiotic must have good *H. influenzae* coverage; because of the frequency of ampicillin-resistant strains, chloramphenicol or a cephalosporin like cefuroxime or cefotaxime should be give at age-appropriate doses.

In some cases, epiglottitis will be complicated by infections in other sites. Otitis media, pneumonia, and adenitis are relatively common complications, whereas meningitis and septic arthritis are quite rare. These possibilities should be investigated, but only after airway management has been undertaken.

Epiglottitis is thus an illness that strikes fear in the hearts of pediatricians. Fortunately, early recognition and appropriate airway management now allow for a good outcome in most cases, and the use of *H. influenzae* type b vaccines now available for routine use may substantially reduce the incidence of the disease in future years.

WHEEZING

Wheezing is a high-pitched sound created by linear airflow through a narrowed airway. The narrowing may be focal or diffuse and involve large or small air passages. Wheezing is typically heard during expiration, but in some cases, there may be an inspiratory component as well. It may or may not be associated with dyspnea, although commonly there is at least mildly increased expiratory effort. It is critical to localize approximately the site of obstruction, particularly if there is a focal tracheal narrowing, by auscultating over the neck as well as the chest. Note the presence or lack of rales and rhonchi. Then, perform a careful general physical examination, observing for any diagnostic clues such as evidence of atopic disease (*e.g.*, eczema, allergic "shiners"), congenital heart disease, or other chronic illnesses (*e.g.*, growth failure, digital clubbing).

The old adage, "All that wheezes is not asthma," deserves emphasis. The differential diagnosis for the wheezing child is quite broad and encompasses causes of obstruction in the trachea, major bronchi, smaller bronchi, and bronchioles. Obstructive lesions in the trachea that may produce wheezing include tracheal webs, vascular rings, tracheomalacia, and aspirated foreign bodies. In the large bronchi, there may be obstruction due to foreign bodies or to external compression by tumors or mediastinal adenopathy. Narrowing of the small airways may occur as the result of asthma, bronchiolitis, tracheoesophageal fistula, cystic fibrosis, pulmonary edema, and α_1-antitrypsin deficiency.

The evaluation of the wheezing child must include a thorough history and physical examination. The following information should be obtained: In what timeframe has the illness developed? Is this a recurrent problem? Has the child been on bronchodilator therapy in the past? Is there an associated cough? What factors seem to precipitate or exacerbate the wheezing? Is there an associated upper respiratory infection? Does the child or anyone in the family have a history of atopic disease? Is the child otherwise healthy? These data will provide a framework for additional questioning and the formulation of a differential diagnosis.

In the physical examination, first assess the degree of respiratory distress and the potential need for immediate intervention. Evaluate the adequacy of air movement, as well as the use of accessory muscles, the prolongation of the expiratory phase, the degree of hyperinflation, the pulsus paradoxus, and the presence of cyanosis. The measurement of a peak expiratory flow rate is an additional tool that is of great value in assessing the degree of obstruction and monitoring the response to therapy.

Further evaluation will depend on the particular situation. A chest x-ray is generally warranted in the assessment of any child's first episode of wheezing. Airway x-rays may also be indicated, especially if a foreign body is suspected. An arterial blood gas evaluation should be done if impending respiratory failure is suspected.

Although "all that wheezes is not asthma," asthma is certainly the most common cause of wheezing in infants and children. The following is an approach to the emergency management of asthma. A more in-depth discussion of asthma and its long-term management may be found in Chapter 58.

Acute Asthma Attacks

When a child presents with an acute asthma attack, it is important to initiate therapy quickly, after taking a brief, carefully directed history and performing a physical examination. Historical data should include the child's past history of wheezing and response to therapy, the precipitants and duration of this attack, the medications that already have been taken, and the presence of any other significant illnesses. The examination is done as described above, to assess quickly the degree of respiratory distress and the adequacy of air movement.

The first line of therapy for an acute asthma attack is administration of a beta-adrenergic agonist. Although the subcutaneous injection of aqueous epinephrine (0.01 ml/kg/dose) is traditional and highly effective, more effective drugs and delivery systems are available and should be used. These allow for the delivery of more specific β_2-adrenergic agents (*e.g.*, metaproterenol, albuterol, isoetharine) by an aerosol route, providing rapid onset of effect with fewer side effects and significantly prolonged duration of action as compared with epinephrine. Even most young children may be treated in this manner by allowing them to sit in a parent's lap with a mask attached to the nebulizer, although some infants and toddlers who are in severe distress or otherwise unable to cooperate will benefit most from an initial injection of epinephrine.

If the wheezing has not cleared after the first dose of an adrenergic agonist, a second dose may be given. Then, if wheezing still persists, the addition of theophylline usually will be required. This may be given either orally or intravenously, depending on the severity of the attack. A dose of 6 mg/kg is usually recommended, although this should be adjusted downward if the child already is receiving a theophylline preparation. A serum theophylline level should be obtained if there are any questions about dosing, aiming for the thera-peutic range of 10 to 20 μg/ml. Another dose of the beta-adrenergic agonist may be given while waiting for the theophylline to take effect.

Corticosteroids are not indicated for all patients but should be given to those children who are steroid dependent (including those on long-term therapy with inhaled steroids), those with impending respiratory failure, and those who show no improvement after 6 to 8 hours of therapy. Other therapy is largely supportive, with special attention paid to adequate oxygenation and hydration.

Common complications of acute asthma include atelectasis, pneumomediastinum, and pneumonia. A chest x-ray is indicated if these conditions are suspected or if the attack is otherwise atypical. Little other evaluation is required, except for blood gas measurements in any child in severe distress. Peak expiratory flow measurements should be repeated at regular intervals throughout the course of therapy.

If the wheezing clears or at least resolves significantly, the child may be discharged. It is important to realize, however, that no matter how clear the chest may sound on auscultation, there commonly is some degree of airway obstruction and increased airway hyperreactivity for 1 to 2 weeks after an acute attack. Hence, the child should be managed during this period through administration of an oral bronchodilator, usually theophylline and/or metaproterenol. In addition, if the attack was a recurrence or if the patient has been on long-term steroids therapy, a short course of prednisone should be given, usually 0.5 to 1.0 mg/kg/day for 5 to 7 days. All patients should then be seen in follow-up after 10 to 14 days to assess the need for further therapy.

If a patient's wheezing has not cleared sufficiently after several hours of treatment in the emergency room, hospitalization will be required. In the hospital, the therapy that was begun initially should be continued: adrener-gic agonists should be given every 2 to 4 hours, a therapeutic theophylline level should be maintained, corticosteroids are frequently given, adequate oxygenation is ensured, and the child is carefully monitored. In the most severe cases, this regimen will be insufficient, and the child will require intensive care, at times needing intravenous administration of isoproterenol and even mechanical ventila-tion.

Once the wheezing has subsided, the patient may begin to receive medication oral-ly and may be discharged, again with a follow-up visit 10 to 14 days after discharge and daily oral administration of medication in the inter-im. The final critical step is a careful review of the asthma attack by both the physician and the patient/family, examining both the pre-cipitating events and the response to therapy and aiming to prevent future acute attacks.

The Wheezing Infant

Wheezing in infancy deserves special consid-eration. It is a common problem, with an esti-mated incidence of about 10%, and is distinct from wheezing in older children in several respects. Infants are particularly prone to wheezing because of their airway anatomy and are much less responsive to bronchodila-tor medications than are older children. In addition, many congenital anomalies of the airway present with wheezing in infancy. Here a general approach to the wheezing infant will be provided. A more detailed dis-cussion of the major causes of wheezing in infancy, asthma and bronchiolitis, can be found in Chapter 14.

It has been postulated that infants have dis-proportionately narrow peripheral airways, placing them at increased risk of developing airway obstruction. While this concept has come under some debate, it is clear that infant airways are of smaller absolute caliber than those of older children. Because resistance to

airflow in a tube is inversely proportional to the fourth power of the radius, narrowing of a small tube results in significantly more obstruction than an equal narrowing of a larg-er tube. Thus, resistance to airflow in infants may be dramatically increased by a process (e.g., edema, bronchospasm, mucus produc-tion) that might have only a minimal effect on airway resistance in an older child or adult.

The evaluation of the wheezing infant is essentially the same as that noted previously for wheezing in general. Additional points that deserve attention, however, include any evidence of feeding difficulties, fatigue, or apnea. While those difficulties are possible at any age, they are particularly relevant for infants, who may possess less reserve and poorer control of the respiratory musculature. Any infant who is gagging or choking with feeding, usually secondary to tachypnea, is at significant risk for aspiration.

Although the differential diagnosis for the wheezing infant is very much the same at that described previously, several critical points should be noted. First, this is the age when congenital anomalies of the airway and car-diovascular system (e.g., tracheal webs, vascu-lar rings) most commonly present, and one must maintain a high level of suspicion in order to diagnose these conditions. Second, bronchiolitis is by definition a disease of infancy and early childhood and is a very com-mon cause of wheezing in this age-group. Third, cystic fibrosis must be considered in the wheezing infant, especially if it is a recur-rent problem. Finally, for too long physicians have taught that reactive airway disease (asth-ma) is uncommon in infancy. This is clearly not the case, although it is true that the diag-nosis may be difficult to establish, especially on the first episode of wheezing, and that the response to bronchodilators may be poor. In fact, however, it has been shown that more than 30% of asthmatics developed their ini-tial symptoms in the first year of life.

The most appropriate therapeutic approach

to the wheezing infant remains controversial. Most important is establishing an accurate diagnosis. Too often the patient with a congenital anomaly is treated with multiple courses of bronchodilators before the correct diagnosis is made. Further, there is little data to support the efficacy of bronchodilators in this age-group under any circumstances, presumably because of lesser amounts and altered responsiveness of the bronchiolar smooth muscle, although some patients do appear to improve clinically. If the child has only mild wheezing and is in no significant distress, no medication need be given. If there is significant respiratory distress, a trial of a beta-adrenergic agonist such as epinephrine or metaproterenol is warranted. One study suggested that the combination of a beta-adrenergic agonist and corticosteroid might be most efficacious, and this combination might be recommended for the patient whose condition requires hospitalization. Theophylline might also be added for those sickest infants, as long as great caution with dosing is observed; theophylline is metabolized slowly and, at times, erratically by infants, and overdose is not uncommon.

For the infant with recurrent wheezing, the diagnosis of asthma is made once other conditions, such as anatomic abnormalities and cystic fibrosis, have been ruled out. These patients may respond better to bronchodilators than those with bronchiolitis, although that is not always the case. For these patients, nebulized cromolyn sodium on a long-term basis may be a useful adjunct to the medications noted above, with oral administration of beta-adrenergic agonists probably being the most useful and safest first-line therapy.

BIBLIOGRAPHY

Croup and Epiglottitis

Bates JR: Epiglottitis: Diagnosis and treatment. Pediatr Rev 1:173, 1979

Battaglia JD: Severe croup: The child with fever and upper airway obstruction. Pediatr Rev 7:227, 1986

Davis HW, Gartner JC, Galvis AG et al: Acute airway obstruction: Croup and epiglottitis. Pediatr Clin North Am 28:859, 1981

Denny FW, Murphy TF, Clyde WA et al: Croup: An 11-year study in pediatric practice. Pediatrics 71:871, 1983

Nelson WE: Bacterial croup: A historical perspective. J Pediatr 105:52, 1984

Tunneson WW, Feinstein AR: The steroid-croup controversy: An analytic review of methodologic problems. J Pediatr 96:751, 1980

Asthma

Ben-Zvi Z, Lam C, Hoffman J et al: An evaluation of the initial treatment of acute asthma. Pediatrics 70:348, 1982

Fischl M, Pitchenik A, Gardner L et al: An index predicting relapse and the need for hospitalization in patients with acute bronchial asthma. N Engl J Med 305:783, 1981

Howard WA: The differential diagnosis of wheezing in children. Pediatr Rev 1:239, 1980

Kunland G, Leong A: The management of status asthmaticus in infants and children. Clin Rev Allergy 3:37, 1985

Leffert F: The management of acute asthma. J Pediatr 96:1, 1980

Lulk S, Newcomb R: Emergency management of asthma in children. J Pediatr 97:346, 1980

Ownby D, Abarzua J, Anderson J et al: Attempting to predict hospital admission in acute asthma. Am J Dis Child 38:1012, 1984

Stempel D, Mellon M: Management of acute severe asthma. Pediatr Clin North Am 31:879, 1984

Wheezing in Infants

Eigen H: Clinical pharmacology of the wheezing infant. Pediatr Ann 14:325, 1985

Fireman P: The wheezing infant. Pediatr Rev 7:247, 1986

Nickerson BG: Approach to the wheezing infant. Pediatr Ann 15:99, 1986

9

Fever

Fever is the most common presenting complaint in the pediatric emergency room, as well as the most common reason for telephone calls and unscheduled visits to the pediatrician. In most cases, a careful history and physical examination will lead to a specific diagnosis. In others, however, no obvious source or focus of infection will be evident, in which case it becomes the physician's responsibility to identify the few children presenting with fever who may have a significant illness, particularly meningitis or septicemia. The following discussion will deal with the evaluation and management of the infant or child who presents with a fever without an obvious source. The discussion will be divided into three separate age-groups, because although there may be significant overlap among them, they are sufficiently distinct to warrant separate consideration.

FEVER IN INFANTS AGED 1 TO 8 WEEKS

Fever in the first 2 months of life deserves special consideration for several reasons. Infants in this age-group are unusually susceptible to pathogens against which they have not received passive protection and tend to localize infections poorly. In addition, the signs and symptoms of meningitis or sepsis in young infants may be very subtle, especially early in the course of an illness and during the first month of life. Thus, all febrile infants in the first 2 months of life must be considered at high risk for bacterial infection.

The pathogens encountered in this age-group are quite unique. In the first 4 weeks of life, the most common pathogens are those acquired perinatally, including group B *Streptococcus*, *Escherichia coli*, other enteric gram-negative bacilli, *Listeria monocytogenes*, and herpes simplex virus. The second month of life brings a wider variety of pathogens, including both those acquired perinatally and those commonly affecting older infants, such as *Streptococcus pneumoniae*, *Haemophilus influenzae* type b, *Neisseria meningitides*, and *Salmonella*. As will be discussed later, this diversity in possible pathogens presents significant therapeutic challenges.

The work-up of the febrile infant is relatively straight forward. A careful history should assess all potential perinatal risk factors (*e.g.*, maternal infections, premature rupture of membranes), any exposures to infections in the household, and any clues to a possible source of infection. A judgment should be made as to how "ill" the infant appears, based on factors such as feeding, irritability, consolability, interaction with the observer, looking about the room, reaching for objects, vocalizing, and smiling. The examination should further assess the degree of fever and any evidence of ear, soft tissue, pulmonary, or skeletal infection.

Unfortunately, because neither the height of the fever nor the appearance of the infant will identify all infants with or without a significant illness, any infant in this age-group with a temperature higher than 38° C deserves a complete laboratory evaluation, including a complete blood count with differential, a blood culture, a lumbar puncture, a urinalysis, a urine culture, and, frequently, a chest x-ray. Some physicians also advocate the use of the erythrocyte sedimentation rate and C-reactive protein to help assess the risk of bacterial illness.

The physician will now have compiled a significant body of data on which a therapeutic decision may be based. For the infant who appears profoundly ill, the decision to hospitalize and institute parenteral antibiotic therapy is clear-cut. Most febrile infants, however, appear well or only mildly ill and have no source of fever on physical examination; their management is more controversial. It is clear that if a specific diagnosis, such as meningitis, pneumonia, or a urinary tract infection has been made, the infant should be admitted for therapy. It has also been shown, however, that 20% to 50% of infants younger than 8 weeks of age selected only for a temperature greater than 38° C will be shown to have a significant illness on further evaluation. These diagnoses include osteomyelitis, meningitis, pneumonia, and, in 4% to 15% of such infants, bacteremia. Both infants with a focus and without a focus of infection are at risk for bacteremia.

Many investigators have sought to develop criteria to identify those infants with or without bacteremia or other significant illness. In general, particularly in infants over 4 weeks of age, the risk of significant illness increases with higher fever, an ill appearance, total white blood cell counts greater than 15,000, and band counts greater than 1500. Each of these criteria is less useful in infants under a month of age, however, and no system is predictive in 100% of cases. This dilemma places the physician in a difficult position.

The end result is that in most centers all febrile infants under 8 weeks of age receive the full work-up described above. Then, realizing our limitations and the possible consequences of missing a significant diagnosis, all infants less than 4 or 6 weeks of age are admitted to the hospital. Most then receive intravenous antibiotic therapy, although some felt to be at lowest risk of bacterial illness may be admitted only for observation. It is important to realize, however, that these regimens are not ideal, since hospitalization is often not a benign procedure and truly adequate observation of the infant is often not done well in the hospital.

Infants in the second month of life are managed somewhat differently in some centers. While all still generally receive a complete evaluation, including a lumbar puncture, those without any of the risk factors noted above (i.e., fever >39° C, white blood cell count >15,000, band count >1500) and who appear clinically well, exhibiting a social smile and normal interactions with the environment, may at times be managed as outpatients. This may be done safely, however, only if the family is reliable and careful follow-up is arranged. The advantage of this outpatient management of the febrile infant 4 to 8 weeks of age is that the hazards of hospital admission (e.g., intravenous sloughs, side effects of antibiotics) may be avoided in those patients deemed to be at lowest risk for significant illness.

Antibiotic therapy for those infants admitted to the hospital must be directed at the pathogens noted previously. In the first 4 weeks, ampicillin and an aminoglycoside (*e.g.*, gentamicin, amikacin) are usually regarded as the first-line agents for empiric therapy. A third-generation cephalosporin, such as cefotaxime, may be used in place of the aminoglycoside and is generally preferred in cases of meningitis in this age-group. In the second (and third) month of life, empiric therapy must be directed at a wide variety of pathogens and is probably best done using a combination of ampicillin and a third-generation cephalosporin, providing coverage for perinatally acquired group B streptococci, coliforms, and *Listeria*, as well as *H. influenzae* and *S. pneumoniae*.

Once antibiotic therapy has been initiated, the infant should remain hospitalized for a minimum of 2 or 3 days. If no source for the fever has become evident and all cultures are negative, the antibiotic may be discontinued and the infant discharged from the hospital. A similar regimen of close observation while culture results are pending should be used for those infants not receiving antibiotics as well.

Hopefully, new advances in the coming years will provide the means for more rapid identification of those infants with a significant illness. Rapid viral diagnostic techniques will certainly contribute in that regard. Until that time, however, we are obligated to accept our limitations and exercise great caution in the care of the febrile infant.

FEVER IN THE CHILD AGED 2 MONTHS TO 2 YEARS

The approach to the febrile patient is quite different after the first 2 or 3 months of life. Febrile illnesses are extremely common and generally self-limited. Immunologic development allows the infant to localize infection more effectively and to eliminate the vast majority of pathogens encountered. Furthermore, their evaluation is greatly facilitated by an increasing ability to display specific signs referable to a particular site of infection and to appear "ill" when they have a significant infection.

The infant in this age-group is exposed to a wide variety of viral and bacterial pathogens. For the child without an obvious source of infection, the primary diagnostic concerns that must be addressed are meningitis and bacteremia. The vast majority of children with meningitis declare themselves as significantly ill and are managed accordingly. It can be more difficult, however, to separate those with bacteremia from the much larger group of patients who have a benign, self-limited illness.

Although much has been written in recent years about the occurrence of bacteremia in children with fever and no obvious source of infection, there is still a great deal of controversy about their management. The incidence of occult bacteremia in such patients has been reported to be between 3% and 7% in various studies. *Streptococcus pneumoniae* accounts for about 75% of cases, followed by *Haemophilus influenzae*, *Salmonella*, and *Neisseria meningitidis*. The occurrence of bacteremia more reliably correlates with specific risk factors in this age-group than in infants younger than 2 months of age. That is, fever above 38.9° C, a white blood cell count >15,000, an erythrocyte sedimentation rate >30 mm/hr, and an ill or toxic appearance are all associated with bacteremia and may be used to identify patients at risk. Unfortunately, however, while the sensitivity of these risk factors is high, their specificity is low; thus, the majority of children with these risk factors do not have bacteremia, whereas nearly all children with bacteremia exhibit at least one of these features. It should be emphasized that in this age-group the most important predictive factor is the physician's clinical impression.

Thus, most pediatrician's would agree that infants in this age-group with a temperature higher than 39° C and no obvious source of infection are at some real risk of having bacteremia. If any other risk factors are present, particularly an ill appearance, a blood culture and possibly even a lumbar puncture are indicated. This approach is particularly true in the emergency room situation, in which close observation and follow-up may not be ensured. In this circumstance, the blood culture at least guarantees that the sickest children will be identified and may then be brought back by whatever means for appropriate management. The private pediatrician may be able to take a very different approach, realizing that certain parents will be able to recognize their child as significantly ill long before a blood culture might be shown to be positive.

Much has been written about the generally benign nature of pneumococcal bacteremia. While it is true that it may be a transient condition that often resolves without therapy, soft tissue complications such as otitis media and pneumonia develop in 10% to 25% of cases, and up to 4% of patients have been reported to develop meningitis. Systemic complications are much more common in *H. influenzae* and meningococcal bacteremia, conditions that should never be regarded as benign. Thus, when a blood culture is found to be positive, all patients should be called back for reevaluation. Those with cultures positive for *H. influenzae*, *N. meningitidis*, and most other pathogens should be admitted for parenteral administration of antibiotics pending repeat cultures, while those with pneumococcal bacteremia may be treated differently. If they are febrile or otherwise ill, they should also be admitted, whereas if they appear completely well and careful observa-

tion at home is ensured, they may generally be sent home with no therapy, their bacteremia considered truly transient.

Finally, controversy persists about the use of outpatient antibiotic therapy in patients felt to be at high risk for bacteremia. While only a small body of data currently exists, it would appear that the complications of bacteremia may be significantly reduced by such antibiotic use. Orally administered amoxicillin, often along with a dose of ampicillin injected intramuscularly, is generally recommended in this circumstance. It is critical that this therapy be used judiciously, being reserved for infants at highest risk and with all necessary cultures, including spinal fluid, obtained prior to antibiotic administration. Further, oral therapy should never be used as a substitute for parenteral administration of antibiotics in infants felt sick enough to warrant hospitalization, for whom broad-spectrum coverage with a second- or third-generation cephalosporin is usually recommended.

CHILDREN OLDER THAN 2 YEARS OF AGE

Immunologic maturation and accumulating antigenic exposures result in less frequent occurrence of serious infections as the child approaches school age. While bacteremia and meningitis certainly still occur, the ability to communicate with the patient and perform a complete physical examination lessens the chance of missing these and other significant diagnoses. As with younger children, the height of fever, elevation of the white blood cell count and erythrocyte sedimentation rate, and degree of toxicity are all predictive of bacteremia and dictate the need for blood cultures and antibiotic therapy. Thus, while the physician should not be lulled into a sense of false security, the evaluation of the febrile child in this age-group should be more straightforward and less anxiety provoking than the evaluation of the febrile infant.

BIBLIOGRAPHY

Bratton L, Teele DW, Klein JO: Outcome of unsuspected pneumococcemia in children not initially admitted to the hospital. J Pediatr 90:703, 1977

Carroll WL, Farrell MK, Singer JI et al: Treatment of occult bacteremia: A prospective randomized clinical trial. Pediatrics 72:608, 1983

DeAngelis C, Joffe A, Wilson M et al: Iatrogenic risks and financial costs of hospitalizing febrile infants. Am J Dis Child 137:1146, 1983

Dershewits RA, Wigder HN, Wigder CM et al: A comparative study of the prevalence, outcome, and prediction of bacteremia in children. J Pediatr 103:352, 1983

Klein JO, Schlesinger P, Karasic R: Management of the febrile infant 3 months of age or younger. Pediatr Infect Dis 3:75, 1984

Long SS: Approach to the febrile patient with no obvious focus of infection. Ped Rev 5:305, 1984

Lorin MI: Fever without localizing signs. In Lorin MI: The Febrile Child, 1982, John Wiley and Sons, p. 69.

Roberts K: The management of young, febrile infants: Primum non nocere revisited. Am J Dis Child 137:1143, 1983

10   Loss of Consciousness

The child with an altered state of consciousness often presents significant diagnostic and therapeutic challenges to the emergency room physician. True loss of consciousness, particularly if prolonged, represents a medical emergency. While in some cases a clear-cut etiology may be evident, in many others no cause is revealed by the initial history and physical examination. Such cases require a careful, systematic approach to ensure an optimal outcome. A general approach to the patient with an altered state of consciousness is outlined here, with the focus primarily on the unconscious patient.

Clinically, several levels of altered consciousness may occur. *Delirium* is characterized by confusion, disorientation, and, often, excitability. *Lethargy* is marked by drowsiness and disinterest in one's surroundings. The *stuporous* patient is difficult to arouse and when aroused, will generally respond irrationally. In *coma*, the patient is unarousable and may or may not still have demonstrable reflex reactions (*e.g.*, corneal reflexes).

ETIOLOGIC CLASSIFICATION OF LOSS OF CONSCIOUSNESS

There are numerous causes of altered consciousness in children. The following etiologic classification is by no means complete but should nevertheless serve to provide a framework on which a comprehensive evaluation may be based.

1. Disorders of the central nervous system
   A. Head trauma
   B. Intracranial hemorrhage
   C. Cerebrovascular accident
   D. Brain tumor
   E. Hydrocephalus/shunt obstruction
   F. Status epilepticus/postictal coma
2. Systemic or metabolic disorders
   A. Infections (meningitis, encephalitis, brain abscess)
   B. Reye's syndrome
   C. Diabetic ketoacidosis
   D. Hepatic encephalopathy
   E. Urea cycle defects
   F. Organic acidemia

G. Hypoglycemia

H. Uremia

I. Hypoxemia

J. Cardiac arrhythmias

K. Hypertensive encephalopathy

3. Poisoning/drugs

EVALUATION OF LOSS OF CONSCIOUSNESS

The physical examination of an unconscious child must first focus on basic airway and cardiovascular assessment. An unobstructed airway should be ensured and supplemental oxygen provided. Pulse and blood pressure should be checked and if inadequate, external cardiac massage should be instituted. Once this initial evaluation has been completed, a meticulous examination should be done to seek possible causes for the altered consciousness. In ideal circumstances, a team approach may be used, with one colleague obtaining a history and another working to begin the laboratory evaluation that will be discussed later.

Carefully inspect the child to discern any evidence of external trauma, particularly about the head and neck. Examine the skin for the presence of petechiae, purpura, or needle marks. Assess the respiratory pattern and cardiac rhythm. In performing the neurologic examination, devote special attention to the eye grounds (rule out papilledema), localizing neurologic signs, and corneal and pupillary reflexes. Note the presence of nuchal rigidity as well as any evidence of blood or spinal fluid leakage from the nose or ears.

Key points in the history should include any recent trauma, possible ingestions (including all medications present in the home), infectious illnesses, and seizure activity. The possibility of child abuse should be addressed. The past medical history should elicit any history of a seizure disorder, hydrocephalus, metabolic disease, or other systemic illness. It should be determined whether the onset of the altered state of consciousness was sudden or gradual and if any intervening signs or symptoms might have been noted.

Several emergency laboratory tests should be performed on any child with altered consciousness. These include the following:

1. Urinalysis, including examinations for ketones, protein, glucose, salicylates, red blood cells, white blood cells, and bacteria.
2. Serum/plasma chemistries, including electrolytes, glucose, ammonia, hepatic enzymes, urea nitrogen, creatinine, and calcium.
3. Complete blood cell count with differential, examination of a blood smear (for sickling, stippling, etc.), and coagulation studies.
4. Blood cultures if any concern regarding infection exists.
5. Toxicology screens of the blood, urine, and gastric aspirate.
6. Computed tomography of the head (indicated in most cases, particularly in coma of uncertain etiology).
7. Examination of the spinal fluid, including glucose, protein, gram stain, and culture. This must be done only after increased intracranial pressure has been ruled out and, even then, with extreme caution.

Other tests, such as electroencephalograms and specialized metabolic studies, should be used as the particular case may dictate.

With the framework provided here, the physician should be able to assimilate data from the history, physical examination, and laboratory evaluation to discern quickly the cause of the altered consciousness in the vast majority of cases. Therapy will then depend largely on the specific etiology suspected, although it should be noted that in addition to the basic steps in stabilization noted previously, other early measures should include the administration of intravenous fluids, dextrose, and frequently, naloxone (Narcan).

BIBLIOGRAPHY

Mafenson HC, Greensher J: The unknown poison. Pediatrics 54:336, 1974

Plum F, Posner JB: The Diagnosis of Stupor and Coma. Philadelphia, F.A. Davis, 1980

Raphaely RC, Swedlow DB, Downes JJ et al: Management of severe pediatric head trauma. Pediatr Clin North Am 27:715, 1980

Sabin TD: The differential diagnosis of coma. N Engl J Med 290:1062, 1974

11 Poisoning

Poisonings are extremely common in pediatrics, with over 1 million episodes in the United States each year, accounting for approximately 3000 deaths. Most reported poisonings involve children younger than 5 years of age, are accidental, and occur within the home. Ideally, the vast majority of poisonings could be prevented, and it is the physician's responsibility to provide detailed information to parents on methods of reducing the risk of an accidental ingestion, a task that requires a great deal of thought and organization.

Because of the vast number of potential poisons that may be present in the child's environment, no physician will be familiar with the specific toxicities of each substance. For this reason, regional poison control centers have been established throughout the United States to provide detailed, up-to-date information on the thousands of drugs and household products that a child might ingest. These centers are an absolutely invaluable resource and should be used fully. Here, a general approach to the poisoned child is provided, along with specific information on several of the most common ingestions encountered in the pediatric emergency room.

In most cases, the diagnosis of poisoning is quite straightforward, since the child will have been observed taking the poison, or an open container will have been found. In these cases, attempt to quickly identify the substance that was ingested and estimate the maximum quantity that might have been taken. In other cases, however, such as in adolescent suicide attempts or the child presenting with an altered mental status but no history of an ingestion, the poison will be unknown. Characteristic signs and symptoms may be present in such cases, allowing the physician to make a tentative diagnosis while awaiting laboratory confirmation. (For an excellent review of toxicologic syndromes, see the article by Mofenson and Greensher listed in this chapter's bibliography). It should also be emphasized that any puzzling clinical case should at least suggest the possibility of poisoning, even if any possibility of an ingestion is denied by the patient or family.

In general, the principles of management of any poisoning are the same: absorption of the poison should be minimized while general supportive care measures are maintained. Unfortunately, few specific antidotes are available, although they should certainly be used when appropriate.

The first step in the treatment of most significant ingestions is to empty the stomach. This is usually done most effectively by inducing vomiting with syrup of ipecac (15 ml for children 1 to 10 years and 30 ml for patients over 10). This step may often be done while the patient is still at home, and all families should be encouraged to have ipecac available at home. The induction of emesis is contraindicated, however, in the presence of coma or convulsions or when a caustic substance or hydrocarbon has been ingested.

If ipecac administration is unsuccessful or if the patient is obtunded or convulsing, gastric lavage is the preferred method of emptying the stomach. If the gag reflex is felt to be insufficient, then the patient must first be intubated with a cuffed endotracheal tube to protect the airway from aspiration. Gastric lavage is also contraindicated in the ingestion of caustic substances or hydrocarbons. Once a lavage tube is in place, a syringe is attached and the stomach contents are emptied. To maximize emptying, 1/2 normal saline solution is then instilled and suctioned out for several cycles, ensuring that the aspirate is completely clear before stopping.

Once the stomach has been emptied, activated charcoal should be given at a dose of 0.5 to 1.0 g/kg to bind any poisons remaining in the gastrointestinal tract. Since the charcoal binds ipecac as well, it should be given only after emesis has been completed. It may be given either orally or *via* the lavage tube. After charcoal, cathartics (*e.g.*, magnesium citrate, 1 ml/kg) are usually recommended to hasten passage of any remaining poison through the intestinal tract and further reduce systemic absorption.

Regardless of the poison involved, general supportive care should be provided as the particular situation dictates. Initial assessment and stabilization of the airway and cardiovascular status are absolutely critical. Fluids should be administered intravenously as needed. Further, the patient should be carefully monitored for the development of signs and symptoms that may not have been present initially. Specimens of blood, urine, and gastric aspirate should be collected for toxicology screens and specific drug levels as indicated.

In some cases, the excretion of a poison may be enhanced through diuresis or alkalinization/acidification of the urine. These are not routine measures and should be used only when specifically indicated. Finally, in severe cases of some types of poisoning, dialysis may be of benefit; hemodialysis, charcoal hemoperfusion, and peritoneal dialysis all may be used in certain situations. The regional poison control center will be of great assistance in selecting these and other measures.

Several of the more serious and common types of ingestions will now be described briefly.

POISONING WITH CAUSTIC SUBSTANCES

This category includes both strong acids and alkalis, materials that, unfortunately, are contained in many household products (*e.g.*, lye, drain cleaners, oven cleaners). The major toxicity arises from chemical burns of the esophagus, frequently leading to chronic scarring and stricture formation. Emesis should not be induced. All patients with mouth burns and/or a history of a significant caustic ingestion should be given nothing by mouth and administered intravenous fluids, antibiotics (ampicillin, 100 to 200 mg/kg/day), and corticosteroids (hydrocortisone, 10 mg/kg/day). Endoscopy should then be performed to identify esophageal burns conclusively. If no burns are present, antibiotic and corticosteroid administration may be stopped. If esophageal burns are present, the child will require antibiotics for at least 5 to 7 days, steroids for at least 3 weeks, gradual reinstitution of oral nutrition, and follow-up esophagoscopy and barium swallow studies to evaluate for strictures formation. The road to recovery may be a very long one for the child with a significant caustic ingestion.

POISONING WITH HYDROCARBONS

Hydrocarbon ingestions account for 5% to 7% of all reported poisonings of children younger than 5 and are the second most common cause of hospital admission for accidental poisoning. Hydrocarbons are found in many household products and, unfortunately, are frequently stored in unmarked containers. Products commonly ingested include petroleum solvents, furniture polish, stains, preservatives, lighter fluids, gasoline, kerosene, and fuel oil.

A chemical pneumonitis secondary to aspiration is the most common toxicity in hydrocarbon poisoning. Common presenting symptoms include cough, tachypnea, dyspnea, grunting, and, occasionally, cyanosis. The physical examination may also show fever, retractions, and rhonchi or rales on auscultation. Chest x-ray abnormalities may appear within 30 minutes of ingestion and in most cases are present within 6 to 8 hours; these abnormalities include perihilar densities, basilar consolidation, and, at times, pleural effusion.

Other less common toxicities include central nervous system depression from systemic absorption (may be complicated by seizures as well), cardiac arrhythmias, renal damage, hepatomegaly, and hypoglycemia.

Treatment consists primarily of supportive care, including intravenous fluids, oxygen, and more aggressive respiratory support in severe cases. There is generally considered to be no benefit from induced vomiting or gastric lavage, unless very large quantities are ingested or the hydrocarbon contains another toxic substance (*e.g.*, a pesticide). There is no role for prophylactic antibiotic therapy or corticosteroids. Any child who is symptomatic with an abnormal chest x-ray should be hospitalized. Hospitalization is generally not required if a child remains asymptomatic for a 6-hour observation period, even if the chest x-ray is abnormal.

POISONING WITH SALICYLATES

Salicylate overdose continues to be one of the most commonly reported poisonings. Doses greater than 150 mg/kg generally produce toxicity; classic presenting symptoms include hyperpnea, an altered state of consciousness (lethargy, delirium, coma), hyperthermia, dehydration, and metabolic acidosis. In severe toxicity, cardiovascular collapse may occur.

Salicylate poisoning increases the metabolic rate of the body and interferes with carbohydrate metabolism, leading to ketosis, organic acid production, and hypoglycemia. This primary metabolic acidosis may be particularly or even completely compensated by a respiratory alkalosis produced by hyperventilation. Also common are electrolyte imbalances, resulting from vomiting, fever, excessive sweating, and hyperventilation. Although coagulation may be mildly impaired, significant bleeding is unusual.

Initial therapy should consist of stabilization followed as quickly as possible by administration of ipecac or gastric lavage; then activated charcoal is given. Blood should be drawn for determination of pH, electrolytes, blood urea nitrogen (BUN), creatinine, prothrombin time, and salicylate levels. Fluids should be given intravenously to maintain hydration, and sodium bicarbonate may be needed to correct acidosis. In very severe cases, alkalinization of the urine may be used to increase salicylate removal, and, in a very few, hemodialysis is required.

POISONING WITH ACETAMINOPHEN

Acetaminophen poisoning has become increasingly common in recent years. Doses in excess of 150 mg/kg frequently produce hepatotoxicity and are potentially fatal if management is not optimal.

Early symptoms in acetaminophen overdose are nonspecific and do not predict hepatotoxicity. These occur within 4 hours of ingestion and include nausea, vomiting, diaphoresis, and lethargy. These symptoms usually resolve over a 24-hour period, and for the next 24 hours the patient is generally asymptomatic. The development of liver necrosis may then become evident approximately 48 hours after ingestion. Right-upper-quadrant tenderness is common during this phase, as is elevation of hepatic enzymes (serum glutamic-oxaloacetic transaminase [SGOT], serum glutamic-pyruvic transaminase [SGPT]), bilirubin, and prothrombin time. In severe cases, hepatic encephalopathy and renal failure may develop, occasionally leading to death. The liver will generally recover completely, however, in patients who survive the acute hepatic injury.

Treatment of acetaminophen poisoning includes minimizing gastrointestinal absorption, using specific compounds containing sulfhydryl (N-acetylcysteine [Mucomyst]) to prevent hepatotoxicity, monitoring hepatic function, and providing supportive care. Administration of ipecac or gastric lavage is recommended, but activated charcoal should not be given to patients in whom N-acetylcysteine may be needed. Early measurements of plasma acetaminophen levels are mandatory because they are the only accurate means of predicting hepatotoxicity. If the plasma level taken no earlier than 4 hours after the ingestion indicates a risk of hepatic damage (consult local poison control center for reference values), therapy with N-acetylcysteine should be instituted. This antidote is highly efficacious in preventing hepatic damage if administration is begun within 12 hours of ingestion.

POISONING WITH IRON

More than 2000 cases of iron poisoning are reported annually in the United States. The toxicity of iron is related to effects on the gastrointestinal, cardiovascular, and central nervous systems. The lethal dose of iron is generally considered to be about 200 mg/kg of elemental iron (5 g ferrous sulfate supplies 1 g elemental iron) although lethal doses as low as 500 mg have been reported. Mortality from iron overdose may be as high as 2% to 3%.

The clinical manifestations of iron poisoning are generally divided into four phases. The first phase is related primarily to damage to the gastrointestinal mucosa, with symptoms including abdominal pain, nausea, vomiting, hematemesis, and melena. In severe cases there may also be lethargy, acidosis, shock, and coma. This phase lasts for 1 to 12 hours and is followed by a latent period, during which clinical symptoms improve. A third phase may begin 12 to 48 hours after ingestion and may include shock, coma, liver failure, acidosis, hypoglycemia, and death. A fourth phase, characterized by late complications such as pyloric stenosis, cirrhosis, or central nervous system sequelae, may occur.

Initial management includes emptying the stomach, obtaining a serum iron level (if possible), and performing a deferoxamine challenge test (give 2 g IM deferoxamine; presence of "vin rose" color of urine indicates a significant iron ingestion). Then, all patients felt to have had a significant ingestion should have gastric lavage with 2 g deferoxamine in 1 liter of 5% sodium bicarbonate. An abdominal x-ray should be obtained, and any patient with significant symptoms, a positive deferoxamine challenge test, or evidence of iron tablets on x-ray should be admitted to the hospital and treated intravenously with deferoxamine (10 to 15 mg/kg/hr) until the urine is clear and the patient is free of symptom for 24 hours. Follow-up for all patients, monitoring for late complications, should then be arranged.

POISONING WITH LEAD

Although lead poisoning rarely results from an acute overdose and a discussion of its management is beyond the scope of this book, it should be noted that lead intoxication remains a significant health problem among children in the United States, particularly in urban areas. It usually results from prolonged, excessive exposure and leads to the deposition of toxic levels of lead in bones, the brain, and the kidneys. Children at highest risk are those from 1 to 5 years of age who reside in dwellings built prior to World War II. A history of pica imparts even greater risk.

Ideally, children with lead poisoning will be diagnosed by routine screening of high-risk populations before symptoms have developed. Early symptoms may include loss of appetite, vomiting, irritability, and clumsiness. Encephalopathy may develop in severe cases and be characterized by lethargy, ataxia, seizures, and coma.

A presumptive diagnosis of lead poisoning may often be made based on the presence of iron deficiency anemia, basophilic stippling, and "lead lines" on long bone x-rays. A definitive diagnosis is based on blood lead and free erythrocyte protoporphyrin levels. The degree of elevation of these levels, combined with the patient's symptoms, dictates the therapeutic regimen that will be recommended. The major drugs used in lead poisoning include CaEDTA and BAL (British anti-Lewisite). In addition to these agents, it is critical that adequate supportive care be provided and, most important, that the child be permanently removed from lead sources and carefully monitored on a long-term basis.

BIBLIOGRAPHY

Anas N, Namasonthi V, Ginsburg C: Criteria for hospitalizing children who have ingested products containing hydrocarbons. JAMA 246:840, 1981

Kilham HA: Hospital management of severe poisoning. Pediatr. Clin North Am 27:603, 1980

McGuigan MA: Poisoning in childhood. Emerg Med Clin North Am 1:187, 1983

Mofenson HC, Greensher J: The unknown poison. Pediatrics 54:336, 1974

Piomelli S, Rosen JF, Chisolm JJ et al: Management of childhood lead poisoning. J. Pediatr 105:523, 1984

Robotham JL, Lietman PS: Acute iron poisoning. Am J Dis Child 134:875, 1980

Rumack BH, Peterson RG: Acetaminophen overdose. Pediatrics 62:898, 1978

12 Child Abuse and Neglect

The physical, sexual, or emotional maltreatment of a child is known as *child abuse.* Failure to provide a proper environment, adequate nutrition, clothing, medical care, or nurturance is known as child neglect. In any given year, 1.25% to 1.5% of U.S. children are reported for suspected abuse; if 18 years of age is the upper age cutoff for reporting, 1 million children are reported annually. Of these, 70% are new cases and 30% are repeats; 25% are reported for physical abuse, 55% for neglect, 10% for sexual exploitation, and 10% for unknown reasons. These figures are only approximately representative of the actual abuse that occurs and, as such, are underestimates. Studies that have questioned young adults about their own childhood experiences have revealed that 20% to 30% of interviewees recall some type of personal abuse. Several studies have reported that as many as 10% of males and 20% of females recall being sexually exploited as a child.

Child abuse and neglect occur among all races and at all socioeconomic strata. The average age of the abused child is 7 years, but 33% of abused children are younger than 6 years and 15% to 20% are adolescents. In 95% of reported cases, "parental" persons were the perpetrators. It is estimated that 5% of abuse results in fatalities and another 5% results in permanent physical damage to the victims.

The phenomenon is certainly not new. Reports of child maltreatment abound in myths, legends, fairy tales, and literature. Children have been abandoned and left to die because they were of the wrong sex or of the wrong parentage. They have been sold into slavery, beaten, and forced to earn a living for adults. They have also been the sexual playthings of several civilizations. Interestingly, a society to prevent cruelty to animals existed before there were services to prevent cruelty to children. Currently, most states have laws that mandate the reporting of any child or adolescent in whom abuse or neglect is suspected. Physicians are provided with immunity from suit if the reports are made in good faith, even if the charge of abuse is eventually proven to be unfounded.

ETIOLOGY

Three factors may contribute to child abuse: parental, child, and situational. The parent who abuses his child may himself have been abused as a child. He may be insecure, immature, dependent, lonely, or helpless. He frequently demonstrates poor impulse control, a low tolerance for frustration, unrealistic expectations of the child, and a lack of understanding of child development or behaviors such as crying. He may have a rigid attitude toward corporal punishment of children.

There may be marital strife with physical and verbal abuse between spouses. The abusing parent may attempt to hurt the spouse by abusing the child ("batterer-by-proxy"). There may also be financial stresses on the family or recent loss of employment.

Thus, the abusing parent may be stressed to his limit and may have developed few personal techniques to deal with such stresses. In frustration, he vents his stress on the one who is least likely to resist.

Child factors operant in abuse have been described. A child who was a low birth weight, premature, the product of a difficult pregnancy or delivery, separated from mother for a prolonged period after birth because of illness, or who has physical deformities, slow development, emotional problems, chronic medical problems, or a "difficult" temperament is more likely to be abused. Frequently, the child does not meet the parent's stringent expectations. He may not be cuddly or "lovable." He may act out to attract parental (negative) attention because that is the only way he can get it. He may have been the product of an unwanted pregnancy or may serve as a constant reminder to the mother of the child's father, whom she now despises.

Thus, the child who is abused may have certain characteristics that lead to parental anger or disappointment, which, in turn, leads to his maltreatment.

Not every parent or child with the characteristics discussed above are involved in abuse. Sometimes situational factors precipitate the abuse. A relentlessly crying infant with colic may frustrate a parent. Employ-ment termination may result in a lack of parental self-esteem. During an alcohol or drug binge, the parent may lose control of his faculties and act according to whim. A parent who recently has been abused or who currently is being abused by the spouse may take out frustrations on the child.

In the case of sexual exploitation, several vulnerability factors have been elucidated. Female victims frequently have mothers who are aloof, are divorced and remarried, have unsatisfactory marital relations, demonstrate an attitude of sexual "punitiveness" toward spouses, have few friends, or have a low educational level. Male victims frequently have seductive mothers (rather than aloof mothers) in addition to the other factors enumerated.

Thus, the sexually abused child may be the "chosen companion" of a weak, ineffectual parent or may be the object of anger, scorn or ridicule if the parent displaces these feelings toward the opposite sex onto the child.

EVALUATION

History

If the child presents with an injury, the circumstances of occurrence should be elucidated. What happened to the child? When did it happen? If the injury is old, why was there a delay in seeking treatment? Was the injury witnessed by anyone? Who? Was the child supervised at the time of the injury? If so, by whom? Is the history compatible with the injury? Is the mother concerned by the injury? Is she angry or defensive? Does she seem stressed? What is the child's past medical history with regard to birth history, chronic medical problems, hospitalizations, injuries, or "difficult temperament"? Who else cares for the child?

If a child presents for well-child care or for a specific complaint, and neglect seems likely, the history must include questions pertinent to health maintenance (or to the specific injury) and questions regarding diet, activity, past medical history, family history of the sizes of family members, and social history. Especially important social questions are the following: How many siblings are there? How many people live in the house? Is the child's father at home? Who else lives there? Who tends the child when the mother is away? Does the mother have support systems? Which ones? Is the family receiving public assistance? Is there always food in the house? Is the mother, patient, or other sibling being abused? By whom?

If the child presents with the possibility of sexual exploitation, inquiry must be made into (1) who is doing it and that person's relationship to the child, (2) when it occurs, (3) how long it has been occurring, and (4) exactly what has been happening. *Sexual misuse* is the exposure of a child to inappropriate sexual stimuli. *Sexual abuse* is forced sexual contact. *Incest* is sexual abuse by a parent, sibling, or close relative, whereas *molestation* is sexual abuse by a stranger. *Sexual assault* (including rape and sodomy) is the forced penetration of the penis into the victim's vagina, mouth, or anus.

Frequently, sexually abused children do not present in a straightforward fashion. They may be brought to medical attention for enuresis, encopresis, hyperactivity, fearfulness, sleep disorders, compulsive masturbation, sexualized play, or genital injury. When any of these nonspecific complaints are prominent, the possibility of abuse should be raised and appropriately investigated.

Whenever abuse of any kind is suspected, the child and parent should be questioned separately. However, a child reluctant to be interviewed alone should not be forced to do so. Abused children are frequently more comfortable discussing what happened to them and their feelings about it by use of drawings or play with anatomically correct dolls.

Physical Evaluation

Whenever abuse is suspected, a complete physical examination is mandatory. The examination begins with an observation of parent–child interaction. Is it one of love and trust or one of fear or antagonism? How does the child appear? Is he dirty or well-kept? Scrawny or well-nourished? Fearful or friendly? Appropriately frightened of the examiner or overly friendly? Does the child stare blankly or avert his gaze? Does he smile, talk, or laugh?

Examine the child's skin for evidence of abuse. Are burns present? If so, do they have the shape of the hot object (such as the circular burn of a cigarette)? Are they immersion burns (*i.e.,* is there a doughnut-shaped burn of the lower back and thighs with sparing of the central buttocks)? Does the child have abrasions, belt-marks (linear bruises), rope/cord marks, handprints, or teeth marks on his skin? An estimation of the age of the child's bruises is possible because the bruise's color changes as it ages. Red-blue or violet bruises are 1 to 2 days old, blue-brown or purple bruises are 3 to 4 days old, yellow-green bruises are 5 to 7 days old, and yellow-brown bruises are 7 to 10 days old. Does the child have evidence of multiple types of injuries of different ages? Are there choke marks on the neck, pinch marks on the ears, or swelling of any body parts? Is there hair missing from his scalp?

Does the child have superficial marks, swellings, or distortion of his extremities? If so, an x-ray may be in order.

Are the chest and abdomen covered with bruises? If so, suspect fractured ribs or internal organ injury in the abdominal cavity, especially if abdominal distress is present. An abdominal film or scan may be in order.

Because cranial injuries are the most common causes of death or permanent injury, a careful skull examination is mandatory. Does the child have bruises, linear marks, or depressions on his head? Are any teeth fractured (mouth blows)? Is the frenulum torn (forced bottle or pacifier in the mouth)? Is the tympanic membrane ruptured (blow to the head)? If the patient is an infant, is his fontanelle bulging? Is there evidence of retinal hemorrhage? If yes to either of the last two questions, suspect a shaking injury. Because of the infant's large head size and weight, weak neck muscles, and thin cerebral vasculature, he is particularly susceptible to develop serious complications, such as a subdural hematoma, with head or shaking injuries. In addition to checking for retinal hemorrhages or detachment, look for evidence of hyphema, corneal abrasion, subconjunctival hemorrhage, or lens dislocation.

Whenever visible injuries are present, photographs should be taken and coded with the patient's name, history number, date, and body part (if not obvious).

If sexual abuse is suspected, the genitalia/anal examination must be carefully and sensitively performed. The physician should gently explain all procedures to the child before they occur and should permit him to touch any instruments that might be necessary to the examination. Evidence of genital lesions (ulcers, vesicles, warts, pustules, papules, bruises), inappropriately lax anal sphincter tone, or an abnormally large vaginal introitus should be sought. The presence of hairs, blood, or semen should be noted and collected for forensic evidence. Gonorrhea cultures of the throat, anus, and urethra/vagina and ELISA for evidence of chlamydial infection (using genital secretions) should be performed. If there is a vaginal discharge, the presence of *Trichomonas* should be ruled out by a wet prep examination microscopically. The child should have a Venereal Disease Research Laboratory (VDRL) determination; a pubertal girl should also have a serum pregnancy test.

MANAGEMENT

The physician must care for the child's immediate injuries and ensure his safety by preventing further abuse.

The child's wounds or burns are cleaned, lacerations are sutured, and fractures are set. If sexual abuse has occurred, the child may receive therapy for sexually transmitted diseases. These physical injuries are much easier to treat than the accompanying emotional injuries. On this initial visit, the child should be supported and allowed to cry, vent anger, talk, or remain silent.

To prevent further abuse, the physician must determine if the nonhospitalized child should return to his home, go to a relative's house, or go to foster care. This decision is made in consultation with a social worker, who also interviews the family and observes their interactions. The case must be reported as suspected abuse to Protective Services. This report should be made even if one wants to give the parent the benefit of the doubt or if it is unclear who the actual abuser is. The parent should be made aware of this reporting process and be permitted to voice opposition or fears.

The child's placement may eventually be determined by the court. If the child returns home, the court may mandate home visits by a social worker, or visiting nurse, or may recommend psychiatric counseling for the victim and his family. Even with the best of community services, the severely or chronically abused child may bear long-term emotional scars.

BIBLIOGRAPHY

Altemeier W et al: Antecedents of child abuse. J Pediatr 100:823–829, 1982

Fontana V: The maltreatment syndrome of children. Pediatr Ann 13:736–744, 1984

Helfer R: The epidemiology of child abuse and neglect. Pediatr Ann 13:745–51, 1984

Woollcott P et al: Doctor shopping with the child as proxy patient—A variant of child abuse. J Pediatr 101:297–301, 1982

13

Sudden Infant Death Syndrome

Sudden infant death syndrome (SIDS) is the sudden death, usually during sleep, of a healthy infant. Although infants with cardiac, neurologic, or other congenital anomalies may die suddenly, they are not usually considered to be victims of SIDS; nor are infants who have overwhelming infections at the time of their deaths. The definition, then, of SIDS is the sudden death of any infant or young child, which is unexpected by history, and in which a thorough postmortem examination fails to demonstrate an adequate cause for death.

SIDS is not a new entity. There are references to "overlaying" of an infant by an adult in the Bible (I Kings 3:19–20) and in early textbooks of pediatrics indicating that death of an infant during sleep was a known entity. For many years, sudden infant death was attributed to an enlarged thymus. However, this explanation for SIDS was refuted in the mid 1950s, when it was pointed out that infants dying of SIDS had thymuses that were no larger than those of similarly aged children dying accidentally. The notion of the majority of SIDS cases being the result of either malicious or accidental suffocation was finally put to rest in the 1940s and 1950s by forensic pathology investigations in New York.

INCIDENCE

The incidence of SIDS is approximately 2 to 3 per 1000 live births. This means that approximately 10,000 infants die of SIDS each year in the United States. The incidence of SIDS does not vary by parental age, site of domicile (urban vs. rural) or type of feeding (breast milk vs. formula). Some investigations have found higher rates of SIDS in infants with histories of (1) stays in neonatal intensive care units, (2) low birth weight, regardless of gestation, (3) poor social situations and poor living standards, and (4) maternal narcotic addiction during pregnancy. Several investigations have noted a higher incidence of SIDS in colder temperatures, but others have not.

Age Distribution

The peak age of SIDS incidence is 2 to 4 months of age. Half of SIDS cases occur before 3 months, and more than 90% occur by 6 months.

Sex

Virtually every study has demonstrated a male predominance, perhaps reflecting the overall male predominance in mortality from all causes in early infancy.

Circumstances of Death

SIDS is a phenomenon that is almost universally associated with sleep. When adults have been in the same room as the victim, they report no outcry before the terminal event. There may be signs of silent struggle, such as the blanket being clutched by the infant or unusual positioning (face pressed between crib slats, face oriented directly downward into the mattress, etc.).

Genetic Predisposition

Although there have been a number of reports of SIDS in siblings or first-degree cousins, the exact mechanism of inheritance of polygenic risk factors is unknown. Indeed, many investigators postulate that it is the common environment of the siblings and not a common genetic complement that leads to familial clustering of cases.

Infectious Disease

Although viral agents have been isolated from the victims' nasopharynx or stools, there has been no evidence for overwhelming viremia or multiple organ involvement.

Relationship to Immunizations

In the period between 2 and 6 months, infants are scheduled to receive three immunizations: diphtheria–pertussis–tetanus (DPT). Pertussis has been associated with several severe side effects (see Chapter 1). Since the peak incidence of SIDS is between 2 and 4 months, some investigators have sought evidence for a causal relationship between a DPT immunization and a SIDS event. Although early studies had suggested that such a rela-

tionship existed, other studies using a strict case-control (*i.e.*, DPT immunization vs. no DPT immunization) method and strict definitions of post-DPT exposure time have found no relationship between DPT immunizations and SIDS.

Previous History of Central Nervous System or Respiratory System Dysfunction

Both retrospective and prospective studies of SIDS victims have found a greater incidence of anoxic/hypoxic conditions at or shortly before birth in these infants than in controls. Some of the victims demonstrated abnormalities in respiration, feeding, temperature regulation, and the quality of their cries. However, possession of one of these physiologic risk factors does not mean SIDS will occur.

PATHOLOGIC FINDINGS

External examination usually reveals a well-nourished child with blood-tinged frothy fluid in the mouth and nose. The face may also have vomitus on it. The infant's diaper will be full of urine and/or stool as if a massive agonal event occurred. Depending on the length of time between death and discovery, and if the child's face was against the slats or oriented downward, the face may be purplish with pressure indentations.

Internal findings are intrathoracic petechiae (covering the surfaces of lungs, pericardium, and thymus) attributed to intrathoracic negative pressure with agonal capillary rupture, pulmonary edema and congestion, microscopic inflammatory pulmonary infiltrates (insufficient on their own to cause death), and, occasionally, areas of inflammation and fibrinoid necrosis in the vocal cords. The other organs are usually normal. However, there may be gliosis of the brain stem. This is significant, since respiration centers are located in this area of the brain.

POSSIBLE ETIOLOGIES

There is probably no one single etiology of SIDS: different victims may have different causes of the common terminal event. Possible etiologies include child abuse, suffocation, aspiration, abnormal nasal-occlusion aversion reflex, hyperacute vasovagal reflex, diving reflex, laryngospasm, apnea (see section on "near-miss SIDS") and miscellaneous abnormalities of cardiac conduction or serum electrolyte concentrations. Many other proposed etiologies have been popular at one time but, with careful research into SIDS, have been refuted.

CLINICAL PRESENTATION

Typically, the infant presents to the emergency room already dead. Various stages of rigor mortis may be present. The parents usually report that the infant was entirely well or had a minor upper respiratory infection when they last saw him alive. Typically, the child had been fed and put to sleep in his crib; the parents discover their infant's condition when he does not awaken for his next feeding or sleeps past his usual hour of waking. The infant may be in any position and may be clutching his blanket. Resuscitation efforts are generally unsuccessful at the time of discovery because the victims have usually been dead for some time.

The entity known as "near-miss SIDS" will be discussed in the next section.

TREATMENT

There is no way to treat a SIDS victim, but there is one important way to treat his family: through compassionate counseling. The parents (and siblings) may feel extremely guilty and responsible for the death. Siblings may have wished that the new baby, who required so much parental time, would die so that they would have the parents all to themselves. When the baby does die, the siblings feel intense guilt and may demonstrate behavior problems. Since deaths of young infants are questioned by legal authorities, the parents may feel like criminals. They may also feel that they should have known the baby was "sick," should had taken him to a doctor, should have checked him more carefully during sleep—should have done something that they did not do or should not have done something that they did do. Parents may blame one another or medical personnel.

Treatment of the family begins in the emergency room, where a social worker or clergyman is often of great help. The possibility of SIDS should be discussed and, if possible, printed material on SIDS given to the parents. The feelings that the parents and siblings have and will have should be discussed openly. An autopsy is mandatory both for medicolegal reasons and the family's peace of mind. If the autopsy reveals findings compatible with SIDS, the family can be reassured that they were not at fault.

"NEAR-MISS SIDS"/INFANTILE APNEA

Occasionally an infant is found pale or cyanotic, apneic, and apparently lifeless in his crib and is successfully resuscitated. The supposition is that had not the infant been found and resuscitated in a timely fashion, he, too, would have been a SIDS victim. Thus, he has experienced "near-miss SIDS" or symptomatic infantile apnea. Although SIDS and apnea are not synonymous, the child with infantile apnea is at high risk for SIDS.

Apnea–cyanosis episodes have been described in young relatives of SIDS victims and sometimes in the victims themselves prior to their deaths. In prospective studies of infants, such apneic episodes were associated with rapid-eye-movement (REM) sleep and were prolonged during respiratory illnesses. These apnea–cyanosis episodes are subject to recurrence. The apnea may be central (secondary to brain-stem dysfunction), peripheral (nasopharyngeal), or mixed central–peripheral. Bradycardia also occurs both in combination with the apnea and in isolation. An abnormal autonomic nervous system responsiveness has been postulated as the common pathway for these events.

Significant apnea is defined as respiratory cessation of 20 seconds or more or of any duration when bradycardia, cyanosis, pallor, or oxygen desaturation are present. Periodic breathing, which is present in all infants to a greater or lesser degree, is defined as three or more respiratory pauses of 3 seconds' duration with the respiration interrupting the apnea less than 20 seconds.

Historical Information

When the infant who has been a "near-miss SIDS" victim presents to medical attention, the parents should be asked about the event and any precipitating factors (such as the presence of infectious illness), any prior history of such events or periodic breathing in the infant, a family history of death in early infancy, and the child's past medical (including birth) and development history.

Physical examination

A thorough physical examination should be performed, noting, in particular, abnormalities in the infant's respiratory or neurologic function. Frequently, however, results of the physical examination are entirely normal.

Diagnostic evaluation

The evaluation of an infant with near-miss SIDS must address the most likely causes of the episode (see below). In the emergency room, the infant should be evaluated for sepsis/meningitis, electrolyte abnormalities, anemia, pneumonia, and trauma. The infant should then be hospitalized both for further evaluation and for continuous electronic cardiopulmonary monitoring.

Differential diagnoses. Entities that can cause (an) acute or recurrent apnea episode(s) include cardiac defects, especially shortened Q-T intervals, airway obstruction secondary to infection or congenital anomalies, infections, trauma, inborn errors of metabolism, seizures, severe anemia, gastroesophageal reflux, tumors, chronic pulmonary diseases with resultant chronic hypoxia, and respiratory control abnormalities.

Treatment

If no cause is found for the near-miss SIDS event, the issue of recurrence must be considered. The parents should be taught cardiopulmonary resuscitation, and the child's primary physician should be apprised of the situation. The child should be sent home on an apnea monitor after his cardiopulmonary responses are studied during sleep. The parents must be taught about the monitor's operation, what to do if the monitor sounds, and to record such alarms. The use of the monitor has been criticized as disrupting family life and parent–child bonding, and creating anxious parents. Hence, parents whose children require monitoring must be supported. Apnea monitors are *not* for all infants. Infants who have experienced near-miss SIDS or apnea are certainly candidates for monitoring; infants who are siblings of SIDS victims or infants with apnea are probable candidates. Monitoring is continued until the child (1) has been free of apnea or near-miss SIDS episodes requiring resuscitation for 3 months, (2) has not had a monitor alarm for at least 2 months, (3) has had an upper respiratory illness or DPT immunization without problems or alarm sounding, *and*

(4) the ongoing evaluation of the child is normal (or has normalized if the initial evaluation was abnormal).

Another suggested therapy for infants with idiopathic recurrent apnea is theophylline in a dosage of 20 to 24 mg/kg/day to achieve a serum concentration of 10 to 20 μg/dL. Theophylline is felt to be efficacious by its action of stimulating the brain's respiratory center. Because theophylline pharmokinetics are highly variable during infancy, during viral illnesses, and while receiving other medications, serum levels of the drug must be closely monitored.

BIBLIOGRAPHY

Ariagno R: Evaluation and management of infantile apnea. Pediatr Ann 13:210-217, 1984

Ariagno R et al: "Near-miss" for sudden infant death syndrome infants—A clinical problem. Pediatrics 71:726-730, 1983

Beckwith JB: The Sudden Infant Death Syndrome. DHEW Publication #(HSA) 76-5137, 1976

Fulginiti V: Sudden infant death syndrome, diphtheria-tetanus toxoid-pertussis vaccination and visits to the doctor: Chance association or cause and effect. Pediatr Infect Dis 2:5–6, 1983

Merritt TA, Valdes-Dapena M: SIDS research update. Pediatr Ann 13:193–207, 1984

Valdes-Dapena M: Sudden Infant death syndrome—A review of the medical literature, 1974–79. Pediatrics 66:597–614, 1980

Part V: Neonatology

14

Respiratory Distress Syndrome

Acute neonatal *respiratory distress syndrome (RDS)*, or hyaline membrane disease (HMD), occurs in about 1% of all live births and is the most common pulmonary disease in the newborn. Improved obstetric and neonatal care has reduced the mortality associated with HMD (from 2.68 to 0.97 deaths per 1000 live births between 1971 and 1984) as it has changed the clinical expression of the disease. More common assessment of fetal pulmonary maturity before elective cesarean section, more conservative management of premature rupture of the fetal membranes, and more aggressive monitoring and delivery of the 24- to 28-week fetus are three of the trends that have dramatically shifted the distribution of HMD toward smaller and more immature infants. Because a general decline in neonatal mortality has paralleled the improved outcome of infants with HMD, the disease still impacts significantly on neonatal mortality and morbidity. In 1984, HMD was associated with 13.8% (3600 infants) of all neonatal deaths. Not only does the case-fatality ratio for HMD rise as gestational age falls, but also the likelihood of significant HMD-associated morbidity (*e.g.,* chronic lung disease) is greater among more immature survivors.

The primary risk factor for HMD is prematurity. From a rate of 0.05% in term infants, the incidence of HMD increases with decreasing gestational age, and rises rapidly below a gestational age of 33 to 34 weeks. Table 14-1 lists other factors that modify the risk of HMD at a given gestational age. Maternal diabetes, maternal hemorrhage before or during delivery, and mode of delivery (cesarean section without labor vs. vaginal delivery) are well-established risk factors for HMD. An appropriate course of maternal steroid therapy enhances lung maturity in certain groups of infants. It has been stated but not yet unequivocably demonstrated that certain conditions associated with chronic fetal stress (*e.g.,* prolonged rupture of membranes, maternal toxemia, maternal heroin abuse) reduce the incidence of HMD.

This chapter will concentrate on the clinical features and current concepts of the pathogenesis of HMD and on newer strategies to prevent or treat the disease. Only the most general principles of current conventional management will be reviewed.

Table 14–1. Risk and Protective Factors for HMD

Risk	Protective
Definite	
Prematurity > term	Maternal steroid therapy
Male > female	
White > black	
Twin B > twin A	
Infant of diabetic mother	
Cesarean section (without labor) > vaginal delivery	
Maternal bleeding	
Asphyxia	
Controversial	
If premature: history of premature	Chronic fetal stress:
siblings with HMD	Prolonged rupture of membranes
	Maternal toxemia
	Maternal heroin abuse

PATHOLOGY

Infants dying with HMD in the first several days of life have characteristic lung pathology. On gross examination, the lungs are firm and dark and often sink when placed in water, even when fixed in inflation. Inspection of cut sections reveals striking atelectasis and dilatation of proximal airways. Under light microscopy, the alveolar saccules (the immature terminal gas exchange units) demonstrate a combination of the following three findings: atelectasis, pulmonary edema, and hyaline membranes. A lining of hyaline membranes may also extend up to the respiratory bronchioles (the terminal conducting airways). Depending on the age of the infant, hyaline membranes are composed of varying proportions of necrotic alveolar epithelial debris, plasma proteins such as fibrin, and plasma transudate. If an infant dies in the first several hours of life, these membranes may be lacking or inconspicuous. If the infant recovers, the hyaline membranes are resorbed with the help of pulmonary macrophages, and the alveolar epithelium regenerates. These membranes are not specific for neonatal HMD but occur uncommonly outside of this clinical setting. Other pathologic findings of HMD may include pulmonary arteriolar constriction with dilatation of pulmonary capillaries, venules, and lymphatics; interstitial edema; interstitial, perivascular, or peribronchial air dissection; and pulmonary hemorrhage.

PATHOPHYSIOLOGY

Building on insights dating back to 1929 when von Neergaard postulated the existence of pulmonary surface active material, Avery and Mead in 1959 performed seminal studies demonstrating that the lungs of premature infants who died of HMD were deficient in surfactant. Although recent clinical trials (see below) have confirmed that surfactant deficiency is the principal factor in the pathogenesis of HMD, other abnormalities associated with prematurity contribute to the clinical expression of the disease. These include (1) anatomic and physiologic immaturity of the pulmonary airways, interstitium, and vascular bed; (2) an underdeveloped chest wall; and (3) immaturity of the patent ductus arteriosus.

Immaturity of the pulmonary parenchyma

The development of the fetal lung is a complicated but orderly process. At approximately 24 weeks of gestation, the third and final (alveolar) stage of lung development begins. During this stage, many structural changes take place to adapt the lung for its postnatal function as a respiratory organ. The following are some of the more important changes:

1. A progressive increase in the number of gas exchange units (alveolar ducts and saccules) that branch off the terminal bronchioles. This proliferation increases the surface area available for gas exchange.
2. A simultaneous increase in the surface area of the pulmonary capillary bed.
3. A thinning of the interstitium, resulting in a closer approximation of the pulmonary capillaries to the gas exchange surface. These first three features have clear implications for respiratory function.
4. Increased deposition of interstitial elastic elements, which contribute to normal respiratory mechanics and incidentally protect against pulmonary air leak complications of HMD.
5. Differentiation of the alveolar epithelium into type I and type II pneumocytes. The type II cell is important because it synthesizes and releases surfactant.
6. A gradual decrease in pulmonary vascular permeability. This protects the lungs from edema as pulmonary perfusion rises after birth.

Especially in the most premature infants, it is likely that these anatomic and functional immaturities contribute as much to the clinical spectrum of HMD as surfactant deficiency itself. Moreover, severe pulmonary immaturity will undoubtedly impose limitations on the survival of the 22- to 23-week fetus even with surfactant replacement therapy.

Surfactant deficiency

Surfactant is a complex mixture of a variety of phospholipids, proteins, and other compounds. The phospholipids and proteins are synthesized by the type II pneumocyte and can be detected in lung assays as early as 16 to 18 weeks of gestation. As surfactant synthesis increases during the third trimester, the composition of surfactant changes; specifically, phosphatidylglycerol (PG) and phosphatidylinositol (PI) are synthesized and the percentage of saturated dipalmitoylphosphatidylcholine (DPPC), or lecithin, increases. Recently, even more subtle maturational changes involving the distribution of the fatty acid moieties has been described. A rise in the concentration of active steroid hormone (cortisol or cortisol-equivalent) stimulates the synthesis of fibroblast pneumocyte factor (FPF) by the pulmonary fibroblasts. FPF in turn directly enhances choline synthetic pathways in the type II cell and leads to a rapid increase in the concentration of phosphatidylcholine. Surfactant is released into the airways *in utero* and eventually can be detected in the amniotic fluid. This forms the basis of the prenatal assessment of pulmonary maturity by amniocentesis. If the amniotic fluid sample is not contaminated by blood or meconium, a ratio of lecithin to sphingomyelin (L/S ratio) greater than 2:1 or certain minimum concentrations of DPPC or PG give excellent assurance that the infant will not develop HMD after delivery. A higher L/S ratio or DPPC concentration seems to be necessary to ensure pulmonary maturity if the mother is a gestational or insulin-dependent diabetic.

Native surfactant has a number of properties important for gas exchange. Most widely known is the capability of surfactant to lower surface tension at the air-liquid interface of the alveolar surface. In the absence of surfactant, surface tension forces would tend to collapse the alveoli, much as air bubbles are observed to shrink as they rise in an aquarium. Surfactant spreads out over the alveolar surface and resists compression (by exerting a surface pressure in the opposite direction of surface tension) more and more forcefully as alveolar surface area decreases; in physiological terms, surfactant inhibits atelectasis. Native surfactant is also easily adsorbed to the alveolar surface under normal *in vivo* conditions and is dynamically respreadable—in other words, surfactant maintains its ability to lower surface tension over repeated cycles of inflation and deflation. Finally, surfactant may inhibit the formation of pulmonary edema.

Functional surfactant deficiency (whether due to abnormalities of quantitative or qualitative synthesis or secretion, or to surfactant inhibition by endogenous substrates) decreases lung compliance and promotes alveolar atelectasis. These abnormalities contribute to the increased work of breathing, the reduction in functional residual capacity (FRC), and the profound hypoxemia (*via* severe ventilation–perfusion mismatch) that typify the clinical picture of HMD (see below).

Underdeveloped chest wall

Functional residual capacity is reached when an equilibrium develops between the forces that drive lung deflation and chest wall recoil. In the immature chest wall, a predominance of cartilaginous rather than bony support decreases elastic recoil. A reduction in FRC in infants with HMD results from the unhappy union of decreased compliance of the surfactant-deficient lungs and increased compliance of the chest wall. In combination, these two factors produce a fixed retraction of the chest wall (akin to pectus excavatum). Large negative transpulmonary pressures during labored respiration are apt to distort the more compli-

ant chest wall further until, literally, "the breastbone touches the backbone." Stabilization of the chest wall by placing the infant in the prone rather than in the supine position frequently improves oxygenation.

Immaturity of the ductus arteriosus

In the full-term infant, the ductus arteriosus constricts postnatally under the influence of a rise in arterial pO_2. Functional closure occurs by 24 to 48 hours of life. This process is less likely to be successful in the premature infant, especially in the setting of HMD. Symptoms of a PDA vary depending on the gestational age of the infant. In some very immature infants, pulmonary overperfusion *via* a net left-to-right shunt through the PDA with attendant pulmonary edema is thought to be responsible for much of the pulmonary dysfunction from the first hours of life. Pulmonary edema (interstitial and alveolar) decreases lung compliance and interferes with gas exchange. In older infants (gestational age 31 to 36 weeks), symptomatic ductal shunting arrests and often reverses clinical improvement at 2 to 4 days of age coincident with a fall in the pulmonary vascular resistance.

CLINICAL FEATURES

Initial presentation

Beginning immediately after birth, a transient period of respiratory distress (tachypnea, hyperpnea, retraction of chest wall muscles, nasal flaring, and/or expiratory grunting) frequently can be observed. Usually these symptoms resolve rapidly so that the newborn is breathing room air comfortably and is centrally pink with an arterial pO_2 of 75 mm Hg or better by 1 hour of age; further cardiopulmonary transition is likely to be uncomplicated. Infants who develop HMD have, at birth, abnormal pulmonary findings that fail to improve, although a temporary abatement in grunting may be misleading. The rate of clinical deterioration is variable. In general, significant signs of respiratory distress are recognized earlier in smaller and more premature infants, often in the delivery room. In contrast, larger infants may have a more insidious course, with symptoms worsening over hours. Diagnosis of HMD in this group may be delayed, especially if an appropriate degree of clinical suspicion is not entertained.

The cardinal sign of HMD is respiratory distress, manifested by some combination of an expiratory grunt, retractions, flaring of the nasal alae, and tachypnea. Each finding can be understood in pathophysiologic terms. The expiratory grunt is generated by exhalation of air against a partially closed glottis. The added resistance decreases end-expiratory flow rate and results in the maintenance of positive pressure at end-expiration (PEEP). This "physiologic PEEP" partially counteracts the tendency of surfactant-deficient alveoli to collapse and thereby promotes gas exchange.

Retractions in HMD reflect two abnormalities; the first is a consequence of surfactant deficiency, whereas the second is a function of prematurity *per se*. The fundamental abnormality is a marked decrease in pulmonary compliance (dV/dP), which can be demonstrated in the isolated, excised lung (static compliance) as well as *in vivo* (dynamic compliance). As compliance decreases, the infant must generate an increasing amount of transpulmonary pressure to effect the same tidal volume. This increases the work of breathing and brings accessory respiratory muscles (intercostal and supersternal muscles) into use. The second abnormality contributing to retractions is the increased compliance (decreased elastic recoil) of the underdeveloped chest wall (see above).

Newborns are predominately but not exclu-sively nose-breathers. A large portion of total inspiratory airway resistance resides in the nasal passages. Nasal flaring in infants with HMD decreases the inspiratory resistance to air flow by dilating the nasal canals.

Infants with HMD are almost invariably tachypneic (*e.g.*, respiratory rate greater than 60 to 70 breaths/minute). Tidal volume is usually low, thereby minimizing the pressure–volume work of each breath. Respiratory rate must increase to sustain an adequate effective minute ventilation. Actual measurements of minute ventilation are supranormal because of the increased percentage of physiological dead space in a tidal respiration. Occasionally a larger, stronger infant with HMD is not tachypneic but hyperpneic. Often these infants have loud and consistent expiratory grunting with prolongation of the expiratory phase. Progression to an irregular respiratory pattern signals impending fatigue. Any infant with HMD may tire and become apneic. Very premature infants may fail to initiate spontaneous respiration at delivery; larger infants may experience a life-threatening apnea at several hours of age.

Other findings complete the clinical picture. Auscultation verifies decreased air entry; fine to coarse rales are audible, especially with deep inspiration. As pulmonary function deteriorates, central cyanosis becomes obvious. Early, the infant's color improves with an increase in the inspired oxygen concentration, but eventually cyanosis may persist despite an F_iO_2 of 1.00. Mottling and pallor of the skin are signs of peripheral vasoconstriction in response to decreased cardiac output; mesenteric and renal blood flows may also be reduced. The mental status of the infant predictably changes as the disease worsens. Initially, the infant is quite reactive to stimuli. He later appears worried or anxious. Without appropriate intervention, his eyes close and he becomes unresponsive even to noxious stimuli.

Diagnosis

The diagnosis is usually straightforward and is made in a high-risk infant with the typical clinical, radiologic, and laboratory findings. The characteristic chest x-ray reveals lung hypoinflation, diffuse (possibly asymmetric) reticulogranular pulmonary infiltrates with a ground-glass texture, and prominent air bronchograms (Fig. 14-1). The infiltrates are due to acinar atelectasis and edema. Lung hypoinflation may not be present in the stronger, more mature infant with HMD who is hyperpneic and whose chest wall has greater elastic recoil. Also, nasal continuous positive airway pressure (CPAP) or mechanical ventilation with PEEP decreases alveolar atelectasis and edema, so that x-rays obtained shortly after initiation of either therapy may show only subtle abnormalities. Arterial blood gas analysis typically reveals hypoxemia with a large calculated alveolar–arterial oxygen gradient (AaDO$_2$), hypercarbia, and a mixed respiratory and metabolic acidosis.

The differential diagnosis is limited. The clinical features are inconsistent with most congenital cyanotic heart diseases (see Chapter 20). In the first few hours, the hyperoxia test is usually positive (*i.e.*, the pO$_2$ rises to 150 mm Hg or greater on an F$_i$O$_2$ of .95 to

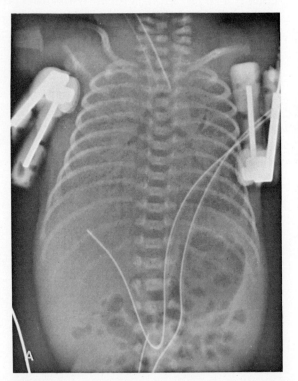
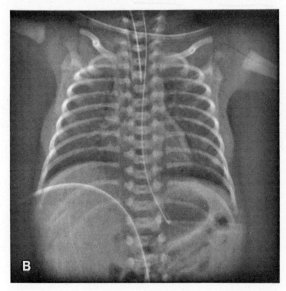

FIGURE 14–1 *(A)* Chest x-ray taken shortly after birth of premature infant (birth weight, 650 g; gestational age, 24 weeks) shows bilateral reticulogranular infiltrates and air bronchograms consistent with hyaline membrane disease. Note the presence of an endotracheal tube, an umbilical arterial catheter with its tip at L3–L4 interspace, and an umbilical venous catheter advanced into the portal venous system. *(B)* Chest x-ray taken a few hours after birth of another premature infant (birth weight, 930 g; gestational age, 27 to 28 weeks) contrasts with 1A and demonstrates normal lungs.

1.00) and rules out congenital cyanotic heart disease with a large fixed right-to-left shunt (see Chapter 20). Congenital pneumonia is often difficult to exclude except in retrospect. The early clinical and radiographic findings of group B streptococcal disease may be indistinguishable from HMD. Moreover, many premature infants are born after prolonged rupture of the membranes, placing them at risk for both HMD and group B streptococcal infection. Indeed, the two diseases may coexist. For these reasons, a premature infant with respiratory distress in our nursery routinely receives a short course of antibiotics until sepsis is excluded by negative cultures, unless the membranes are intact and the infant is delivered by cesarean section because of maternal indications (e.g., severe toxemia).

Subsequent course and complications

Classically, HMD in the larger premature infant worsens over the first 2 days of life before stabilization and then rapid improvement occur by days 3 to 4. The more immature infant occasionally requires maximal support on the first day of life and experiences consistent but gradual recovery. In either case, clinical disease is present for at least 48 hours. Infants who initially require assisted ventilation and high inspired oxygen concentrations but who wean to room air before 48 hours of life do not have HMD but some other process (e.g., persistent postnatal pulmonary edema, asphyxia, patent ductus arteriosus [PDA]).

Diuresis precedes and predicts recovery from HMD. In infants with low insensible water losses, a sustained urine output equal to 80% or greater of fluid intake suggests that a fall in $AaDO_2$, a rise in FRC, and an increase in dynamic compliance are imminent. In cases of uncomplicated HMD, this diuresis is usually noted between 24 and 48 hours of age. Delayed onset of maximal diuresis beyond 72 hours may be predictive of chronic lung disease. Pharmacologic stimulation of an early diuresis with furosemide probably improves pulmonary function acutely (perhaps by a direct effect on decreasing interstitial lung water) allowing a reduction in ventilatory support, but it is not clear that this treatment improves survival or decreases morbidity.

Several events may complicate recovery from HMD. Significant left-to-right shunting through a PDA should be suspected when physical examination reveals typical findings (hyperdynamic precordium, bounding pulses, systolic or continuous murmur, gallop rhythm, increased rales, hepatomegaly), when ventilatory or oxygen requirements increase, or when urine output falls and serum creatinine increases. In some infants, a murmur may be lacking (the silent ductus). Chest x-ray shows an increase in heart size and haziness of the lung fields. Judicious fluid management may decrease the incidence of symptomatic PDA. Treatment with indomethacin, a prostanglandin synthetase inhibitor, closes the ductus successfully in three of four cases. Occasionally, surgical ligation is necessary.

Pulmonary barotrauma can greatly complicate the treatment of HMD. The ventilator is not responsible for all barotrauma; before artificial ventilation was common, 25% of infants with HMD developed pneumothoraces. Air leak may take several forms: pulmonary interstitial emphysema, pneumothorax, pneumomediastinum, or, more rarely, pneumopericardium or pulmonary venous air embolus. Air leaks may develop gradually and initiate an insidious deterioration, or they may occur precipitously and cause catastrophic symptoms or even sudden death related to lung atelectasis and/or tamponade of cardiac output.

The frequency of chronic lung disease, defined as a persistent oxygen requirement at 28 days of life, varies among institutions (see Chapter 15). The incidence is likely influenced by the patient population and by different obstetric and neonatal care practices.

Intraventricular hemorrhage is associated with HMD in part because the primary risk factor for both conditions is prematurity. There is an additional association between symptomatic pneumothoraces and significant intraventricular hemorrhages (grades III and IV).

MANAGEMENT

The intensive care of the infant who develops HMD properly begins with careful fetal monitoring during labor to recognize and treat fetal asphyxia, and continues in the delivery room to ensure optimal resuscitation and stabilization of the newborn infant. The overall care of the premature infant is very complex and demands scrupulous attention to matters such as temperature homeostasis, volume status, fluid and electrolyte balance, and nutrition.

The specific management of HMD aims to support adequate gas exchange while minimizing the risks of acute (*e.g.,* barotrauma) and chronic lung disease, hypoxic pulmonary vasoconstriction, and retinopathy of prematurity. It is generally agreed that maintainence of arterial pO_2 between 50 and 70 mm Hg achieves sufficient fetal hemoglobin saturation to prevent systemic hypoxia and to avoid a significant rise in pulmonary vascular resistance. Recently, a trend has developed toward accepting higher arterial pCO_2 levels (45 to 60 mm Hg) as long as oxygenation is adequate and *pH* is maintained above 7.20 to 7.25, with the hope of decreasing the incidence and/or severity of subsequent chronic lung disease. The method by which these blood gas levels are attained, including the criteria for endotracheal intubation and initiation of artificial ventilation, varies from practitioner to practitioner and even from infant to infant for the same clinician. Similar results may be obtained by strikingly different clinical practices. The one unifying principle is that continuous application of positive pressure, either with (PEEP) or without (continuous positive airway pressure [CPAP]) intermittent mandatory ventilation, is helpful in stabilizing alveoli, reducing atelectasis, increasing FRC, and improving oxygenation and CO_2 exchange. Very recently, the experience of the Columbia group (see Bibliography: Avery, 1987) has renewed interest in the dedicated use of nasal CPAP to minimize chronic lung disease.

PREVENTION AND NEWER METHODS OF TREATMENT

There is no longer any question that prenatal maternal administration of steroids that begins 48 hours before delivery decreases the incidence of HMD. Results of the large perinatal collaborative study (see Bibliography: Collaborative Group on Antenatal Steroid Therapy) show that the effect is more pronounced in females than males. Moreover, at least two recent studies suggest that prenatal steroid administration is helpful at a lower gestational age (*e.g.,* 24 to 28 weeks). Steroid therapy has many effects on the fetal lungs other than augmentation or surfactant production. These include stimulation of pulmonary anatomic maturation, induction of pulmonary anti-oxidant enzymes, and reduction of pulmonary vascular permeability. In addition, the incidence of PDA may be decreased among male recipients of prenatal steroid therapy. A careful, detailed collaborative follow-up study of the neurologic outcome of steroid-treated infants detected no abnormalities in comparison to a control population at 3 years of age.

Two new therapies are under evaluation for the treatment of HMD. One is high-frequency ventilation; although initial results are encouraging, it is too early to say whether this mode of ventilation will provide consistent therapeutic or outcome advantages over conventional ventilation in uncomplicated HMD. Clinical use at this time is limited to infants with severe pulmonary interstitial emphysema or meconium aspiration.

A second experimental therapy for HMD is the use of surfactant replacement. Extensive studies in a variety of mammalian species have proven that appropriate surfactant therapy is safe and effective. Figure 14-2 demonstrates the histologic disparity between lung tissue of control and surfactant-treated premature lambs. Clinical human trials, using either artificial surfactant (derived from bovine lungs and supplemented with phospholipids) or homologous human surfactant (derived from human amniotic fluid), show great promise. Preliminary combinational analysis of data from several randomized, controlled studies of prophylactic surfactant administration (e.g., surfactant is given by endotracheal bolus immediately after birth) demonstrates

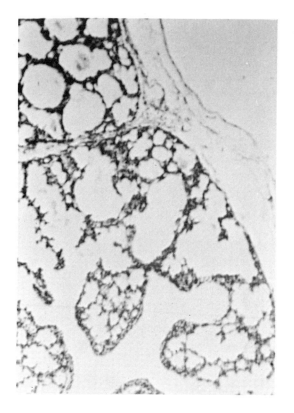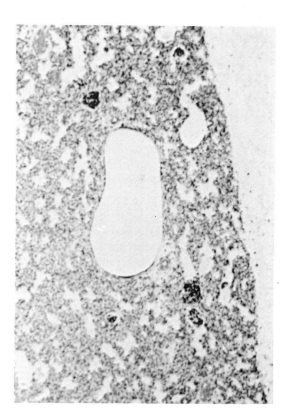

FIGURE 14–2. The left panel shows even expansion of bronchioles and alveoli and normal airway epithelium in a premature lamb that received surfactant therapy at birth. In contrast, the right panel was taken from a control lamb delivered at the same gestation. Marked atelectasis with dilatation of a proximal airway as well as plugging of airways with necrotic epithelial debris is obvious. Both photomicrographs were taken at 35× magnification. (Used by permission, from Adams FH, Towers B, Osher AB et al: Effects of tracheal instillation of natural surfactant in premature lambs. I. Clinical and autopsy findings. Pediatr Res 12:841–848, 1978)

both significant immediate improvement in pulmonary function as well as a significant reduction in mortality and subsequent chronic lung disease. The clinical issues under investigation at this time include the optimal dose, timing, and frequency of surfactant administration (*e.g.*, rescue from HMD vs. prophylaxis of HMD, single vs. multiple doses); identification of short-term and long-term (immunogenicity) side effects; and specification of the optimal composition of surfactant, the method of preparation, and the mode of delivery. It is reasonable to suppose by the early to mid-1990s that surfactant replacement therapy will be a standard of care.

BIBLIOGRAPHY

Avery ME, Mead J: Surface properties in relation to atelectasis and hyaline membrane disease. Am J Dis Child 97:517–523, 1959

Avery ME, Tooley WH, Keller JB et al: Is chronic lung disease in low birth weight infants preventable? A survey of eight centers. Pediatrics 79:26–30, 1987

Collaborative Group on Antenatal Steroid Therapy: Effect of antenatal dexamethasone administration in the prevention of respiratory distress syndrome. Am J Obstet Gynecol 141:276–287, 1981

Engle WD, Arant Jr BS, Wiriyathian S et al: Diuresis and respiratory distress syndrome: Physiologic mechanisms and therapeutic implications. J Pediatr 102:912–917, 1983

Gersony WM, Peckham GJ, Ellison RC et al: Effects of indomethacin in premature infants with patent ductus arteriosus: Results of a national collaborative study. J Pediatr 102:895–906, 1983

Gluck L, Kulovich MA, Borer RC Jr et al: The interpretation and significance of the lecithin/sphingomyelin ratio in amniotic fluid. Am J Obstet Gynecol 120:142–155, 1974

Gregory GA, Kitterman JA, Phibbs RH: Treatment of the idiopathic respiratory-distress syndrome with continuous positive airway pressure. N Engl J Med 284:1333–1340, 1971

Heaf DP, Belik J, Spitzer AR et al: Changes in pulmonary function during the diuretic phase of respiratory distress syndrome. J Pediatr 101:103–107, 1982

Jacob J, Gluck L, DiSessa T et al: The contribution of PDA in the neonate with severe RDS. J Pediatr 96:79–87, 1980

Langman CB, Engle WD, Baumgart S et al: The diuretic phase of respiratory distress syndrome and its relationship to oxygenation. J Pediatr 98:462–466, 1981

Notter RH, Shapiro DL: Lung surfactant in an era of replacement therapy. Pediatrics 68:781–789, 1981

Perelman RH, Farrell PM: Analysis of causes of neonatal death in the United States with specific emphasis on fatal hyaline membrane disease. Pediatrics 70:570–575, 1982

Spitzer AR, Fox WW, Delivoria-Papadopoulos M: Maximum diuresis—a factor in predicting recovery from respiratory distress syndrome and the development of bronchopulmonary dysplasia. J Pediatr 98:476–479, 1981

Stark AR, Frantz ID III: Respiratory distress syndrome. Pediatr Clin North Am 33:533–544, 1986

Strang L: Neonatal Respiration. Oxford, Blackwell Scientific, 1977

Wegman ME: Annual summary of vital statistics—1985. Pediatrics 78:983–994, 1986

Yeh TF, Shibli A, Leu ST et al: Early furosemide therapy in premature infants (≦2000 gm) with respiratory distress syndrome: A randomized controlled trial. J Pediatr 105:603–609, 1984

15 Chronic Lung Disease

HISTORICAL BACKGROUND

The typical infant with chronic lung disease was born prematurely and required treatment with supplemental oxygen and mechanical ventilation for an acute lung injury (usually hyaline membrane disease). However, chronic lung disease has also developed in full-term infants ventilated for other reasons (heart disease, pneumonia, meconium aspiration) and in preterm infants without initial clinical or radiologic signs of acute lung disease who are ventilated for apnea of prematurity. Three types of neonatal chronic lung disease have been described in the past 30 years.

Wilson-Mikity syndrome

Wilson-Mikity syndrome was first reported in 1960, when it was observed in premature infants who usually had little or no acute respiratory symptomatology after birth, but who later experienced the insidious onset of tachypnea, retractions, and cyanosis on room air. Some infants had frequent and severe apneic episodes. Initially, the chest radiograph was normal, but over a period of weeks, bilateral streaky infiltrates became prominent. Eventually, small, regular (1- to 4-mm) cysts outlined by reticular radiodensities evolved, imparting a bubbly, honeycombed appearance to the lungs. With clinical resolution of the disease, the lungs became hyperlucent and hyperinflated coincident with growth and consolidation of the cysts. Histologic findings on lung biopsy or at autopsy were not striking; uneven aeration with large, underdeveloped air spaces was characteristic. Occasionally, septae were thickened but interstitial fibrosis was minimal or lacking. It has been proposed that an arrest in lung maturation decreased the alveolar surface area enough to interfere with normal gas exchange.

When this syndrome was described, aggressive therapy with mechanical ventilation was not customary. In addition, oxygen therapy was often restricted because retrolental fibroplasia leading to blindness had recently been linked to the use of high inspired oxygen concentrations. Wilson-Mikity syndrome is now infrequently recognized, probably because routine ventilatory intervention has altered the natural history of the disease.

Bronchopulmonary dysplasia

Today, the term bronchopulmonary dysplasia (BPD) is synonymous with chronic lung disease in infants, even though chronic lung disease in most nurseries today bears little resemblance to the syndrome of BPD as it was first described by Northway and associates in 1967. These workers catalogued an orderly progression of clinical, radiologic, and pathologic chronic pulmonary disease that developed in premature infants with hyaline membrane disease who were treated with high inspired oxygen concentrations and mechanical ventilation. Stage 1 disease was seen in the first few days of life and was radiologically indistinguishable from hyaline membrane disease. Diffuse reticulogranular infiltrates with superimposed air bronchograms were ascribed to generalized edema and acinar atelectasis. By the end of the first week, total lung opacification defined stage 2. The evolution of diffuse small cysts marked stage 3 disease and signaled the onset of chronic pulmonary disease. By 1 month of life, stage 4 disease was evident radiographically. Lung hyperinflation, sometimes severe, was invariable. The small cysts present in stage 3 disease had enlarged or coalesced to produce focal areas of emphysema. These areas were surrounded by streaks of increased density, which were attributed to fibrosis and atelectasis.

Pathologically, stage 1 disease was equivalent to hyaline membrane disease. Overdistention of alveolar ducts and distal airways accompanied collapse of the alveolar saccules. Interstitial and alveolar edema was present. Hyaline membranes lined the distended distal airways and usually overlay desquamated and necrotic epithelium. In later stages of BPD, obliterative bronchiolitis, cystic dilatation of the airways, epithelial metaplasia, and interstitial fibrosis denoted advanced pulmonary injury. Bronchiolar smooth muscle hypertrophy was common. Medial hypertrophy of the pulmonary arterial smooth muscle and of the right ventricle was consistent with the clinical picture of cor pulmonale. Detailed morphometric analysis has been reported in one infant with stage 4 disease at autopsy. Alveolar number was decreased and average alveolar volume increased compared to full-term infants without lung disease.

Chronic pulmonary insufficiency of prematurity

The third form of chronic lung disease described in premature infants is known as chronic pulmonary insufficiency of prematurity (CPIP). The original series reported infants with birth weights less than 1250 g who were apparently well at birth but by 5 to 10 days of age developed apnea and hypoxia. Chest radiographs typically showed either hypoinflation or diffuse mild haziness as the only abnormalities. Gradual improvement occurred at 3 to 4 weeks of age, with clinical resolution of pulmonary symptoms by about 2 months. The histopathology of this form of chronic lung disease is unknown. Proposed etiologies for CPIP have included delayed surfactant deficiency (due to inadequate postnatal synthesis or secretion of surfactant) with consequent microatelectasis, respiratory muscle fatigue, and persistent fetal lung fluid secretion.

Current Definition

Dramatic changes in both the prenatal and postnatal care of premature infants have occurred since these three types of neonatal chronic lung disease were first described. For example, there have been major advances in prenatal obstetric management (e.g., electronic fetal monitoring, maternal steroid therapy to induce fetal lung maturity, tocolytic agents to prevent premature labor), improvements in respiratory technology (new ventilatory equipment and strategies), development of potent pharmacologic tools (indomethacin to treat patent ductus arteriosus), and acquisition of a vast amount of experience in the nonrespiratory care of tiny babies. Consequently, infants of younger gestational ages with less-mature lungs and different responses to therapies are surviving. It is not surprising that the pattern of lung disease in these infants does not conform to one of the classic descriptions. Because of the difficulty and inutility of classifying lung disease, the more general term "chronic lung disease" is often favored. Differences in the definition of chronic lung disease among institutions have complicated the interpretation of a vast descriptive literature on the subject, but the following functional definition has achieved wide acceptance. Chronic lung disease may be said to be present in any infant with (1) an abnormal chest radiograph and (2) an arterial PO_2 ≤60 torr or an arterial PCO_2 ≥45 torr on room air, or a supplemental oxygen requirement. This functional definition embraces a heterogeneous group of infants.

INCIDENCE

Comparison of the incidence of chronic lung disease among institutions has historically been complicated by differences in both the definition of chronic lung disease (the numerator) and the population of infants considered to be at risk (the denominator). Nonetheless, it is clear from more recent studies that the incidence of chronic lung disease varies greatly among institutions. One survey of 16 centers found that the mean incidence of chronic lung disease was 7% of all premature admissions (range, 3% to 33%) or 20% of all infants with hyaline membrane disease (range, 6% to 50%). The most current retrospective analysis sampled eight centers and included 1625 infants with birth weights between 700 and 1500 g. The incidence of chronic lung disease, defined simply as oxygen dependence at 28 days of age, ranged from 6% to 32% of live-born infants. Although the risk of chronic lung disease increases substantially with each 100-g decrement in birth weight and is also greater in the male sex, these factors did not explain the greater than fivefold difference in incidence that was observed. Chronic lung disease is uncommon in infants who weigh more than 1500 g at birth.

ETIOLOGY AND PATHOGENESIS

Chronic lung disease truly has a multifactorial etiology. This has been obvious to all clinicians who have ever tried to predict whether a given infant requiring treatment of acute lung disease with oxygen and mechanical ventilation will develop long-term clinical and radiologic pulmonary abnormalities.

It is generally agreed that pulmonary immaturity is the single most important risk factor for chronic lung disease; the likelihood of chronic lung disease increases dramatically as gestational age decreases. It must be emphasized that lung maturity refers not only to surfactant sufficiency but also to the capability of the lung to heal and grow normally following an acute injury as well as to anatomic maturity. The cytology of the tracheal aspirate may provide an early indication whether the lungs of infants with hyaline membrane disease are healing or undergoing progressive damage. Compared to infants who recover from hyaline membrane disease, infants destined to develop chronic lung disease have more acute inflammatory cells in their tracheal aspirates. Because polymorphonuclear leukocytes produce free radicals and secrete proteases, a vicious cycle of continued lung injury is easily conceivable. Anatomic differences in lung maturity have not been defined histopathologically but can be inferred on clinical grounds. Otherwise, the fact that some infants develop severe pulmonary interstitial emphysema or pneumothoraces on minimal peak ventilator pressures is not readily explained.

Other factors contributing to continued lung injury include abnormalities of surfactant composition, secretion, or function; prolonged exposure to high inspired oxygen concentration; mechanical ventilation; and pulmonary edema. Many of these factors are interrelated.

Abnormal surfactant function, regardless of etiology, contributes to the collapse of alveolar saccules with secondary dilatation of distal alveolar ducts, promotes necrosis of the bronchiolar epithelium, and probably contributes to pulmonary edema. Adequate synthesis and secretion of surfactant during recovery does not guarantee normal surfactant function: plasma surfactant inhibitors have been identified in the airways of infants recovering from hyaline membrane disease.

Studies in animals and in adult humans have demonstrated that oxygen is a potent pulmonary toxin. Exposure to a high inspired oxygen concentration impairs ciliary motility, alters airway mucus production, and produces airway epithelial metaplasia within a few days. Oxygen also interferes with normal lung growth and development, including the pulmonary capillary bed, and stimulates inflammation. Nonetheless, oxygen probably does not initiate lung injury but rather exacerbates existing pulmonary damage caused by other factors.

The assessment of oxygen toxicity has usually been confounded by the simultaneous use of mechanical ventilation. Positive pressure ventilation contributes to airway distention and barotrauma, and also has more subtle and possibly equally important effects. These include denudation of tracheal epithelium by the endotracheal tube, bronchial injury secondary to suctioning, and impairment of ciliary function and mucociliary transport by inadequate heating and humidification of inspired gases.

Pulmonary edema is a pathologic *sine qua non* of hyaline membrane disease, but excessive pulmonary edema has been linked to an increased risk of chronic lung disease. An imbalance in the Starling forces that regulate transcapillary flux, an increase in pulmonary blood flow or perfused capillary surface area, or an increase in capillary permeability favor the development of pulmonary edema. For several reasons, premature infants are more likely than full-term infants to develop pulmonary edema. Decreased colloid osmotic pressure in preterm infants secondary to lower concentrations of serum proteins increases transcapillary flux. The ductus arteriosus is commonly patent in premature infants with hyaline membrane disease and increases pulmonary blood flow *via* a left-to-right shunt. Capillary permeability to proteins and solutes is elevated in infants with hyaline membrane disease. The failure of permeability to return to normal has been linked to development of chronic lung disease. The combination of pulmonary interstitial edema and inflammation stimulates fibrosis. It is not clear whether pulmonary edema is a primary cause of chronic lung disease or instead a marker of pulmonary injury. There is some evidence, however, that high levels of fluid intake are more likely to be associated with patent ductus arteriosus and chronic lung disease.

CLINICAL MANIFESTATIONS

Typically, the infant with chronic lung is born at less than 34 weeks of gestation weighing less than 2000 g and is treated with supplemental oxygen and mechanical ventilation for hyaline membrane disease. The infant does not have the spontaneous diuresis at 2 to 4 days of age that augurs a successful recovery.

In addition, the early clinical course is likely complicated by air leaks and/or a symptomatic patent ductus arteriosus. By 1 week of age, significant oxygen and ventilatory support is still required, and the chest radiograph may show early chronic changes. As the disease progresses, the infant works harder to breathe and exhibits subcostal and intercostal retractions. Increased physical exertion, feeding, or a decrease in inspired oxygen concentration lead to tachycardia, tachypnea, and cyanosis. On auscultation, rales are usually present; audible wheezing and prolongation of the expiratory phase of respiration are also common. In severe disease, a right ventricular heave, a loud prominent P_2, and increased hepar signify development of cor pulmonale. Digital clubbing develops in infants with prolonged hypoxia.

Laboratory studies reflect the chronicity of pulmonary disease. Arterial blood gases demonstrate an elevated pCO_2 but normal *pH*. Hypoxia becomes profound without supplemental oxygen. Electrolyte abnormalities include a hypochloremic metabolic alkalosis (secondary to diuretic therapy and/or renal compensation for a primary respiratory acidosis), and hyponatremia and hypokalemia (exacerbated by diuretic therapy). Radiologic findings are variable but generally include hyperinflation and migratory areas of atelectasis and emphysema (Fig. 15-1). ECG and echocardiogram are consistent with right ventricular hypertrophy and pulmonary hypertension. Abdominal x-rays or renal sonogram may show renal calculi or nephrocalcinosis due to the calciuretic effects of certain diuretics (*e.g., furosemide*).

Pulmonary function studies have been performed in relatively few neonates during the early stages of chronic lung disease. Studies are difficult to compare for two principal reasons: the use of different techniques and differences between the patient populations reported (with regard to birth weight, gesta-

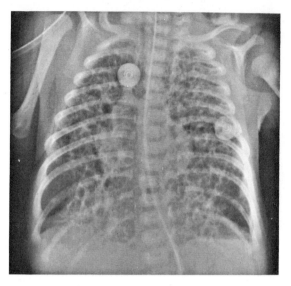

FIGURE 15–1. Infant with severe chronic lung disease showing hyperinflation, coarse infiltrates, and cystic changes. Note that emphysematous areas are confined to both lung bases.

tional age, etiology, and severity of disease). Nonetheless, the following conclusions can safely be drawn:

1. The most striking and consistent finding is that airway resistance is markedly increased compared both to normal controls and to infants recovered from uncomplicated hyaline membrane disease.
2. Functional residual capacity (as assessed by either helium dilution or nitrogen washout) is decreased or normal. Tidal volume is decreased, the rate of respiration is increased, and total minute ventilation is usually increased.
3. Specific dynamic pulmonary compliance is decreased.
4. The work of breathing is significantly increased.
5. Expiratory flow-volume curves generated by rapid chest compression demonstrate a significant decrease in maximal flow at

FRC even after correction for FRC. This test is analogous to the forced expiratory flow velocity test in older cooperative patients.

6. Elevated pCO_2s support maldistribution of ventilation.

MANAGEMENT

As with most diseases, prevention of chronic lung disease is the best therapy. In the last decade, prophylactic measures have centered primarily on decreasing the number of premature births (improved general prenatal care, tocolysis of premature labor) or lessening the risk of hyaline membrane disease if premature delivery appears imminent (antenatal steroid therapy). Current studies suggest that optimal use of exogenous surfactant will decrease the severity of acute lung disease and minimize chronic pulmonary sequelae. Finally, a recent multi-center retrospective analysis of the incidence of chronic lung disease has suggested that tolerance of lower pO_2s and higher pCO_2s, use of nasal continuous positive airway pressure (CPAP), less aggressive ventilation, and early extubation may significantly reduce the risk of chronic lung disease. This hypothesis has not yet been evaluated in a controlled prospective trial.

During the course of hyaline membrane disease, it is reasonable to limit exposure to high inspired oxygen concentrations and to adopt the ventilatory approach least likely to result in barotrauma. Fluids are generally restricted with the intent of minimizing pulmonary edema and the risk of patent ductus arteriosus. There is some evidence that dexamethasone therapy may be effective in preventing the development of chronic lung disease in ventilator-dependent infants who have not developed chronic changes on chest x-ray at 2 weeks of age. Again, a recommendation for the routine use of steroids must await further clinical trials.

The transition from hyaline membrane disease to chronic lung disease requires changes in the therapeutic approach. Efforts are directed toward augmenting pulmonary function, preventing cor pulmonale, and attaining normal growth and development.

Cardiorespiratory management

Adequate oxygenation is essential to prevent life-threatening cor pulmonale. Traditional invasive monitoring of arterial blood gases provides only an intermittent and frequently misleading assessment of oxygenation. Newer technologies that provide continuous measurements of transcutaneous pO_2 or arterial hemoglobin saturations (pulse oximetry) are preferable. These methods allow adjustment of inspired oxygen concentration during care and feedings, when hypoxia often occurs. $TcPO_2$ should be maintained greater than 60 mm Hg or 50 mm Hg in infants less than or greater than 3 months of age respectively. Hemoglobin saturations should be maintained between 90% and 95%.

When mechanical ventilation is required, pCO_2s between 50 and 70 mm Hg can be tolerated. Uneven patterns of alveolar gas exchange (air trapping) are treated with slower ventilatory rates and longer expiratory times. Ventilator dependency is best managed by gradual weaning. In institutions proficient in its use, nasal CPAP can be helpful during the weaning process.

Pulmonary edema frequently complicates the management. Fluid restriction is limited because of high caloric requirements. Diuretics improve lung compliance and decrease airway resistance; however, chronic diuretic therapy with furosemide can result in electrolyte derangements and renal disease (e.g., nephrocalcinosis). Addition of chlorothiazide to furosemide lowers the risk of renal complications, and the combination of chlorothiazide and spironolactone lessens electrolyte abnormalities.

Infants with chronic lung disease have increased bronchial smooth muscle and clinical reactive airway disease. Both nebulized beta-2 agonists and theophylline can be useful in their pulmonary management. Inhaled isoproterenol 0.1% decreases airway resistance. Similarly, subcutaneous administration of terbutaline (5 μg/kg) improves lung compliance and decreases airway resistance. Theophylline has several potentially beneficial actions, including smooth muscle dilation, improved diaphragmatic contractility, central respiratory stimulation, and mild diuretic activity.

Steroid therapy for chronic lung disease is controversial. Several studies have shown marked short-term improvement with steroid treatment. These improvements were not always maintained once therapy was discontinued. In some studies, mortality rates of the steroid-treated infants were greater than for the placebo group. Actual and theoretic risks of chronic steroid use include infection, hyperglycemia, hypertension, and peptic ulcer with bleeding.

Nutrition

Infants with chronic lung disease have higher oxygen requirements and therefore greater caloric needs than healthy, size-matched controls, at least in part due to an increased work of breathing. Caloric density can be increased safely to 24 to 30 calories per ounce with special infant formulas while limiting fluid intake. Calcium and phosphorus status must be monitored carefully in infants receiving chronic diuretic therapy.

General care and discharge planning

Infants hospitalized with chronic lung disease should receive immunizations per the recommendation of the American Academy of Pediatrics. Periodic follow-up by a developmentalist and occupational therapist are useful in some infants for both therapeutic and prognostic purposes. Serial echocardiographic evaluation of right-ventricular function and regular screening for chemical evidence of rickets (hypocalcemia, hypophosphatemia, and elevated alkaline phosphatase) may also be indicated.

Older babies should have their daily routine normalized. When possible, parents should be involved in the daily care of their child to foster infant–parent bonding and to prepare for discharge. Often oxygen can be discontinued before discharge. Our experience with home oxygen therapy shows that it can be a safe alternative to prolonged hospitalization. The need for home cardiorespiratory monitoring must be decided on an individual basis but is recommended for all infants discharged home on oxygen. Instruction in cardiopulmonary resuscitation is essential for all parents and caretakers.

OUTCOME

The prognosis for infants with chronic lung disease depends on the nature and severity of their pulmonary disease and other associated medical conditions. Although most of the patients originally described by Northway died, more recently mortality rates of 23% to 39% are reported. Most deaths are related to sepsis and cardiopulmonary failure. The risk of sudden death in infants with chronic lung disease following hospital discharge is approximately 1%. After discharge, infants with chronic lung disease are more likely than normal infants to be rehospitalized, usually secondary to respiratory tract infections.

Increased airway resistance and airway reactivity are more common in survivors with chronic lung disease followed through 10 years of age. Cor pulmonale has developed following discharge when adequate oxygenation was not maintained. Pulmonary function tests in survivors of chronic lung disease usually show different rates of resolution of most of the abnormalities cited in the neonatal studies. That airway resistance declines less rapidly than FRC increases suggests that there is continued abnormal growth and development of the airways.

The independent contribution of chronic lung disease to neurodevelopmental outcome is uncertain. Some analyses have suggested that chronic lung disease, independent of other variables, is associated with a poorer cognitive outcome. Other studies have related developmental outcome to perinatal–neonatal events other than chronic lung disease.

BIBLIOGRAPHY

Avery ME, Fletcher BD, Williams RG: The Lung and Its Disorders in the Newborn Infant. Major Problems in Clinical Pediatrics, vol I. Philadelphia, WB Saunders, 1981

Bancalari E, Gerhardt T: Bronchopulmonary dysplasia. Pediatr Clin North Am 33:1–23, 1986

Bronchopulmonary Dysplasia and Related Chronic Respiratory Disorders: Report of the Ninetieth Ross Conference on Pediatric Research. Ross Laboratories, 1986

Escobedo MB, Gonzales A: Bronchopulmonary dysplasia in the tiny infant. Clin Perinatol 13:315–326, 1986

Koops BL, Abman SH, Accurso FJ: Outpatient management and follow-up of bronchopulmonary dysplasia. Clin Perinatol 11:101–122, 1984

Krauss AN, Klain DB, Auld PAM: Chronic pulmonary insufficiency of prematurity (CPIP). Pediatrics 55:55–58, 1975

Northway WH Jr, Rosan RC, Porter DY: Pulmonary disease following respiratory therapy of hyaline-membrane disease. N Engl J Med 276:357–368, 1967

O'Brodovich HM, Mellins RB: Bronchopulmonary dysplasia: Unresolved neonatal acute lung injury. Am Rev Respir Dis 132:694–709, 1985

Wilson MR, Mikity VG: A new form of respiratory disease in premature infants. Am J Dis Child 99:489–499, 1960

Workshop on bronchopulmonary dysplasia. J Pediatr 95(suppl):815–920, 1979

16 Neonatal Jaundice

Nothing has vexed caretakers of newborns more than the management of hyperbilirubinemia. Perhaps no other topic in neonatology has been studied so intensively in proportion to the yield of clear and useful information acquired. Although there is no doubt that an excessively high level of indirect bilirubin in the newborn in association with certain conditions (*i.e.*, erythroblastosis fetalis, Crigler-Najjar disease) carries a high risk of permanent neurologic damage (kernicterus) or death, basic questions remain unanswered about more common clinical situations. For instance, is there a population of infants at risk for subtle but permanent neurologic injury due to "modest" elevations (10 to 20 mg/dl) of serum bilirubin? If so, what factors determine risk? What is the optimal therapeutic approach to jaundice in the tiny sick premature infant? In the absence of firmly grounded data that answer these questions satisfactorily, clinicians have relied instead on empirical algorithms for the management of jaundice.

Nonetheless, the pediatrician must be able to evaluate neonatal hyperbilirubinemia carefully and thoughtfully. An abnormality of bilirubin metabolism can be the first sign of a more serious disorder that may benefit from early intervention. This chapter considers how a basic knowledge of bilirubin metabolism can provide a working framework for a logical differential diagnosis and subsequent evaluation of neonatal hyperbilirubemia.

BILIRUBIN METABOLISM

The metabolism of bilirubin can be divided into five topics: derivation, transport, uptake, conjugation, and excretion.

Bilirubin derives from the catabolism of heme, a protoporphyrin found predominantly in hemoglobin and myoglobin and in small quantities in other heme proteins such as cytochrome. Heme breakdown occurs in two steps. First, a microsomal heme oxygenase opens the protoporphyrin ring to form biliverdin IXα. In this reaction, the heme-associated iron is liberated, and one molecule of carbon monoxide (CO) is formed. Because this reaction is the only known source of CO production in the human, the rate of bilirubin production can be determined accurately by measurement of pulmonary CO excretion. In the second reaction, biliverdin IXα is reduced to bilirubin IXα.

115

In the normal newborn infant, the degradation of hemoglobin from senescent red cells accounts for three-fourths of the production of bilirubin. One gram of hemoglobin yields 34 mg of bilirubin. Breakdown of other heme proteins and the degradation of red blood cells before they are released from the bone marrow (ineffective erythropoiesis) are responsible for the remaining bilirubin production. The total rate of production in a newborn (6 to 11 mg/kg/day) is two or three times greater than in an adult; this is true for three reasons. First, the neonate has a larger red cell mass per kilogram; both the mean hematocrit (55%) and the blood volume (80 to 110 ml/kg) are greater than the adult levels. Second, the half-life of red cells is only 90 days in the neonate, compared with 120 days in the adult. Third, ineffective erythropoiesis does not contribute significantly to adult bilirubin production.

The bilirubin isomer formed after heme degradation is poorly soluble in water and is transported to the hepatocyte bound to albumin.

Uptake of bilirubin into the hepatocyte is probably facilitated by a carrier. In the hepatocyte, bilirubin is bound by several proteins. The concentration of some of these proteins may be increased by phenobarbital.

An enzyme associated with the smooth endoplasmic reticulum conjugates bilirubin with a glucuronide moiety, forming a water-soluble compound. This monoglucuronide is likely changed to the diglucuronide form by another enzyme associated with the canalicular membrane as it is excreted by active transport into the bile canaliculus. In the adult, bacteria convert bilirubin diglucuronide into stercobilin, which ultimately is excreted; only a small fraction of the diglucuronide is deconjugated to bilirubin and resorbed through the intestinal mucosa into the blood. In the newborn, however, the latter enterohepatic circulation may predominate, especially under circumstances of decreased intestinal motility, because of a large native con-

centration of B-glucuronidase.

In the fetus, unconjugated bilirubin is taken up across the placenta and processed by the maternal liver. Only a small amount is metabolized and excreted by the fetal liver. Thus, at birth, the newborn is not prepared to metabolize bilirubin efficiently.

PHYSIOLOGIC HYPERBILIRUBINEMIA

Almost without exception, every newborn has a period of hyperbilirubinemia (bilirubin ≥ 2 mg/dl). It is said that only 50% of newborns will have detectable jaundice; in the neonate, jaundice is more difficult to detect than in the adult, requiring a level of 5 to 7 mg/dl. A graph of the mean level of bilirubin in a group of full-term newborns during the initial 2 weeks of life is shown in Figure 16-1. The rapid rise in bilirubin over the first 3 to 4 days is known as phase I; it has been attributed to a gradual induction of the enzyme responsible for bilirubin conjugation. The cause of the remaining period of hyperbilirubinemia (phase II), from day 4 to day 10 to 14, is not completely understood. It is possible that hepatic concentrations of the bilirubin binding proteins are decreased.

The curve of bilirubin concentration versus time is quantitatively different in the preterm infant. The peak level is higher and occurs later. In addition, phase II is prolonged. These differences increase with the degree of prematurity.

This transient hyperbilirubinemia, if clinically detectable, is termed "physiologic jaundice." The clinician must distinguish physiologic from nonphysiologic, or pathologic, jaundice.

BREAST-MILK–ASSOCIATED JAUNDICE

Surprisingly, normal values of bilirubin have only recently been described over the intitial several weeks of life in breast-fed infants.

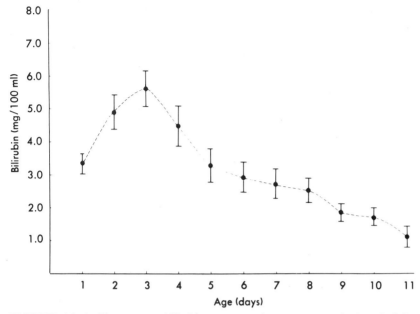

FIGURE 16–1. Mean serum bilirubin concentration versus age in days in full-term infants.

Classic breast-milk jaundice, on the other hand, is a well-recognized entity, which probably represents the extreme end of the spectrum of breast-milk–associated jaundice. In the former condition, which occurs in perhaps 2% of breast-fed infants, bilirubin levels continue to rise after 3 days of age and can peak at 20 to 30 mg/dl by 10 to 20 days of age. Thereafter, the level declines slowly but jaundice may persist for months. The infants are healthy (there have been no published reports of kernicterus due to breast milk jaundice) and have no evidence of liver dysfunction. A cardinal feature of this condition is that the bilirubin level falls sharply over 1 to 3 days when formula is temporarily substituted for breast milk. Upon resumption of breast-feeding, serum bilirubin is either stable or rises only slightly.

Breast-milk–associated jaundice refers to a prolonged elevation of serum bilirubin found in breast-fed compared to formula-fed infants. Mild jaundice is evident for weeks; bilirubin levels average less than 10 mg/dl. In formula-fed infants, physiologic jaundice has resolved by 7 to 10 days.

The mechanism of breast-milk–associated jaundice has been the subject of much debate. It now appears likely that it is due to an increase in the enterohepatic circulation of bilirubin. Previously postulated mechanisms, such as inhibition of the hepatic enzyme responsible for conjugation of bilirubin, have been invalidated for the vast majority of breast-fed infants.

PATHOLOGIC JAUNDICE

Definition

Jaundice as an isolated clinical finding should be carefully evaluated if it deviates significantly from the "physiologic" course. Maisels has suggested that the following aberrations warrant attention:

1. Clinical jaundice prior to 24 hours of age.
2. A peak bilirubin level that is greater than 13 mg/dl. In the National Collaborative Perinatal Project of 1959–1966, peak bilirubin levels were obtained in 35,307 infants. The peak level was 13 mg/dl or greater in only 6.2% and 4.5% of white and black infants, respectively. In the preterm infant, a peak level of 15 mg/dl has been somewhat arbitrarily chosen as an upper limit of the physiologic.
3. A bilirubin level that rises too quickly (*i.e.*, more than 5 mg/dl/day).
4. In formula-fed infants, prolonged jaundice (more than 7 to 10 days in the full-term or 14 days in the preterm infant).
5. Any elevation of the direct, conjugated fraction of total serum bilirubin.

Prospective studies of all infants with any of the above abnormalities of the indirect component of serum bilirubin have shown that an etiology of the hyperbilirubinemia can be found in about 50% of the cases. Other studies have indicated that up to 80% of the unexplained cases have been associated with breast-feeding. Therefore, not all cases of jaundice that fall outside the "physiologic" range are due to pathologic causes.

Etiologies

In general, the etiologies of pathologic hyperbilirubinemia can be divided into two groups: those that result from an increased bilirubin load and those due to decreased bilirubin clearance. An increase in bilirubin load, in turn, may result either from an abnormally high rate of heme catabolism or from an increase in or persistence of the enterohepatic circulation. Specific causes are listed in Table 16-1.

Conditions that increase heme catabolism include hemolytic disorders, an elevated circulating red cell mass, and significant extra-

Table 16–1. Etiologies of indirect hyperbilirubinemia

Increased Bilirubin Production
Hemolysis
  Isoimmune
    Rh
    ABO
    Other red cell antigens
  Red cell membrane abnormalities
    Hereditary spherocytosis
    Elliptocytosis
    Stomatocytosis
  Red cell enzyme deficiencies
    Pyruvate kinase
    Glucose 6-phosphatase
    Other
  Abnormal hemoglobins
    α-Thalassemia
    β-Thalassemia
  Drug-induced hemolysis
    Vitamin K_3
Polycythemia
Extravasated blood
Increased enterohepatic circulation

Decreased Bilirubin Clearance
Inborn errors of bilirubin conjugation and excretion
  Crigler-Najjar types I and II
  Gilbert's syndrome
Other inborn errors of metabolism
  Galactosemia
  Tyrosinemia
  Hypermethionemia
Endocrine disorders
  Hypothyroidism
  Hypopituitarism

vascular collections of blood. The enterohepatic circulation of bilirubin may be increased or prolonged in association with small or large bowel obstruction, intestinal ileus, or large quantities of swallowed maternal blood. Situations that increase bilirubin load much more commonly cause pathologic hyperbilirubinemia than do conditions that decrease bilirubin clearance.

Hemolysis is the most frequently encountered cause of increased bilirubin load. Table 16-1 lists five mechanisms of hemolysis in the newborn. The isoimmune category will be discussed in greater detail.

ABO incompatibility. With rare exceptions, ABO incompatibilities occur when type A or type B infants are born to type O mothers. Type O mothers generally have IgG anti-A and anti-B antibodies, since the A and B red cell antigens are similar to common environmental antigens. These IgG antibodies cross the placenta and can initiate hemolysis *in utero* by binding to the fetal red blood cells. Fifteen percent of pregnancies are ABO incompatible, but of these only one-fifth result in postnatal hyperbilirubinemia outside the physiologic range. Prenatal hemolysis rarely produces anemia or hyperbilirubinemia at birth. Fetuses are probably protected by a relatively low concentration density of A and B antigens on the fetal red cell membrane. Interestingly, there is no predictable familial pattern; the same incompatibility may present with hyperbilirubinemia requiring treatment in one infant but not even cause jaundice in a subsequently born infant. Kernicterus has occurred in association with hyperbilirubinemia secondary to ABO incompatibility. Early treatment with phototherapy (see below) in selected high-risk cases can almost always prevent an indirect hyperbilirubinemia ≥20 mg/dl and obviate exchange transfusion. Even after hyperbilirubinemia has resolved, continued hemolysis may place these infants at risk for an exaggeration of "physiologic anemia" at 2 to 3 months of age.

Implication of an ABO incompatibility as the cause of hyperbilirubinemia requires, as a minimum, demonstration of a positive direct Coombs' test result on the infant red cells (*i.e.*, a demonstration of maternal antibody on the red cell membrane). Documentation of specific anti-A or anti-B antibody in an eluent of the infant red cells (an indirect Coombs' test) is a more specific test. Spherocytes and polychromasia are typically seen on the peripheral smear. As noted in Table 16-1, many other incompatibilities of maternal–fetal red cell antigens (Kell, Duffy, etc.) can lead to neonatal hyperbilirubinemia.

Rh incompatibility. With rare exceptions, prenatal isoimmune hemolytic disease is due to incompatibility of the Rh antigen system. Three antigens are involved: (C,c), (D,d) and (E,e). Of these, the D antigen evokes the most intense antibody response. Seventeen percent of white and 10% of black women are Rh(D) negative. Maternal–fetal Rh(D) incompatibility occurs in about 10% of pregnancies. Before effective prophylaxis of Rh hemolytic disease existed, maternal sensitization (*i.e.*, maternal production of anti-D antibody) developed in only 15% of pregnancies at risk. Prophylaxis has driven down this rate in susceptible pregnancies by a factor of 10. The sensitization rate was only 15% for two reasons. First, sensitization required maternal exposure to the fetal Rh antigen significant enough to cause an antibody response. If this occurred, for instance due to a large fetal–maternal bleed, a small exposure to the fetal Rh antigen in a subsequent pregnancy induced an amnestic antibody response, which could then result in a spectrum of fetal disease, ranging from mild anemia and hyperbilirubinemia at birth to fetal hydrops and death *in utero*. However, significant maternal exposure to fetal Rh antigen was not a universal event. Second, in some instances of maternal exposure, a concurrent ABO incompatibility presumably removed circulating fetal red cells and prevented Rh sensitization.

One of the principal reasons kernicterus has become so rare that many current neonatologists have never encountered a case is the improvement of obstetric care to women at risk of delivering an Rh-incompatible infant. Prenatally, mothers are screened for their Rh blood type; if a woman is negative, antibody titers to the C and D Rh antigens are evaluated in the first trimester. If these initial titers are lacking, this is presumptive evidence of a lack of previous sensitization. These titers can be followed periodically throughout the pregnancy; if sensitization occurs, the titers become positive, and the absolute levels correlate with the severity of fetal disease. A known history of previous sensitization or a presumption of past sensitization on the basis of positive initial titers mandates more careful attention to the fetus. Amniocentesis can be performed, beginning at approximately 22 weeks' gestation, and amniotic fluid bilirubin levels can be determined by spectrophotometry. These levels at a given gestational age correlate with the severity of fetal disease. The fetus also can be regularly followed by ultrasound looking for evidence of fetal hydrops (scalp edema, ascites, pleural effusions), which signals fetal anemia and cardiovascular compromise. An attempt to treat a severely affected previable fetus can be made by an intrauterine transfusion of Rh negative blood. Typically, this is performed by infusing a quantity of packed red cells (based on the estimated fetal weight) into the fetal peritoneal cavity under ultrasonic guidance; the red cells are gradually absorbed into the fetal bloodstream *via* the subdiaphragmatic lymphatics. In some centers, blood is directly infused into the umbilical vein. Such transfusions repair fetal anemia and temporarily improve some of the abnormalities associated with fetal hydrops; unfortunately, helpful effects persist no longer than 2 weeks. Since the mortality risk to the fetus secondary to an intrauterine transfusion is on the order of 5%, at some point, the fetus is better served by early elective delivery and intensive postnatal care.

Prophylaxis of Rh sensitization was initiated in 1968 by giving Rh-negative mothers who delivered Rh-positive infants intramuscular anti-Rh immune globulin (Rhogam) immediately postpartum. This prevented sensitization that might otherwise have occurred during labor and delivery. Treatment "failures" followed instances of large fetal–maternal transfusions around the time of delivery or smaller transfusions earlier in pregnancy. In some institutions, the latter event has prompted administration of the initial dose of Rhogam to Rh-negative mothers at 28 weeks' gestation. Rhogam also is frequently administered following amniocentesis. Currently, many cases of Rh sensitization are attributable to missed abortions with consequent unsuspected sensitization.

Diagnosis of an affected infant is straightforward. Peripheral blood smear shows evidence of hemolysis, polychromasia, and nucleated red blood cells. Infants born with a cord hemoglobin of less than 14 g/dl and/or bilirubin greater than 4 mg/dl should be treated initially with phototherapy; an exchange transfusion should be performed if the peak indirect bilirubin level rises above 20 mg/dl. Most authors have advocated earlier exchange transfusions if the rate of rise of bilirubin suggests that a level of 20 mg/dl is likely despite phototherapy, or if the infant's condition is complicated by perinatal asphyxia, hypoalbuminemia, or acidosis. In some cases, a small transfusion of washed O-negative cells may correct the anemia and, by decreasing the stimulus for bone marrow production of Rh-positive red cells, ward off an exchange transfusion.

Other hemolytic processes. Abnormalities of red cell membranes, red cell enzyme deficiencies, abnormal hemoglobins, and a variety of drugs given prenatally to the mother or postnatally to the infant may cause or exacerbate hemolysis. In these cases, evidence of isoimmune disease is lacking; a diagnosis can frequently be made by careful examination of the peripheral smear and appropriate ancillary tests.

Miscellaneous causes of increased bilirubin load. Polycythemia results in an increased circulating red cell mass; it can occur in macrosomic infants of diabetic mothers or in association with intrauterine growth retardation secondary to uteroplacental insufficiency. Delayed cord clamping with the infant held below the placenta or an *in utero* placental transfusion secondary to fetal asphyxia can also cause neonatal polycythemia. In monochorionic twin gestations complicated by arteriovenous anastomoses, a twin–twin transfusion syndrome can produce a plethoric infant (recipient) at the expense of the anemic donor twin.

Extravasation of blood, generally as a result of birth trauma, may lead to prolonged hyperbilirubinemia. The classic example is cephalohematoma, or subperiosteal bleeding. This occurs gradually, so that even loss of a significant volume of blood does not produce neonatal shock. Other occult bleeds (*i.e.*, subgaleal hematoma, intraventricular hemorrhage, hepatic subcapsular bleeding, retroperitoneal hemorrhage) are likely to present with more acute symptoms.

The enterohepatic circulation (EHC) of bilirubin will be elevated when anatomic or functional small or large bowel obstruction is present. The etiology of the prolonged hyperbilirubinemia associated with pyloric stenosis is poorly understood; in some cases, a decreased activity of hepatic glucuronyl transferase has been observed. Increased EHC is one of the mechanisms responsible for the association of hyperbilirubinemia with decreased caloric intake.

Decreased bilirubin clearance. As a group, these are uncommon causes of hyperbilirubinemia. They include a spectrum of inborn errors of bilirubin conjugation and excretion, other inborn errors of metabolism that cause hepatic injury (*i.e.*, galactosemia, tyrosinemia), and certain endocrine abnormalities. Although uncommon, this group is very important to consider; for example, prolonged hyperbilirubinemia in a formula-fed infant may be the only early clue to hypothyroidism, which can cause irreversible neurologic damage if not treated early.

EVALUATION OF HYPERBILIRUBINEMIA

A careful evaluation of neonatal hyperbilirubinemia should first consider relevant points of the maternal medical history, the neonatal history of other siblings, events during labor and delivery, and other findings of the newborn examination. For example, microcephaly, purpuric or petechial rash, hepatosplenomegaly, or chorioretinitis may suggest a congenital infection; a large umbilical hernia, hypothyroidism. After this initial evaluation, selected laboratory tests (fractionated bilirubin levels, hematocrit, blood types of the mother and infant, direct and indirect Coombs' tests on infant, evaluation of peripheral smear, urinary non-glucose reducing substances) may suggest or confirm a diagnosis.

BILIRUBIN TOXICITY

Kernicterus

The term *kernicterus* was first used in 1904 to describe yellow staining of the basal ganglia, putamen, globus pallidus, caudate nuclei, and, less frequently, other cranial and bulbar nuclei in jaundiced infants dying of erythroblastosis fetalis. Symptoms of kernicterus were quite distinctive. Initially, they included hypotonia and a poor Moro's reflex, lethargy, poor feeding and/or vomiting, and a high-pitched cry. Shortly thereafter, opisthotonus (a posture characterized by hyperextension of the back and neck; see Figure 16-2) and hypertonia developed, accompanied by paralysis of upward gaze and possibly by seizures and hyperpyrexia. Many infants died at this stage; survivors had a triad of choreoathetoid cerebral palsy, nerve deafness, and dental dysplasia. Some survivors also had mental retardation.

By the 1950s, two points were clear: (1) The chance of kernicterus complicating hemolytic disease of the newborn (due to Rh or ABO

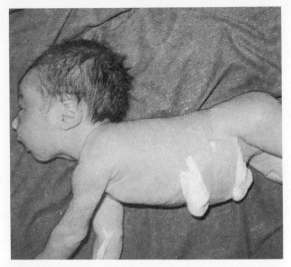

FIGURE 16–2. Infant with kernicterus. Note the characteristic opisthotonic posture.

incompatibility) increased in relation to the level of serum bilirubin. The risk was low for total bilirubin levels less than 20 mg/dl (whence the current exchange level is derived) but uncertain even when the level exceeded 30 mg/dl. (2) Exchange transfusions performed to maintain serum bilirubin levels less than 20 mg/dl in hemolytic disease or less than 24 mg/dl in preterm infants with nonhemolytic disease almost completely eliminated the risk of kernicterus.

Today both the putative mechanism by which bilirubin is toxic to neural tissue and the necessary conditions for bilirubin to cross the blood–brain barrier are disputed. Some authors have even argued that hyperbilirubinemia is only a marker for other pathologic events and does not by itself cause neurologic injury; however, infants with Crigler-Najjar syndrome have developed kernicterus with hyperbilirubinemia presumably the sole abnormality. Moreover, in this population, the incidence of kernicterus has been reduced by judicious use of phototherapy and agents that decrease the EHC.

Autopsy of some premature infants has identified bilirubin staining of neural tissue. These infants have died with peak bilirubin levels well below 20 mg/dl. This finding by itself does not mean that these infants would have developed kernicterus had they lived, especially in light of recent evidence suggesting that the staining is reversible in animal models. It is, however, one factor that has motivated clinicians to perform exchange transfusions in sick premature infants with peak bilirubin levels as low as 10 mg/dl.

Bilirubin and subtle neurodevelopmental impairment

Conflicting evidence exists whether mild levels of hyperbilirubinemia are associated with a risk of subtle neurodevelopmental handicap. The safest interpretation of all the data is that for levels less than 20 mg/dl, peak bilirubin level does not correlate with neurodevelopmental outcome.

Recent evidence has demonstrated that brain stem auditory evoked potentials become progressively abnormal as bilirubin levels rise. The potentials revert to normal as the bilirubin concentration falls during exchange transfusion. It is not yet clear whether this finding has any implications for long-term auditory function.

TREATMENT OF HYPERBILIRUBINEMIA

Phototherapy

Exposure of the naked infant skin to blue light (wavelength range, 425-475 nanometers [nm]) with an irradiance of 4 to 12 microwatts/cm^2/nm effectively reduces the serum bilirubin level. This treatment was suggested by an old clinical observation that jaundice resolved more rapidly in infants placed in bright, sunlit areas of the nursery. The mechanism by which phototherapy increases bilirubin clearance has only recently been elucidated. Bilirubin deposited in the subcutaneous tissue absorbs light in the blue spectrum and undergoes photoisomerization to a water-soluble form. This photobilirubin isomer is assimilated into the bloodstream, passes through the hepatocyte without undergoing conjugation, and is excreted in the bile. It can be resorbed into the vascular compartment by the EHC. Phototherapy also causes photodegradation of bilirubin into a number of nontoxic compounds, which are then excreted in the urine. Contrary to previous dogma, this mechanism contributes little to net bilirubin clearance.

A large collaborative study has failed to demonstrate significant short-term or long-term morbidities of phototherapy. Nonetheless, it is prudent to shield the infant's eyes and gonads with opaque patches. Phototherapy increases insensible water losses, although the mechanism is not understood. It can also increase gastrointestinal motility and cause loose stools. Occasionally, phototherapy causes skin bronzing (the bronze-baby syndrome) and a mild direct hyperbilirubinemia; these effects are a relative contraindication to continuing phototherapy as they are readily reversible.

A widely used rule-of-thumb is to initiate treatment with phototherapy when the bilirubin level rises to within 5 mg/dl of the "exchange" level. Phototherapy is often begun "prophylactically" in situations where it will likely be employed in any case (*i.e.*, in premature infants with substantial bruising from delivery, or in infants with hemolytic disease in the hope of obviating an exchange transfusion).

Exchange transfusion

Occasionally, exchange transfusions are necessary to maintain bilirubin levels at less than 20 mg/dl (or lower levels in premature infants presumed to be at greater risk for kernicterus). A double-volume exchange transfusion can remove nearly 90% of circulating intravascular bilirubin and result in a transient fall in bilirubin level; however, a "rebound" is inevitable as bilirubin from the interstitial compartment equilibrates with the intravascular space. An exchange transfusion in a newborn infant must be performed with great caution and monitored intensively to avoid potential complications. An isovolemic procedure (*i.e.*, slow withdrawal of blood from an umbilical vessel or a peripheral artery as fresh whole blood is infused simultaneously at the same rate) is preferred whenever possible.

BIBLIOGRAPHY

Auerbach KG, Gartner LM: Breastfeeding and human milk: Their association with jaundice in the neonate. Clin Perinatol 14:89–107, 1987

Cashore WJ, Stern L: Neonatal hyperbilirubinemia. Pediatr Clin North Am 29:1191–1203, 1982

DeCarvalho M, Robertson S, Klaus M: Fecal bilirubin excretion and serum bilirubin concentrations in breast-fed and bottle-fed infants. J Pediatr 107:786–790, 1985

Lascari AD: "Early" breast-feeding jaundice: Clinical significance. J Pediatr 108:156–158, 1986

Maisels MJ: Hyperbilirubinemia. In Nelson NM (ed): Current Therapy in Neonatal–Perinatal Medicine 1985–1986, Philadelphia, BC Decker, 1985

Maisels MJ: Jaundice in the newborn. Pediatr Rev 3:305–319, 1982

National Institute of Child Health and Human Development Randomized, Controlled Trial of Phototherapy for Neonatal Hyperbilirubinemia. Pediatr 75(suppl):385–441, 1985

Watchko JF, Oski FO: Bilirubin 20 mg/dL = Vigintiphobia. Pediatrics 71:660–663, 1983

17

Necrotizing Enterocolitis

Necrotizing enterocolitis (NEC) is an acquired disease of the newborn infant characterized by intestinal necrosis in the absence of predisposing anatomic (e.g., malrotation with midgut volvulus, incarcerated inguinal hernia) or functional (e.g., Hirschsprung's disease) factors. Necrosis may extend the full thickness of the bowel wall or be limited to the mucosa; the disease may involve random patches throughout the small and large bowel or affect continuous segments of intestine. The most frequently involved areas of bowel are the terminal ileum, ascending colon, and cecum. NEC is the most common neonatal medical and surgical emergency, occurring in an estimated 4000 to 8000 infants per year in the United States alone. The incidence of NEC has increased as aggressive treatment of the very low birth weight infant (<1000 g) has become more widespread. Ninety percent of infants who develop NEC are born prematurely.

EPIDEMIOLOGY, ETIOLOGY, AND PATHOGENESIS

NEC afflicts between 1% and 5% of all admissions to neonatal intensive care units (NICUs). Depending on the number and the gestational age distribution of admissions, most NICUs can anticipate 5 to 25 sporadic cases per year of endemic NEC. Superimposed on this background rate may be "mini-epidemics" of NEC, which in large part account for the variation in reported incidence among NICUs. Epidemic NEC tends to occur later and in seemingly healthier and more mature infants than endemic NEC. The only consistent significant risk factor for either variety of NEC is prematurity. Sex, race, maternal socioeconomic status, geography, and season fail to influence the incidence of NEC. NEC generally presents between 3 and 10 days after birth, but may present as early as the first day or as late as 3 to 4 months of life. There is a roughly inverse relationship between gestational age and postnatal age at onset of NEC such that the disease is uncommon once an infant attains a postconceptional age of 35 to 36 weeks.

No single etiology or pathogenesis for NEC has been identified. At this point, NEC is best considered to be a multifactorial disease that represents the common clinical expression of critical ischemic, infectious, immunologic, and/or other unknown insults to an immature gastrointestinal tract. In many cases, enteral substrate may potentiate mucosal injury.

Early clinical descriptions of NEC documented a high incidence of certain obstetric and neonatal complications such as fetal distress, low Apgar scores, respiratory distress syndrome, patent ductus arteriosus, and the use of umbilical vessel catheters. These findings led to the speculation that NEC was a consequence of gut ischemia; however, this became untenable as a unifying hypothesis when these same perinatal risk factors were found in similar percentages of case-controlled infants who did not develop NEC. Moreover, in perhaps 10% of cases of NEC, no "ischemic" risk factor is present, and in another 10% of cases, presentation is late enough that intestinal recovery from perinatal ischemia can reasonably be presumed to have occurred. The observation that NEC is more likely to occur in the firstborn rather than the secondborn of twins also implicates factors other than ischemia. Nonetheless, asphyxia can produce pathologic changes consistent with NEC in several experimental immature animal models. Current clinical evidence cannot exclude the possibility that ischemia precipitates NEC in a subset of infants.

Most recent work has attempted to establish an infectious etiology for NEC. In support of this hypothesis are the frequent epidemic outbreaks of NEC that appear to be contained by strict infection control measures, and the high incidence of positive blood and/or peritoneal cultures (30% to 40%). Although epidemics have been associated with a variety of enteric bacteria (*Escherichia coli, Klebsiella, Enterobacter, Clostridia*) and some viruses (corona-, rota-, pararota-, and enterovirus), in most instances no common agent is found. The identification of one predominant agent may only signify opportunistic infection by the prevailing nursery flora following mucosal disruption by another initiating event. Breech of local gastrointestinal defenses by even nonpathogens may lead to systemic signs and symptoms of sepsis that are out of proportion to the initial intestinal injury.

The role of feeding in the pathogenesis of NEC remains controversial. It is probable that enteral substrate acts synergistically with other factors in the pathogenesis of NEC. The fact that NEC has developed in the unfed infant, however, demonstrates that enteral feedings are not a prerequisite for NEC. Retrospective analyses have incriminated rapid advancement of enteral feedings as a causative factor for NEC, but as yet no properly randomized controlled trials have evaluated the prophylactic benefit of cautious feeding regimen recommendations. In our experience, prudent advancement of enteral substrate in the very low birth weight infant is advisable to reduce the incidence of feeding intolerance, characterized by large gastric residuals and/or abdominal distention. Feeding intolerance may be benign, but also may be the first clinical sign of NEC. It was once hoped that breast milk feedings would prevent NEC; however, NEC has developed in infants fed pooled, pasteurized, refrigerated, and frozen human milk. Nonetheless, a controlled clinical trial using fresh homologous breast milk has not yet been reported.

CLINICAL FEATURES

The clinical presentation of NEC in the preterm infant varies widely both in severity and in the rate of progression. Usually the onset is insidious. Signs and symptoms of ileus or obstruction (gastric residuals, mild abdominal distention, diminished bowel sounds, vomiting) and, frequently, occult or frank blood in the stools or gastric aspirate may focus attention early on the gastrointestinal tract. On the other hand, systemic signs such as increasing apnea and bradycardia, hypothermia, and lethargy may be the only initial indications of NEC. Abdominal radiographs at this point usually reveal only nonspecific changes, including gaseous distention or bowel wall edema. Under the Bell classification, these findings represent stage I, or suspected, NEC. The diagnosis of definite (stage II) NEC requires some of the clinical findings of stage I disease plus radiographic demonstration of pneumatosis intestinalis or hepatic portal venous air. Persistent abdominal tenderness or abdominal wall erythema may herald transmural necrosis and peritonitis. Cardiovascular collapse, respiratory failure, oliguria, and/or coagulopathy signal advanced, or stage III, disease. Full-thickness intestinal necrosis may cause bowel perforation, which may be documented by a pneumoperitoneum on abdominal x-ray. Fulminant NEC is stage III disease, which develops within hours in a previously asymptomatic infant. This presentation of NEC may be confused with a primary sepsis if the usual clinical and radiographic features of NEC are not carefully sought.

The clinical staging of NEC is used not only to guide therapy (see below), but also to predict the subsequent course. Infants who remain stable on conservative management 2 days after becoming symptomatic rarely progress to stage III disease. In one review, intestinal perforation in advanced NEC cases occurred at mode, median, and mean times of 12, 24, and 36 hours after initial symptoms.

Ten percent of cases of NEC occur in full-term infants. Most cases occur in infants with well-defined risk factors, including growth retardation and polycythemia, hypoglycemia, or respiratory distress. Full-term infants with cyanotic congenital heart disease (especially those who have undergone diagnostic angiography with high doses of hyperosmolar contrast) or chronic enteritis are also at risk to develop NEC. Occasionally, NEC strikes a seemingly healthy full-term infant with no obvious risk factors.

The laboratory findings of NEC are nonspecific. Thrombocytopenia with or without disseminated intravascular coagulation, leukopenia, refractory metabolic acidosis, and hyponatremia secondary to third spacing are often present.

The diagnosis of NEC is not always straightforward. Neither pneumatosis intestinalis (Fig. 17–1) nor pneumoperitoneum

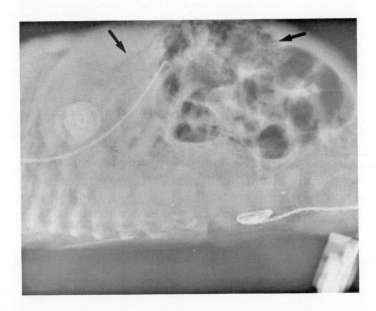

FIGURE 17–1. Pneumatosis intestinalis (*arrows*) in an infant with necrotizing enterocolitis as seen on a cross-table lateral film. Both linear and bubbly patterns of gas are visible.

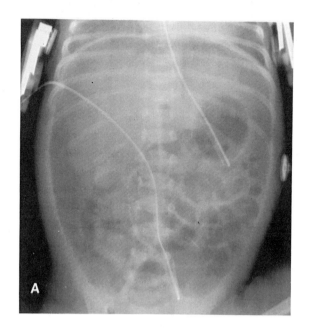 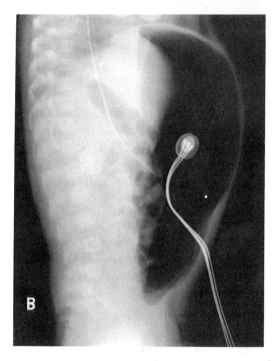

FIGURE 17–2. Large pneumoperitoneum is conspicuous on both anteroposterior (A) and cross-table lateral (B) views.

(Fig. 17–2) may be found prior to pathologic confirmation of NEC at laparotomy or at autopsy. For instance, analysis of submucosal (manifested by "bubbly" pneumatosis) or subserosal ("streaky" pneumatosis) air at autopsy has disclosed a 30% hydrogen gas component. Because only fermentation of enteral feedings by enteric bacteria can generate hydrogen, one cannot exclude a diagnosis of NEC in the unfed infant with the typical clinical syndrome solely on the basis of a lack of pneumatosis. Indeed, radiographic evidence of pneumatosis has been reported to be lacking in 15% to 35% of cases of confirmed pathologic NEC. Similarly, a pneumoperitoneum will not be apparent if perforation occurs in a fluid-filled, gasless segment of bowel. Adding to the diagnostic difficulty is that air bubbles mixed in meconium or in intraluminal blood can be indistinguishable from pneumatosis. Conversely, neither pneumatosis nor pneumoperitoneum is pathognomonic of NEC. Pneumatosis intestinalis may be seen in bowel infarction secondary to malrotation with midgut volvulus or in the enterocolitis of Hirschsprung's disease, and a pneumoperitoneum may be consequent to gastric perforation by a feeding tube or rectal perforation by a thermometer. In particular, the differentiation of midgut volvulus from NEC is sometimes difficult but must be done promptly to secure the proper surgical treatment and optimal outcome.

THERAPY

The goals of the medical therapy for suspected or confirmed NEC are three: to prevent further intestinal injury, to support vital functions, and to anticipate progression of disease. Initial management includes discontinuation of enteral feedings, effective bowel decompression by straight gastric drainage or intermittent suction, and institution of appropriate parenteral nutrition. Blood, stool, and cerebrospinal fluid (CSF) (meningitis complicates at least 2% of cases of NEC) cultures should be obtained before broad-spectrum antibiotic therapy is provided. Coverage should be tailored to treat gram-negative enteric bacteria, *Pseudomonas*, and anaerobes. Enteral antibiotics do not improve the prognosis significantly. Blood gases, electrolytes, and hematologic and coagulation parameters are followed as necessary. In stage I or stage II disease, these measures alone are usually successful. The optimal duration of antibiotic therapy and bowel rest has not been determined prospectively, but it is common clinical practice to pursue a 3- to 7-day or a 7- to 14-day course for stage I and II disease, respectively.

Progression to advanced disease without pneumoperitoneum is an ominous development. Continuous monitoring and aggressive support of respiratory and cardiovascular function is required. Third spacing and endotoxemic shock may combine to produce an enormous fluid requirement. Assessment of peripheral perfusion (or the relationship of transcutaneous to arterial Po_2), urine output, blood pressure, acid–base status, hematocrit, and clotting functions will help determine the relative need for crystalloid, fresh frozen plasma, or packed red cell repletion. Pharmacologic agents such as dopamine or dobutamine may be used to increase peripheral vascular tone, enhance cardiac function, or improve renal or mesenteric perfusion. Cross-table and left lateral decubitus abdominal x-rays should be obtained to screen for evidence of intestinal perforation. Despite all these measures, hypotension, metabolic acidosis, thrombocytopenia and disseminated intravascular coagulation may not respond to treatment.

Surgical consultation is necessary once NEC is suspected. The most widely accepted indication for laparotomy is intestinal perforation. A minority of surgeons recommend exploration if full-thickness intestinal necrosis is suspected on the basis of abdominal wall erythema, suggestive findings on paracentesis, persistence of a dilated bowel loop on serial x-rays, a fixed abdominal mass on physical examination, or deterioration despite aggressive medical management. When gangrenous bowel can be clearly delineated, surgical repair consists of a diversion by proximal jejuno-, ileo-, or colostomy and creation of a distal mucous fistula. If so much bowel is diseased at the first laparotomy that total resection would be incompatible with future enteral nutrition, a second-look operation 24 to 48 hours later is justifiable if the infant's condition stabilizes.

OUTCOME

Mortality varies with the size of the infant and the severity of disease, but averages 20% to 40% during the acute course. There is also a significant late mortality among survivors of advanced disease. Morbidity may include intestinal (usually colonic) strictures (20%) that present 1 to 8 weeks after the onset of symptoms such as obstruction, gastrointestinal (GI) bleeding, or recurrent NEC; adhesions; abscesses; enteric fistulae; short-gut syndrome; and multiple complications secondary to central venous alimentation. The developmental outcome of survivors treated by medical management alone does not differ from that of control infants. The prognosis of infants requiring surgical treatment is poorer.

Although prenatal maternal glucocorticoid therapy may decrease the incidence of NEC, there are no effective postnatal prophylactic measures. The unpredictable epidemiology of NEC renders suspect any recommendation for prophylaxis not founded on a prospective clinical trial. Arrest or prevention of NEC by earlier detection is a worthwhile goal that is so far unrealized.

BIBLIOGRAPHY

Barnard J, Green H, Cotton R: Necrotizing enterocolitis. In Kretchmer N, Minkowski A (eds): Nutritional Adaptation of the Gastrointestinal Tract of the Newborn. New York, Nestle, Vevey/Raven Press, 1983

Bauer CR, Morrison JC, Poole WK et al: A decreased incidence of necrotizing enterocolitis after prenatal glucocorticoid therapy. Pediatrics 73:682–688, 1984

Brown EG, Sweet AY: Neonatal necrotizing enterocolitis. Pediatr Clin North Am 29:1149–1170, 1982

Kliegman RM, Hack M, Jones P et al: Epidemiologic study of necrotizing enterocolitis among low-birth-weight infants. Absence of identifiable risk factors. J Pediatr 100:440–444, 1982

Kliegman RM, Walsh MC: Neonatal necrotizing enterocolitis: Pathogenesis, classification, and spectrum of illness. Curr Probl Pediatr 17:213–288, 1987

Marchildon MB, Buck BE, Abdenour G: Necrotizing enterocolitis in the unfed infant. J Pediatr Surg 17:620–624, 1982

Ostertag SG, LaGamma EF, Reisen CE et al: Early enteral feeding does not affect the incidence of necrotizing enterocolitis. Pediatrics 77:275–280, 1986

Samm M, Curtis-Cohen M, Keller M et al: Necrotizing enterocolitis in infants of multiple gestation. Am J Dis Child 140:937–939, 1986

Stoll BJ, Kanto WP Jr, Glass RI et al: Epidemiology of necrotizing enterocolitis: A case control study. J Pediatr 96:447–451, 1980

Thilo EH, Lazarte RA, Hernandez JA: Necrotizing enterocolitis in the first 24 hours of life. Pediatrics 73:476–480, 1984

Wilson R, del Portillo M, Schmidt E et al: Risk factors for necrotizing enterocolitis in infants weighing more than 2,000 grams at birth: A case-control study. Pediatrics 71:19–22, 1983

18

Surgical Emergencies
of the Newborn

Neonatal surgical emergencies can be divided into three categories: conditions that present with symptoms of gastrointestinal (GI) obstruction, those that present with respiratory distress, and major anomalies that are obvious immediately after birth. In the past few decades, the prognosis for many of these conditions has improved markedly because of advances in both surgical and medical neonatal intensive care. This chapter will outline a general approach to the recognition and diagnosis of surgically treatable causes of GI obstruction and respiratory distress and discuss a few of the more common anomalies in greater detail.

GASTROINTESTINAL OBSTRUCTION

General principles

Obstruction of the GI tract may be suspected prior to birth if polyhydramnios develops during pregnancy or if abdominal calcifications, dilated bowel loops, or ascites are discovered on fetal ultrasonography.

Polyhydramnios is defined as an excessive volume of amniotic fluid (≥2 liters). The fetus

participates in the formation of amniotic fluid by excreting urine and by secreting pulmonary fluid. The fetus also swallows amniotic fluid, which is absorbed by the fetal GI tract. The differential diagnosis of polyhydramnios includes conditions that increase the rate of amniotic fluid production (abdominal wall defects, fetal anemia, inability of the fetus to concentrate urine), conditions that interfere with fetal swallowing (CNS disorders: *e.g.,* anencephaly; neuromuscular disorders: *e.g.,* congenital myotonic dystrophy; extrinsic esophageal compression: *e.g.,* tight nuchal cord); or high (generally at or above the ligament of Treitz) intestinal obstructions (esophageal, pyloric, duodenal or high jejunal atresias, or malrotation with *in utero* volvulus). Polyhydramnios is also associated with maternal diabetes and twin pregnancies. In many cases, polyhydramnios is idiopathic.

Abdominal calcifications suggest meconium peritonitis. This condition is usually due to meconium ileus, an intestinal obstruction secondary to inspissation of abnormally thick, viscous meconium. Infants who present with meconium ileus must be presumed to have cystic fibrosis until proven otherwise. When perforation of the GI tract occurs *in utero*, the meconium that spills into the peritoneal cavity later calcifies. Often, the intestinal perforation seals by the time of delivery. Meconium peritonitis has also been reported in association with other congenital intestinal obstructions as a result of antenatal bowel perforation.

Fetal ultrasonography sometimes shows *dilated, fluid-filled loops* of bowel. Usually, this signifies an upper GI tract obstruction. *Fetal ascites* occasionally is found in association with meconium peritonitis or *in utero* volvulus. More frequently, however, it is caused by urinary tract anomalies, severe anemia or cardiac failure, congenital infection, or storage diseases.

The first clue to intra-abdominal pathology sometimes occurs during labor and delivery when abdominal dystocia is unexpectedly encountered. Abdominal distention at birth is most likely due to meconium peritonitis, ascites, or genitourinary tract anomalies such as hydronephrosis or hydrometrocolpos (uterine distention secondary to an imperforate hymen).

The majority of intestinal obstructions present postnatally after the infant begins to feed. The four cardinal signs of neonatal GI obstruction uncomplicated by necrosis are increased salivation, abdominal distention, vomiting, and obstipation (failure to pass meconium, or failure to pass transitional stools after initially passing meconium). Two additional signs are more ominous. Abdominal tenderness suggests regional bowel ischemia or peritonitis. GI bleeding in the setting of an ileus or obstruction usually indicates intestinal necrosis.

Abdominal distention and vomiting may also occur in the newborn in such diverse clinical settings as sepsis, congenital heart disease, inborn errors of metabolism, and digestive disorders. Even bilious vomiting is not specific for intestinal obstruction, especially in premature infants, who have de-

creased pyloric sphincter tone. Nonetheless, because some anatomic or functional abnormalities (*e.g.,* malrotation with volvulus, Hirschsprung's disease) can be fatal if surgical intervention is delayed, all infants with distention or vomiting must be evaluated promptly and carefully to rule out intestinal obstruction.

A logical approach to the differential diagnosis of gastrointestinal obstruction entails consideration of the maternal history, the nature and progression of clinical signs in the infant, the physical examination, and appropriate plain and contrast radiologic studies of the GI tract. Any infant thought to have a GI obstruction should have feedings discontinued, reliable intravenous access established, and an orogastric or nasogastric tube placed for bowel decompression and aspiration and analysis of gastric contents (*e.g.,* for bile).

Certain lesions should be obvious at birth or on the first newborn physical examination. The significance of abdominal distention present at birth has already been noted. If the abdominal x-ray reveals free intraperitoneal calcifications, meconium peritonitis is present. An additional triad of radiologic findings, which include disparity in the degree of distention of individual loops of bowel, a "bubbly" or "soapy" appearance of intraluminal meconium, and the lack or paucity of air–fluid levels on upright or decubitus examinations, supports the diagnosis of meconium ileus (the most common cause of meconium peritonitis). When the typical radiologic findings of meconium ileus are not seen, an *in utero* perforation secondary to a small bowel atresia and/or malrotation with volvulus should be considered. Hydrometrocolpos, which may cause extrinsic bowel obstruction, is readily discriminated by palpation of a uterine mass and by discovery of an imperforate hymen on vaginal inspection. An imperforate anus would be an obvious cause of generalized abdominal distention.

The infant with esophageal atresia is sometimes identified before the first feeding by excessive oral secretions. Invariably, there is difficulty with the first feeding, which may precipitate coughing, choking, and cyanosis. There is often a history of maternal polyhydramnios. The diagnosis is supported if resistance to passage of a nasogastric tube occurs at about 7 to 8 cm. A plain film of the neck, chest, and abdomen confirms the diagnosis if the nasogastric tube ends or coils at the approximate level of the third thoracic vertebra. A fistula from the trachea to the distal esophageal segment is present if any abdominal gas is seen.

The neonate who presents with nonbilious vomiting in the absence of distention most likely suffers from overfeeding or achalasia with gastroesophageal reflux. Sepsis, central nervous system (CNS) lesions, and metabolic errors must be considered but usually can be distinguished because other clinical signs are prominent. Localized epigastric distention raises the possibilities of pyloric stenosis, pyloric atresia, or upper duodenal obstruction. Pyloric stenosis is a partial obstruction that classically presents with postprandial projectile vomiting in the 3rd to 6th week of life but may occur (rarely) as early as the 1st week. Palpation of an olive-sized mass in the right upper quadrant supports the diagnosis but requires a calm, relaxed infant, much patience, and some skill. An upper GI contrast or ultrasound study can be confirmatory, but negative studies do not rule out the diagnosis. Pyloric atresia is very rare. Plain abdominal film will show a dilated stomach but no other intestinal gas. This lesion is more common in infants with epidermolysis bullosa. Duodenal obstructions proximal to the ampulla of Vater (annular pancreas, duodenal webs, duodenal stenosis) are uncommon but may be suggested by a plain abdominal x-ray that demonstrates a prominent "double-bubble" with (incomplete) or without (complete obstruction) distal intestinal gas and confirmed by upper GI contrast study.

Development of abdominal distention after birth that is accompanied by bilious vomiting must be considered a surgical emergency until proven otherwise. This remains true despite a recent study showing that the majority of bilious vomiting in the newborn lacks surgically treatable causes. Physical examination may suggest the level of obstruction. If distention is limited to the epigastric area or to the upper abdomen, a proximal small bowel obstruction is likely; generalized distention may result from obstruction at or distal to the midjejunum. Plain abdominal films help localize the degree and site of the obstruction even in the first few hours of life; in the normal newborn infant, air reaches the duodenum within the first few breaths, the cecum by 3 to 6 hours after birth, and fills most of the colon by 8 to 12 hours. A double-bubble sign with complete obstruction is classically described in association with duodenal atresia and less commonly with annular pancreas, but does not exclude a malrotation with midgut volvulus. Surgical laparotomy should be performed expediently; if a malrotation is responsible for the obstruction, progressive bowel distention after birth can initiate or exacerbate a volvulus and cause or extend intestinal gangrene.

If plain abdominal films suggest a partial duodenal obstruction, then intrinsic duodenal stenosis, extrinsic duodenal compression by an annular pancreas, preduodenal portal vein, or an aberrant superior mesenteric artery, and malrotation are the diagnostic possibilities. If indicated by the clinical status of the infant, a barium study of the upper GI tract will usually identify a malrotation. In a normally rotated GI tract, a contrast study shows the ligament of Treitz (which marks the duodenal–jejunal transition) to the left of the vertebral column. An abrupt termination of contrast in the distal duodenum is characteristic of a malrotation with volvulus. The diagnosis of malrotation can also be reliably established if a barium enema reveals that the cecum lies either to the left of the midline or in the midline of the upper abdomen; however, a lower GI contrast study is less specific because "normal" cecal position in the right lower quadrant does not rule out a malrotation. The safe rule is to operate if a malrotation with volvulus cannot confidently be excluded.

Generalized abdominal distention is consistent with obstruction at or distal to the midjejunum. Plain abdominal films confirm distention of multiple bowel loops, but are often not helpful in localizing the site of obstruction, since differentiation of dilated small vs. large bowel usually cannot be made with confidence. Diagnostic possibilities include atresia or stenosis of the small bowel or colon, meconium plug syndrome, small left colon syndrome, Hirschsprung's disease, or functional obstruction secondary to maternal drugs (e.g., hypermagnesemia secondary to antenatal treatment of preeclampsia). An inguinal hernia must be ruled out as the cause of obstruction that presents after gastrointestinal patency has been established, especially in the growing premature infant. With some small bowel atresias, the infant may feed normally on the first day and even pass meconium. Later, the infant becomes distended, vomits and fails to pass transitional stools. However, Hirschsprung's disease may present with the same history. If the infant is born to a gestational or insulin-dependent diabetic, small left colon syndrome is the most likely possibility. Unless rectal air is unambiguously seen in plain films, a lower GI study with a high osmolar water-soluble contrast agent should be performed for diagnostic and therapeutic reasons. The infant must have reliable intravenous access for rehydration because the hyperosmolar contrast causes third-spacing into the intestinal lumen and can result in intravascular hypovolemia with hypoperfusion. Findings in small intestinal atresia may

include diminished caliber of the colon ("microcolon") as a result of disuse atrophy, and abrupt cessation of reflux of contrast into the small bowel. The outline of meconium plugs delineates the syndrome; the high osmolar agent is therapeutic as well as diagnostic because it loosens and helps expel the obstructive plugs. In small left colon syndrome, the colon has a normal caliber up to the splenic flexure. The classic findings in Hirschsprung's disease are a dilated rectosigmoid that narrows over a short transition zone. Often, however, the diagnosis of aganglionosis cannot be made by barium enema in the neonate and instead requires rectal biopsy or anal manometry. In addition, the possibility of Hirschsprung's disease should be seriously considered in all infants with an initial diagnosis of meconium plug syndrome or small left colon syndrome.

Specific entities

This section describes in more detail three of the more important disorders of the neonatal GI tract that are surgically treatable. Necrotizing enterocolitis, the most common GI emergency of the premature infant, is discussed in Chapter 17.

Esophageal atresia/tracheoesophageal fistula. This anomaly occurs in approximately 1 in 4000 live births. There are five anatomic variants: the most common (85%) is esophageal atresia with distal tracheoesophageal fistula (EA/TEF). Isolated esophageal atresia (EA:8%) and isolated tracheoesophageal fistula (TEF:4%), also known as an H-type fistula, are the other variants seen with appreciable frequency.

In EA/TEF, the esophageal fistula connects to the trachea just above the carina; occasionally, the fistula is so large that it can be seen clearly on a lateral chest x-ray. EA/TEF is associated with other anomalies such as congenital heart disease, duodenal atresia, and imperforate anus. Infants with EA/TEF are at risk for pneumonia not only from aspiration of feedings, but also from reflux of gastric secretions through the TEF into the lungs. The latter is the more significant problem; gastric distention due to a continual flux of air through the fistula increases gastric acid secretion. Special aspects of preoperative care include continuous suction of the blind esophageal pouch by a multiple-lumen (Repogle) tube and placement of the infant in the prone semi-upright position to minimize reflux. When possible, optimal surgical therapy includes division of the TEF and end-to-end esophageal anastomosis via an extrapleural approach and gastrostomy placement. Premature infants with hyaline membrane disease may require a staged surgical repair, with division of the fistula and gastrostomy preceding the reanastomosis. Survival is excellent in infants without other significant congenital anomalies. Postoperative complications include leak at the esophageal anastomosis (usually transient and adequately controlled by an extrapleural chest tube) and gastroesophageal reflux. In some infants, severe gastroesophageal reflux requires a Nissen fundoplication. All patients have some degree of esophageal dysmotility.

Isolated EA has a somewhat greater association with other congenital defects and certain chromosomal abnormalities (trisomies 13 and 18). As with EA/TEF, a careful review for other components of the VATER syndrome (V = vertebral anomalies, A = imperforate anus, TE = tracheoesophageal atresia, R = renal or radial anomalies) is warranted. Obviously, infants with EA are not at risk for reflux aspiration. The preferred surgical repair is an end-to-end esophageal anastomosis and a gastrostomy placement. Unfortunately, the proximal and distal esophageal segments may not be approximated closely enough to permit an immediate primary reanastomosis. In

VATER

some cases, cautious serial dilatation and stretching of the esophageal segments permit a later primary repair. Because of the increased risk of sepsis and meningitis with esophageal dilatations, the infant should receive appropriate antibiotic therapy prior to each procedure. In other instances, a primary anastomosis is impossible, and other means of connecting the esophageal segments are tried (e.g., a colonic interposition).

H-type TEF usually presents later in infancy. This variant is not associated with other anomalies. The usual symptoms include recurrent coughing or cyanosis (especially during feedings), abdominal distention, frequent pneumonias, and increased flatus ("gassy" babies).

Malrotation with volvulus. Between the 10th to 12th weeks of gestation, the embryonic intestine rotates 270° about the axis of the superior mesenteric artery as it assumes its final position within the abdominal cavity. This rotation leads to a fixed retroperitoneal duodenum which is traversed anteriorly by the superior mesenteric artery, stabilization of the mesentery by its fusion with the posterior peritoneum over a broad line extending from the ligament of Treitz to the cecum in the right lower quadrant, and ultimately to firm adhesion of the right colon in the peritoneal gutter.

Malrotation refers to the failure of normal rotation to proceed beyond a given point and thus embraces a range of anatomic abnormalities. In its most complete expression, malrotation results in a complete lack of mesenteric support (e.g., the entire mesentery is free to twist around the superior mesenteric vessels) and adhesive bands (Ladd's bands), which stretch from the right colon over the duodenum to the hepatic area. The first abnormality predisposes the infant to intestinal ischemia and/or necrosis because of the likelihood that volvulus will compromise bowel perfusion;

the second abnormality may cause intestinal obstruction secondary to extrinsic duodenal compression. Malrotation commonly presents in the first few months of life but may not become symptomatic until late in adulthood. Certain conditions are nearly always accompanied by malrotation (abdominal wall defects, diaphragmatic hernia). Other intestinal lesions (duodenal stenosis or atresia, small bowel atresia, imperforate anus) as well as extraintestinal abnormalities (particularly cardiac and renal lesions) occur in association with malrotation.

The clinical presentation may range from intermittent episodes of intestinal obstruction to an acute fulminant illness with shock and sepsis. Malrotation with or without volvulus heads the list of possible diagnoses of obstructions that present after intestinal patency has been clearly established.

In some cases, the patient may be stable enough to allow diagnostic contrast radiologic studies. With severe illness, urgent surgical laparotomy is required. Surgical treatment includes untwisting of the mesentery and lysis of Ladd's bands. Frankly necrotic intestine must be resected, but marginal bowel may be left in place pending a "second-look" laparotomy 24 to 48 hours later. The duodenum and small bowel must be carefully probed to exclude coexisting atretic segments. Postoperatively, total parenteral nutrition is essential.

If diagnosis and/or surgical therapy is delayed, mortality is high. Postoperative morbidity may arise from a "short-gut" syndrome if insufficient viable bowel (<40 cm) remains.

Aganglionic megacolon (Hirschsprung's disease). *Hirschsprung's disease* is a functional intestinal obstruction caused by the congenital lack of ganglion cells in the myenteric plexus of the distal colon. It occurs in 0.2% of live births (predominantly in males), and

more frequently in infants with trisomy 21 and in infants with a family history of Hirschsprung's disease. The etiology is unknown.

Because innervation of the intestine proceeds distally during early gestation, it is not surprising that in Hirschsprung's disease ganglion cells are absent in continuity a variable (but usually short) distance proximal to the distal rectosigmoid colon. Only rarely is total colonic aganglionosis present. In contrast to normally innervated colon, the failure of aganglionic colon to relax with distention causes functional obstruction with proximal colonic dilatation (hence the term, *megacolon*).

Most infants with Hirschsprung's disease present in early infancy. The usual scenario is an infant with marked constipation that results in poor feeding, vomiting, and failure to thrive. An oft-quoted statistic is that 95% of infants with Hirschsprung's disease fail to pass meconium in the first 24 hours after birth (in contrast, 98% of full-term infants stool on the first day of life). In desperation, many interventions (including neonatal enemas!) may be tried with variable success before the diagnosis is entertained. Less frequent but more dangerous is the development of a foul and/or bloody diarrhea secondary to a severe enterocolitis. Abdominal films may demonstrate pneumatosis coli suggestive of neonatal necrotizing enterocolitis in addition to bowel distention. Finally, unusual delayed presentations include ascites and generalized edema secondary to a protein-losing enteropathy and urinary tract infection secondary to ureteral obstruction.

A barium enema that shows an abrupt funneling of a dilated colon over a short "transition zone" in combination with a subsequent plain film that demonstrates abnormal retention of barium is highly suggestive of the diagnosis. Unfortunately, a barium enema alone is not reliable in the early neonatal period. Lack of ganglion cells on an adequate rectal biopsy specimen has been the standard diagnostic test. Recently, some centers have preferred rectal manometry. With aganglionosis, the internal sphincter does not relax with balloon dilatation; thus, recorded intraluminal pressure rises.

Immediate treatment includes colonic decompression with a soft rubber rectal tube or saline enemas, and antibiotic therapy for gram-negative and anaerobic organisms if enterocolitis is present. Initial surgical management is a colostomy proximal to the aganglionic segment. Later during childhood, the colostomy is taken down and one of a variety of procedures is attempted to achieve rectal continence. At our institution, the Soave procedure is usually chosen. This operation involves excision of the submucosa of the aganglionic colon with "pull-through" of the proximal normally innervated bowel.

RESPIRATORY DISTRESS REQUIRING SURGICAL TREATMENT

The differential diagnosis of respiratory distress in the newborn is lengthy and touches on many organ systems other than the lungs and heart. Statistically, most cases of respiratory distress in the newborn are not caused by surgically remediable etiologies but by parenchymal lung pathology such as hyaline membrane disease, transient tachypnea, aspiration syndromes, and pneumonia. It is nonetheless important to recognize promptly the surgically remediable conditions (Table 18-1).

Significant congenital airway obstruction presents in the delivery room. Infants may labor intensely to breathe but soon become fatigued, apneic, and bradycardiac. With a complete laryngeal or tracheal web, no lung aeration is possible. The lesion obstructs intubation. Survival is rare, since urgent tracheostomy or tracheal cannulation with a large-gauge angiocatheter is necessary in the

Table 18–1. Surgically Remediable Causes of Neonatal Respiratory Distress

Airway obstruction
Intrinsic
    Choanal atresia
    Pierre-Robin anomalad
    Laryngeal webs
    Congenital subglottic stenosis
    Tracheal stenosis
    Laryngeal or tracheal hemangioma
Extrinsic
    Vascular rings or aberrant innominate artery
    Neck masses
Lung parenchymal compression
    Diaphragmatic hernia
    Eventration of the diaphragm
    Congenital lobar emphysema
    Cystic adenomatoid malformation of the lung
    Bronchogenic cyst
    Pneumothorax
    Chylothorax
    Pleural effusions
    Massive ascites

delivery room. Such complete airway obstruction is, fortunately, rare. Conditions with incomplete airway obstruction present with stridor or abnormal phonation. Tracheal intubation relieves symptoms, and tracheostomy may be required electively. Choanal atresia is a bony or membranous obstruction of one or both nasal choanae. This lesion should be suspected in any cyanotic infant whose color improves with vigorous crying. Failure to pass a #8 French nasogastric tube into the oropharynx confirms the diagnosis. Symptoms are relieved by placement of an oral airway. Neck masses such as teratomas and large cystic hygromas are obvious on inspection. Symptoms due to extrinsic compression by vascular rings or an aberrant innominate artery are more subtle and insidious in their onset. Often, symptoms relating to esophageal compression, such as vomiting and dysphagia, are also present.

Diaphragmatic hernias originate during embryogenesis. Severe hernias usually result from migration of intestine and often liver and spleen through a defect in the left posterolateral diaphragm (the foramen of Bochdalek). As many as 50% of infants with diaphragmatic hernias have coexisting major congenital anomalies. In those infants in whom the hernia is an isolated abnormality, the time of onset of respiratory symptoms is variable and depends on the size and location of the hernia. Many present in the delivery room with severe respiratory distress that does not respond well even to intubation and artificial ventilation. Others have a gradual evolution of respiratory symptoms over hours to days. The diagnosis is usually not made until the initial chest x-ray. The classic diagnostic clue of a scaphoid abdomen often disappears because of vigorous attempts at ventilation with bag and mask in the delivery room.

Herniation that occurs *in utero* is associated with a reduced number of generations of the tracheobronchial tree (lung hypoplasia) and with extensive medial hypertrophy of the pulmonary vascular bed. These abnormalities are most severe in the ipsilateral lung but have been described in the "normal" contralateral lung as well. It is not surprising that the management of diaphragmatic hernia is complicated by a high incidence of both pneumothorax and persistence of the transitional circulation. Infants who are symptomatic early have a high rate of mortality. Usual therapy consists of early surgical repair of the defect, carefully controlled artificial ventilation to minimize the risk of pneumothorax, and other adjunctive measures to decrease pulmonary vascular resistance. Some centers are now performing clinical trials using extracorporeal membrane oxygenation (ECMO) in conjunction with surgery.

Other mass-occupying lesions that cause respiratory distress include pneumothorax (present in 1% and symptomatic in 0.1% of live births), pleural effusions, and chylothorax. Congenital lobar emphysema, usually involving an upper lobe, tends to present insidiously; the emphysematous lobe may cause a marked mediastinal shift and atelectasis of healthy lung.

BIBLIOGRAPHY

Anderson KD: Congenital diaphragmatic hernia. In Pediatric Surgery, 4th ed. Chicago, Year Book Medical Publishers, 1986

Filston HC, Izant RJ Jr.: The Surgical Neonate: Evaluation and Care. Norwalk, CT, Appleton-Century-Crofts, 1985

Grosfeld, JL (ed): Pediatric surgery. Surg Clin North Am 61(5), 1981

Grosfeld JL, Ballantine TVN (eds): Surgical respiratory distress in infancy and childhood. Curr Prob Pediatr 6(7), 1976

Lilien LD, Srinivasan G, Pyati SP et al: Green vomiting in the first 72 hours in normal infants. Am J Dis Child 140:662–664, 1986

Rowe MI (ed): Neonatal surgery. Clin Perinatol 5(1), 1978

19 Neonatal Infections

The fetus and newborn are uniquely susceptible to many infectious agents with potentially devastating consequences. An infection that develops in the fetus as a consequence of transplacental transmission is termed a *congenital infection*. Transmission of certain agents during the period of embryogenesis or early fetal development may result in some combination of growth retardation, central nervous system (CNS) damage, congenital heart disease, and other defects. Later fetal infection may be asymptomatic in the neonatal period or may present at birth as a characteristic clinical syndrome. *Perinatal infection* may be either natal (acquired shortly before or during birth) or postnatal (acquired shortly after birth). Natal infections are acquired either by ascending spread of an organism from the genital tract (usually but not always in the presence of ruptured maternal membranes) or by direct innoculation of the infant during a vaginal delivery. Postnatally, the neonate is still at risk for serious infectious diseases, some of which are caused by agents that are not pathogens in normal adult hosts.

One factor that increases the neonate's risk of infection is his relative immunologic immaturity compared with the older child or adult. The premature infant is even less immunologically competent. He is especially at risk when skin and respiratory defenses are disrupted by the necessities of intensive care (e.g., vascular catheters, endotracheal tubes) and is therefore predisposed to infection by unusual agents such as *Staphylococcus epidermidis* and *Candida albicans.*

The epidemiology of neonatal infectious disease has changed substantially over the past several decades. Improved maternal prenatal and/or intrapartum care has reduced the incidence of certain congenital infections (e.g, rubella, syphilis). The spread of human immune virus (HIV) to heterosexual women has resulted in an increasing incidence of congenital HIV. Finally, whereas bacterial sepsis in the newborn was once commonly caused by the group A streptococcus (1940s) and *Staphylococcus aureus* (1950s to 1960s), these pathogens have been supplanted more recently by the group B streptococcus (1970s), *Streptococcus viridans*, and *Haemophilus influenza* (1980s). In contrast, the incidence of bacterial sepsis due to gram-negative organisms (in particular, *Escherichia coli*) has not changed significantly over the same interval.

CONGENITAL INFECTIONS

In 1974, Nahmias concocted the acronym TORCH as a mnemonic for the more common pathogens purportedly responsible for congenital infection (T = toxoplasmosis, O = other, R = rubella, C = cytomegalovirus [CMV], H = herpes simplex virus [HSV]). More recently, the acronym CROTCHS (CMV, rubella, other, toxoplasmosis, Coxsackie, herpes simplex virus, syphilis) has been (facetiously) suggested. The incidences of selected maternal and fetal infections are summarized in Table 19–1. Either acronym is misleading on two accounts: (1) HSV is rarely responsible for fetal infection; instead, it is usually transmitted perinatally (Tables 19–2 and 19–3). Moreover, HSV has a strikingly different clinical presentation than the other congenital infections. (2) The importance of CMV relative to the other agents is masked by either acronym.

Cytomegovirus

Cytomegalovirus (CMV) is a member of the herpesvirus family and resides exclusively in the human species. CMV is excreted from the

Table 19–1. Incidence of Maternal and Fetal Infections

Infectious agent	Maternal infection or colonization (per 1000 pregnancies)	Fetal infection (per 1000 live births)
Cytomegalovirus	40–150	5–25
Toxoplasmosis	2–7	1–2
Syphilis	0.2	0.1
Rubella (interepidemic)	0.03	0.01
Herpes simplex virus	6–40	Rare
Enterovirus (Coxsackie, ECHO)	5–35	Rare
Hepatitis B	1–5	Rare
Varicella-zoster	<0.1	Rare

Table 19–2. Incidence, Symptoms, and Diagnosis of Congenital Infections

Infectious Agent	Maternal Symptoms (%)	Neonatal Symptoms (%)	Distinctive Clinical Findings
Cytomegalovirus	Rare	10	Microcephaly with periventricular calcifications Petechial/purpuric rash with thrombocytopenia
Toxoplasmosis	10–20	30	Hydrocephalus with generalized intracranial calcifications Chorioretinitis
Syphilis	Variable	50	Osteochondritis and periostitis Mucocutaneous lesions (snuffles) Eczematoid skin rash
Rubella	50	35	Blueberry muffin rash Cataracts Patent ductus arteriosus, pulmonic stenosis
Varicella-zoster	100	?	Cicatricial skin lesions in dermatomal distribution Limb atrophy and/or paresis Chorioretinitis

Table 19–3. Incidence of Maternal and Perinatal Infections

Infectious agent	Maternal infection or colonization (per 1000 pregnancies)	Perinatal infection (per 1000 pregnancies)
Chlamydia trachomatis	20–250	12–100
Cytomegalovirus	40–150	10–70
Group B streptococcus	50–300	1–4
Escherichia coli	50–300	0.5–2
Enterovirus (Coxsackie, ECHO)	5–35	0.5–2.5
Hepatitis B	1–5	1–2
Herpes simplex virus	6–40	0.1–0.4

oropharynx (*via* saliva), from the genitourinary system (*via* urine, cervical and vaginal secretions, semen), and in tears, breast milk, and blood. Viral shedding may persist for weeks to years following a primary infection, and may recur following either reactivation of a latent infection or reinfection with a different genetic strain. Transmission of CMV to children and adults occurs secondary to close interpersonal contact (including sexual intercourse) or to transfusion of contaminated blood. With the exception of a heterophile-negative mononucleosis-like illness in young adults, such primary CMV infection in the immune competent host is almost always asymptomatic. CMV seropositivity tends to be greater in lower socioeconomic classes or in populations in which prolonged (>1 month) breast-feeding is common. In the United States, up to 80% and 50% of women belonging to low and middle-to-high socioeconomic classes, respectively, are seropositive by the time they reach child-bearing age.

Congenital CMV usually results from a primary maternal infection during pregnancy and less often from a recurrent infection. The rate of seroconversion during pregnancy ranges from 1% to 4%, depending primarily on maternal socioeconomic status. Fetal infection occurs in 30% to 50% of primary maternal infections. In the U.S., it is estimated that congenital CMV complicates 1% of all live births; however, only 5% of cases will have generalized symptomatic disease at birth. In another 5%, milder symptoms will be present. Fully 90% of cases of congenital CMV will be asymptomatic at birth.

The severe form of congenital CMV, which is clinically evident at birth, is sometimes called cytomegalic inclusion disease (CID). Petechiae and purpura ("blueberry muffin" rash), hepatosplenomegaly, jaundice, and microcephaly are found in more than 50% of affected infants. Intrauterine growth retardation, prematurity, cerebral periventricular calcifications (demonstrated by cranial x-rays, computed tomography (CT) scan), chorioretinitis, and microphthalmia occur in approximately 10% to 50% of cases. Laboratory studies may reveal some combination of a mixed hyperbilirubinemia (the significant component of which is an elevated level of direct bilirubin), mild hepatitis, thrombocytopenia, and hemolytic anemia. Mortality among infants with CID averages 30%. Neonatal mortality is usually due to hepatic failure with disseminated intravascular coagulation (DIC) and bacterial superinfections. Between 1 month and 1 year of age, death may be consequent to cirrhosis and severe failure to thrive; after 1 year, most deaths occur among infants with profound neurologic sequelae due to aspiration pneumonia, malnutrition, or infection. Among survivors, 90% have neurologic handicaps, which range from mild expressive language disability, visual–motor dysfunction, and/or learning disability on the one hand to mental retardation (intelligence quotient [IQ] or developmental quotient [DQ] <70), cerebral palsy, unilateral or bilateral progressive sensorineural hearing loss, postnatal onset of microcephaly, and chorioretinitis with optic atrophy on the other. According to one recent study, chorioretinitis is highly predictive; microcephaly and neonatal neurologic abnormalities are somewhat predictive; and other isolated systemic disease (rash, hepatosplenomegaly) is not predictive of subsequent severe handicap (DQ and/or IQ <70).

Among infants with congenital CMV who are asymptomatic at birth, a small proportion (5% to 15%) will develop one or more of the same neurologic deficits catalogued for infants with CID. In particular, sensorineural hearing loss, often bilateral, may progress even after the first year of life to reach a degree (50 to 100 dB) sufficient to hinder normal language development.

The diagnosis of congenital CMV is best made by isolation of the virus by tissue culture from urine or saliva within the first two weeks of life (to discriminate congenital from perinatal infection). Alternatively, verification of specific IgM antibody to CMV within the same time interval is suggestive of a congenital infection. Even this result may be ambiguous; for instance, the immunofluorescent IgM test is only 75% sensitive and 80% specific. Greater accuracy may be achieved in the future by a radioimmunoassay. Paired assays for specific anti-CMV IgG (using acute and convalescent sera) are helpful only in excluding a diagnosis. Not only may the titer fall with culture-proven congenital infection, but a stable or increasing titer does not exclude perinatal acquisition of infection, which is even more common than congenital CMV (see Table 19–3).

At the present time, there are no effective means of treating or preventing congenital CMV infections.

Other Congenital Infections

Congenital infections due to agents other than CMV occur very uncommonly in the U.S. (Table 19–1). The diagnosis of congenital infection is complicated by a high incidence of asymptomatic disease in both mother and newborn (Table 19–2). Even when symptomatic disease is present in the newborn, it is often impossible on clinical grounds to differentiate among bacterial sepsis, congenital infection, and other noninfectious diseases, much less to incriminate a specific agent. Nonetheless, certain combinations of findings suggest specific etiologies and warrant careful diagnostic study (Table 19–2).

Congenital toxoplasmosis is the second most common congenital infection. Acute maternal toxoplasmosis, usually acquired by ingestion of toxoplasma cysts in undercooked meat, complicates approximately 0.5% of pregnancies in the U.S. Fewer than one in five mothers are symptomatic; moreover, the lack of specificity of symptoms (fever, malaise, hepatosplenomegaly, lymphadenopathy) rarely leads to a prenatal diagnosis. The risk of fetal infection varies directly, but the morbidity to the fetus varies inversely with the time in gestation during which maternal infection is acquired. Similar to CMV, an average of 40% of primary maternal infections results in fetal infection. Seventy percent of infected infants are asymptomatic at birth; infants infected early in gestation are likely to demonstrate significant CNS disease (microcephaly, hydrocephalus, seizures, scattered intracerebral calcifications, chorioretinitis) as well as hepatosplenomegaly, lymphadenopathy, and rash. Again, similar to CMV, a small percentage of infants asymptomatic at birth are at risk for developing CNS lesions, including auditory and visual deficiencies, after birth. It is recommended that suspected or confirmed congenital toxoplasmosis be treated with a 3-week course of pyrimethamine, sulfadiazine, and folinic acid. Diagnosis is made by demonstration of specific IgM in cord or neonatal serum, by a rising titer of specific IgG, or by documentation of recent acute maternal disease together with the typical congenital syndrome. The prognosis for infants symptomatic at birth is poor despite chemotherapy.

A common clinical question concerns how aggressively a diagnostic workup for congenital infection should be pursued on the strength of an isolated clinical finding (e.g., intrauterine growth retardation, microcephaly, conjugated hyperbilirubinemia, hepatomegaly, splenomegaly, thrombocytopenia, hydrocephalus). Current evidence discourages such an evaluation for isolated growth retardation at birth. On the other hand, infants with unexplained isolated hydrocephalus should be evaluated for congenital toxoplasmosis. It is also reasonable to screen infants with hepatomegaly and/or splenomegaly associated with hepatitis for congenital infection. Insufficient information is available to guide the work-up for isolated hepatomegaly or splenomegaly in the absence of hepatitis, or for isolated microcephaly.

PERINATAL INFECTIONS

Bacterial infections

As shown in Table 19–3, bacterial agents account for a minority of perinatal infections. Nonetheless, they are responsible for the majority of infectious mortality and morbidity in the neonate.

The incidence of neonatal bacterial infection (defined as infection occurring within 28 days after birth) has remained relatively constant over the past several decades (1 to 10 per 1000 live births depending on the population studied), but the distribution of organisms has changed over the same time period. The case fatality ratio ranges from .20 to .75. Much of this latter variability is due to two factors: (1) different distributions and/or virulences of causative organisms and (2) differences in the profiles of gestational age and postnatal age at onset of infection among study populations.

In the United States, up to 60% of bacterial infections are caused by the group B β-streptococcus and *E. coli*. However, in some areas, the incidence of the viridans α-hemolytic streptococcus rivals or exceeds that of the group B organism. *Staphylococcus aureus*, other gram-negative enteric bacilli, and *Pseudomonas* account for 15% to 30% of bacterial infections. The incidence of *Listeria monocytogenes* infection shows marked regional and temporal variation in the U.S., although it has been the most common organism in Spain. In the past decade, non-typeable *H. influenzae* has become an increasingly important cause of mortality and morbidity. Unusual bacterial pathogens such as *Staphylococcus epidermidis* and *Serratia marcescens* are common in the sick compromised premature infant.

Risk factors for neonatal infection can be subdivided into three large categories: (1) obstetric complications, (2) virulence of the organism, and (3) impaired host defenses. Obstetric complications include prolonged rupture of membranes (>20 hours), especially when complicated by clinical chorioamnionitis (otherwise unexplained maternal fever, fetal tachycardia, uterine irritability), maternal urinary tract infection, and the use of invasive devices such as intrauterine pressure transducers or fetal scalp electrodes during labor. In general, for every 1000 pregnancies, 100 will be complicated by prolonged rupture of the membranes and 10 by clinical *chorioamnionitis*. One of ten infants born to mothers with chorioamnionitis will develop bacterial sepsis. Exposure to an especially virulent organism can also change the risk and clinical expression of disease. For example, among infants colonized after birth with the group B streptococcus, 30% to 40% are positive for type III, whereas type III is responsible for 80% of neonatal group B streptococcus infections that are complicated by meningitis. similarly, *E. coli* sepsis and meningitis are typically due to strains with the K1 antigen. Finally, host factors such as prematurity, male sex, and low type-specific antibody titers (*e.g.*, vs. type III group B streptococcus) are important risk factors for infection.

The signs and symptoms of bacterial sepsis in the neonate may be few and relatively nonspecific. For instance, temperature instability may be the only early sign. In the full-term infant during the first 4 days of life, a rectal temperature greater than 37.8° C (when unrelated to maternal fever) is highly sensitive (up to 91%) for bacterial sepsis but has a lower positive predictive value (10%). In the preterm infant, sepsis is more likely to cause hypothermia rather than hyperthermia. Tachypnea and other evidence of respiratory distress such as retractions and grunting are common. These signs may be secondary to a pneumonia or may represent compensation for a profound metabolic acidosis secondary to overwhelming systemic disease. Gastrointestinal related findings may include poor feeding (poor suck), vomiting, and diarrhea. Frequently, an ileus is responsible for gastric aspirates and abdominal distention. Sepsis may also cause CNS symptoms such as lethargy or irritability, hypotonia, apnea, or seizures, even in the absence of meningitis. Jaundice and petechiae may be present. In the older neonate, refusal to move an extremity may be the only clue to an underlying osteomyelitis. Bacterial sepsis may also present fulminantly with shock and disseminated intravascular coagulation.

A minimal laboratory screen for infants strongly suspected of bacterial infection consists of a complete blood count with differential and chest x-ray. Leukopenia, absolute neutropenia, or an elevated ratio of immature to mature neutrophils is highly suggestive of infection. Leukocytosis is less reliable. Thrombocytopenia may be an early clue to DIC. The chest x-ray is mandatory in infants with respiratory symptoms even if auscultation fails to disclose any abnormalities. Findings compatible with pneumonia range from a discrete pulmonary infiltrate to a generalized reticulogranular pattern consistent with hyaline membrane disease to prominent vascular markings, pulmonary edema, and small pleural effusions consistent with transient tachypnea of the newborn. Many other screening tests have been proposed but have not been superior either singly or in combination to the white count and differential.

Any infant with clinical sepsis who is started on antibiotics should have a lumbar puncture performed. If the infant is judged too unstable, cerebrospinal fluid (CSF) examination should be performed 1 to 2 days after antibiotic therapy is started. A pleocytosis provides evidence for a preexisting meningitis even if the CSF culture is subsequently negative and may affect the choice of antimicrobials and/or the duration of therapy. It should be cautioned, however, that the lack of a pleocytosis does not rule out meningitis; the CSF white cell count as well as the glucose and protein concentrations may be within the normal range in culture-positive neonatal meningitis.

Group B streptococcus. Neonatal disease due to the group B streptococcus has been studied intensively and serves as a prototype for other bacterial infections. The organism may be recovered from the rectum, vagina, and/or cervix. At some time during pregnancy, between 5% and 30% of women asymptomatically harbor group B streptococcus in the genitourinary tract. Sexual partners of colonized women have a 60% rate of positive urethral cultures and can reintroduce the organism into the maternal genitourinary tract following spontaneous regression or eradication by antibiotic therapy. Within 72 hours of birth, about 70% of infants born to colonized mothers are themselves colonized at one or more skin and mucous membrane sites with the identical maternal type of group B streptococcus. Of these infants, only 1% to 2% will develop systemic disease within the first 5 days of life.

There are two different clinical syndromes of group B streptococcal infection: early-onset and late-onset disease. Early-onset disease results from vertical transmission from mother to infant. Maternal obstetric complications are present in more than half of the cases. Clinically, the infants present with pneumonia and respiratory symptoms at or shortly after birth (mean age of onset, 20 hours). Meningitis complicates 30% of cases. Mortality is high, especially in the premature infant. Late-onset disease has a mean age of onset of 3 to 4 weeks. The organism is probably acquired in most instances from the mother, but some cases result from nosocomial or horizontal transmission. A minority of cases are associated with an obstetric complication. The usual clinical presentation includes fever, lethargy, and a disturbed feeding pattern. Seventy percent of cases are complicated by meningitis. Mortality is lower than in early-onset infection, but morbidity among survivors of meningitis is high and may include hypothalamic dysfunction with temperature instability and diabetes insipidus, deafness and other cranial nerve deficits, cortical blindness, cerebral palsy, and/or mental retardation. Some infants with late-onset disease will present with a localized infection following clearance of a bacteremia. Osteomyelitis of a single bone with or without an adjacent pyarthrosis is the second most common localized site of infection after the CNS; group B streptococcal otitis media, cellulitis, breast abscess, endocarditis, and pericarditis have also been reported.

As for any bacterial infection, a definitive diagnosis of group B streptococcal infection requires a positive culture from blood, CSF, or other infected site (e.g., aspirate from bone, joint, or soft tissue abscess). Prior antibiotic therapy can interfere with the growth of the organism in culture. In this circumstance, a presumptive diagnosis can be made if a latex particle agglutination (LPA) test is positive for group B streptococcal polysaccharide antigen in urine and/or CSF. This test is both highly sensitive and specific; it is available only for the group B streptococcal antigen. After early enthusiasm, neither the presence of polymorphonuclear leukocytes and/or bacteria on stained smear of the gastric aspirate nor a positive gastric aspirate culture has proven reliable in most centers for diagnosis.

In addition to supportive care, specific treatment is with intravenous penicillin G. The recommended dose is 250,000 units/kg/day for sepsis and 400,000 units/kg/day for meningitis. Duration of therapy is usually 10 to 14 days for sepsis and 2 to 3 weeks for meningitis. Some clinicians recommend simultaneous treatment with an aminoglycoside, at least initially, because of in vitro synergism with penicillin.

Other therapies that are less commonly employed are transfusion with irradiated granulocytes (in the presence of documented bone marrow depletion of neutrophil precursors), exchange transfusion with whole blood, and administration of hyperimmune gamma globulin.

Viral infections

Cytomegalovirus. Perinatal CMV infection may result from exposure to the virus during birth, from breast-feeding, or from blood transfusions. The incubation period ranges from 4 to 12 weeks. Perinatal CMV infection is more common than congenital CMV infection and, with few exceptions, has only minor short- or long-term clinical consequences. Because infants with congenital infection may excrete virus for months to years after birth, the diagnosis of perinatal CMV infection requires exclusion of viral excretion during the first 2 weeks of life.

Most perinatal CMV infections are acquired during reactivation of a maternal infection, are asymptomatic, and carry no risk for later neurologic sequelae. The clinical expression of infection is likely modified by fetal acquisition of maternal antibody. In a small percentage of infants, perinatal CMV infection causes an afebrile pneumonitis characterized clinically by disturbances of respiratory pattern (tachypnea and/or apnea), retractions, cough, and coryza. Chest x-ray suggests lower airway obstruction with scattered areas of hyperexpansion and atelectasis. Acutely, some infants require supplemental oxygen and assisted ventilation. Mortality is low (<5%), but pulmonary morbidity (recurrent wheezing and hospitalizations, persistence of abnormal chest x-rays and pulmonary function tests) is frequent among survivors. CMV has been implicated alone or together with another agent in up to 20% of infants hospitalized with pneumonitis.

Transfusion-acquired CMV infection is potentially a serious infection, especially in small (<1500 g) preterm infants born to CMV-seronegative mothers. The complete post-transfusion clinical syndrome consists of pneumonitis with need for increased oxygen or ventilatory support, hemolytic anemia with thrombocytopenia and lymphocytosis, hepatosplenomegaly, and mild direct hyperbilirubinemia. Mortality may be as high as 20%. Transfusion of seronegative preterm infants with seronegative donor blood almost eliminates the risk of this syndrome.

Herpes simplex virus. Perinatal HSV infections, in contrast to CMV infections, are almost always symptomatic and can devastate the neonate. HSV-1 and HSV-2 produce identical clinical syndromes and are isolated in the same 20%/80% ratio in the newborn as they are found in the maternal genitourinary tract. Infection may be acquired by the following four routes: (1) transplacentally; (2) as an ascending infection, usually in the presence (but possibly in the absence) of ruptured membranes; (3) during passage through the birth canal; and (4) by postnatal contact with an active skin lesion (e.g., an orolabial or breast lesion). Of these, the most common is infection during a vaginal delivery.

In 1973, it was reported that primary maternal HSV infection during pregnancy is associated with certain congenital malformations (hydranencephaly, chorioretinitis) and later that primary infection during the first 20 weeks of pregnancy is associated with up to a 25% rate of spontaneous abortion. Recently, it has been estimated that perhaps 5% of culture-positive neonatal HSV infections represent true congenital infections. The clinical syndrome includes skin (vesicles at or shortly after birth, bullae, skin scarring without limb atrophy), CNS (microcephaly, hydranencephaly, brain atrophy), and ophthalmic (chorioretinitis, microophthalmia) abnormalities. Death or severe neurologic impairment is invariable.

Infants born to mothers with primary, recurrent, or asymptomatic HSV infection are at risk for disease. The risk is higher for infants born by vaginal delivery to mothers with primary genital HSV (40% to 50%) than for infants delivered of mothers with recurrent infection (perhaps 5%). Exposure to a lower titer of genital HSV and transplacental transmission of specific antibody probably combine in recurrent maternal infections to reduce the risk to the infant. The risk for perinatal HSV infection in the setting of an asymptomatic genital HSV infection is undefined but probably low. Delivery by cesarean section may not prevent ascending spread of a primary infection if performed too long after membranes have ruptured. Because obstetric management dictates cesarean delivery in the setting of documented active primary infection or suspicious genital herpetic lesions, most cases of neonatal HSV follow asymptomatic maternal infection.

Neonatal HSV disease may be either disseminated (50%) or localized (50%) to one organ system (CNS: 50%; skin and mucous membranes: 50%). This differentiation can be made only retrospectively; the first clinical manifestations do not always predict the subsequent clinical course. For example, although skin involvement is the first clinical manifestation in 70% of infants, fully 70% of these develop disseminated infection. The onset of symptoms ranges from 3 days to 4 weeks after birth, with a mean of 7 days for disseminated disease and of 11 days for localized CNS disease. The first sign of disseminated disease is often the evolution of a crop of vesicular or pustular lesions, frequently on a presenting part (*e.g.*, scalp) or around skin abrasions due to scalp electrodes or forceps. Mucous membrane (including conjunctival) lesions are common. Fulminant systemic disease may ensue with hepatic, renal, and pulmonary failure. CNS involvement occurs in two-thirds of cases and manifests as encephalitis or seizures. Death may result from hypotension and liver dysfunction with DIC. Disease localized to the CNS presents with lethargy and seizures. This latter form is difficult to diagnose promptly because of the lack of cutaneous or ocular findings.

Diagnosis is made by recovery of HSV in tissue culture from vesicular fluid, skin or conjunctival scrapings, throat or rectal swabs, and urine or CSF specimens. Typical cytopathic changes are generally seen by 2 days. A positive Tzanck preparation or a fluorescent antibody stain of skin or conjunctival scrapings can establish a diagnosis earlier, but these tests are only 50% to 75% sensitive. CSF examination of the late-onset localized CNS infection reveals red cells, a lymphocytosis, and an elevated protein, but culture of the CSF for HSV is usually negative. In that case, diagnosis requires a brain biopsy.

Prompt antiviral therapy of neonatal HSV infections with vidarabine or acyclovir has decreased mortality substantially (from 70%–80% to 15%–20%). Unfortunately, even with treatment, half of the survivors suffer significant neurologic sequelae.

BIBLIOGRAPHY

Alkalay AL, Pomerance JJ, Rimoin DL: Fetal varicella syndrome. J Pediatr 111:320–323, 1987

Alpert G, Plotkin SA: A practical guide to the diagnosis of congenital infections in the newborn infant. Pediatr Clin North Am 33:465–479, 1986

Baker CJ: Group B streptococcal infections in neonates. Pediatr Rev 1:5–15, 1979

Conboy TJ, Pass RF, Stagno S et al: Early clinical manifestations and intellectual outcome in children with symptomatic congenital cytomegalovirus infection. J Pediatr 111:343–348, 1987

Hutto C, Arvin A, Jacobs R et al: Intrauterine herpes simplex virus infections. J Pediatr 111:97–101, 1987

Prober CG, Sullender WM, Yasukawa LL et al: Low risk of herpes simplex virus infections in neonates exposed to the virus at the time of vaginal delivery to mothers with recurrent genital herpes simplex virus infections. N Engl J Med 316:240–244, 1987

Siegel JD: Neonatal sepsis. Semin Perinatol 9:20–28, 1985

Spigelblatt L, Saintonge J, Chicoine R et al: Changing pattern of neonatal septicemia. Pediatr Infect Dis 4:56–58, 1985

Stagno S: Cytomegalovirus infection: A pediatrician's perspective. Curr Probl Pediatr 16:630–667, 1986

Stagno S, Whitley RJ: Herpesvirus infections of pregnancy. Part II. Herpes simplex virus and varicella-zoster virus infections. N Engl J Med 313:1327–1330, 1985

St. Geme JW, Murray DL, Carter J et al: Perinatal bacterial infection after prolonged rupture of amniotic membranes: An analysis of risk and management. J Pediatr 104:608–613, 1984

Vollman JH, Smith WL, Ballard ET et al: Early onset group B streptococcal disease: Clinical, roentgenographic, and pathologic features. J Pediatr 89:199–203, 1986

Voora S, Srinivasan G, Lilien LD et al: Fever in full-term newborns in the first four days of life. Pediatrics 69:40–44, 1982

Wilson CB: Immunologic basis for increased susceptibility of the neonate to infection. J Pediatr 108:1–12, 1986

20

Cyanosis

Central cyanosis—always abnormal in a neonate—is clinically evident in the newborn when the amount of unsaturated hemoglobin in the arterial circulation exceeds 3 to 4 g/dl. In contrast, mild peripheral cyanosis, or acrocyanosis, is a common finding on the first day of life. Marked or prolonged peripheral cyanosis is caused by conditions in which decreased systemic blood flow leads to a compensatory increase in the peripheral extraction of oxygen. Hypothermia, hypoglycemia, hypovolemia, hypotension, acidosis, sepsis, polycythemia, and heart failure can cause peripheral cyanosis in the newborn.

The first part of this chapter will discuss the physiological causes of central cyanosis and outline some general principles that guide the initial clinical evaluation. The latter half will describe several of the more common cyanotic congenital heart lesions in more detail.

PHYSIOLOGY OF CENTRAL CYANOSIS

Almost without exception, central cyanosis results from a low arterial pO_2. In an adult with a hematocrit of 45%, an arterial pO_2 of 45 mm Hg achieves an 80% hemoglobin satu-

ration (equivalent to 3 g/dl of unsaturated hemoglobin). Because most of the hemoglobin in a neonate is fetal hemoglobin, which has a greater affinity for oxygen than does adult hemoglobin, the arterial pO_2 must decrease to approximately 35 mm Hg at the same hematocrit to produce the same concentration of unsaturated hemoglobin. Therefore, significant arterial desaturation can be more difficult to detect in the neonate than in the adult. Central cyanosis can also, rarely, be present at a normal pO_2. This occurs during methemoglobinemia because there is an abnormally high percentage of heme-associated iron in the oxidized state (thereby making hemoglobin unavailable for O_2 binding), either due to a toxin or to an enzyme deficiency. Failure of a drop of dark, desaturated blood to become bright red in color when allowed to dry on filter paper exposed to room air supports this diagnosis.

Three abnormalities can produce arterial hypoxia in the neonate; in order of frequency, these are pulmonary ventilation–perfusion mismatch, shunting of blood from the systemic venous to arterial circuit, and hypoventilation. Inequalities of pulmonary ventilation–perfusion relationships are usually caused by primary parenchymal lung disease or by atelectasis secondary to compression of lung tissue (*e.g.*, by a pneumothorax, pleural effusions, chylothorax, diaphragmatic hernia, or pulmonary interstitial emphysema). Right-to-left shunting is responsible for systemic arterial hypoxia in cyanotic congenital heart disease and in persistent pulmonary hypertension of the newborn (PPHN, also known less accurately as PFC, or persistent fetal circulation). Finally, upper airway obstructions and a variety of neurologic or neuromuscular disorders can produce cyanosis due to hypoventilation. Several mechanisms may operate in concert; for instance, severe pneumonias may be complicated by hypoventilation and intrapulmonary shunts (functional right-to-left shunts) in addition to ventilation–perfusion mismatch.

CLINICAL EVALUATION OF CYANOSIS

When an infant presents with cyanosis, proper therapy depends critically on prompt establishment of an accurate diagnosis. Careful attention to the history and physical examination and thoughtful use of a few laboratory tests will narrow the diagnosis to a category of disorders even if a specific diagnosis requires more sophisticated tests.

Certain causes of airway obstruction are obvious on inspection (*e.g.*, macroglossia and neck masses). Choanal atresia is the likely diagnosis if cyanosis diminishes with crying and is confirmed by failure to pass a tube through either or both nasal choanae to the oropharynx. Other airway obstructions present with respiratory distress and/or stridor. Symptoms resolve once the obstruction is bypassed by tracheal intubation or tracheostomy. Infants with tracheomalacia improve when placed in the prone position. Arterial pO_2 will exceed 150 mm Hg when the infant breathes 100% oxygen; arterial pCO_2 may be

elevated. Chest x-ray is usually normal, but a right aortic arch suggests a vascular ring, and enlargement or calcification of the mediastinum suggests intrathoracic airway obstruction secondary to a mass such as a teratoma.

Congenital anomalies (encephalocele, hydranencephaly) and acquired disorders (cerebral asphyxia, meningoencephalitis, intracranial bleeding) of the central nervous system also cause cyanosis secondary to hypoventilation. In addition, the presentation of certain neuromuscular disorders such as neonatal myasthenia gravis may include cyanosis. On examination, diminished respiratory effort, apnea, or a markedly irregular respiratory pattern is apparent. Similar to hypoventilation secondary to airway obstructions, pO_2 significantly increases and cyanosis resolves when adequate supplemental oxygen is administered. Chest x-ray is normal unless the course is complicated by aspiration pneumonia or atelectasis. An exception to this clinical mold is phrenic nerve paralysis. Profound cyanosis can result despite intense respiratory effort. Other signs of birth injury (*e.g.*, brachial plexus palsy, Horner's syndrome) often accompany this lesion. Sonography provides the best confirmation of the diagnosis by demonstrating paradoxical motion of the hemidiaphragm. The chest x-ray eventually shows elevation of the paralyzed hemidiaphragm, but this may not be apparent early in the course.

The usual clinical problem is differentiation of congenital cyanotic heart disease, persistent pulmonary hypertension of the newborn, and lung disease. Certain historical features favor lung disease. These include prematurity, prolonged rupture of membranes, and meconium staining with acute fetal distress. Evidence of sustained fetal compromise before delivery, on the other hand, suggests persistent pulmonary hypertension. No specific historical features (other than a positive family history) favor congenital cyanotic heart disease, but it is important to remember that a history of prematurity or asphyxia does not exclude heart disease.

Physical examination may suggest a diagnostic category. The presence of other malformations increases the chance of coexisting heart disease. Heart disease is especially likely in certain syndromes and chromosomal abnormalities. Significant dyspnea supports lung disease or PPHN, whereas intense cyanosis with relatively little respiratory distress favors heart disease. Differential cyanosis (cyanosis that spares the face, right upper extremity, and upper thorax) is evidence for a large right-to-left ductal shunt and may be found in PPHN, interrupted aortic arch, or critical coarctation. Reversed differential cyanosis suggests transposition of the great vessels with associated coarctation and patent ductus arteriosus (PDA). The presence of a murmur usually but not always indicates heart disease; for instance, tricuspid insufficiency may complicate PPHN. The lack of a murmur, however, does not rule out heart disease. Careful auscultation of the heart sounds can be rewarding. A split S_1 in a cyanotic infant accompanied by a holosystolic regurgitant murmur and cardiomegaly implicates Ebstein's anomaly. A single second heart sound is a *sine qua non* for some types of cyanotic heart disease; however, splitting of S_2 may not be heard in the normal infant until the second day. S_2 also tends to be single or narrowly split in PPHN. A widely split S_2 may be heard in pulmonary stenosis and in anomalous pulmonary venous return due to a prolonged right ventricular ejection time. Palpation of the peripheral pulses is essential. Decreased femoral pulses or more than a 20-mm blood pressure differential between the upper and lower extremities suggests an abnormality of the aortic arch. Pulses are symmetrically decreased in the hypoplastic left heart syndrome. Widening of the pulse pressure is responsible for bounding pulses

and is found in conditions with a large systemic run-off. It occurs most commonly with PDA, but may indicate truncus arteriosus in the cyanotic full-term infant. If abnormal situs is suspected by auscultation or by palpation of the liver below the left coastal margin, complex heart disease is highly probable.

Potentially helpful laboratory tests include anteroposterior (AP) and lateral chest x-rays, a twelve lead electrocardiogram (ECG), and arterial blood gas analysis. The chest x-ray is extremely useful in diagnosing parenchymal lung disease and in confirming pneumothorax, pleural effusion, and diaphragmatic hernia. When cardiac disease is suspected, evaluation of the heart size, silhouette, and degree of pulmonary vascularity is essential. A cardiothoracic ratio greater than 0.60 on an end-inspiratory, nonrotated chest radiograph is a criterion of cardiomegaly in the neonate and frequently accompanies many of the congenital cyanotic lesions. A narrow mediastinum is often noted in transposition of the great vessels. A boot-shaped heart suggests tetralogy of Fallot (TOF) but may not develop until later in infancy. Twenty-five percent of infants with TOF have a right-sided aortic arch. Right atrial enlargement implies tricuspid regurgitation (*e.g.,* Ebstein's anomaly), but identification of dilatation of other chambers is difficult on an AP film. The pulmonary vasculature may be prominent secondary to increased pulmonary blood flow (*e.g.,* some forms of transposition of the great vessels [TGV] and truncus arteriosus) or pulmonary venous obstruction (total anomalous pulmonary venous return with obstruction, hypoplastic left heart syndrome). Oligemia of the lung fields, as demonstrated by diminished prominence of the hila and lack of vessels in the middle third of the lungs, is seen with pulmonary atresia, TOF, pulmonary stenosis with or without transposition, tricuspid atresia, and type IV truncus arteriosus.

Some normal ECG findings in the full-term

neonate are listed in Table 20-1, together with criteria for atrial and ventricular enlargement or hypertrophy. Most forms of cyanotic congenital heart disease have ECG findings that are, strictly speaking, within the normal range; however, a QRS axis of −30 to −90 in the absence of rhythm disturbances is common in tricuspid atresia, as is left ventricular dominance or hypertrophy. Less marked left axis deviation (0 to +90) is the norm for pul-monary atresia with an intact ventricular septum.

Arterial blood gas analysis after the infant breathes 100% oxygen for 15 minutes (hyperoxia test) usually rules out congenital heart disease if the pO_2 rises above 150 mm Hg. The test discriminates cyanosis due to hypoventilation and ventilation–perfusion mismatch from cyanosis due to significant right-to-left shunts. False-positive test results may occur

---

TABLE 20–1. Interpretation of the Neonatal Electrocardiogram

1. QRS axis (degrees)

0–24 hours	Mean 135	Range 60–180
1–7 days	Mean 125	Range 80–160
8–30 days	Mean 110	Range 60–160

2. T wave orientation in V_1

0–4 days	Upright *or* inverted
> 4 days	Inverted only

3. Voltage amplitudes (mm*) in precordial leads (5th–95th percentiles)

	RV_1	SV_1	RV_5	SV_5	RV_6	SV_6
30 hours	4.3–21.0	1.1–19.1	3.1–16.6	2.4–18.5	1.5–11.3	1.0–13.8
1 month	3.3–18.7	0.0–12.0	3.8–24.2	2.6–18.3	1.0–16.2	0.0–9.5

4a. Right atrial enlargement (RAE)

   i. Peaked P wave (>2.5 mm), best seen in leads II, III, V_3R, or V_1
   ii. P/PR segment† ratio <1 in the absence of conduction abnormalities

b. Left atrial enlargement (LAE)

   i. P wave >0.08 seconds
   ii. Terminal inversion of P wave in V_3R or V_1
   iii. P/PR segment† ratio <1.6 in the absence of conduction abnormalities

c. Right ventricular hypertrophy (RVH)

   i. R in V_1 >95%
   ii. S in V_5, V_6 >95%
   iii. Upright T in V_1 after 4 days
   iv. qR in V_3R or V_1

d. Left ventricular hypertrophy (LVH)

   i. R in V_5, V_6 >95%
   ii. S in V_1 >95%
   iii. R in V_1 <5%
   iv. q in V_5, V_6 >4 mm

---

*10 mm = 1 mvolt
†PR segment defined as the interval between the end of the P wave and the beginning of the q wave
(Adapted from the Harriet Lane Handbook)

in PPHN and in parenchymal lung disease, especially if the test is delayed and lung disease is severe. PPHN can still be implicated if a 15-minute period of hyperventilation with 100% oxygen achieves a significant rise in arterial pO_2 (Table 20-2). Elevation of pCO_2 is more consistent with lung disease.

Despite careful attention to the history, physical examination, and easily available laboratory studies, occasionally this differentiation requires two-dimensional echocardiography and/or cardiac catheterization with angiography.

CYANOTIC CONGENITAL HEART DISEASE

The incidence of congenital heart disease (not including bicuspid aortic valve) is estimated to be approximately 8 in 1000 live births. For the purpose of this chapter, a more meaningful figure can be gleaned from the data of the New England Regional Infant Cardiac Program. This collaborative study demonstrated that heart disease severe enough to require hospitalization, cardiac catheterization, or surgery in the first year of life occurred in approximately 2 per 1000 live births in New England. These data are further broken down by diagnosis in Table 20-3 and by diagnosis

and age of presentation in Table 20-4. The seven specific heart defects discussed below comprise 30% of this total (the majority of the remainder present with signs and symptoms of congestive heart failure). TGV is the most common congenital heart lesion that presents in the first week of life and the most common congenital *cyanotic* heart lesion in the initial 2 weeks of life. After the first 2 weeks, TOF becomes the most likely diagnosis of a cyanotic heart defect.

Transposition of the Great Vessels

As implied by its name, the origins of the aorta and pulmonary artery are reversed in TGV. Hence, the aorta arises from the right ventricle, and its root lies anterior, superior, and to the right of the root of the pulmonary artery, which in turn derives from the left ventricle. Associated defects are not uncommon and may include one or more of the following: atrial or ventricular septal defects, PDA, subpulmonic stenosis, and coarctation.

In utero, this arrangement preserves the basic elements of fetal circulation. Systemic venous blood, which includes the oxygenated umbilical venous return, enters the right atrium. Most of the inferior vena caval return is shunted across the foramen ovale to the left atrium to be ejected with the pulmonary

TABLE 20–2. Differentiation of Heart Disease, Lung Disease, and PPHN

	F_iO_2*	PCO_2 (mm Hg)	PO₂ (mm Hg)		
			PPHN	*Lung disease*	*Heart disease[†]*
Room air	21	40	40	40	40
Hyperoxia test	100	40	40	>100	40
Hyperoxia–hyperventilation test	100	20–25	>100	>150	40

*Inspired fractional oxygen concentration
[†]Cyanotic congenital heart disease with fixed right-to-left shunting
(Adapted from Fox WW, Duara S: Persistent pulmonary hypertension in the neonate: Diagnosis and management. J Pediatr 103:505, 1983)

Table 20–3. Distribution of Heart Disease* by Diagnosis†

Diagnosis	Incidence (%)
Ventricular septal defect	16.2
Tetralogy of Fallot	
Simple	**7.0**
With pulmonary atresia	**2.2**
D-TGV	**8.9**
Coarctation of the aorta	8.1
Hypoplastic left heart syndrome	6.6
Patent ductus arteriosus	5.6
Endocardial cushion defect	5.5
Malposition	3.8
Severe pulmonic stenosis	**3.2**
Pulmonic atresia	**2.7**
Atrial septal defect	2.7
Single ventricle	2.5
Tricuspid atresia	**2.1**
Total anomalous pulmonary venous return	**2.1**
Myocardial disease	2.1
Truncus arteriosus	**1.5**
Other	16.2

*Heart disease requiring hospitalization or surgery in the first year of life
†Defects likely to present with cyanosis in bold type
(Adapted from Cloherty JP, Stark AR [eds]: Manual of Neonatal Care, 2nd ed. Boston, Little, Brown and Co, 1985.)

Table 20–4. Percentage Distribution of Cardiac Disease by Age at Presentation

0–6 Days		7–13 Days		14–28 Days		180–365 Days	
TGV	15	COA	20	VSD	18	VSD	20
HLH	12	VSD	14	TOF	17	PDA	14
TOF	8	HLH	9	COA	12	TOF	14
COA	7	TGV	9	TGV	10	ASD	10
VSD	6	TOF	7	PDA	5	ECD	7

ASD = atrial septal defect
COA = coarctation of the aorta
ECD = endocardial cushion defect
HLH = hypoplastic left heart syndrome
PDA = patent ductus arteriosus
TGV = transposition of the great vessels
TOF = tetralogy of Fallot
VSD = ventricular septal defect
(Adapted from Cloherty JP, Stark AR [eds]: Manual of Neonatal Care, 2nd ed. Boston, Little, Brown & Co, 1985; and Fyler DC et al: Pediatrics 65[suppl]:375, 1980)

venous return by the left ventricle into the pulmonary artery. Most of this left ventricular output flows through the PDA into the descending aorta secondary to the high intrauterine pulmonary vascular resistance and perfuses the lower body. Systemic return reaching the right ventricle is ejected into the aorta and perfuses the heart, brain, and upper body. The adverse physiologic consequences of this defect are not apparent until after birth when the placenta has been removed and the pulmonary vascular resistance falls. The transposition of the aorta and pulmonary artery leads to two parallel circulations with oxygenation of the systemic side dependent on the amount of shunting that occurs at the atrial, ventricular, and ductal levels.

At presentation, cyanosis may vary from minimal to profound; duskiness becomes more obvious as the PDA constricts. Unless hypoxia is severe enough to cause metabolic acidosis, respiratory distress is lacking, although shallow tachypnea may be noted. Because the pulmonary artery is posterior to the aorta, the normally soft P_2 is usually inaudible with a resultant single second heart sound. Typically, no murmur is heard with an isolated transposition. In defects with a ventricular septal defect (VSD), a holosystolic murmur gradually develops at the lower left sternal border. If subpulmonic stenosis also is present, a second systolic ejection murmur may be heard at the upper left sternal border. Heart size and pulmonary vascularity are normal to increased on the chest x-ray except when significant subpulmonic stenosis is present. In the latter case, the lungs fields are oligemic. Typically, the mediastinum is narrow, and the heart silhouette may resemble an "egg-on-side." EKG usually shows a normal degree of right ventricular predominance. Echocardiography confirms the diagnosis.

Without treatment, one-third of infants with transposition will die in the first week of life. Life-saving palliative measures include administration of intravenous prostaglandin E_1 to maintain ductal patency and a Rashkind balloon atrial septostomy to increase atrial shunting. The latter procedure has recently been performed using echocardiographic rather than fluoroscopic guidance. There are two corrective surgical techniques. The older Mustard or Senning procedure reestablishes normal blood flow patterns at the atrial level by creation of an interatrial baffle. Complica-

tions have included baffle obstruction, bundle branch block, arrhythmias, and right heart failure. For these reasons, an early arterial switch operation (performed before left ventricular pressure falls) is now preferred at a number of institutions. Centers experienced with this procedure have reported an improved outcome over several years relative to the baffle techniques; however, evaluation of longer-term outcome awaits further follow-up.

Tetralogy of Fallot

TOF derives its name from a tetrad of anatomical findings that include a variable degree of right ventricular outflow tract (RVOT) obstruction (infundibular stenosis, usually accompanied by hypoplasia of the pulmonary valve annulus and/or pulmonary valve abnormalities), a ventricular septal defect, right ventricular hypertrophy, and an aorta that "overrides" the interventricular septum. Associated cardiac abnormalities include right aortic arch, origin of the anterior descending from the right coronary artery, lack of the pulmonic valves, and atrial septal defect. As with transposition, the *in utero* blood flow pattern in this lesion does not interfere with fetal growth and places no pressure or volume overload stresses on the fetal heart. Physiologic consequences of this defect after birth depend directly on the degree and progression of the RVOT obstruction, which varies from mild pulmonic stenosis to frank pulmonary atresia. Right-to-left shunting through the VSD is responsible for cyanosis.

Not surprisingly, the clinical expression of TOF is variable. Infants with severe RVOT obstruction present as early as the first day of life with severe cyanosis and worsen as the ductus constricts. TOF with mild pulmonic stenosis and a large VSD may present initially with congestive heart failure as the pulmonary vascular resistance declines. Most patients with TOF present somewhere between these two extremes and develop cyanosis between 1 week and 6 months of life. Older infants may present with "tet" spells in which an acute increase in RVOT obstruction causes cerebral hypoxia; there may be a history of squatting.

Findings on examination are also variable. In the neonatal period, S_2 is almost always single (due to a combination of a malpositioned pulmonary artery and stenotic valves). A systolic ejection murmur at the upper left sternal border characterizes the RVOT obstruction. Acute diminution of the murmur is ominous, since it suggests an acute decrease in pulmonary blood flow. Ejection clicks are usually lacking, but may be present later in infancy with progressive dilatation of the aortic root. Chest x-ray shows decreased pulmonary vascularity; over time, enlargement of the right heart and diminished prominence of the pulmonary root lead to the classic "boot-shaped" cardiac silhouette. The neonatal ECG demonstrates right ventricular predominance within the normal range. Definite right ventricular hypertrophy (RVH) is usually found in later-presenting defects.

Medical palliation with PGE_1 is invaluable in certain cases presenting with early cyanosis. The traditional surgical approach has been two-pronged, with initial palliation by creation of a systemic vein-branch pulmonary artery shunt preceding definitive repair. More recently, early total correction has been attempted.

Pulmonary Atresia with an Intact Ventricular Septum

The primary lesion in pulmonary atresia with an intact ventricular septum (PA with IVS) is an imperforate pulmonary valve. Total obstruction to the RVOT results in right ventricular hypoplasia, and dilatation and hypertrophy of the right atrium. All blood flow must pass right-to-left across the foramen ovale; consequently, the left atrium and ventricle are also dilated. Postnatally, pulmonary blood flow is supplied exclusively by left-to-right ductal shunting. As a result, infants present early with intense cyanosis.

The physical examination is notable for a single second heart sound. Frequently, there is also a murmur of tricuspid insufficiency. Chest x-ray shows cardiomegaly with reduced pulmonary vascularity. ECG typically reveals a leftward axis (0 to +90 degrees), right atrial enlargement and left ventricular predominance on precordial leads.

The surgical approach to this defect depends partly on the extent of right ventricular hypoplasia. With mild hypoplasia, a pulmonary valvotomy can produce good results. Significant hypoplasia requires shunt placement from a systemic vessel or the right atrium to a pulmonary artery. Prognosis remains grim for the lesions with severe right ventricular hypoplasia.

Pulmonary Stenosis with Intact Ventricular Septum

Pulmonary stenosis (PS) with IVS is similar in many respects to PA with IVS. The fundamental difference is that the pulmonary valve, though abnormal, permits a variable amount of pulmonary blood flow. As a result, right ventricular hypoplasia and right atrial and left heart dilatation tend to be less than in PA with IVS. Consequently, cyanosis is less obvious at birth; some infants with relatively mild PS even tolerate ductal closure. Possible findings that distinguish this defect from PA with IVS include a softly split S_2, a systolic ejection murmur at the upper left sternal border, and a pulmonary click. Recently, balloon angioplasty of the pulmonary valve during cardiac catheterization has successfully supplanted surgical therapy in selected cases.

Tricuspid Atresia

Tricuspid atresia is the unifying feature of a spectrum of anatomic abnormalities. Most lesions with tricuspid atresia have normally related great vessels (type I: 70%); in the remainder (type II: 30%), the great vessels are transposed. In either category, there may be (1) PA with IVS; (2) PS with small VSD; or (3) large VSD. In type I, the majority of patients have PS and a small VSD; in type II, most have a large VSD without PS. Anatomically, right ventricular hypoplasia is the rule, even in infants with VSDs.

Clinically, tricuspid atresia presents with profound cyanosis when it is complicated by PA or significant PS. Alternatively, when tricuspid atresia and a large VSD coexist, cyanosis is minimal and congestive heart failure is the prominent symptom. Physical examination is not specific for this lesion. Similarly, depending on the subclass of tricuspid atresia, the chest x-ray may demonstrate findings ranging from a small heart with decreased pulmonary vascularity (1 and 2) to cardiomegaly with pulmonary vascular prominence (3). Left axis deviation ($-30°$ to $-90°$) or left ventricular predominance or LVH independently secure the diagnosis in the cyanotic infant. In the infant with congestive heart failure, a superior axis raises the possibility of an endocardial cushion defect, which can usually be discriminated by the relative lack of left ventricular predominance.

Total Anomalous Pulmonary Venous Return

Total anomalous pulmonary venous return (TAPVR) is another cardiac lesion with a range of anatomic expression. As the name implies, the common feature of TAPVR is that pulmonary blood flow returns to the right atrium. Anatomic variants include drainage of a common pulmonary vein to the right atrium (1) via a vertical vein into the innominate vein and the superior vena cava; (2) via the coronary sinus; and (3) via the portal vein through the ductus venosus and inferior vena cava. Less commonly, four pulmonary veins may drain directly into the right atrium. Each of these variants may occur with or without obstruction.

Since pulmonary blood flow represents only 7% of combined ventricular output *in utero*, fetal development is normal. TAPVR with obstruction invariably presents early in the neonatal period, usually with cyanosis; however, with lesser degrees of obstruction, cyanosis may be minimal and congestive failure predominant instead. Physical examination is not usually helpful in infants with marked obstruction and cyanosis; however, S_2 tends to be widely split in infants with minimal obstruction and congestive failure. In TAPVR with obstruction, the heart size is normal or small, and pulmonary plethora secondary to venous congestion is seen on chest x-ray. Right ventricular predominance on ECG is within normal limits for a newborn.

Nonetheless, this lesion has proven difficult to distinguish from PPHN even with two-dimensional echocardiography. This is well-illustrated by the inclusion of infants with TAPVR in many large series in which presumed PPHN is treated by extracorporeal membrane oxygenation. Usually, cardiac catheterization and angiography are necessary to establish the diagnosis and define the precise anatomy of pulmonary venous return. Surgical outcome, once almost assuredly fatal, is improving.

Truncus Arteriosus

In truncus arteriosus, one major arterial trunk supplies both the systemic and pulmonary circuits. Four types of truncus arteriosus have been defined, depending on the anatomy of the pulmonary branch vessels. Usually, sufficient pulmonary blood flow exists so that cyanosis is minimal and the primary symptoms are secondary to congestive heart failure, which develops in concert with the postnatal fall of the pulmonary vascular resistance. In type IV truncus (branch pulmonary arteries arise from the descending aorta), pulmonary blood flow is diminished and cyanosis predominates. A bicuspid or quadricuspid truncal valve occurs in approximately 40% of cases; the valve may be thickened and cause both stenosis and regurgitation. DiGeorge's syndrome should be considered in all infants with truncus arteriosus.

In infants with truncus arteriosus and congestive failure, the second heart sound is single. Multiple pulmonary clicks may be heard, giving the erroneous impression of a split S_2. Murmurs are variable. The precordial impulse is striking, and peripheral pulses are bounding due to a rapid aortic run-off through the lower resistance pulmonary vascular bed. Chest x-ray shows cardiomegaly and pulmonary vascular congestion. A right aortic arch may be visualized. ECG may suggest biventricular hypertrophy. In type IV truncus, cyanosis is profound; bounding pulses are absent, chest x-ray reveals diminished pulmonary vascularity, and evidence of left ventricular hypertrophy is lacking on ECG.

CONCLUSION

This short account of congenital cyanotic heart disease has purposefully and necessarily erred on the side of simplicity. Many complex defects (heterotaxies, single ventricle, etc.) have not been described nor mentioned in the differential diagnosis. Relatively common defects that present primarily with congestive failure or myocardial dysfunction and only secondarily with cyanosis (*e.g.*, hypoplastic left heart syndrome) are considered briefly elsewhere. Nonetheless, the reader should now have some idea of the variability of the clinical expression of heart disease. Perhaps some solace may be achieved upon reflecting that even experienced pediatric cardiologists make an accurate pre-echocardiographic diagnosis in no more than three of four cases!

BIBLIOGRAPHY

Fink BW: Congenital Heart Disease: A Deductive Approach to Its Diagnosis, 2nd ed. Chicago, Year Book Medical Publishers, 1985

Fox WW, Duara S: Persistent pulmonary hypertension in the neonate: Diagnosis and management. J Pediatr 103:505–514, 1983

Fyler D et al: Report of the New England Regional Infant Cardiac Program. Pediatrics 65(suppl):377–461, 1980

Kitterman J: Cyanosis in the newborn infant. Pediatr Rev 4:13–23, 1982

Philips JB III (ed): Neonatal Pulmonary Hypertension. Clin Perinatol 11(3), 1984

Part VI: Infection and Immunity

21

Recurrent Infections in Childhood

Virtually all children have recurrent infections. In fact, the average preschool-aged child has six upper respiratory infections a year, in addition to occasional episodes of otitis media and gastroenteritis. It is the responsibility of the pediatrician to differentiate the few children with an immunodeficiency disorder from the vast majority of children with recurrent infections who are immunologically normal. Ideally, this task will be accomplished in such a fashion that all children with an immunodeficiency disease are diagnosed as early in life as possible without evaluating an inordinate number of children for immunodeficiency.

Fortunately, in the great majority of children, a careful history and physical examination will provide sufficient information to effectively rule out an immunodeficiency. As outlined in Table 21-1, the immunodeficient child usually not only has an increased number of infections, but will also has infections that are unusually severe, complicated, or prolonged. Infections with unusual organisms (e.g., Pneumocystis carinii) are also frequently seen. While upper respiratory infections are seen most commonly in all children, in the immunodeficient child they are usually ac-

companied by infections of the lower respiratory tract and other organ systems (e.g., skin, gastrointestinal [GI] tract, blood, bones, or joints).

On physical examination, the immunodeficient child commonly appears chronically ill with evidence of both recurrent infection and failure to thrive. A normal growth pattern speaks strongly against the diagnosis of a significant, long-standing immunodeficiency. Other signs of immunodeficiency may in-

Table 21–1. Common Clinical Manifestations of Immunodeficiency

1. Recurrent sinopulmonary infections
2. Infections characterized by
   - Increased frequency
   - Unusual severity
   - Prolonged course/persistence
   - Unusual organisms (at times)
3. Failure to thrive
4. Persistent thrush
5. Diarrhea/malabsorption
6. Associated conditions may include
   - Skin lesions (e.g., rash, eczema, pyoderma)
   - Autoimmune disease
   - Hematologic abnormalities (anemia, neutropenia, thrombocytopenia)
   - Hepatosplenomegaly

clude the lack of tonsillar tissue or lymph nodes, hepatosplenomegaly, oral candidiasis, and a variety of dermatologic conditions. Certain findings on examination may even point to a specific immunodeficiency syndrome, such as eczema in Wiskott-Aldrich syndrome or telangiectasias in ataxia–telangiectasia.

A variety of noninfectious conditions may also be associated with immunodeficiency, including hematologic abnormalities (aplastic anemia, hemolytic anemia, neutropenia, thrombocytopenia), autoimmune disorders, arthritis, and chronic diarrhea. While none of these conditions are universally associated with immunodeficiency, their presence in a child with recurrent infections should be taken very seriously.

Since many immunodeficiency diseases are genetically determined, a family history is critical in the evaluation of a child with recurrent infections. A history of severe infections, recurrent infections, or early neonatal deaths in near or distant relatives should be explored carefully, as should a history of autoimmune or rheumatic disease.

Finally, a careful history of the pattern of infections is also useful in evaluating the child with recurrent infections. Infections localized to a single organ system or specific

area of the body, such as the urinary tract, generally indicate a mechanical abnormality rather than an immunologic defect. Similarly, any break in the integument predisposes to infection. These and other nonimmunologic mechanisms that may underlie recurrent infections are outlined in Table 21-2.

CLASSIFICATION OF IMMUNODEFICIENCY DISEASES

Immunodeficiency diseases may be either primary or secondary. Secondary immunodeficiencies are considerably more common than primary immunodeficiencies and include all cases in which a previously normal individual develops an impairment in immunologic function as a result of some illness, drug, or other condition. A few of the more common causes of secondary immunodeficiencies are listed in Table 21-3.

The primary immunodeficiencies are clas-

Table 21–2. Nonimmunologic Causes of Recurrent Infections

1. Integumental breaks
   • Eczema, burns, sinus tracts
2. Obstructive disorders
   • Ureteral or urethral stenosis, asthma, eustachian tube obstruction
3. Foreign bodies
   • Ventricular shunts, artificial heart valves, central venous catheters
4. Circulatory disorders
   • Edema, angiopathy, infarction
5. Unusual microbiologic flora
   • Alterations by antibiotic therapy (overgrowth, resistance)

Table 21–3. Causes of Secondary Immunodeficiencies

1. Immunosuppressive agents
   • Chemotherapy
   • Radiation
   • Corticosteroids
2. Infectious diseases
   • HIV infection (AIDS)
   • Infectious mononucleosis
3. Malignancy
4. Hematologic diseases
   • Sickle cell disease
5. Infiltrative diseases
   • Sarcoidosis
   • Histiocytosis
6. Surgery/trauma
   • Burns
   • Splenectomy
7. Metabolic diseases
   • Malnutrition
   • Uremia
   • Nephrotic syndrome
   • Diabetes mellitus

sified according to the component of the immune system in which the deficiency lies. These include deficiencies of B cells, T cells, phagocytic cells, or complement. Many primary immunodeficiency diseases involve defects in two or more components of the immune system, particularly T-cell defects with associated B-cell (antibody) deficiency. In all, more than 70 separate primary immunodeficiency diseases have been described, the most common of which are listed in Table 21-4.

Defects in humoral immunity (B cell, antibody mediated) are the most common class of immunodeficiency, composing 50% to 75% of the symptomatic primary immunodeficiencies. This figure does not include selective IgA deficiency, which may occur in up to 1 in 300 individuals and be asymptomatic. Combined B-cell and T-cell deficiencies make up another 15% to 20% of the primary immunodeficiencies, with the remainder comprised of isolated T-cell defects (5% to 10%), phagocytic defects (1% to 2%), and complement deficiencies (1% to 2%).

Because most primary immunodeficiencies are hereditary and congenital, they occur predominantly in pediatric patients. The overall incidence is estimated to be about 1:10,000, resulting in about 400 new cases a year in the United States. About 70% of cases occur in males because of the X-linked inheritance of many of these diseases.

LABORATORY EVALUATION

In the patient with recurrent infections in whom immunodeficiency is suspected, several screening laboratory tests should be performed (Table 21-5). These include a complete blood count with differential and platelet count, serum immunoglobulin levels (IgG, IgA, IgM) and specific antibody titers. If abnormal, these tests should be followed up by

Table 21–4. Classification of Primary Immunodeficiencies

1. B-cell deficiencies
   - X-linked agammaglobulinemia
   - IgA deficiency
   - IgG subclass deficiencies
   - Common variable immunodeficiency
2. T-cell deficiencies
   - DiGeorge's syndrome
   - Chronic mucocutaneous candidiasis
   - Nezelof's syndrome
3. Combined T-cell and B-cell deficiencies
   - Severe combined immunodeficiency
   - Ataxia-telangiectasia
   - Wiskott-Aldrich syndrome
4. Phagocytic disorders
   - Hyper IgE syndrome
   - Chronic granulomatous disease
   - Chédiak-Higashi syndrome
5. Complement disorders

more specific tests. In general, tests for disorders in phagocytosis or complement are not part of the initial evaluation. They should be pursued if strongly suggested by the clinical history or if there is a convincing history of immunodeficiency but normal T- and B-cell function.

The CBC may reveal anemia, thrombocytopenia, neutropenia, or lymphopenia, all highly significant in children with suspected immunodeficiency. In particular, the presence of lymphopenia (lymphocyte count less than 2000/mm^3) is suggestive of a T-cell immunodeficiency. The peripheral smear should also be examined for the presence of Howell-Jolly bodies or other evidence of impaired splenic function.

The quantitation of serum immunoglobulin (IgG, IgA, IgM) levels is critical in any patient with suspected immunodeficiency. Because of dramatic age-dependent variation, it is important that all levels be interpreted using age-appropriate standards. Neonates begin with adult quantities of IgG acquired transplacentally and then produce very little

Table 21–5. Laboratory Evaluation of Suspected Immunodeficiency

Screening Tests	Advanced Tests
B-cell deficiency	
Immunoglobulin levels	B-cell enumeration
Antibody titers	Vaccination/antibody response
IgG subclasses	
T-cell deficiency	
Lymphocyte count	T-cell enumeration
Skin tests for delayed hypersensitivity	T-cell subsets
	Mitogenic stimulation
Phagocytic deficiency	
WBC count	Chemotaxis assays
Nitroblue tetrazolium dye test	Phagocytic and antimicrobial activity
IgE level	
Complement deficiency	
Ch_{50} activity	C3, C4 levels
	Other component assays

IgG for several months. Serum IgG levels during this period frequently drop as low as 200 mg/dl (low normal for an adult is 600 mg/dl). IgA and IgM do not cross the placenta and are usually present in very low quantities at birth, gradually increasing over the first several months of life.

The initial evaluation of the humoral immune system should also include tests of antibody function. These tests are particularly important in patients with low total immunoglobulin levels, since they allow one to differentiate the patient with normal antibody function in spite of low total immunoglobulin levels from the patient with a true deficiency in humoral immunity. Ideally, specific antibody titers to diphtheria and tetanus may be checked to evaluate response to protein antigens, while titers to *Haemophilus* influenza and/or pneumococcus may be assayed to study response to polysaccharide antigens, realizing that even normal children may not respond to polysaccharide antigens until after the age of 2.

While the matter is still not entirely clear, one may argue that for any child with a significant history of recurrent infection, IgG subclass values should be obtained in the initial

evaluation. Unfortunately, a normal total serum IgG does not rule out the possibility of a subclass deficiency, and low levels of IgG2 and IgG3 are clearly associated with increased susceptibility to infection. Possible subclass deficiency should be evaluated in all patients with IgA deficiency.

If these initial laboratory tests are completely normal, the possibility of an immunodeficiency, particularly an antibody deficiency, becomes quite unlikely. If, however, any of these tests is abnormal or if the clinical history is unusually worrisome, further testing must be done. For suspected antibody deficiency, B-cell enumeration studies should be performed, and the child should be re-immunized to further assess specific antibody response. If a defect in cellular (T-cell) immunity is suspected, further studies should include skin tests for delayed hypersensitivity, enumeration of total T-cell numbers and T-cell subsets (helper/suppressor ratio), and in vitro mitogenic stimulation. For suspected complement deficiency, measurement of the total serum complement activity (CH_{50}) is an excellent screening test. If results are abnormal, it should be followed up with assays for C3, C4, and, possibly, other individual complement components. Finally, for suspected defects in phagocytosis, tests may include the nitroblue tetrazolium dye reduction test (for chronic granulomatous disease), measurement of IgE level (to rule out the hyper IgE syndrome), tests of chemotactic activity, and other highly specialized tests of cell movement, phagocytosis, or microbial killing.

SPECIFIC IMMUNODEFICIENCY DISEASES

As described in the section on classification (see Table 21-4), immunodeficiencies may be divided into disorders with predominantly B-cell defects, T-cell defects, combined B- and T-cell defects, phagocytic defects, or complement defects. Here, several of the more common and/or representative immunodeficiency diseases will be discussed briefly.

B-cell Deficiency

The most important example of an immunodeficiency involving B cells is X-linked (congenital, Bruton's) agammaglobulinemia. This disorder is characterized by recurrent pyogenic infections beginning in infancy or early childhood, panhypogammaglobulinemia, inability to synthesize antibodies, and the lack of plasma cells in lymphoid tissues. As the name implies, only males are affected. Although sinopulmonary infections are seen most frequently, bacterial sepsis, meningitis, and arthritis are not uncommon. Further, although pyogenic infections are a hallmark of the disease, affected children are also frequently plagued by persistent viral or parasitic infections (e.g., rotavirus and *Giardia lamblia* gastroenteritis).

Common variable immunodeficiency is a condition of acquired agammaglobulinemia that may have its onset at any age. The disorder is often familial, but no specific mode of inheritance has been discerned, and males and females are affected equally. In contrast to congenital agammaglobulinemia, this disorder is characterized by normal numbers of B cells. The clinical presentation is quite similar, however, with most patients presenting with chronic progressive bronchiectasis.

While any immunoglobulin class may be selectively deficient in a given person, IgA deficiency is most noteworthy because of its high incidence. In fact, about 1 in 700 people are IgA deficient (although some reports estimate the incidence to be as high as 1 in 300). It appears from retrospectively screening large numbers of blood donors that a majority of IgA-deficient individuals are entirely well. When symptomatic, patients may present either with recurrent infections, predominantly of the sinopulmonary and gastrointestinal tracts, or with autoimmune disease.

Finally, deficiency of one or more IgG subclasses deserves note. While accurate data are lacking, it is now clear that recurrent infections may be associated with a specific deficiency of an IgG subclass; IgG2 appears to be of particular importance in this regard. Further, it has also been reported that symptomatic IgA deficiency is not infrequently associated with an IgG subclass deficiency. Ongoing studies may further clarify this somewhat confusing area.

The treatment of all immunodeficiency states relies on careful attention to infection and aggressive antibiotic therapy. For defects in humoral immunity, however, gammaglobulin replacement therapy is also of tremendous benefit (except in selective IgA deficiency). While such therapy cannot match the specific antibody function of an intact immune system, it does significantly reduce the number and severity of infections when used appropriately.

T-cell Antibody

Isolated T-cell defects are quite uncommon. The best example is DiGeorge's syndrome, a disease characterized by thymic and parathyroid hypoplasia. Clinical manifestations include neonatal tetany and hypoclacemia, midline facial defects, cardiac outflow abnormalities, and a variable T-cell deficit. Common infections include recurrent candidiasis, severe viral infections, occasional pyogenic infections, and *Pneumocystis carinii* pneumonia. Frequently, the immunologic defect is correctable by fetal thymic implants.

Combined B- and T-cell Deficiency

The class of combined B- and T-cell deficiency is best represented by the disease known as severe combined immunodeficiency (SCID). This disorder is inherited either as an autosomal-recessive or X-linked trait; hence, about 75% of affected patients are male. Infants with SCID usually become ill in the first 2 to 3 months of life and most commonly present with persistent oral thrush, chronic diarrhea, and pneumonia, often due to *Pneumocysitis carinii*. Growth is generally very poor, and overwhelming bacterial or viral infections are common. There is usually profound lymphopenia, low T-cell numbers, and panhypogammaglobulinemia. Gammaglobulin replacement therapy and aggressive antimicrobial support may help the child temporarily, but the disease is still considered universally fatal in the first few years of life. A cure is possible, however, through bone marrow transplantation; this is recommended for all patients, even if only a haploidentical donor is available.

Phagocytic Defects

As noted, phagocytic defects may include deficiencies in neutrophil numbers (neutropenia), opsonization, phagocytosis, or microbial killing. The best example of this class is chronic granulomatous disease (CGD), a syndrome characterized by recurrent purulent infections secondary to the inability of neutrophils and monocytes to kill bacteria and fungi that do not produce hydrogen peroxide. Microorganisms are actually ingested normally but then not killed appropriately because of an inability of the phagocyte to produce the microbicidal metabolites superoxide anion, hydrogen peroxide, and hydroxyl radical. Abscesses of the skin, lungs, lymph nodes, and liver are common, with most infections caused by *Staphylococcus aureus*, *Candida albicans*, enteric bacteria, and *Aspergillus*. Bacteria that produce hydrogen peroxide, including pneumococci and *Haemophilus influenzae*, are not problems for patients with CGD.

Complement Disorders

The types of infections experienced by patients with a congenital deficiency of a complement component vary, depending on the particular component that is missing. For example, patients deficient in C3, an important component for opsonization, are plagued by recurrent pyogenic infections. Alternatively, patients deficient in the terminal complement components (C5-C9), have dramatically increased risk of developing neisserial infections, particularly *N. meningitidis* sepsis or meningitis and gonococcal arthritis. These disorders are rare but should be suspected in any patient with significant recurrent bacterial infections.

BIBLIOGRAPHY

Gotoff SB: The secondary immunodeficiencies. In Stiehm ER, Fulginiti VA (eds): Immunologic Disorders and Children, 2nd ed, pp 399–430. Philadelphia, WB Saunders, 1980

Johnston RB: Recurrent bacterial infections in children. N Engl J Med 310:1237, 1984

Rosen FS, Copper MD, Wedgwood RJP: The primary immunodeficiencies. N Engl J Med 311:235, 298, 1984

Stiehm ER: Clinical and laboratory evaluation of lhe child with unsuspected immunodeficiency. Pediatr Rev 7:53, 1985

22

Infections in the Immunocompromised Host

As described in Chapter 21, children with impairments in immunologic function are prone to infections that are characterized by both increased frequency and unusual severity. Further, unusual organisms, often of very low pathogenicity (*e.g., Pneumocystis carinii, Staphlycoccus epidermidis*), may produce significant infections in the immunocompromised host. Any evidence of infection in an immunodeficient patient must therefore be evaluated promptly and treated aggressively. Frequently, broad-spectrum antibiotic therapy will be used until a specific pathogen can be identified. This coverage must be designed to treat not only the usual childhood pathogens, but also any other infectious agents associated with the particular immunodeficiency at hand.

The primary immunodeficiencies were described in some detail in Chapter 21. It should be stressed that while these diseases are important, it is patients with secondary immunodeficiencies (see Table 21-3) who make up the bulk of immunocompromised patients in both the inpatient and outpatient settings. In this section, three common secondary immunodeficiency states and their associated infections will be described briefly.

FEVER AND NEUTROPENIA

Children with neoplastic diseases may be affected by a variety of immunologic defects, resulting both from the therapies used and the disease processes themselves. The most common of these is neutropenia. Fever and neutropenia is the phrase used to describe the clinical situation in which the oncology patient presents with fever and an absolute neutrophil count (ANC) of less than 1000/mm^3. This situation has become increasingly common because of the more aggressive chemotherapy protocols being used to treat both leukemias and solid tumors. It is of tremendous clinical importance because of the potential for significant morbidity and even mortality secondary to infections in the neutropenic host.

While it is clear that there are many noninfectious etiologies for fever in the patient with cancer (*e.g.,* tumor necrosis, chemotherapy reactions), it is generally advisable to consider all patients with fever and neutropenia to be infected and to institute early empiric antibiotic therapy in an attempt to avoid the potentially devastating consequences of a significant infection. In several large studies, it has been shown that an infectious etiology of the

167

fever can be proven in approximately 50% of febrile, neutropenic patients. The actual incidence may be somewhat higher, since many infections may be missed because of the lack of a normal inflammatory response or by virtue of the early antibiotic therapy itself. This possibility is supported by data showing that if antibiotics are discontinued in patients in whom no infection could be proven but who are still neutropenic, infectious complications will become evident in about 50%. Thus, overall infections appear to be responsible for about three-fourths of the fevers seen in neutropenic patients.

When infection is proven, the most common sites involved are the upper and lower respiratory tract, with pneumonia accounting for approximately 25% of infections in most series. Although the incidence of sepsis varies somewhat from center to center, overall between one-fourth and one-third of all proven infections in the setting of fever and neutropenia will be due to sepsis. The remainder of documented infections may involve the skin, gastrointestinal tract, genitourinary system, and rarely, the musculoskeletal or central nervous systems.

The organisms most frequently isolated from blood cultures in febrile neutropenic patients are *Staphlycoccus aureus*, *Staphylococcus epidermidis*, *Streptococcus viridans*, and gram-negative enteric bacilli, including *Pseudomonas aeruginosa*, *Escherichia coli*, and *Klebsiella*. Fungal infections account for only 1% to 2% of infections overall but are significantly more common than that in patients with prolonged periods of neutropenia. The true incidence of viral infections is unknown, with various studies reporting documented viral infections in zero to 29% of all febrile neutropenic children.

The need for early empiric antibiotic therapy is underscored by reported mortality rates of over 50% for gram-negative sepsis in the neutropenic patient. Current recommendations for antibiotic therapy generally include a combination of antibiotics designed to cover those pathogens encountered most frequently. Gram-negative coverage is commonly provided by a combination of an aminoglycoside and a semisynthetic penicillin (*e.g.*, ticarcillin), whereas gram-positive coverage may be provided by vancomycin, nafcillin, or cephalothin. Protocols are currently under study comparing these agents to newer cephalosporins with very promising results. There is even some suggestion that a single third-generation cephalosporin (*e.g.*, ceftazidine) may provide equal efficacy as the first-line empiric agent.

As a general rule, antibiotic therapy should be continued as long as the patient remains significantly neutropenic. If a specific pathogen is identified, antibiotic therapy should be adjusted to its sensitivities, but broad-spectrum coverage should not be discontinued while the neutropenia persists. If no organism is identified, antibiotics may need to be adjusted if new or persistent fevers are encountered. The possibility of a fungal superinfection must always be considered as well.

In summary, while the aggressive use of chemotherapeutic agents has improved the overall outcome for children with cancer, it has also increased the risk of serious infectious complications. Empiric antibiotic therapy with broad-spectrum antibiotics for all patients with fever and neutropenia is the best means currently available to limit the potential risks of these infections.

Sickle Cell Disease

Children with sickle cell disease are at a dramatically increased risk of developing overwhelming bacterial infections, particularly sepsis and meningitis caused by *Streptococcus pneumoniae*. Their risk of pneumococcal sepsis is, in fact, between 400 and 600 times that of normal controls. Up to 30% of all deaths among individuals with sickle cell anemia occur before the age of 5 years, and the majority of these are due to bacterial sepsis and meningitis. Although pneumococcal infections are of paramount importance, an increased risk of serious *Haemophilus influenzae* infections has also been demonstrated. This susceptibility to infection with encapsulated bacteria is the result of a combination of impaired splenic function and deficient serum opsonizing activity.

The onset of splenic dysfunction (secondary to splenic infarction) occurs between several months and several years of age and is generally regarded as the major risk factor for serious infection. Under ideal circumstances, all children with sickle cell disease will be identified in the neonatal period and then prospectively followed for the onset of splenic dysfunction. In the absence of this information, all children with sickle cell anemia should be regarded as significantly immunocompromised. While no strict rules exist for the management of the child with sickle cell anemia and fever, most experts agree that those children with a temperature over 39° C should be treated for possible infection with *S. pneumoniae* or *H. influenzae*. This usually means hospitalization and intravenous administration of antibiotics (*e.g.,* cefuroxime) pending results of cultures. While those children with lesser degrees of fever may usually be observed without antibiotic administration, any clinical suspicion of a more serious illness (*e.g.,* lethargy, irritability, meningismus) should be pursued and treated aggressively.

Unfortunately, fevers are common in children with sickle cell anemia; they not only contract all of the usual viral illnesses of childhood but also frequently become febrile with their vaso-occlusive crises. It is unfortunate that each febrile episode must be taken so seriously, but nonetheless special treatment is absolutely critical, since the risks of ignoring a significant fever are completely unacceptable. Although improvements in prophylactic antibiotic therapy and bacterial vaccines have clearly reduced these risks, they currently are not sufficiently effective to influence the decision-making process outlined above.

HIV INFECTION

Although many viral infections may lead to mild, usually transient impairments in immunologic function, none can compare with the human immunodeficiency virus (HIV) in terms of the immunologic compromise it produces. The syndromes associated with HIV infection, AIDS and AIDS-related complex (ARC), are characterized by profound, generalized dysregulation of the immune system. The cellular immune system, particularly T-helper cells, is most severely affected, but abnormalities have been demonstrated in B-cells and monocytes as well. In fact, in spite of marked hypergammaglobulinemia in most patients, specific humoral immune responses are usually inadequate. These patients are therefore at greatly increased risk of developing serious infections. While the incidence of HIV infection in children is still relatively low, it is rapidly increasing and consuming an ever-growing proportion of health care expenditures.

The most common infections seen in pediatric AIDS are chronic oral candidiasis and recurrent bacterial infections, including otitis media, sinusitis, pneumonia, and septicemia. *Haemophilus influenzae* and *Streptococcus pneumoniae* are the organisms most frequently encountered. Sepsis is seen in pediatric AIDS much more commonly than with adult AIDS, and, consequently, children with AIDS who present with significant fever should be examined carefully, samples should be taken for culture, and administration of appropriate antibiotics should be begun. If pneumonia or interstitial pneumonitis is diagnosed, the possibility of an opportunistic infection (*e.g.,* *Pneumocystic carinii, Mycobacteria* species) must be considered. In that situation, bronchoscopy or open lung biopsy may be required to make a definitive microbiologic diagnosis. Severe viral and fungal infections are also commonly seen in AIDS patients and must always be considered in the differential diagnosis.

Finally, it is obvious that the infections encountered in pediatric AIDS cannot be appropriately treated until the disease itself is diagnosed. Establishing a diagnosis early in the course of the disease requires a high index of suspicion. All children should be evaluated for possible risk factors and any clinical evidence of the disease. Having a parent with, or at risk for, HIV infection is clearly the most important risk factor, with approximately 75% of all pediatric AIDS patients having an infected mother. If a mother is infected, there is approximately a 50% chance that each of her children will become infected, with transmission occurring either *in utero*, perinatally, or, occasionally, postnatally. The second most important risk factor is that of transfusion, with approximately 15% of cases being due to the receipt of infected blood or blood products, primarily prior to the institution of routine HIV screening in March, 1985.

In addition to recurrent infections, clinical features suggestive of AIDS include failure to thrive, chronic diarrhea, hepatosplenomegaly,

Table 22–1. Clinical Features of Pediatric AIDS

Recurrent bacterial infections
Persistent oral thrush
Failure to thrive
Chronic diarrhea
Hepatosplenomegaly
Interstitial pneumonitis
Encephalopathy

lymphadenopathy, interstitial pneumonitis, and encephalopathy (Table 22-1). A specific dysmorphic syndrome associated with intrauterine HIV infection may also be seen. It is critical that all children with these symptoms be evaluated for HIV infection, bearing in mind that the laboratory diagnosis of AIDS in infants may be made more difficult by the possible presence of transplacentally acquired HIV antibody until the age of 15 months.

BIBLIOGRAPHY

Brown, AE: Management in the febrile, neutropenic patient with cancer: Therapeutic considerations. J Pediatr 106:1035, 1985

McIntosh S, Rooks Y, Ritchey AK, et al: Fever in young children with sickle cell disease. J Pediatr 96:199, 1980

Pizzo PA, Robichaud KJ, Wesley K, et al: Fever in the pediatric and young adult patient with cancer. Medicine 61:153, 1982

Shannon KM, Amman AJ: Acquired immune deficiency syndrome in childhood. J. Pediatr 106:332, 1985

23

Meningitis

Meningitis is one of the most common serious infections of childhood. Although the term meningitis refers to all causes of inflammation of the pia and arachnoid meninges, the overwhelming majority of meningitis cases among children are caused by bacteria and viruses, while fungi, amoebae, and noninfectious causes account for rare cases.

BACTERIAL MENINGITIS

The spectrum of bacterial species that cause meningitis varies with the age of the child and, to a lesser degree, with other host factors. Up to 2 months of age, group B streptococci, *E. coli*, and *Listeria monocytogenes* are most commonly associated with meningitis, although *Haemophilus influenzae* (both type B and untypeable strains), *Streptococcus pneumoniae* (pneumococci), *Streptococcus viridans*, group D streptococci (enterococci), and *Citrobacter divirsus* are well known to cause meningitis in neonates. Infants who are premature or who are born following maternal amnionitis or prolonged rupture of membranes are at much higher risk for meningitis

than are infants who do not have one or more of these risk factors.

Beyond the age of 2 months, *H. influenzae*, type B, pneumococci, and *Neisseria meningitidis* (meningococci) are responsible for virtually all cases of bacterial meningitis among normal children. *H. influenzae*, type B, which accounts for approximately 80% of all cases of bacterial meningitis beyond the neonatal period, is usually restricted to children between the ages of 2 months and 5 years. Pneumococcal and meningococcal meningitis may occur at any age, but are both most common during the first 5 years of life. In each case, bacteria reach the subarachnoid space during a bacteremia which occurs in some children who become colonized in the nasopharynx. Each of these three organisms has a polysaccharide capsule which is thought to enhance virulence by resisting phagocytosis, and perhaps by other mechanisms. Serum antibody to each capsular polysaccharide is protective against disease, but children less than 24 months old are generally unable to make antibody to bacterial polysaccharides, which accounts, in part, for the high incidence of bacterial meningitis in this age-group. Children with hypofunctioning spleens or anatomic abnormalities of the base of the skull, and children with deficiencies of certain complement components, have a higher risk of meningitis with encapsulated bacteria, and sometimes experience recurrent bacterial meningitis. Recurrent meningitis with skin flora, or with gram-negative enteric bacilli, may indicate the presence of a neurocutaneous fistula at the base of the vertebral column. Meningitis with *Staphylococcus aureus*, *Staphylococcus epidermidis*, gram-negative bacilli, and several other species is, unfortunately, a frequent complication following placement of ventricular drainage shunts for obstructive hydrocephalus.

Clinical Manifestations and Diagnosis

Meningitis may present abruptly or following nonspecific prodromal symptoms of a few days' duration. The characteristic symptoms and signs include fever, irritability, headache, anorexia, nausea, and vomiting. Seizures occur in 30% to 40% of cases, and are more common in infants under 18 months. The presence of a petechial or purpuric rash is characteristic of meningococcal disease, but may also occur with *H. influenzae* type B infection.

On examination, older infants and children usually appear listless and irritable. Coma on presentation is a poor prognostic sign. Resistance to flexion of the neck (Brudzinski's sign) and to extension of the knee with the hip flexed (Kernig's sign) are characteristic physical signs that result from painful stretching of the spinal nerve roots as they exit the inflamed subarachnoid space. Papilledema is unusual in early bacterial meningitis. Focal neurologic abnormalities are present in 5% to 15% of children. The presence of papilledema should prompt the clinician to consider other causes of central nervous system (CNS) disease and obtain an emergency CT scan of the head before attempting a lumbar puncture.

Neonates and infants up to 6 to 12 months of age present with listlessness, pallor, hypotonia, anorexia, poor suck, and a weak cry but otherwise do not display the physical findings characteristic of meningitis in older children. The presence of a full anterior fontanelle or opisthotonus (hyperextension of the vertebral column) may be an important clue to the presence of meningitis in this age-group.

The key to the diagnosis of bacterial meningitis is early and complete examination of the cerebrospinal fluid (CSF), including measurement of the opening and closing CSF pressures, visual inspection, Gram's stain and culture, and measurement of the CSF white blood cell (WBC) count, WBC differential, glucose, and protein. In pyogenic bacterial meningitis, the normally clear CSF is usually cloudy to visual inspection and contains an elevated number of WBC (normal $\leq 5/mm^3$) and predominance of polymorphonuclear leukocytes (usually >90%) among the WBC counted. The protein content is generally elevated above 45 mg/dl, and the glucose is characteristically lower than the normal value of 50% to 60% of the simultaneous blood glucose level. Gram's stain of the CSF will demonstrate the organism in approximately 80% of cases of bacterial meningitis previously untreated with antibiotics.

Growth of the organism from CSF in the bacteriology laboratory within 1 to 3 days remains the definitive means of making the diagnosis of bacterial meningitis. Blood cultures are also positive in approximately 50% of cases. The use of rapid, simple, commercially available tests for the polysaccharide antigens of *H. influenzae* type B, group B streptococci, meningococci, and many types of pneumococci in CSF and serum will often speed the recognition and diagnosis of a specific type of meningitis. Because antigen detection methods are neither entirely sensitive nor entirely specific, important therapeutic decisions should not be based on data obtained from these methods alone.

Management

Intravenous administration of antibiotics, careful fluid management, and frequent reassessment are the cornerstones in the initial management of suspected bacterial meningitis.

The choice of antibiotics is guided primarily by the child's age. Ampicillin and gentamicin (dosages depend on the infant's age and birth weight) are our drugs of choice for the initial therapy of meningitis in the child under 1 month of age, because this combination provides the optimal coverage for the group B *Streptococcus*, the most common pathogen in this age-group, and also ensures excellent coverage for most of the other pathogens (except *H. influenzae*) that cause neonatal meningitis. If a gram-negative enteric organism such as *E. coli* is suspected on the basis of a Gram's stain or subsequent growth on culture, most clinicians would prefer to use a broad-spectrum β-lactam agent such as cefotaxime or aztreonam, which achieve CSF levels well in excess of the minimal inhibitory concentration (MIC) for most gram-negative bacilli; however, the use of these agents has not been shown to be superior to ampicillin plus an aminoglycoside antibiotic. Neonatal meningitis should be treated for 3 weeks with appropriate intravenous antibiotics. Group B streptococcal meningitis is adequately treated with ampicillin (or penicillin) alone, if the organism is sufficiently susceptible to this agent. Approximately 5% of group B streptococci recovered from septic newborns demonstrate tolerance to ampicillin (*i.e.*, the minimal bactericidal concentration [MBC] of ampicillin exceeds the MIC by eightfold or more). Although definitive studies are lack-

ing, it is prudent to treat infants with tolerant isolates with both ampicillin (or penicillin) and gentamicin for 3 weeks.

For infants between 1 and 2 months of age, we prefer the combination of ampicillin (200 mg/kg/day qid) and cefotaxime (150 mg/kg/day, qid) as initial therapy because both group B streptococci and *H. influenzae* type B must be covered.

After 2 months of age, chloramphenicol (75 mg/kg/day, qid, with close monitoring of drug levels) is our preferred initial therapy because *H. influenzae* type B is the dominate pathogen. Many physicians add ampicillin (200 mg/kg/day) as well, although there is no compelling clinical reason to add ampicillin to chloroamphenicol. Some pediatricians choose to use a cephalosporin with good CSF penetration, such as cefuroxime, cefotaxime, or ceftriaxone, alone. When β-lactamase producing strains of *H. influenzae* type B are recovered, the child must be treated with chloramphenicol or one of the cephalosporins. β-Lactamase-negative strains of *H. influenzae* type B can be treated with ampicillin alone. The standard duration of antibiotic treatment for *H. influenzae* type B meningitis is 10 days, but current studies indicate that 7 days of treatment is sufficient. In addition, many physicians are now using orally administered chloramphenicol to complete a course of treatment once the patient is afebrile and able to take oral medication.

Pneumococcal meningitis and meningococcal meningitis are treated with penicillin (100,000 U/kg/day q4h) alone. Pneumococcal isolates should be tested in the laboratory for their ability to be inhibited (MIC) and killed (MBC) by penicillin, since some institutions are now experiencing a 2% to 5% recovery rate of pneumococci that are relatively resistent to penicillin; such infections will require the addition of vancomycin, rifampin, or chloramphenicol. Pneumococcal meningitis should be treated for 10 days, whereas meningococcal meningitis requires only 7 days of treatment.

Because inappropriate secretion of antidiuretic hormone can be demonstrated in the majority of children with bacterial meningitis, and because cerebral edema is thought to contribute significantly to an adverse outcome, careful assessment of the child's state of hydration on admission and special attention to fluid and electrolyte management is critical. Fluid losses and electrolyte disturbances from vomiting may require judicious replacement therapy. As a general rule, fluid intake is restricted to 75% of normal (or about 1200 ml/M^2/day) for the first 2 to 4 days of hospitalization. Once noticible neurologic improvement occurs, fluid intake can be gradually liberalized.

Complications and Prognosis

Persistent or recurrent fever is a common problem in managing children with bacterial meningitis. It is not uncommon for fever to persist for 5 to 7 days or longer after starting antibiotics or to recur after the patient has become afebrile. Persistent and recurrent fever is often found to be due to drug fever, nosocomial infection, or the presence of an otherwise insignificant subdural effusion. Pleural effusion, arthritis, or pericarditis occurring during therapy is usually noninfectious in origin and responds to anti-inflammatory agents such as indomethacin. Relapse of appropriately treated meningitis is rare.

Cerebral edema, cerebral arteritis, and cortical venous thrombosis account for many of the neurologic complications that accompany or follow acute bacterial meningitis. Generalized and focal seizures do not, by themselves, portend a poor prognosis. Cranial nerve dysfunction (12%), sensorineural deafness (10%), cerebral infarction (4%), hydrocephalus, coma, and herniation are among the complications of acute meningitis. Although mortality is only about 5%, 20% to 30% of survivors are left with significant neurologic sequelae, including hemiparesis, cortical blindness, deafness, persistent seizures, and varying degrees of mental retardation. Ongoing assessment, consisting of neurologic examination, hearing evaluation, and developmental testing, is an important part of the management of meningitis patients following discharge from the hospital.

VIRAL MENINGITIS

Viruses are the most common cause of the aseptic meningitis syndrome, a term that technically refers to meningitis not caused by pyogenic bacteria or fungi. Aseptic meningitis resembles bacterial meningitis clinically, but is generally considered to be less severe and less likely to result in permanent neurologic sequelae. Aseptic meningitis may occur in the setting of a recognized clinical syndrome such as mumps, herpes zoster, Rocky Mountain spotted fever, Kawasaki disease, cat scratch disease, or leptospirosis or more frequently as the cause of acute illness in which the CNS signs and symptoms predominate in the absence of involvement of other organ systems. In the latter case, prospective studies have shown that the non-polio enteroviruses account for 70% or more of cases in which an etiologic agent can be defined. Given the difficulty of isolating some enteroviruses (especially coxsackie A viruses) and the control of mumps by widespread use of mumps vaccine in the United States and Canada, it is likely that enteroviruses cause more than 90% of cases of aseptic meningitis in children. The remaining cases are due to lymphocytic choriomeningitis virus, arboviruses, adenoviruses, Epstein-Barr virus, and rare cases of mumps.

Aseptic meningitis occurs principally from

June through October, reflecting the seasonal activity of the enteroviruses. All age-groups are affected, but in many outbreaks of enteroviral disease, the age-specific attack rates of aseptic meningitis have been highest in infants less than 2 years of age. Males have a slightly higher incidence than females.

Clinical Manifestations

Although the presenting signs and symptoms of aseptic meningitis are generally less severe than those of acute bacterial meningitis, there is sufficient overlap in the clinical spectrum so that the etiology cannot be distinguished reliably by clinical features alone. Frank meningismus is usually present in children more than 12 months of age. In younger infants, especially those less than 3 months of age, the diagnosis is often made on the basis of a lumbar puncture performed because of fever, lethargy, poor feeding, or excessive irritibility. Serious signs such as seizures, coma, paresis, sensory deficits, or cranial nerve dysfunction occur in fewer than 5% of patients with aseptic meningitis.

Diagnosis and Management

Aseptic meningitis is a self-limited disease that requires little therapy other than fever control and attention to hydration status. The principal task of the physician is to exclude the more serious, treatable causes of meningitis, primarily pyogenic bacteria, fungi, and tuberculosis.

In most cases of viral meningitis, the CSF white cell count is less than 2000/mm^3 in aseptic meningitis. The WBC differential may show a predominance of polymorphonuclear leukocytes early in the course, but the count very rarely exceeds 90% of the total WBC count, and the characteristic predominance of lymphocytes is seen within 2 to 3 days after onset of illness. The CSF protein does not

often exceed 100 mg/dl and at least one-third of patients have a protein concentration that falls in the normal range of less than 45 mg/dl. The CSF glucose concentration may be low in a minority of patients but very rarely falls below 20 mg/dl. Gram's stain and culture of the CSF for bacteria, and tests for bacterial antigens in CSF, blood, and urine show negative results.

Although viral meningitis can usually be separated from bacterial meningitis on the basis of these laboratory studies, the clinician inevitably encounters patients in which the distinction cannot be made with comfort. This is especially true when the ill child has received oral antibiotics prior to the diagnostic lumbar puncture, possibly reducing the chance of obtaining a positive CSF culture if the patient has bacterial meningitis. Even though the other CSF values are rarely obscured by prior antibiotic therapy, most pediatricians choose a conservative path and treat with a full course of antibiotics.

In previously untreated cases of suspected viral meningitis in patients who (1) are less than 12 months old, (2) are toxic appearing, or (3) have any CSF values that suggest bacterial meningitis, antibiotics should be administered until the CSF bacterial cultures are reported negative, usually at 48 to 72 hours. Other patients may be observed in hospital without administration of antibiotics. Frequently, a second lumbar puncture is performed on untreated patients 6 to 12 hours after the first to ensure that the CSF has evolved towards a "viral" profile. This strategy has the advantage of allowing early discharge for those children with clear evidence of viral meningitis.

Prognosis

The prognosis of viral meningitis is generally considered good, although about 5% of children will experience acute neurologic complications or require prolonged hospitalization. Long-term neurologic sequelae are not thought to be a problem, except perhaps for a minority of infants who become infected very early in life (*i.e.*, at less than 12 months of age).

OTHER TYPES OF MENINGITIS

Tuberculous meningitis

Mycobacterium tuberculosis is a rare cause of meningitis, but important because the diagnosis is often difficult or altogether unsuspected, and because specific treatment is life saving. Tuberculous (TB) meningitis is predominantly a disease of young children, occurring when the meninges are seeded by tubercule bacilli during the bacillemia of primary tuberculous infection. CNS infection results in both a vasculitis with ischemia, infarction, and cerebal edema and also in progressive meningeal inflammation, which is often most marked at the base of the brain, involving the cranial nerves. Early clinical symptoms are often nonspecific; signs indicative of CNS involvement such as meningismus, alterations of mental status, and cranial nerve palsies develop insidiously. The diagnosis is further confounded by the observation that only half of children with TB meningitis will have a chest x-ray suggestive of pulmonary tuberculosis, and the tuberculin skin test (PPD) may be negative in 25% to 50% of children. Recent studies indicate that prolonged therapy with isoniazid and rifampin is as effective as strategies that employ more than two drugs, when there is little risk that the organisms have primary drug resistance. Even with treatment, mortality rates of 30% to 40% are common, and residual neurologic abnormalities are frequent.

Fungal meningitis

Fungal meningitis is largely limited to newborn infants and children who are severely debilitated or immunocompromised. *Candida* sp. and *Cryptococcus neoformans* are the most common fungi that cause meningitis. Although treatment with antifungal agents such as amphoteracin B and 5-fluorocytosine are useful, the outcome of fungal meningitis often depends on the status and the management of the underlying illness.

BIBLIOGRAPHY

Lepow ML, Carver DH, Wright HT et al: A clinical, epidemiologic and laboratory investigation of aseptic meningitis during the four-year period, 1955–1958. N Engl J Med 266:1181–1187, 1962

Lepow ML, Coyne N, Thompson LB et al: A clinical, epidemiologic and laboratory investigation of aseptic meningitis during the four-year period, 1955–1958. N Engl J Med 266:1188–1193, 1962

Smith DH, Ingram DL, Smith AL et al: Bacterial meningitis. Pediatrics 52:586–600, 1973

Swartz MN, Dodge PR: Bacterial meningitis—A review of selected aspects. N Engl J Med 272:725–731, 779–787, 842–848, 898—902, 954–960, 1003–1010, 1965

Wilfert CM, Nusinoff Lehrman S, Katz SL: Enteroviruses and meningitis. Pediatr Infect Dis 2:333–341, 1983

24

Pneumonia is one of the more common problems seen by the pediatric practitioner, being recognized annually in 30 to 40 per 1000 children from 1 to 5 years of age and in slightly lower numbers in younger and older children. Both bacterial and nonbacterial infectious agents are common causes of pneumonia, the former causing an estimated 10% to 30% of cases in normal children. Noninfectious causes such as aspiration and hydrocarbon ingestion must also be considered in many settings. Both bacterial and nonbacterial pneumonias often occur simultaneously with other forms of acute lower respiratory tract disease, including bronchiolitis and laryngotracheobronchitis (croup). In practice, it is often difficult to differentiate bacterial from nonbacterial pneumonia in children, particularly in an outpatient setting; moreover, most childhood pneumonias are managed without a specific laboratory diagnosis.

The etiologic spectrum of childhood pneumonia is strongly influenced by age and by host factors such as prematurity, congenital anomalies, hereditary diseases, and acquired immunodeficiency disorders.

PNEUMONIA IN NORMAL INFANTS AND CHILDREN

Nonbacterial Pneumonias

At least 70% of normal children with pneumonia are infected by respiratory viruses, *Mycoplasma pneumoniae,* or *Chlamydia trachomatis.* The virus most commonly associated with childhood pneumonia is respiratory syncytial virus (RSV), although pneumonia is well known to occur in the course of infection with parainfluenza viruses (especially type 3), influenza A and B viruses, rhinoviruses, adenoviruses, enteroviruses, and measles virus. Studies looking specifically at the etiology of pneumonia have demonstrated two or more pathogens in a substantial number of young children.

Chlamydia trachomatis is an important cause of pneumonia in children 1 to 3 months of age. Transmission of this agent to children occurs exclusively *via* the maternal genital tract at parturition, and thus chlamydial respiratory disease is limited to this narrow age-group. Nonetheless, *Chlamydia tracho-*

matis accounts for 30% to 50% of lower respiratory tract disease in this age-group. The clinical picture of chlamydial pneumonia in this age-group is rather distinctive, with onset of a dry cough at 3 to 6 weeks of age, tachypnea, lack of fever, eosinophilia, hypergammaglobulinemia, and hyperexpansion of the lungs on chest x-ray with a variable degree of perihilar and interstitial infiltration. Although the illness is generally mild and self-limited, as many as 25% of infants will have illness severe enough to require hospitalization. Treatment with erythromycin or a sulfa-containing antibiotic for 14 days seems to limit the duration of symptoms.

RSV is the most common cause of pneumonia in children under 5 years of age. Although RSV has been recovered in all seasons, disease due to RSV reaches epidemic proportions in temperate climates each year between December and February. Infants under 6 months of age are most severely affected, with a rate of hospitalization for bronchiolitis and pneumonia of 5 per 1000. Onset of pneumonia with RSV and other respiratory viruses usually follows a brief prodrome of coryza, fever, and refusal to feed normally. Examination reveals tachypnea, productive cough, fever, nasal flaring, congestion, wheezing, and retractions. Apnea and cyanosis may be apparent in very young infants. The chest x-ray in younger infants shows hyperexpansion with air trapping, streaky perihilar infiltration, and patchy areas of consolidation or atelectasis in both lungs. Lobar consolidation and pleural effusions may occur, but their presence should raise the possibility of a bacterial pneumonia. Arterial blood gas determination in hospitalized infants inevitably indicates some degree of oxygen desaturation. The course of infants hospitalized with viral pneumonia is variable; severe cases may require several weeks for complete resolution. Overall mortality for hospitalized infants is 1% to 2%, but infants with chronic pulmonary disease (*i.e.*, bronchopulmonary dysplasia) or congenital heart disease with increased pulmonary blood flow may have considerably higher mortality. Postmortem examination of infants dying of viral pneumonia shows destruction of the ciliated epithelium of small airways and mononuclear inflammatory infiltration of the alveolar and peribronchial interstitial spaces.

Adenoviruses are responsible for 5% to 10% of childhood pneumonias. A particularly severe type of lower respiratory tract illness characterized pathologically by necrosis of bronchiolar epithelium is associated with adenovirus types 3, 4, 7, and 21. Survivors of necrotizing bronchiolitis may develop chronic obstructive pulmonary disease due to fibrosis of small airways.

Mycoplasma pneumoniae infections occur at all ages but become an increasingly important relative to other pathogens after age 5. Beyond age 10, mycoplasma accounts for 30% to 50% of all pneumonia cases. Mycoplasma spreads slowly but thoroughly within households, but transmission without such close contact is much less likely. Studies have shown that about 80% of children become infected when exposed to close family members who are ill, and as many as 70% of infected children so exposed will develop symptoms. Mycoplasma produce disease by adherence to the surface membranes of columnar respiratory epithelial cells. Clinical pneumonia is recognized in as many as 3% to 10% of infected persons. Gradual onset of fever, malaise, and headache is characteristic, with a nonproductive cough appearing 2 to 5 days later. Rales, rhonchi, and diminished breath sounds on examination indicate the presence of pneumonia; other findings may include pharyngitis, cervical adenopathy, and otitis. Some patients have extrapulmonary manifestations of mycoplasma infection, including rash, joint involvement, neurologic manifestations, and mild hemolytic anemia. Chest x-ray findings are variable. Unilateral lower lobe infiltration is the rule, with patchy areas of consolidation or atelectasis. Pleural effusions can be seen in approximately 20% of patients with a lateral decubitus film. Slow recovery over a 3 to 4-week period is the rule. Treatment with erythromycin or tetracycline enhances resolution of symptoms, although not dramatically. Patients with sickle cell disease, B-cell immunodeficiency, and chronic cardiac or pulmonary diseases may have especially severe and prolonged infections.

Bacterial Pneumonia

Pyogenic bacteria account for less than one-third of pneumonia cases in children. Most bacterial pneumonias acquired by normal children are caused by one of three organisms: *Streptococcus pneumoniae* (pneumococcus), *Haemophilus influenzae* type B, and *Staphylococcus aureus*. Rare cases are caused by group A streptococci, meningococci, anaerobes, *Legionella* sp., and *Klebsiella pneumoniae*. Bacterial pneumonia is most common in the cold-weather months. Attack rates are highest in the first year of life after the expected decline in passively acquired maternal antibody, which protects against pneumococci and *H. influenzae* during the first 2 to 4 months of life.

The mechanism of transmission and development of invasive pneumonia by pyogenic bacteria is not completely understood, in part because these organisms are often found in the upper respiratory tract of healthy children. Presumably, pneumonia results from aspiration of small amounts of saliva containing the organism. Many cases of bacterial pneumonia follow an antecedent viral infection of the upper respiratory tract, which may temporarily alter local and cellular host defenses.

The pathologic hallmark of bacterial pneumonia is segmental or lobar consolidation and acute, inflammatory infiltration of alveolar spaces of the involved segment. Clinically, disease is manifest by abrupt onset of fever, chest pain, dyspnea, cough and tachypnea. Unlike adults young children may not produce large amounts of sputum. Physical examination will generally reveal some signs of respiratory disress, splinting, and decreased breath sound over the involved lung.

Streptococcus pneumoniae remains the most common cause of bacterial pneumonia at all ages. Of the 84 known serotypes, types 1, 3, 6, 7, 14, 18, 19, and 23 are the most common cause of pneumonia in children, which differs slightly from the spectrum of serotypes that cause pneumonia in adults. Pleural effusion occurs in a minority of cases that may or may not contain viable pneumococci; frank empyema is now unusual, and pneumatocele formation is quite rare. Positive blood cultures occur in 30% to 50% of children and are associated with more severe disease. Abrupt resolution with appropriate antibiotic therapy is the rule, but prolonged courses occur, especially with extensive lung involvement and empyema. Pericarditis, meningitis, endocarditis, arthritis, and bursitis are unusual conplications. The mortality in children is approximately 10%; there is little or no residual impairment of lung function.

Haemophilus influenzae type B causes disease that is clinically and radiographically indistinguishable from pneumococcal pneumonia, is nearly as common as pneumococcal pneumonia in children under 2 years of age. Blood cultures are positive in 75% to 90%, and 40% to 75% will have accompanying pleural effusions. Importantly, 10% to 30% of children with pneumonia due to *H. influenzae* type B also have purulent meningitis, epiglottitis, or other site of infection. Counterimmunoelectrophoresis or latex agglutination tests for *H. influenzae*, type B capsular (PRP) antigen should be performed on the serum and urine of all young children with suspected bacterial pneumonia. Mortality is 5% to 10%.

Staphylococcus aureus is an uncommon but important cause of pneumonia, especially in infants less than 6 months of age. Staphylococcal pneumonia initially presents like other types of pneumonia, but characteristically progresses rapidly to pneumatocele formation and empyema, even in the presence of appropriate antibiotic therapy. Although recovery of staphylococci from the blood occurs in only 10% of infants, organisms are usually present in large numbers in a gram-stained tracheal aspirate. Mortality due to staphylococcal pneumonia is significant, and recovery may take weeks.

Diagnosis and Management. The history, physical examination, complete blood count (CBC), and chest x-ray remain the cornerstones of evaluation of the child with suspected pneumonia. The diagnosis of chlamydial pneumonia is often suspected on the basis of characteristic signs in the 1 to 3-month-old infant. Otherwise, the differentiation between viral, mycoplasma, and bacterial pneumonia is less often clear. A specific diagnosis of viral pneumonia is best made by virus culture of a nasopharyngeal aspirate, or by FA or enzyme immunoassay where these techniques are available. The diagnosis of mycoplasma infection requires recovery of the organism on special cell-free media, a process that may require up to 3 weeks, or a fourfold rise in specific antibody titers.

Because young children with pneumonia do not produce sputum readily, the time-honored methods of sputum Gram's stain and culture used to diagnose adult bacterial pneumonias are often unrewarding for the pediatrician. A specimen obtained by tracheal aspiration *via* direct laryngoscopy is usually feasible in hospitalized infants; these specimens are best interpreted when *both* Gram's stain and culture are performed on the same specimen. Blood culture and pleural effusion specimens obtained by thoracentesis should be obtained from all children ill enough to be hospitalized. Although not widely performed, a direct needle aspiration of a consolidated lobe is practical for seriously ill children who do not have a

bleeding disorder or other contraindication. Adjunctive laboratory tests on serum, including C reactive protein and specific antigen detection tests (*i.e.*, latex agglutination or CIE) for pneumococcal and *H. influenzae* type B antigens are also helpful. All children with pneumonia should have a purified protein derivative (PPD) skin test applied.

For children who are hospitalized, attention should first be directed to stabilization of vital signs and symptomatic care. This will often include administration of humidified oxygen by mask, or by intubation and positive pressure ventilation for children with severe arterial hypoxemia or respiratory failure (*i.e.*, $pCO_2 > 50$ torr). Pleural effusions may be drained by needle aspiration alone, but purulent empyema fluid generally requires the surgical placement of a thoracotomy tube. Antibiotics are usually administered intravenously to hospitalized children. The initial choice should be a drug combination of drugs that will cover each of the common pathogens (*i.e.*, pneumococci, *H. influenzae*, and *Staphylococcus aureus*). We recommend cefuroxime or a combination or nafcillin and chloramphenicol.

Many children with pneumonia do not require hospitalization. Although most children treated as outpatients are likely to have viral or mycoplasma pneumonia, most physicians prefer to administer oral antibiotics. Erythromycin is probably the drug of choice, especially for children over 5 years of age. The pediatrician must keep in mind that a small percentage of pneumococci are resistant to erythromycin.

NEONATAL PNEUMONIA

The group B streptococcus is the dominant cause of pneumonia in the first month of life, but *Haemophilus influenzae, E. coli, Listeria monocytogenes, Staphlyococcus aureus,*

Pseudomonas aeruginosa, and *Streptococcus pneumoniae* also cause occasional cases. These organisms are usually acquired from the mother during parturition, but also occur as nosocomial pathogens acquired from the hospital environment. In either case, prematurity, maternal amnionitis, and perinatal distress are significant risk factors for development of neonatal pneumonia.

Group B streptococcal pneumonia occurs in the setting of "early-onset" sepsis with this organism in infants during the first 5 days of life. Infected infants are often severely ill with meningitis, generalized sepsis, and hypotension. The pneumonia of group B streptococcal sepsis is clinically and radiologically similar to respiratory distress syndrome, with marked tachypnea, apnea, hypoxia, diffuse pulmonary opacification, and air bronchograms. The mortality of this disease is as high as 50%.

PNEUMONIA IN ABNORMAL AND IMMUNOCOMPROMISED CHILDREN

Certain congenital anatomical defects, inherited diseases, severe mental retardation, coma, and congenital and acquired immune deficient states each are associated with an increased risk of pneumonia, often with pathogens that pose no risk to normal children.

Congenital Abnormalities and Severe Central Nervous System Deficiency

Aspiration of oral and upper pharyngeal secretions into the lower airway may lead to pneumonia in infants with congenital anomalies such as cleft palate or tracheoesophageal fistula, or in children with weakness or paresis of pharyngeal musculature such as those with muscular dystrophy, seizure disorders, severe motor retardation, or coma. In these cases, bacteria that inhabit the oral cavity (mixed aerobic and anaerobic bacteria) are usually the causitive agents, and lung abscess formation is a common sequela. Treatment with penicillin or erythromycin is generally sufficient in these cases.

Congenital and Acquired Immune Deficiency States

Pneumonia is one of the most common infections occurring in children with congenital immunodeficiency syndromes (*i.e.,* congenital agammaglobulinemia, severe combined immune deficiency, DiGeorge syndrome) and with acquired immune deficiency states such as corticosteroid therapy, chemotherapy for malignancy, or pharmacologic immunosuppression for organ transplantation. A wide range of opportunistic viral, fungal, bacterial, and protozoan pathogens causes pneumonia in these patients, which, unfortunately, is a common cause of severe morbidity and death.

BIBLIOGRAPHY

Chartrand S, McCracken G: Staphylococcal pneumonia in infants and children. Pediatr Infect Dis 1:19, 1982

Denny F, Clyde W, Glezen W: Mycoplasma pneumoniae disease: Clinical spectrum, pathophysiology, epidemiology, and control. J Pediatr Dis 123:74, 1971

Dworsky M, Stagno S: Newer agents causing pneumonitis in early infancy. Pediatr Infect Dis 1:188, 1982

Ginsburg C, Howard J, Nelson J: Report of 65 cases of *Haemophilus influenzae* B pneumonia. Pediatrics 64:283, 1979

Long S: Treatment of acute pneumonia in infants and children. Pediatr Clin North Am 30:297, 1983

Murphy T, Henderson D, Clyde W et al: Pneumonia: An eleven year study in a pediatric practice. Am J Epidemiol 113:12, 1981

25

Otitis Media

Otitis media refers to inflammation of the epithelium of the middle ear, usually with the presence of fluid in the middle ear cavity. Otitis media represents one of the diseases most commonly diagnosed by pediatricians. The highest incidence is during the first 2 years of life, when approximately two-thirds of all infants experience at least one episode. Otitis media also occurs in high frequency up to 6 years of life, with an overall incidence of 10% to 20% annually. The increased risk of otitis in young children is probably secondary to differences in eustachian tube anatomy and function as well as to the high prevalence of respiratory tract infections in this age-group. Middle ear infections are slightly more common during autumn and winter.

Several types of otitis media are recognized on the basis of clinical or pathologic findings. For the purpose of this chapter, we will distinguish acute (suppurative) otitis media, chronic otitis media, and serous (or secretory) otitis.

ANATOMY AND PHYSIOLOGY OF THE EUSTACHIAN TUBE AND MIDDLE EAR

The eustachian tube is composed of two contiguous portions joined at a narrow isthmus. The lateral portion, which transverses the

temporal bone, contains the same low cuboidal and squamous epithelium as the middle ear cavity. The anteromedial two-thirds of the tube is supported by cartilage and lined with the columnar epithelial mucosa of the respiratory tract.

The medial orifice of the tube is periodically opened by contraction of the tensor palatini muscle during swallowing, maintaining patency of the tube and allowing for drainage of secretions into the nasopharynx. The patent eustachian tube maintains atmospheric pressure within the middle ear, allowing ventilation of the middle ear cavity and normal mobility of the tympanic membrane.

In young infants, it may be more difficult to maintain normal middle ear ventilation because of the anatomic orientation of the eustachian tube and perhaps because of increased compliance of the tubal wall.

PATHOPHYSIOLOGY OF OTITIS MEDIA

Otitis media begins with impairment of eustachian tube ventilatory function. In the normal child, tubal dysfunction is usually secondary to viral respiratory tract infection, especially with respiratory syncytial virus, influenza viruses, and adenoviruses. Less commonly, tubal dysfunction may be associated with allergic rhinitis. Tubal obstruction results in negative pressure in the middle ear cavity because of absorption of O_2 and CO_2 into surrounding mucosal capillaries and subsequent transudation of serous fluid into the middle ear leading to *serous otitis*. Progressive serous otitis is characterized by metaplasia of the mucosa, a thick, mucoid middle ear effusion, and, sometimes, the presence of inflammatory cells.

When pathogenic bacteria are present in the nasopharynx, *acute suppurative otitis* may develop as a result of serous fluid accumulation, poor drainage through the obstructed eustachian tube, and, possibly, aspiration of nasopharyngeal secretions into the middle ear during intermittant opening of the tube. When children with suspected acute otitis have undergone diagnostic tympanocentesis, pathogenic bacteria are recovered in about two-thirds of cases. *Streptococcus pneumoniae* is the most common pathogen, accounting for about 65% to 75% of isolates. *Haemophilus influenzae* (usually nontypeable strains) and *Brahmanella catarrhalis* are each recovered from 5% to 25% of cases, and *Staphylococcus aureus, Staphylococcus epidermidis*, group A streptococci, gram-negative bacilli, and anaerobic bacteria represent unusual isolates. More than one bacterial pathogen is sometimes cultured. Although several types of viruses have been recovered from the middle ear fluid of children with acute otitis, it is unlikely that they are a direct cause of suppurative otitis.

Bottle-feeding of infants in a supine position is known to predispose to development of acute otitis because of reflux of nasopharyngeal secretions into the middle ear during swallowing. Otherwise, children with cleft palate, hypertrophied adenoids, dental malocclusion, and Down's syndrome are quite susceptible to tubal dysfunction and thus are at risk of recurrent or persistent otitis media.

Newborn infants who require assisted ventilation *via* a nasotracheal tube have a very high risk of otitis media. Several small scale studies suggest that otitis occurring in infants requiring intensive care is often secondary to *S. aureus* or to gram-negative enteric bacilli. In contrast, when otitis occurs in normal infants less than 6 weeks of age, the pathogens are more likely to be the same as those that cause otitis media in older infants and children.

ACUTE OTITIS MEDIA

Clinical Features

The most common symptoms of acute otitis media are fever and ear pain (otalgia). Fever is present in at about 50% of children with acute otitis; younger children and patients with otitis due to *S. pneumoniae* are more likely to be febrile. Otalgia is localized to one or both ears (approximately 40% of children with acute otitis media have bilateral involvement) and may be accentuated by swallowing. Children with severe otalgia may experience sudden relief with perforation of the tympanic membrane. Depending on the age of the child one may observe fretfulness, pulling at the involved ear(s), vomiting, malaise, diminished appetite. Unilateral or bilateral hearing loss occurs, but is often not appreciated by either the child or the parents. Vestibular symptoms may occasionally be present.

The diagnosis of acute otitis media rests on examination of the tympanic membrane with the pneumatic otoscope. The external canal of young children is often partially or completely occluded by cerumen, which must be cleared for an adequate examination by irrigation or with an ear curette. In acute suppurative otitis, the tympanic membrane is usually thickened, red, and dull with little or no light reflex. A fluid level may be visible behind the membrane, and bullae occasionally will be found on the membrane. Bulging of the membrane, present in about half of cases, is a specific sign of acute otitis. Similarly, perforation of the membrane with a seropurulent or purulent drainage is found in about 20% of cases of suppurative otitis. When the pneumatic otoscope is used, diminished mobility of the membrane is the most discrete sign of middle ear effusion but does not distinguish acute suppurative otitis media from other types of otitis media.

When available in an outpatient setting, electroacoustic impedance testing (tympanometry) is a very useful method of determining the compliance of the tympanic membrane.

Although most cases of acute otitis media are managed without a specific bacteriologic diagnosis, diagnostic tympanocentesis can provide important information in some clinical situations, including otitis in a sick neonate or immunocompromised child, otitis complicated by mastoiditis or intracranial infection, and otitis that fails to respond to conventional treatment.

Treatment

Placebo-controlled studies have proven that at least 60% to 75% of cases of untreated acute otitis media resolve within 10 to 14 days. The use of antibiotics that are effective *in vitro* against the common bacterial pathogens produce only marginally better results. More importantly, the use of antibiotics is credited with a dramatic reduction in the occurrence of the suppurative complications of otitis media (see below); this factor defines the major indication for antibiotic therapy of acute otitis media.

Although the conclusions of individual antibiotic trials vary, the combined experience from many studies indicates that essentially equivalent efficacy is shared by several oral agents, including ampicillin, amoxicillin, amoxicillin-clavulanate, trimethoprim-sulfisoxazole, and the combination of either penicillin or erythromycin estolate with a sulfonamide. In most cases, these antibiotics are administered orally for 10 days. The oral cephalosporins, cephalexin and cefaclor, are probably less effective overall. Despite the increasing number of *H. influenzae* and *B. catarrhalis* isolates that produce β-lactamase, there is no evidence that use of a β-lactamase-susceptible agent, such as amoxicillin, provides less than optimal therapy for otitis media.

Drainage of the middle ear by myringotomy can be very effective in relieving the severe pain that occasionally accompanies acute otitis media. Decongestants and antihistamines are often prescribed but appear to have little or no efficacy. Their use should be discouraged for most children.

Prognosis

Even with adequate antibiotic therapy, 20% to 30% of children continue to have an abnormal tympanic membrane when reexamined 14 days later, and a smaller number will continue to have some symptoms of otitis. Furthermore, 6% to 8% of children suffer a relapse of acute otitis within 6 weeks of the first episode. Failure of primary therapy and recurrences are often attributed to inadequate treatment secondary to poor compliance.

Hearing loss in varying degrees represents the major long-term morbidity of acute otitis media. Although deafness and language delay have been associated with a single episode of otitis, the risk is greater with recurrent episodes and with chronic otitis.

CHRONIC OTITIS MEDIA

A minority of infants and children with acute otitis will experience frequent recurrences or chronic otitis media, which is associated with a much higher degree of hearing loss and with suppurative complications. Children with anatomic or immunologic defects and children who are poorly compliant with antibiotic therapy of acute otitis are more susceptible to chronic otitis. Persistent or intermittant suppurative otorrhea is often observed with chronic otitis. The bacterial pathogens recovered from children with chronic otitis are often the same as those with acute otitis, but *Staphylococcus aureus, S. epidermidis*, and anaerobic bacteria are also found, sometimes in mixed culture. Bacteriologic identification of the infecting organism(s), surgical drainage of the middle ear, and long-term antibiotic therapy (sometimes with parenteral antibiotics) are the basis for management of chronic otitis.

Complications of Chronic Otitis

Permanent hearing loss is an unfortunate sequela of many cases of chronic otitis because of fibrosis or destruction of the tympanic membrane or necrosis of the auditory ossicles. Hearing loss may also result from a *cholesteatoma*, an expanding epidermal cyst that forms from growth of epidermis from the external canal into the middle ear *via* a perforation in the tympanic membrane.

Occasional unilateral facial palsies are seen with both acute and chronic otitis because of inflammation of the 7th nerve as it traverses the fallopian canal of the temporal bone. Gradenigo's syndrome represents ipsilateral involvement of the 6th nerve and the ophthalmic and maxillary divisions of the 5th nerve secondary to *petrositis*, an inflammatory condition of the pneumatized areas of the apical portions of the temporal bone.

Labyrinthitis is accompanied by severe nausea, vomiting, complete loss of hearing, and lack of caloric responses. Both acute and chronic *mastoiditis* can accompany otitis and can, in turn, lead to any of several serious

intracranial complications, including meningitis, brain abscess, epidural abscess, lateral sinus thrombosis, otitic hydrocephalus (secondary to lateral or sagittal sinus thrombosis), and (very rarely) cavernous sinus thrombosis.

SEROUS OTITIS MEDIA

The presence of serous or mucoid exudate in the middle ear distinguishes secretory otitis from acute or chronic suppurative otitis. Otherwise, the difference between these entities is often difficult to discern: Obstruction of the eustachian tube is a common underlying factor, the clinical and physical findings do not always predict the type of middle ear exudate, pathogenic bacteria are sometimes found in serous otitis media, and the two types of middle ear disease often occur as part of a continuum in the same patient. Despite the nosologic confusion, it is often clinically useful to distinguish serous otitis from other types of otitis media.

The most common presenting complaint is hearing loss. Younger children may exhibit a poor attention span or apparent disobedience, whereas older children may complain of hearing loss, earache, tinnitus, and bubbling or popping noises in the ear. Diminished mobility of the tympanic membrane is the most common physical finding. Usually the membrane is also retracted and discolored with loss of the normal luster and the wedge-shaped light reflex. A conductive hearing loss may be demonstrated with the tuning fork (Rinne test) or by an audiogram.

The natural history of untreated serous otitis is poorly understood. The precise risk of permanent hearing loss is unknown but appears to be low. Recent prospective studies suggest that young children with prolonged or recurrent middle ear effusions experience delays in language acquisition that are proportional to the duration of the effusion in the first years of life.

In addition, there is considerable uncertainty about what constitutes effective therapy. Initially, the physician may elect to observe only or to prescribe a short course of decongestants or antihistamines, recognizing that such agents are of questionable efficacy. Most experts suggest a trial of antibiotics as well, since infection probably plays a significant role in some cases of serous otitis.

In cases where the middle ear effusion persists beyond 2 or 3 months or where significant degrees of hearing loss are demonstrated, then surgical drainage of the middle ear by myringotomy with or without placement of tympanostomy tubes is often performed to ventilate the middle year. Despite the widespread popularity of tympanostomy tube placement, there are no convincing data, pro or con, that tube placement alters the natural history of serous otitis media.

BIBLIOGRAPHY

Henderson FW, Collier AM, Sanyal MA et al: A longitudinal study of respiratory viruses and bacteria in the etiology of acute otitis media with effusion. N. Engl J Med 306:1377–1383, 1982

Howie V, Ploussard JH, Lester RL: Otitis media: A clinical and bacteriological review. Pediatrics 45:29–35, 1970

Paradise JL: Otitis media in infants and children. Pediatrics 65:917–943, 1980

Rowe DS: Acute suppurative otitis media. Pediatrics 56:285–294, 1975

Senturia BH: Classification of middle ear effusions. Ann Otol Rhinol Laryngol 79:358–370, 1970

26

Streptococcal Infections

The β-hemolytic streptococci are among the most common and most important bacterial pathogens of children. The focus of this chapter is the group A streptococci *(Streptococcus pyogenes)*, which commonly cause infections of the upper respiratory tract and skin, as well as scarlet fever and other less common infections. Although most group A streptococcal infections respond promptly to treatment with a variety of antibiotics, the principal goal of therapy is the prevention of serious nonsuppurative complications, especially acute rheumatic fever.

CLASSIFICATION OF THE STREPTOCOCCI

The streptococci are facultatively anaerobic, gram-positive cocci that grow in chains in laboratory culture. They are traditionally classified according to the type of hemolysis produced by extracellular enzymes that diffuse into the blood agar medium around the growing bacterial colony, which is either a greenish zone (alpha [α]), a clear zone (beta [β]), or lack of hemolysis (gamma [γ]). The α-hemolytic streptococci and nonhemolytic streptococci are sometimes referred to as viridans streptococci. They are subclassified into at least six species according to various biochemical reactions. Viridans streptococci are normal inhabitants of the upper respiratory tract and rarely cause disease except for subacute bacterial endocarditis. They also have an important role in the production of dental caries.

The β-hemolytic streptococci are subdivided according to Lancefield's method, which is based on the antigenic composition of the cell wall carbohydrate. Serogroups A through H and K through U have been distinguished, but only groups A, B, C, D, and G are recognized as definitely causing human disease. Parenthetically, it should be noted that some streptococcal strains, especially those with group D antigen, may be α-hemolytic or nonhemolytic.

Group A streptococci can be further subtyped by antigenic differences in the M protein and T protein, which are cell wall constituents. Characterization of the M protein and T protein type has proven very useful in epidemiologic studies of the group A streptococci.

VIRULENCE FACTORS ASSOCIATED WITH GROUP A STREPTOCOCCI

Laboratory research conducted over many years has identified several bacterial products that contribute to the pathogenicity of group A streptococci. The bacterial cell contains several structural (somatic) components that are independently associated with virulence. These include the capsular hyaluronic acid and cell wall M protein, which each inhibits ingestion by host phagocytes, and the cell wall lipoteichoic acid, which plays a role in adherence of the organism to host epithelial cells. M protein is antigenic, and opsonic antibody against M protein confers long-lasting immunity to M subtype identical strains. Strains without M protein are not virulent. There are at least 61 M types, some of which are specifically associated with poststreptococcal acute glomerulonephritis.

Group A streptococci also produce many extracellular products that contribute to virulence, including erythrogenic toxin (four known types), streptolysin O, streptolysin S, streptokinase, hyaluronidase, and several deoxyribonucleases. Hyaluronidase, streptokinase, and the deoxyribonucleases promote spread of streptococci through connective tissues. Erythrogenic toxin, which is antigenic, is the mediator of the skin rash that occurs with scarlet fever. Streptolysin O is a cytotoxic mediator, which is produced by all strains of group A streptococci, as well as some strains of group C and group G streptococci.

EPIDEMIOLOGY OF STREPTOCOCCAL INFECTIONS

Group A streptococcal colonization of the upper respiratory tract is more prevalent in the winter and spring, while skin colonization is facilitated by a moist, warm climate. Person-to-person transmission is responsible for most disease, and outbreaks within families, schools, and other institutions are well documented. Direct transmission, occurring by direct contact or by spread of large airborne droplets, is favored by crowding and by poor hygienic conditions. Although asymptomatic carriage is common, the relative role of carriers in the transmission of group A streptococci is uncertain. Acutely infected persons harbor a greater number of organisms and appear to be more efficient in transmitting infection.

Most streptococcal infections occur between 3 and 12 years of age. The peak age for group A streptococcal pharyngitis occurs during the early school years. Pharyngitis occurring prior to age 3 years is usually viral in origin, but unusual cases are attributed to streptococci. Furthermore, streptococcal infections of the upper respiratory tract in infants during the first few years of life are sometimes characterized by the syndrome of "streptococcosis," which is described below. Streptococcal pyoderma typically occurs in preschool-aged children, but may be seen at any age. Interestingly, the M serotypes of streptococcal strains associated with pyoderma usually differ from those recovered from children with pharyngitis. The biological basis for this phenomenon is unknown.

CLINICAL FEATURES OF GROUP A STREPTOCOCCAL INFECTION

Pharyngitis

The classic symptoms of streptococcal pharyngitis include abrupt onset of fever, sore throat, headache, and sometimes nausea and vomiting. Some patients experience milder symptoms, and asymptomatic infections are well documented. On physical examination, injection, erythema, and edema of the oropharyngeal mucosa are present in association with a purulent, adherent exudate on the tonsils and sometimes on the posterior wall of the pharynx. Enlarged, tender anterior cervical adenopathy is a sign that may be helpful in distinguishing group A streptococcal pharyngitis from pharyngitis caused by viruses or mycoplasmae.

The *diagnosis* of streptcoccal pharyngitis may be problematic. The detection of group A streptococci in the upper respiratory tract does not always indicate infection because the asymptomatic carriage rate can be 10% to 25% in school-aged children, particularly in the winter and spring. In fact, only about one-half of patients with pharyngitis who harbor group A streptococci in their upper respiratory tracts will demonstrate an immune response indicative of true infection.

Nonetheless, the clinical diagnostic standard is the throat swab cultured on a sheep blood agar plate in the office, clinic, or laboratory. Incubation in a reduced oxygen environment will enhance the recovery of streptococci, and the use of a bacitracin disk on the plate allows reliable differentiation of group A streptococci from aother β-hemolytic bacteria. Although the throat culture represents the standard of sensitivity by which other methods are judged, it requires 1 to 2 days of incubation, sometimes delaying timely therapy. The recent introduction of inexpensive, commercially available kits that detect the group A cell wall carbohydrate antigen on throat swabs now provides an alternative method for the office diagnosis of streptococcal pharyngitis that can be performed in less than 1 hour. When compared with culture, the antigen detection methods are highly specific (very few false-positive results) and have a reported sensitivity of 77% to 95%.

The demonstration of an acute rise in antibody to one or more of the extracellular products of the group A streptococcus is a more specific means of indicating true infection. Elevated antistreptolysin O (ASLO) antibodies can be demonstrated in about 80% of patients with streptococcal pharyngitis, and use of additional tests for other streptococcal antibodies increases the sensitivity to more than 95%. These serologic tests are often very useful in demonstrating recent group A streptococcal infection in patients suspected of having acute rheumatic fever, and they are also helpful in clinical and epidemiologic investigations of streptococcal disease. Serologic tests are rarely helpful in the management of acute streptococcal pharyngitis.

Most children with group A streptococcal pharyngitis become asymptomatic in 3 to 5 days without therapy. Even though *antibiotic treatment* appears to shorten the duration of illness and to reduce transmission of infection to others, the major goal of therapy is prevention of suppurative complications and acute rheumatic fever. Untreated, serologically proven group A streptococcal pharyngitis is associated with a subsequent attack rate of acute rheumatic fever of 0.4%.

The traditional standard of therapy is a single intramuscular injection of the combination of procaine penicillin (300,000 units) with benzathine penicillin (900,000 units), which eradicates the organism from the oropharynx in more than 90% of treated cases. Over the years, many practitioners have preferred to prescribe a 10-day course of oral penicillin V in a dose of 250 mg given twice a day (bid), a regimen demonstrated to have efficacy equivalent to intramuscular (IM) penicillin when given in adequate dosage to the compliant patient. Oral erythromycin estolate (20 to 40 mg/kg/day bid–qid) is the traditional alternative for the penicillin-allergic patient, and clindamycin is also an acceptable alternative. Early studies showed that acute rheumatic fever could be prevented when therapy with either IM penicillin or oral antibiotic therapy was initiated within 9 days of onset of symptoms.

In recent years, the primacy of oral penicillin V has been questioned. Several investigators have found a higher rate of bacteriologic and clinical failures with oral penicillin V than with an oral cephalosporin alone (cephalexin, cefadroxil) or rifampin combined with penicillin V. The reasons for the occasional failure of oral penicillin to treat group A streptococcal pharyngitis effectively are unknown, but some have suggested that either some strains have developed tolerance to penicillin (*i.e.*, are more difficult to kill *in vitro*) or that the presence of β-lactamase-producing bacteria such as *Staphylococcus aureus* or *Branhamella catarrhalis* interferes locally with the activity of penicillin. It also has been suggested that many treatment "failures" occur in children who are merely carriers, and that group A streptococci are more difficult to eradicate from children who are carriers than from children with actual infection. Currently, there are no data to suggest that IM benzathine penicillin is less effective than in the past.

Some children experience a relapse of symptoms shortly after antibiotics are discontinued due to persistent infection. Others may appear susceptible to frequent episodes of group A streptococcal pharyngitis. The reader is referred to the works Dillon, Gerber, and Kaplan (see Bibliography) for excellent discussions of the management of these perplexing patients.

Scarlet Fever

The hallmark of scarlet fever is a diffuse, confluent, erythematous rash that occurs as a result of systemic spread of erythrogenic toxin from a focal group A streptococcal infection, usually pharyngitis. The rash involves the entire body, except the palms and soles, and easily blanches when pressure is applied. The patient may have circumoral pallor of the face and exhibit Pastia's lines, which are lines of more intense erythema within the skin folds of flexor surfaces of the extremities that do not blanch with pressure. Examination of the oropharynx reveals a "beefy red" tongue with hypertrophied papillae and a mucosal enanthem with petechiae on the hard and soft palates.

The rash generally persists for 3 to 7 days and is followed by a fine epidermal desquamation. Fortunately, serious complications of scarlet fever are very rare today.

Streptococcal Infections of the Skin

Streptococcal pyoderma (impetigo) is common among children who live in tropical climates and among socioeconomically disadvantaged children during warm weather in temperate climates. Pyoderma begins as one or more papular lesions on an area of exposed skin, which then rapidly develop into pustular lesions with little or no surrounding erythema. The lesions enlarge and form a thin overlying crust. Regional lymphadenopathy is often present, but children with pyoderma do not have fever or other systemic symptoms.

Proper bacterial cultures require removal or "unroofing" of the overlying crust before swabbing the base of the lesion. When this is done, group A streptococci are easily recovered. Staphylococci may also be recovered from cultured lesions, but these bacteria probably do not play a role in the genesis of streptococcal pyoderma (unlike primary staphylococcal pyoderma, which is characterized by bullous lesions with varnish-like crusts and which produces pure cultures of staphylococci on culture). The ASLO antibody response is often weak following streptococcal pyoderma, but a vigorous rise in anti-DNAse B antibody occurs.

The treatment of pyoderma is the same as that for streptococcal pharyngitis. Topical antibiotic therapy is less effective than administration of systemic antibiotics. Unfortunately, prompt treatment does not appear to affect the risk of subsequent acute glomerulonephritis, which is the major nonsuppurative complication of streptococcal pyoderma.

Erysipelas is an acute, inflammatory solitary skin lesion that often begins on the face as a small papule and expands rapidly in a centrifugal manner with raised, red margins at the periphery and central clearing. Fever and chills may occur. Erysipelas may accompany streptococcal pharyngitis and, untreated, usually resolves in 5 to 10 days. Treatment is similar to that for streptococcal pharyngitis.

Blistering dactylitis is well-described streptococcal lesion characterized by bullae on the palmer surfaces of one of the distal phalanges. Streptococcal *cellulitis* may occur in the perianal region in children or as a secondary infection of a wound site or a burn. Infection of the deeper subcutaneous fascia in the form of a *necrotizing fasciitis* can spread very rapidly and terminate fatally if not recognized and managed appropriately.

Other Types of Streptococcal Infecion

A syndrome of mucopurulent nasopharyngitis occurring in children during the first 4 years of life was widely known in the preantibiotic era. *"Streptococcosis"* was often complicated by cervical adenopathy, streptococcal otitis media, and pyoderma. This clinical entity is rarely diagnosed today.

Purpural sepsis is another disease of streptococcal etiology that, fortunately, is now very rare. Group A streptococci sometimes cause *otitis media, sepsis, meningitis, endocarditis*, and *pneumonia*. Streptococcal pneumonia is associated with a high risk of empyema.

DISEASE CAUSED BY OTHER β-HEMOLYTIC STREPTOCOCCI

Several other of the Lancefield serogroups of β-hemolytic streptococci cause human disease. The most important are the group B

streptococci, which are a dominant cause of serious neonatal infections, and the group D streptococci, which are frequently encountered in patients with endocarditis and in patients with a variety of nosocomially acquired infections. Group D enterococci differ from other streptococcal species in their primary resistance to penicillin.

Streptococcal groups C and G are relatively uncommon human pathogens that have been recovered in patients with several types of illness, including pharyngitis, wound infections, endocarditis, and nosocomial infections. Patients with non-group A streptococcal infections are not at risk of acute rheumatic fever.

BIBLIOGRAPHY

Bass JW: Treatment of streptococcal pharyngitis revisited. JAMA 256:740–743, 1986

Dillon HC: Streptococcal pharyngitis in the 1980s. Pediatr Infect Dis J 6:123–130, 1987

Gerber MA, Markowitz M: Management of streptococcal pharyngitis reconsidered. Pediatr Infect Dis J 4:518–526, 1985

Gerber MA, Randolph MF, Chanatry J et al: Antigen detection test for streptococcal pharyngitis: Evaluation of sensitivity with respect to true infections. J Pediatr 108:654–658, 1986

Kaplan EL: The group A streptococcal upper respiratory tract carrier state: An enigma. J Pediatr 97:337–345, 1980

Kaplan EL: Benzathine penicillin G for treatment of group A streptococcal pharyngitis: A reappraisal in 1985. Pediatr Infect Dis J 4:592–596, 1985

Peter G, Smith AL: Group A streptococcal infections of the skin and pharynx. N Engl J Med 297:311–317, 365–370, 1977

27

Musculoskeletal Infections

OSTEOMYELITIS

Osteomyelitis occurs in about 1 in 5000 children, with males affected slightly more often than females. Most bone infections in children present as acute, hematogenously acquired, bacterial osteomyelitis, which generally responds well to antibiotic therapy when treated in a timely manner. Osteomyelitis also occurs with penetrating trauma or following an open wound involving the bone or overlying soft tissues. Chronic osteomyelitis, which occurs as a consequence of inadequately treated osteomyelitis, is an indolent infection requiring thorough surgical débridement, as well as long-term antibiotic therapy. Most osteomyelitis cases are caused by pyogenic bacteria, although bone infection occurs with disseminated infection due to some fungi such as blastomycosis, cryptococcosis, and coccidioidomycosis.

Pathogenesis

In children, bone infection occurs *via* either the hematogenous route, from direct inoculation of bacteria due to trauma, or, less commonly, as a result of spread from a contiguous focus of infection.

With *hematogenously acquired acute osteomyelitis*, the initial bacteremia usually occurs, unrecognized, days to weeks prior to the onset of symptoms. Many children give a history of blunt trauma to the involved extremity, which often seems minor or insignificant, within the week or two preceding onset of symptoms. Antecedent trauma may produce focal hemorrhage or thrombosis, which would be more accommodative to seeding during an unrelated bacteremia than would healthy bone. Acute osteomyelitis is also known to occur at the site of a previous closed fracture.

Infection usually occurs at a single site in the metaphysis of a long bone; the femur and tibia are more often involved than are the humerus and the radius. In children more than 1 or 2 years of age, the spread of infection is limited by the avascular metaphyseal growth plate, the cortex, and the periosteum. Increased pressure enhances necrosis of bone within the infected focus and produces severe pain and tenderness at the site. In the neonate and young infant, infection is more likely to spread into the adjacent joint space through the vascular growth plate and also to penetrate the thinner cortex, resulting in subperiosteal spread along the diaphysis and penetration of the periosteum into surrounding soft tissues.

Staphylococcus aureus is the organism found in approximately 80% of cases in which a bacterial etiology is established. Gram-negative bacilli (10%), group A streptococci (5%), and *Haemophilus influenzae* (2%) are occasional causes of acute osteomyelitis, whereas anaerobic bacteria and *Streptococcus pneumoniae* are rarely found. As many as 5% of cases of acute osteomyelitis are polymicrobial in origin; multiple organisms can be recovered from 30% to 60% of chronic cases. In addition, group B streptococci are a common cause of hematogenous osteomyelitis among infants under 2 months of age.

Penetrating trauma, such as a puncture wound, may introduce bacteria residing on the instrument of trauma (*i.e.*, splinter, nail) or, more commonly, introduce bacteria found on the skin or apparel worn at the time of the injury. For example, the osteochondritis associated with puncture wounds of the foot can be caused by *Pseudomonas aeruginosa*, which has been cultured from the soles of sneakers. Repeated heelsticks in the newborn infant are another cause. Spread of infection from a primary *contiguous* soft tissue focus to bone is a relatively uncommon process in the pediatric age-group, although this mechanism may be responsible for as many as 50% of cases of osteomyelitis in adults.

Chronic osteomyelitis may develop following any of the mechanisms described above, but tends to be more common following trauma. Poorly perfused bone and necrotic bone sequestra contribute to the persistent infection of chronic osteomyelitis.

Clinical Features

Children with acute osteomyelitis usually present with insidious onset of fever and localized pain; ambulatory children with infection in the lower extremity often limp or refuse to bear weight altogether. Younger infants exhibit irritability and refusal to use the involved extremity (*i.e.*, pseudoparalysis). Edema and erythema of the overlying soft tissues may initially lead to an erroneous diagnosis of cellulitis. In neonates, the entire extremity may exhibit a fusiform swelling in which infection extends beyond the periosteum.

Diagnosis. When symptoms have been present for only a few days, conventional radiographs of the involved extremity may be completely normal or may exhibit only subtle soft tissue swelling adjacent to the infected bone. Bone destruction can be demonstrated within 10 to 20 days of onset, often with periosteal elevation and, later, new bone formation. Radionucleotide bone imaging techniques, which are more sensitive than routine radiographs, will often demonstrate abnormally increased activity when the child first presents. However, bone scans may not distinguish infection from other pathologic processes associated with new bone formation (*i.e.*, infarction, traumatic injury).

Once the diagnosis of osteomyelitis is suspected, determination of the specific etiology depends on recovery of the causative organism from cultures of blood or biopsied bone. Blood cultures are positive in approximately 50% of children with acute osteomyelitis at the time of presentation. Even though the diagnostic yield is higher when specimens are taken directly from the involved bone by needle aspiration or surgical débridement, cultures are negative in as many as 20% to 30% of cases. Cultures of drainage from a sinus tract, if present, correlate poorly with cultures taken directly from the infected bone.

Treatment. The initial management of acute osteomyelitis may include both surgical and medical measures. Cure can be effected by antibiotic therapy alone in many cases, but surgical management is necessary if there is extensive necrosis of bone, if subperiosteal or soft tissue abscesses are present, or if débridement is needed for bacteriologic diagnosis. Chronic osteomyelitis always requires thorough débridement of all necrotic bone.

The choice of antibiotics is guided by the information obtained from the history and physical examination and from a Gram's stain of material obtained by needle aspiration or surgical débridement. When the Gram's stain fails to define clearly a pathogenic bacterium, the clinician should proceed empirically, starting intravenous administration of an antibiotic that will cover the most frequently encountered pathogens (*i.e.*, cefuroxime, or a combination of oxacillin and chloramphenicol). An antibiotic with a more narrow spectrum can be substituted when the culture results are reported. When the blood and bone site cultures are reported as "no growth" and assays of serum and urine for bacterial polysaccharide antigens are negative, it is reasonable to treat with an antibiotic that covers *Staphylococcus aureus*, such as a semisynthetic penicillin or a cephalosporin.

Successful management depends on the duration of antibiotic therapy. Traditionally, acute osteomyelitis has been treated with intravenous antibiotics for a minimum of 4 weeks. However, many pediatric centers now use oral antibiotic therapy to complete 4 weeks of therapy in uncomplicated cases of acute osteomyelitis. The change to oral therapy can be made once the patient is afebrile and all signs of inflammation, including bone pain, have resolved. In order to achieve adequate blood levels, high doses of oral antibiotic must be administered (*i.e.*, 100 mg/kg/day of dicloxacillin qid or 30 mg/kg/day of clindamycin qid). Strict compliance with the oral regimen must be ensured before the patient is allowed to leave the hospital, and careful follow-up is mandatory. The erythrocyte sedimentation rate may be followed as a nonspecific indicator of response to therapy.

Prognosis. The outcome for properly managed acute osteomyelitis is extremely good, with a microbiologic cure achieved in more than 90% of cases. The functional result for the involved extremity depends somewhat on the extent of disease at the time of presentation; however, most children with adequately treated osteomyelitis escape serious functional impairment.

Osteomyelitis Secondary to Penetrating Trauma

Osteochondritis of the *os calcaneus* is a relatively common infection that occurs in children following penetrating injury, often a puncture wound through the sole of the foot by a protruding nail or other sharp object. In a typical case, pain, tenderness, and local swelling develop at the site 2 or 3 days after the initial pain from the injury has subsided, but fever and other systemic symptoms are unusual. *Pseudomonas aeruginosa* is the most common organism isolated, but staphylococci and streptococci are sometimes found. Surgical exploration and débridement are the cornerstones of both diagnosis and management. With adequate surgical débridement, most patients can be treated with an intravenous antibiotic (*i.e.*, gentamicin) for 2 to 3 weeks.

In osteomyelitis of the *patella*, another infectious complication of penetrating trauma, x-ray changes may be very slow to appear. *Staphylococcus aureus* is the organism usually found.

Osteomyelitis in Unusual Locations

While most cases of hematogenous osteomyelitis in children occur in one of the long bones, about 10% involve other skeletal locations, such as the pelvic bones, vertebrae, clavicles, and cranium. *Pelvic osteomyelitis* presents with pain that is often localized by the patient to the hip or buttocks, or mimics the pain of appendicitis. A history of limping is often obtained. The most common site for pelvic osteomyelitis is the ilium.

Children and adolescents are vulnerable to *vertebral osteomyelitis* because the vertebral bodies remain well vascularized for the first two decades of life. The presentation is often quite indolent, with little or no fever and only mild complaints of abdominal pain or back pain. Most cases are due to *Staphylococcus aureus.* Rare cases of vertebral infection with gram-negative bacilli occur in association with chronic obstructive uropathies.

Osteomyelitis in Children with Hemoglobinopathies

Bone infection is second only to pneumonia as a cause of infection in children with sickle cell disease and other hemoglobinopathies. In these disorders, infarcted, poorly perfused bone is susceptible to seeding during a transient bacteremia. There is an increased risk of infection at more than one site. For unknown reasons, *Salmonella* species are responsible for about 50% of bone infections in children with hemoglobinopathies; the remainder of cases are due to staphylococci and other organisms.

Differentiating acute osteomyelitis from the more common syndrome of bone pain due to infarction is a difficult clinical challenge. In general, infection is clinically suspected when fever and bone pain persist after hydration and other management of sickle cell crisis. Despite much interest in several methods of radionucleotide imaging, there is no entirely reliable means of establishing the presence or lack of infection. Because recovery of an organism is important in management, we continue to encourage early needle biopsy or open biopsy in sickle cell patients with suspected osteomyelitis.

Related Diseases

Diskitis results from hematogenous seeding of the intervertebral disk space during an asymptomatic bacteremia, in a similar fashion to osteomyelitis. The disks separating the L3 and L4 vertebrae and the L4 and L5 vertebrae are the most common locations. Diskitis has a predilection to occur in preschool-aged children, who present with a limp, localized back pain, or abdominal pain when thoracic intervertebral disks are involved. Fever is usually lacking, but the sedimentation rate is a good indicator of low-grade infection. Spinal x-rays reveal changes that range from slight narrowing of the intervertebral disk space to erosion of the cartilaginous end-plates of either of the adjacent vertebral bodies. When a diagnostic needle aspiration or open surgical biopsy is performed, about half of cases have cultures positive for staphylococci, pneumococci, or gram-negative bacilli. These cases generally do well with prolonged oral antibiotic therapy. In a minority of cases no organism is recovered. Some authorities believe that culture-negative episodes actually represent aseptic necrosis of the disk, an etiologically unrelated process that responds to prolonged bed rest alone.

Tuberculosis of the vertebral column (Pott's disease) is very rare in developed countries. Spinal tuberculosis presents with pain, limited mobility, and a paravertebral mass on x-ray. A combined antituberculous drug regimen for 18 months is curative in 90% of patients with or without prolonged bed rest. Surgical management is required when the spine is unstable or when there is compression of the spinal cord, but surgery does not enhance the cure rate.

INFECTIOUS ARTHRITIS

Infection of the synovial lining of the joint spaces occurs with a variety of bacteria, fungi, and viruses. Pyogenic bacteria are the most commonly recognized cause of joint space infection in children, especially between 6 and 24 months of age. Bacterial septic arthritis tends to present acutely and to involve a single joint in otherwise healthy infants and children. The major exception to this rule is the disseminated gonococcal infection, which typically causes polyarticular disease. Multiple joints are also sometimes involved during systemic illness with any of several known viruses.

Etiology

Bacterial arthritis in the neonate generally occurs in the setting of systemic bacterial sepsis in the premature newborn. Group B streptococci, gram-negative enteric bacilli, *Staphylococcus aureus,* and *Candida* are the organisms usually found in neonatal arthritis. The disseminated gonococcal syndrome can occur in full-term infants following intrapartum exposure.

The etiologic spectrum for bacterial arthritis among infants and children is markedly dependent on age. Under 24 months, *Haemophilus influenzae* type B is responsible for 80% of cases, whereas *Streptococcus pneumoniae* and *Staphylococcus aureus* are occasional pathogens. Among older children, septic arthritis is usually caused by staphylococci or group A streptococci. In unusual circumstances, gram-negative enteric bacilli, including salmonella, cause pyogenic arthritis in older children. *Pasteurella multocida* has been recovered from septic joints of children with close exposure to dogs or cats. In sexually active adolescents and young adults, *Neisseria gonorrhoeae* is the most prevalent form of bacterial arthritis.

Virtually all clinical studies have found that no organism is recovered in 30% to 35% of children with septic arthritis occurring beyond the neonatal period. Culture-negative cases are clinically indistinguishable from cases in which a bacterial pathogen such as *Staphylococcus aureus* is recovered.

Viral arthritis is most often recognized in association with other clinical manifestations of systemic infection with rubella, mumps, varicella, influenza, Epstein-Barr virus, enterovirus, arbovirus, and lymphocytic choriomeningitis virus infections. Similarly, chlamydia have been recovered from joint fluid in adolescent and adult patients with Reiter's syndrome.

A sterile, reactive arthritis sometimes accompanies infections that occur at other sites. For instance, a postinfectious, monoarthritic arthritis is sometimes observed in patients with gastrointestinal infections due to enteric bacteria such as salmonella, shigella, campylobacter, and yersinia. These cases, which have a distinct predilection for persons with the B27 HLA haplotype, are probably mediated by circulating immune complexes. The inflammation responds to anti-inflammatory therapy. A polyarticular, immune complex-mediated arthritis may precede the development of hepatic inflammation in patients with acute hepatitis B infection.

Pathogenesis

Most cases of acute suppurative arthritis in young children occur *via* hematogenous seeding of the synovium during a transient, often asymptomatic bacteremia. Extension of infection into the joint space from an adjacent focus of osteomyelitis can be demonstrated in some cases, especially those involving neonates. Penetrating trauma may lead to a septic joint in which the offending bacterial pathogen is often one that normally inhabits the skin. Preexisting chronic arthritis from rheumatoid disease or recurrent hemarthroses may predispose to acute septic arthritis.

Animal studies have shown that bacteria adhere to synovial epithelium early in infection, and that synovial edema and inflammation are early pathologic features. Erosion of cartilage and bone are late findings that occur only when appropriate therapy is not begun in a timely manner.

Clinical and Laboratory Features

The young child with suppurative arthritis presents with fever and a swollen, tender joint. There is marked resistance to passive movement of the joint and refusal to use or bear weight on the involved extremity. An effusion can be demonstrated on examination in about 90% of cases of septic arthritis not involving the hip. Septic arthritis of the hip can be a very difficult diagnosis to establish on the basis of the history and examination because pain may be referred and because an effusion is very difficult to demonstrate. The presence of inflammation of the hip may be suspected when there is limited range of motion when the joint is moved passively in all directions.

The presence of systemic symptoms and migratory polyarthritis in a sexually active adolescent should suggest the diagnosis of disseminated gonococcal infection (DGI). The skin lesions occurring with DGI may be papular, petechial, vesicular, pustular, or bullous. Tenosynovitis (inflammation of the tendon sheaths) of the wrist or ankle is characteristic of DGI. Untreated DGI may persist, with symptoms that wax and wane.

The peripheral white blood cell (WBC) count is usually elevated in childhood septic arthritis, with a shift to the left in the differential WBC count. Aspiration of the joint effusion under sterile conditions is central to both the diagnosis and initial management of septic arthritis. The total WBC count of the joint fluid is typically greater than 20,000 and may exceed 100,000 cells/mm^3. More than 90% of the cells are neutrophils, but this finding does not help differentiate septic arthritis from other inflammatory joint diseases such as juvenile rheumatoid arthritis, acute rheumatic fever, and gout. A mononuclear predominance is suggestive of a viral etiology. Elevation of joint fluid protein above 2 g/dL is characteristic of several inflammatory conditions, but a low level of glucose is suggestive of acute bacterial infection or tuberculous arthritis.

Gram's stain of the joint fluid will demonstrate a pathogen in about half of patients with proven bacterial disease. Culture of the joint fluid will indicate the etiology in 50% to 60% of children with a clinical diagnosis of septic arthritis. The blood culture will be positive in as many as 30%. When DGI is under consideration, cultures of the oropharynx, rectum, and cervix or urethra will enhance the recovery of gonococci in culture.

X-rays of an acutely swollen and inflamed joint may help rule out adjacent osteomyelitis or presence of a foreign body following trauma but are not particularly useful in distinguishing infection from other causes of joint effusion. Distension of the capsule and soft tissue swelling is the usual finding. Subchondral destruction of bone is a late manifestation of septic arthritis.

When arthritis of the hip is under consideration, x-rays of both hips should be performed with the child held in the "frog-leg" position. The distance between medial portion of femoral head and the ossified portion of the acetabulum normally will not differ by more than 2 mm when compared with the contralateral hip. Asymmetry greater than 2 mm suggests joint effusion. Unfortunately, hip x-rays may be "normal" when the child first presents with acute illness.

Differential Diagnosis

The differential diagnosis of a single, acutely inflamed joint includes juvenile rheumatoid arthritis, gout, chondrocalcinosis, systemic lupus erythematosus, and other collagen–vascular diseases. When multiple joints are involved, one must consider other disease processes, including acute rheumatic fever, disseminated meningococcemia, Reiter's syndrome, Lyme disease, and rat bite fever.

Treatment

Decompression of the joint by needle aspiration may be required more than once during the first few days of treatment. Multiple needle aspirations are usually preferable to open surgical drainage, except for septic arthritis of the hip or shoulder where placement of a drain is considered mandatory. Immobilization of the joint is unnecessary except to provide comfort to the child.

The choice of intravenous antibiotics depends on the patient's age, the history, and data obtained by Gram's stain of the aspirated joint fluid. For children beyond the neonatal period, the initial regimen should include antibiotics with efficacy against both staphylococci and *H. influenzae,* such as cefuroxime, or the combination of chloramphenicol with a semisynthetic penicillin (oxacillin or nafcillin). Each of these agents penetrates well into synovial fluid. When an organism is recovered from either blood culture or joint fluid, the antibiotic coverage should be narrowed to treat only the offending pathogen. With signs of a response to drainage and antibiotic therapy, physical therapy should be instituted to hasten return of normal joint mobility and function. As in the treatment of acute osteomyelitis, most children with septic arthritis can be managed with oral antibiotics once there is clear evidence of improvement with parenteral therapy. The usual duration of therapy is 3 weeks or more.

Prognosis

The prognosis for acute suppurative arthritis managed early with appropriate drainage and antibiotic is excellent. More than 90% of cases not involving the hip recover normal or near normal function. Unfortunately, the outlook for septic hip disease is less promising, perhaps because of the delay in diagnosis that sometimes occurs. In addition, neonates and patients with gram-negative enteric infections are more likely to have a less than optimal outcome of their joint infection.

Related Syndromes

Tuberculous arthritis is a chronic, slowly progressive disease that usually occurs in a single joint. Carpel tunnel syndrome is characteristic of tuberculous arthritis of the wrist. Although AFB smears of joint fluid are usually negative, cultures of joint fluid are diagnostic. Tuberculosis is a rare cause of primary joint infection in the developed world.

Infectious bursitis is an acute suppurative infection of a bursal sac that often follows nonpenetrating local trauma. The olecranon and prepatellar bursae are the most common locations. *Staphylococcus aureus* is often recovered by aspiration of the inflamed bursa.

BIBLIOGRAPHY

Capitanio M, Kirkpatrick J: Early roentgen observations in acute osteomyelitis. Am J Roentgenol 108:488, 1970

Dan M: Septic arthritis in young infants: Clinical and microbiologic correlations and therapeutic implications. Rev Infect Dis 147–155, 1984

Dich VQ, Nelson JD, Haltalin KC: Osteomyelitis in infants and children. A review of 183 cases. Am J Dis Child 129:1273–1278, 1975

Goldenberg DL, Reed JI: Bacterial arthritis. N Engl J Med 312:764–771, 1985

Waldvogel FA, Medoff G, Swartz MN: Osteomyelitis: A review of clinical features, therapeutic considerations, and unusual aspects. N Engl J Med 282:198–206, 260–266, 316–322, 1970

Waldvogel FA, Vasey H: Osteomyelitis: The past decade. N Engl J Med 303:360–370, 1980

Welkon CJ, Long SS, Fisher MC, Alburger PD: Pyogenic arthritis in infants and children: A review of 95 cases. Pediatr Infect Dis J 5:669–676, 1986

28 Urinary Tract Infections

Urinary tract infections (UTIs) are an extremely common problem in pediatrics. They include a diverse group of conditions that range from asymptomatic bacteriuria to life-threatening sepsis with pyelonephritis. They are a frequent cause of morbidity in children and may lead to chronic renal dysfunction as a result of scarring. A great deal of controversy remains in the pediatric literature regarding the appropriate definition, evaluation, and management of UTIs, a situation that frequently presents the practicing pediatrician with difficult clinical decisions. Here a general approach to the infant or child with a suspected UTI will be outlined.

First, several definitions are important. *Urethritis* refers to infection (or inflammation) localized to the urethra, while *cystitis* defines infection confined to the bladder and *pyelonephritis* refers to infection of the renal parenchyma. *Chronic pyelonephritis* is a confusing term that is most appropriately used to describe a histologic pattern of focal or diffuse renal scarring presumed secondary to chronic or recurrent infection. Finally, *vesicoureteral reflux* refers to the retrograde flow of urine into the ureters from the bladder.

INCIDENCE

The incidence of UTIs varies significantly with age and sex. In neonates, symptomatic UTIs have been reported to occur in approximately 1.4 in 1000 births with a slight male preponderance. Asymptomatic bacteriuria, however, has been demonstrated to occur much more commonly, with prevalence rates of about 1.3% for males and 0.2% for females. By 4 months of age, UTIs are more common in females, and a striking female predominance persists thereafter. The prevalence of bacteriuria (symptomatic plus asymptomatic) after infancy has been reported to vary between 0.5% and 2.5% in females with peak prevalence rates occurring in school-aged girls. Infections are quite rare in males after infancy.

PATHOPHYSIOLOGY

Urinary tract infections are caused by colonic bacteria in the great majority of cases. In females, 75% to 95% of cases are caused by *Escherichia coli*, with *Klebsiella* and *Proteus* species following. The situation in males is somewhat different; although *E. coli* is still a major pathogen, an approximately equal number of cases are due to infection with *Proteus* and gram-positive organisms *(Staphylococcus albus, S. aureus, Enterococcus)*.

Although specific mechanisms remain unclear, the pathogenesis of UTIs also appears to vary significantly with age. In neonates, it is thought that bacteria most commonly reach the urinary tract by a hematogenous route. After infancy, the vast majority of infections are the result of ascending infection *via* the urethra. The preponderance of infections in females is felt to be directly related to their shorter urethra, providing more limited local defense against infection. Many infections are in fact preceded by urethral colonization with the offending organism. Additional risk factors for the development of UTI include poor hygiene, sexual activity, urethral trauma, and, most importantly, any condition that leads to urinary stasis *(e.g.,* obstructive lesions, neurogenic bladder).

Once bacteria gain entrance to the urinary tract, the severity of any given infection is determined by the interplay of multiple factors. These include the virulence of the infecting organism, host defense mechanisms, and anatomic factors such as urinary obstruction, vesicoureteral reflux, and the presence of calculi. The concept of reflux is particularly important. It is a relatively common condition in children that may lead to repeated episodes of pyelonephritis with the potential for significant renal damage (reflux nephropathy). Surgical intervention may be required for severe reflux. It is also important to realize, however, that transient reflux may occur with simple cystitis. This phenomenon is felt to be due to the intense inflammatory reaction that may be seen with such infections, leading to hyperactivity of the detrusor muscle and a decrease in the functional capacity of the bladder.

SIGNS AND SYMPTOMS

The signs and symptoms of UTIs may be quite nonspecific, particularly in infants and younger children. In neonates, the most common symptoms are fever, irritability, lethargy, anorexia, failure to thrive, diarrhea, and jaundice. Bacteremia occurs in about one-third of cases of neonatal UTI. In older infants, nonspecific symptoms still predominate, although the incidence of bacteremia falls significantly by 2 to 3 months of age. By 2 or 3 years of age, more specific symptoms will become evident, including dysuria, frequency, urgency, enuresis, abdominal pain, and foul-smelling urine. Fever is less common in older children with simple cystitis and should always raise suspicion regarding the possibility of pyelonephritis. Other signs and symptoms suggestive of pyelonephritis are chills, costovertebral angle (flank) pain, and abdominal pain and tenderness.

DIAGNOSIS

The diagnosis of UTI first requires the collection of an appropriate (uncontaminated) urine specimen. In pediatrics, this task may actually be quite difficult. Collection of an uncontaminated specimen in an incontinent patient generally requires the use of bladder catheterization or suprapubic bladder aspiration. Both techniques are safe and easily performed by experienced personnel. It is mandatory that these techniques be used for the incontinent patient who is acutely ill and for whom the institution of immediate antibiotics is required. The risk of contamination in samples obtained by collection bags is far too great to justify their use in this situation. For patients who are not acutely ill and for whom no antibiotics are urgently required, it may be acceptable to obtain an initial specimen with a collection bag. However, although a negative culture on a bag specimen is certainly useful, the risk of contamination is so high that repeat specimens frequently have to be obtained by a better method (*e.g.*, catheterization) and the work-up will therefore be delayed by an additional 1 to 2 days. If bag specimens are to be used, whenever possible, two separate samples should be obtained for culture.

Once effective bladder control has been attained, urine samples for culture may generally be obtained by clean-catch, or midstream, collection. Although contamination is still possible, it can be minimized by carefully cleansing the urethral meatus and supervising the collection process. If possible, two separate specimens should also be obtained prior to antibiotic administration in this situation. If this is not possible, particularly if the patient is acutely ill, catheterization or suprapubic aspiration should again be employed.

Once adequate specimens have been obtained, they should be quickly transported to the laboratory for culture (and refrigerated in the interim if any delay is anticipated). Although the laboratory diagnosis of UTI relies primarily on the urine culture, a great deal of information can be obtained while awaiting culture results by performing a careful urinalysis. Chemical tests for protein, blood, *p*H and nitrites should be performed. Nitrite testing is based on the concept that bacteria in the urine will convert naturally occurring (dietary) nitrates to nitrites. While false-negative test results are unfortunately relatively common (sensitivity 70% to 80%), false-positive test results are quite uncommon, and the test has been shown to have a specificity for UTI of over 90%. Hence, nitrite testing may never replace urine cultures for the diagnosis of UTI, but it is certainly a useful addition to "dipstick" technology.

Microscopic examination of the urine may also be very helpful in making a presumptive diagnosis of UTI. This should include inspection of both centrifuged and uncentrifuged urine for bacteria, white blood cells, red blood cells, and cellular casts. Of greatest specificity is the detection of one or more bacteria per high-power (oil immersion) field of unspun urine. This finding has a 80% to 90% correlation with a significant positive urine culture. Examination of centrifuged urine for bacteria may also be useful, although studies have varied with regard to the specific number of bacteria that should be considered significant. In general, greater than 10 organisms per high-power field of spun urine should certainly raise suspicions regarding UTI. The presence of pyuria, commonly defined as more than five WBCs per high-power field of centrifuged urine, may also be indicative of UTI but is far less reliable than the detection of bacteria. This is because up to 65% of cases of UTI may lack pyuria and at least as many cases of pyuria will have a negative urine culture.

The urine culture is of course the single most important test in the diagnosis of UTI. Quantitative culture techniques must be employed, with results generally expressed in colony counts per ml of urine. Quantitative cultures are critical because they serve as the primary means of distinguishing true positive cultures from contaminated specimens. Although important exceptions do exist, a colony count of greater than 100,000/ml is generally considered diagnostic of UTI. It must be remembered, however, that any growth from specimens obtained by catheterization or suprapubic aspiration must be considered potentially significant. Further, a clean-catch specimen with greater than 10,000 colonies/ml of a single organism should also be regarded as potentially significant, particularly if seen on repeated cultures or in the presence of clinical symptoms.

The final step in the diagnosis of UTI must include an attempt to localize the site of infection. This process is important with regard to both antibiotic management and assessing the risk of possible renal damage. At present, we are unfortunately quite limited in our ability to accurately make such a determination and are forced to rely primarily on clinical criteria. Thus, patients with significant fever, chills, and costovertebral angle pain and tenderness are generally assumed to have pyelonephritis. However, while these clinical parameters are useful, it has been shown that they will be lacking in up to 25% of children with pyelonephritis. Multiple laboratory tests, including serum C-reactive protein, urinary lactate dehydrogenase activity, and studies of antibody coating of urinary bacteria, have all been proposed as helpful but none have had adequate sensitivity or specificity. Only the more invasive technique of selective ureteral catheterization and bladder washout will identify all patients with pyelonephritis, but these are clearly unsuitable for routine use.

The Use of Imaging Studies

Studies commonly used for the evaluation of the urinary tract include ultrasonography, voiding cystourethrography (VCUG), and intravenous pyelography (IVP). Their specific use in infants and children with UTI is somewhat controversial. This controversy stems largely from conflicting data regarding the incidence of urinary tract abnormalities in children with UTI. For example, studies have reported abnormalities, including vesicoureteral reflux, in 7% to 75% of males with UTI and in 5% to 63% of females with UTI. In reviewing all available data, most studies indicate a higher incidence of abnormalities in males overall. Further, the incidence of abnormalities in females when evaluated at the time of their first UTI falls significantly with age and is very low by the age of 3 or 4 years.

Bearing these figures in mind, most experts agree with the following recommendations. During an acute febrile infection, particularly if response to therapy is slow, renal ultrason-

ography should be performed to rule out hydronephrosis and renal or perinephric abscesses. In uncomplicated infections, evaluation should be postponed until 2 to 4 weeks after treatment has been completed to allow for the resolution of any changes associated with the acute infection. All males should be evaluated with their first UTI as should all females under the age of 3. With older females, it may be most reasonable to withhold evaluation until the second infection, unless the first infection was particularly severe or complicated. The initial evaluation should consist of a VCUG and either a renal ultrasound or an IVP, depending in part on the experience of the ultrasonographer. Finally, all children with significant reflux should have an IVP to further delineate kidney size, calyceal blunting, and renal scarring if ultrasound was used initially.

TREATMENT

Decisions regarding antimicrobial therapy for presumed UTIs must take into account multiple factors, including the age of the patient, the suspected pathogens, any history of prior infections or urinary tract abnormalities, and the clinical assessment of upper versus lower urinary tract disease. Based on these considerations, it is generally possible to institute appropriate antibiotic therapy while awaiting culture results.

In neonates, in view of the high incidence of bacteremia seen with UTSs, all symptomatic infections should be treated with parenteral antibiotics. A combination of ampicillin and gentamicin (or other aminoglycoside) is usually highly effective in this situation although newer cephalosporins are being used with increased frequency. As with all infections, antibiotics can be altered based on culture and sensitivity results.

In infants and older children with a presumed diagnosis of simple cystitis, oral antibiotics such as ampicillin, amoxicillin, sulfonamides, and trimethoprim-sulfamethoxazole are all generally very effective, as are many oral cephalosporins. Although many experts will recommend a particular favorite drug, studies show approximately equal efficacy for all those listed. Decisions can therefore be made on an individual basis, considering factors such as cost, side effects, and expected compliance.

For children with presumed pyelonephritis or with known urinary tract abnormalities, more aggressive therapy is indicated. Traditionally, a combination of ampicillin and an aminoglycoside has been used with great success. Many new regimens, utilizing both cephalosporins and semi-synthetic penicillins (*e.g.*, piperacillin), are being actively studied and appear very promising.

The appropriateness of the initial antibiotic selection will be evaluated in several ways. As noted, the results of the urine culture and antibiotic susceptibility testing will help guide treatment decisions. However, the clinical response is often very dramatic and may precede any culture results by hours or even days. Further, because most antibiotics are renally excreted and highly concentrated in the urine, a patient may respond very well to a drug that may look far from ideal by susceptibility testing. Next, repeat urine cultures should be obtained on all patients 2 to 3 days after beginning therapy to document clearing. Finally, because recurrence rates of up to 30% have been reported with virtually all antibiotic regimens, all patients need to have follow-up cultures 2 to 3 days and 2 to 3 weeks after the completion of therapy.

One last area of controversy regarding UTIs lies in the decision about the duration of antibiotic therapy. Existing protocols recommend anything from a single large dose to 6 weeks of therapy. Obviously, the answer must not be entirely clear. Although studies of short-course antibiotic therapy for UTI have been promising overall, there are currently insufficient data to support their use on a routine basis. Until further data become available, courses of 7 to 14 days (generally 10 days) should be used for most pediatric UTIs.

The final major aspect of treatment relates to those children with recurrent urinary tract infections and/or significant urinary tract abnormalities. The use of prophylactic antibiotics in these children is an extremely important and effective means of preventing long-term renal damage. Prophylaxis will generally be needed until the anatomic defect can be corrected or until the child is free of infection for a prolonged period of time. Again, although many regimens are available, the drugs most commonly used for prophylaxis are sulfamethoxazole, trimethoprim-sulfamethoxazole, amoxicillin, and nitrofurantoin. A protocol of rotating antibiotics is often necessary to overcome the emergence of resistant organisms, utilizing regular urine cultures at asymptomatic as well as symptomatic periods.

BIBLIOGRAPHY

Durbin WA, Peter G: Management of urinary tract infections in infants and children. Pediatr Infect Dis 3:564, 1984

Ginsburg, CM, McCracken GH: Urinary tract infections in young infants. Pediatrics 69:409, 1982

Hellerstein S, Wald ER, Winberg J, Nelson JD, McCracken GH: Consensus: Roentgenographic evaluation of children with urinary tract infections. Pediatr Infect Dis 3:291, 1984

Rapkin RH: Urinary tract infection. Pediatr Rev 1:133, 1979

Selden RV, Friedman J, Kaplan MR: Managing urinary tract infections in children. Pediatr Ann 10:12, 1981

Shapiro ED: Short course antimicrobial treatment of urinary tract infections in children: A critical analysis. Pediatr Infect Dis 1:294, 1982

Sidor TA, Resnick MI: Urinary tract infection in children. Pediatr Clin North Am 30:323, 1983

29

Infectious Mononucleosis

Infectious mononucleosis is an acute illness resembling typhoid fever that occurs principally in adolescents and young adults. Approximately 80% of cases of infectious mononucleosis are serologically related to infection with the Epstein-Barr virus (EBV) by a positive heterophile reaction. About half of heterophile negative cases of infectious mononucleosis are caused by the human cytomegalovirus (CMV), and the remainder are caused either by EBV or by other agents such as toxoplasmosis or rubella virus.

EPIDEMIOLOGY OF EPSTEIN-BARR VIRUS INFECTIONS

Worldwide, EBV infection occurs at an early age, and most persons are immune by the time they reach adolescence. Most infections in childhood are asymptomatic. In developed countries, there is an inverse relationship between socioeconomic status and prevalence of antibody to EBV. Children from middle and upper income families often escape infection in early childhood and remain susceptible until the second and third decades of life,

when infection is more likely to result in symptomatic disease. The peak age for infectious mononucleosis is 15 to 20 years. College students are particularly susceptible, developing mononucleosis at a yearly rate of 0.5% to 12%.

Most cases of mononucleosis occur sporadically. Both EBV and CMV are thought to be spread directly from person to person by intimate contact, perhaps as a result of exchange of saliva. Persons shedding EBV asymptomatically probably play an important role in transmission. Thus, the reputation of infectious mononucleosis as a "kissing" disease may be well deserved. Both CMV and EBV infections are also transmitted by transfusion of fresh blood (postperfusion syndrome).

PATHOPHYSIOLOGY

Since the host range for EBV is highly restricted, there is no animal model of infection. Furthermore, productive EBV infection can be demonstrated only in human B-lymphocytes. Following oral transmission, there is an incubation period of 30 to 50 days before onset of symptoms. In transfusion-acquired disease, this period is somewhat shorter. During the incubation period, the virus replicates in local lymphoid tissue and then spreads systemically to reticuloendothelial tissue elsewhere. The activation of T cytotoxic/suppressor lymphocytes against infected B-lymphocytes heralds the onset of symptoms, which usually persist for 1 to 4 weeks. These activated T cells are found in the peripheral blood in the form of atypical lymphocytes, which persist for the duration of the illness. Histologic examination of lymph node tissue during the acute phase of mononucleosis shows an increase in lymphoid follicle number and size and active germinal centers. EBV persists in oropharyngeal secretions for 12 to 18 months after clinical recovery and can be recovered intermittently thereafter for the life of the patient. Similarly, following CMV mononucleosis, CMV can be found in the urine for months to years.

CLINICAL FEATURES

EBV and CMV Mononucleosis

More than 90% of diagnosed mononucleosis occurs in the 15-to-25-year age-group. In most patients, illness is characterized by abrupt onset of fever, malaise, sore throat, and tender cervical lymphadenopathy. During the course of the illness, many also complain of chills, anorexia, headache, photophobia, dysphagia, myalgias, or a distaste for cigarettes.

On presentation, the patient with mononucleosis is febrile to a temperature as high as 40°C, and often exhibits periorbital edema, tonsillar enlargement with erythema and exudate, palatine petechiae, cervical lymphadenopathy including the posterior cervical lymph nodes, and splenomegaly. A maculopapular rash (10%), hepatic enlargement (10% to 15%) and jaundice (5% to 11%) are less common findings. Patients given ampicillin during the illness develop a generalized, pruritic rash, which may aid in the diagnosis of mononucleosis.

The CBC can aid greatly in the diagnosis of mononucleosis. The peripheral blood white blood cell (WBC) count will be in the range of 12,000 to 50,000, with most of the increase due to a rise in the number of lymphocytes. Eight percent to 10% or more of the total WBCs will be atypical lymphocytes. If liver function tests are obtained, a mild hepatitis can be demonstrated in more than 80% of cases.

The clinical and laboratory features of illness caused by EBV and CMV are nearly identical, except that CMV mononucleosis is not associated with an exudative pharyngitis or extensive lymphadenopathy.

In practice, the diagnosis of EBV mononucleosis usually depends on the demonstration of heterophile antibodies in the patient's serum. Heterophile antibodies are IgM antibodies, which agglutinate sheep, horse, or ox red blood cells (RBC). They are not specific for EBV infection but occur in association with a variety of other infectious and noninfectious diseases. In 1932, Paul and Bunnell described the occurrence of spontaneous sheep RBC agglutinins in the sera of mononucleosis patients. Davidsohn later showed that these agglutinins could be absorbed by ox RBC but not guinea pig RBC, thus differentiating these heterophile antibodies from those known to occur in serum sickness. This observation forms the basis of the classic "heterophile" test performed for mononucleosis. Many laboratories now perform "slide" or "spot" tests based on agglutination of horse RBC. In general, these newer tests are a bit more sensitive than the classic heterophile procedure.

About 75% of adolescent and adult patients with EBV mononucleosis develop a positive heterophile test result by 7 days after onset of symptoms, and by 3 weeks, 97% are positive.

In these patients, heterophile antibodies may be detected for 6 to 12 months after acute infection. Among preadolescent children however, there is a direct correlation between age and development of heterophile antibodies with symptomatic EBV infection. Under age 6, only about 50% of EBV infections are heterophile positive. Serologic assays for specific antibodies (antibodies to EBV viral capsid antigen) may be required for diagnosis in the unusual cases of mononucleosis that occur in the preadolescent age-group. Unfortunately, these assays are not always readily available. CMV mononucleosis is heterophile negative; diagnosis requires recovery of CMV from the blood, urine, or oropharynx, or demonstration of a rise in CMV-specific antibody titer.

The symptoms of infectious mononucleosis abate slowly, so that 50%, 80%, and 97% of patients are free of symptoms by 2, 3, and 4 weeks, respectively. Complications with protean manifestations are unusual, but well described. They include hemolytic anemia, immune thrombocytopenia, pneumonia, myopericarditis, splenic rupture, severe hepatitis, and bacterial superinfection. Involvement of the central nervous system occurs in less than 1% of cases; encephalitis, aseptic meningitis, transverse myelitis, hearing loss, and peripheral neuropathy (especially Guillain-Barré syndrome) are each associated with EBV mononucleosis. Rare individuals have been reported to develop recurrent fever, malaise, pharyngitis, cervical adenopathy, and neuropsychiatric symptoms for months or years after onset of acute EBV mononucleosis. Proof that these symptoms are due to EBV or CMV infection remains elusive, however.

Mononucleosis-related deaths are very rare, occurring in approximately 1 in 3000 cases. Deaths are usually secondary to central nervous system disease, splenic rupture, or upper airway obstruction from severe tonsillitis.

MANAGEMENT OF MONONUCLEOSIS

Patients with mononucleosis should be advised to curtail activities involving strenuous physical exercise. Because of the debilitating symptoms of acute mononucleosis, most patients will limit their activity spontaneously. The use of corticosteroids to treat mononucleosis is somewhat controversial. Controlled studies have shown that corticosteroids may ameliorate the symptoms of mononucleosis but do not affect the outcome of the disease. These agents may play a role in the management of airway obstruction due to tonsillar enlargement and in rare cases of severe thrombocytopenia.

Acyclovir, an antiviral agent with proven efficacy against diseases caused by other herpesviruses, inhibits the replication of EBV in cell culture. However, clinical trials of acyclovir in mononucleosis have been rather disappointing.

BIBLIOGRAPHY

Horwitz C, Henle W, Henle G et al: Heterophile-negative infectious mononucleosis and momonucleosis-like illnesses. Am J Med 63:947, 1977

Karzon D: Infectious mononucleosis. Adv Pediatr 22:231, 1976

Paul J, Bunnell W: The presence of heterophile antibodies in infectious mononucleosis. Rev Infect Dis 4:1062, 1982

Radetsky M: A diagnostic approach to Epstein-Barr virus infections. Pediatr Infect Dis 1:425, 1982

Rapp C, Hewetson J: Infectious mononucleosis and the Epstein-Barr virus. Am J Dis Child 132:78, 1978

30

Rickettsial Diseases

Most rickettsia that are pathogenic for humans are small (0.3 × 1 to 2μ), obligately intracellular, coccobacillary bacteria that exist in nature in a cycle involving small mammals and birds as natural reservoirs and insects as vectors. Humans are infected with rickettsia *via* seasonal encroachment upon the environment in which this cycle occurs. (An exception is *R. prowazekii*, the agent of epidemic typhus, for which man is the principal reservoir and the common body louse is the principal vector.) Only a small inoculum of rickettsiae are required to cause infection and disease, and all (except Q fever) replicate in the endothelial cells of small blood vessels, causing a systemic vasculitis, the pathologic hallmark of rickettsial infections. With the exception of late-occurring relapses of epidemic typhus due to latency of *R. prowazekii* (Brill-Zinsser disease), rickettsial infections confer lifelong immunity to reinfection with the same organism and, in some cases, cross-protection against other rickettsial species.

Worldwide, there are numerous species of rickettsiae that are pathogenic for man. In North America, the agents of Rocky Mountain spotted fever (*R. rickettsii*), rickettsialpox (*R. akari*), Q fever (*Coxiella burnetii*), murine typhus (*R. typhi*), and epidemic typhus (*R. prowazekii*) are endemic. Rocky Mountain spotted fever is the most important rickettsial disease in North America, with 700 to 1000 cases reported annually in the United States. Approximately 100 to 300 cases of both murine typhus and Q fever are also reported, along with rare cases of rickettsialpox.

ROCKY MOUNTAIN SPOTTED FEVER

Rocky Mountain spotted fever (RMSF) occurs throughout the United States and Canada but is concentrated in regions corresponding to the habitats of *Dermacentor variablilis* (the dog tick) and *Dermacentor andersoni* (the wood tick). In the United States, *D. variablilis* is distributed along the eastern seaboard and in the southeast, whereas *D. andersoni* is found mostly in the northern Rocky Mountain ranges. A variety of small mammals and birds provide the natural reservoir for *R. rickettsii*. Humans are infected when their activities bring them in contact with rickettsia-carrying ticks. Dogs and other domestic animals may also play a role by transporting ticks to humans.

207

Epidemiology

The reported incidence of RMSF rose steadily during the 1970s, peaked in 1981, and has since slowly declined. The states continously reporting the highest disease activity include Oklahoma, North Carolina, Virginia, and South Carolina, but RMSF has been reported from virtually every state in the United States. Reported disease is highly seasonal, reflecting the feeding activity of the vector. In the western states, disease incidence peaks in the early spring; in the east, peak seasons are late spring and early summer. More than 99% of all cases are reported to occur between April and the end of September. School-aged children have the highest rates of infection.

Pathophysiology

The bite of a rickettsia-carrying tick is necessary for transmission of RMSF, even though only half of infected persons give a history of recent tick exposure. The rickettsiae are introduced subcutaneously during a tick feeding and replicate locally. Spread of the organism *via* the bloodstream occurs within 1 to 2 days, leading to development of a systemic vasculitis with replication of rickettsiae in vascular endothelial foci throughout the body. The organism can be isolated from the blood from 2 to 10 days after experimental infection, and then is cleared with the appearance of specific antibody.

Initial symptoms most often occur 4 to 7 days after the tick exposure (range, 3 to 12 days). In children, the severity of illness appears to be inversely related to the length of the incubation period. Asymptomatic infections are common.

Clinical Disease

Onset of symptoms may be abrupt or gradual. Fever and headache are the most prominent early symptoms; many persons with RMSF describe the headache as generalized and severe. Other early signs and symptoms may include periorbital edema, myalgia, muscle tenderness, conjunctivitis, photophobia, nausea, vomiting, and diarrhea. Abdominal pain is a feature of 30% of cases, and meningismus occurs in about 5%. Lymphadenopathy and arthritis are not features of RMSF; the presence of these signs suggests the likelihood of another diagnosis.

The rash of RMSF typically appears 1 to 5 days (range, 1 to 15 days) after the onset of fever and headache. Characteristically, the rash first appears on the distal extremities at the wrists and ankles, and then on the palms and soles. The individual lesions are initially 1 to 3-mm macules that blanch on pressure. As the rash spreads centrally, the lesions become progressively petechial and purpuric. When treatment is begun early, the rash fades quickly with overall recovery of the patient. It is very important to note that 4% to 16% of children with well-documented RMSF never develop a rash.

Most children have an elevated white blood cell (WBC) count with a left-shifted differential WBC count on presentation. Anemia and thrombocytopenia often occur with progression of disease. In addition, a low serum sodium concentration is also characteristic of RMSF; the basis for the hyponatremia has not been satisfactorily explained.

Complications

The natural course of untreated RMSF is a febrile illness of 2 to 3 weeks' duration, often with progressive involvement of multiple organs. Peripheral edema, hypotension, avascular necrosis of digits or the scrotum may occur, along with gastrointestinal bleeding, hepatosplenomegaly, jaundice, pneumonia, myocarditis, or azotemia. Central nervous system (CNS) dysfunction commonly occurs with untreated disease, with lethargy, focal neurologic abnormalities, coma, and seizures reflecting the presence of cerebritis. The mortality of untreated or inappropriately treated disease is 20% to 30%.

Diagnosis

The diagnosis of RMSF is suspected on the basis of clinical grounds alone and is confirmed by serologic means. Both nonspecific and specific antibody tests are now used. The nonspecific Weil-Felix agglutination reactions are based on antigenic cross-reactivity between *R. rickettii* (and other rickettsiae) and the cell wall antigens of certain *Proteus* species, OX-2, OX-19, and OX-K. Although the Weil-Felix tests are widely available, they are less sensitive and less specific than serologic tests based on the use of *R. rickettsii* antigens, which are now standardized in IFA, CF, EIA, and latex agglutination formats. Since neither the Weil-Felix agglutinins nor the specific rickettsial antibodies are normally demonstrable before 7 to 10 days after onset of symptoms, the management of RMSF must be based on clinical grounds alone.

Some centers have reported considerable success in the rapid diagnosis of RMSF by demonstration of *R. rickettsial* antigens by immunofluorescent staining of a biopsied skin lesion. Direct isolation of *R. rickettsii* is sometimes performed as a research technique but is not generally available in clinical laboratories because the live organisms represent a serious risk to laboratory workers.

Management

It is inappropriate to wait for serologic confirmation of a suspected case of RMSF, since therapeutic success depends greatly on early, specific drug therapy. Both chloramphenicol (50 to 75 mg/kg/day) and tetracycline (25 mg/kg/day) are equally effective antibiotics, but

chloramphenicol is usually chosen for young children because of the adverse effects of tetracycline on dental development. Although chloramphenicol and tetracycline both have bacteriostatic activity only on rickettsiae *in vitro*, it is likely that virtually all organisms are eradicated *in vivo* after only a few doses of either antibiotic.

Early therapy generally results in rapid defervescence and clinical improvement. It is customary to continue antibiotic therapy for 5 to 7 days. Antibiotics started after the first few days of illness are less likely to alter the natural course of disease.

The overall mortality among children with RMSF is 2% to 5%. An adverse prognosis is associated with delay in diagnosis and appropriate antibiotic therapy. Delays in diagnosis are often due to an atypical presentation (*i.e.*, lack of rash) or a low index of suspicion on the part of the examining physician.

OTHER RICKETTSIAL DISEASES

Rickettsialpox

Rickettsialpox, a milder disease than RMSF, is caused by *R. akari*, a member of the "spotted fever" group of rickettsiae. The reservoir for *R. akari* is the common mouse, and the agent is transmitted to humans by the painless bite of a mouse mite. Rickettsialpox has been reported infrequently from several urban centers in the eastern United States, and is indigenous to several locations in Asia and Africa. Children from disadvantaged, inner city neighborhoods are most frequently infected.

After an incubation period of 10 to 14 days, the illness is heralded by onset of fever, headache, myalgia, and regional adenopathy. A small papule forms at the site of the mite bite and later develops into a small ulcer that heals with formation of an eschar. Within 2 to 3 days of onset of fever, a generalized papulovesicular eruption develops and then heals with crusting in 3 to 5 days. The lesions can be differentiated from those of varicella by the characteristic small, central vesicle on a wide papular base. Rickettsialpox is usually mild and self-limited; complications are rare.

Weil-Felix serology is unhelpful in the diagnosis, but specific serologic tests are available at reference laboratories. The illness responds quickly to administration of chloramphenicol or tetracycline. Control of house mice is the only method of prevention.

Q Fever

Q fever is a zoonotic disease caused by *Coxiella burnetii*, and organism that, unlike other rickettsiae, survives for long periods outside the intracellular mileu. Spread among animals occurs in nature *via* a tick vector. The organism is transmitted to humans (without a vector) by inhalation of comtaminated aerosols generated in closed environments with infected domestic animals such as goats, sheep, and cattle. Q fever is largely an occupational hazard of persons exposed to livestock; children are rarely infected.

Inhalation of *C. burnetii* results in a systemic "flu-like" illness with fever, chills, headache, and myalgia. Q fever infections are generally self-limited, but a chronic, relapsing form with pneumonia, granulomatous hepatitis, and endocarditis may occur months to years later. It is fatal if not treated with chloramphenical or tetracycline.

Endemic Typhus

The agent of endemic typhus, *R. typhi*, is transmitted to humans by rat fleas. Most cases in the United States occur in children living in urban settings infested by rats, the principal reservoir of *R. typhi*.

The onset of fever, headache, and myalgia

occurs 1 to 2 weeks after the rat flea bite. Unlike rickettsialpox, a local lesion does not develop at the site of the flea bite. The centrally distributed macular or maculopapular rash occurs in approximately 75% of children 3 to 5 days after presentation of illness. Endemic typhus is a relatively mild illness that resolves within 2 to 3 weeks if not treated. The symptoms respond quickly to chloramphenicol or tetracycline. The diagnosis of endemic typhus is serologic. Weil-Felix agglutinins are demonstrable 7 to 10 days after onset of symptoms. *R. typhi* shares considerable antigenic cross-reactivity with *R. prowasekii*, the agent of epidemic typhus.

Epidemic Typhus

Epidemic typhus is a disease associated with famine, war, and other periods of social upheaval, particularly in winter, when some items of clothing may be worn for long periods of time without change. The agent, *R. prowasekii*, is the only known rickettsia that has man as the principal reservoir. It is transmitted by the human body louse directly by close personal contact or indirectly by louse-infected clothing or bedding. The flying squirrel, which may also be a reservoir for *R. prowasekii*, has been implicated in at least one outbreak of epidemic typhus in the United States.

After an incubation period of 5 to 10 days, the patient experiences sudden onset of high fever, chills, headache, and a progressive typhoid-like illness. The rash of epidemic typhus appears 4 to 6 days after presentation as a pink, macular eruption, principally on the torso, that spreads centrifugally as the lesions coalesce and become petechial. The rash usually spares the face and distal extremities. Pneumonia, cranial nerve abnormalities, and a meningoencephalitis are other well-known manifestations of epidemic typhus.

The Weil-Felix agglutination reactions are

usually positive within 7 to 10 days. Specific serologic tests for antibodies to *R. prowasekii* (that cross-react with *R. typhi*) will confirm the diagnosis.

Epidemic typhus is a severe disease with a high mortality under the adverse social conditions in which the disease often occurs. Like other rickettsial diseases, early therapy with either chloramphenicol or tetracycline effects a rapid recovery. Epidemic typhus can be prevented by delousing of affected persons during outbreaks of disease.

Brill-Zinnser disease is a milder illness resulting from reactivation of latent *R. prowasekii* infection years after the original infection. It is rarely diagnosed in the United States today.

REFERENCES

Aikawa JK: Rocky Mountain Spotted Fever. Springfield, IL, Charles C Thomas, 1966

Bell WE, Lascari AD: Rocky Mountain spotted fever. Neurological symptoms in the acute phase. Neurology 20:841–847, 1970

D'Angelo LJ, Baker EF, Scholsser W: Q fever in the United States, 1948–1977. J Infect Dis 139:613, 1979

Hattwick MAW, O'Brien RJ, Hanson BF: Rocky Mountain spotted fever: Epidemiology of an increasing problem. Ann Intern Med 84:732–739, 1976

Helmick CG, Bernard KW, D'Angelo LJ: Rocky Mountain spotted fever: Clinical, laboratory, adn epidemiological features of 262 cases. J Infect Dis 150:480–488, 1984

McDade JE, Shephard CC, Redus MA et al: Evidence of *Rickettsia prowazekii* infections in the United States. Am J Trop Med Hyg 29:277, 1980

Meiklejohn G, Reimer LG, Graves PS et al: Cryptic epidemic of Q fever in a medical school. J Infect Dis 144:107–113, 1981

Wilfert CM, MacCormack JN, Kleeman K et al: Epidemiology of Rocky Mountain spotted fever as determined by active surveillance. J Infect Dis 150:469–479, 1984

Wong B, Singer C, Armstrong D et al: Rickettsialpox: Case report and epidemiologic review. JAMA 242:1998, 1979

31

Viral Syndromes

MEASLES

Measles (rubeola) is a generalized exanthematous disease caused by a virus that is a member of the Morbillivirus genus of the *family* Paramyxoviridae. Primary infection confers lifelong immunity to the disease, although subclinical reinfection probably occurs regularly under conditions of frequent exposure. Measles virus is one of the most highly infectious agents known. Prior to the advent of measles immunization in the 1960s, infection was universal, and 50% of children experienced measles by 4 years of age and virtually all cases of measles occurred in young children. However, the widespread use of measles vaccine in developed countries has allowed many nonimmune persons to escape childhood exposure to measles and remain susceptible as adults. During 1986, nearly 30% of all measles cases reported to the Centers for Disease Control occurred in persons 15 years of age and older. Unlike the prevaccine era, outbreaks of measles now involve adolescents and adults in colleges and other institutional settings. However, most cases continue to occur among unvaccinated pre-school-aged children.

Pathophysiology and Clinical Features

Infected persons shed measles virus from the upper respiratory tract for 1 or 2 days prior the onset of respiratory symptoms until the rash begins to fade. Transmission occurs *via* the respiratory route. After an incubation period of 9 to 11 days, fever occurs with signs of upper respiratory tract infection including cough, coryza, and conjunctivitis. Koplik's spots are diagnostic, blue-white punctuate lesions that appear on the buccal mucosa within 2 to 3 days of onset of symptoms.

The morbilliform rash begins on the face and hairline 3 to 4 days after onset of the fever and respiratory symptoms. Within 2 to 3 days the rash progresses to the trunk and extremities while becoming confluent on the face and neck. In uncomplicated measles, the fever and respiratory symptoms begin to abate rapidly after 4 or 5 days, and the rash fades, sometimes with desquamation.

Complications

Measles is a self-limited disease in most children. Respiratory complications, including otitis media, croup, bronchitis, and bronchiectasis are common. Secondary bacterial pneumonias are caused by pneumococci, *Haemophilus influenzae*, and staphylococci. Pneumonia caused by measles virus (giant cell pneumonia) is a less common but dreaded complication.

Central nervous system (CNS) complications are unusual but serious. Postinfectious encephalitis, which affects 1 child in 1000 with measles, generally appears abruptly during convalescence from the rash illness. The pathogenesis of postinfectious encephalitis is thought to be immunologically mediated, since measles virus cannot be recovered from brain tissue or spinal fluid. The clinical features of measles encephalitis are characterized by recurrence of fever, diminution of consciousness, and generalized seizures. The mortality rate is as high as 20% and about one-third of survivors are left with significant neurologic impairment. Subacute sclerosing panencephalitis (SSPE) is an extremely rare (5–10 cases/10^6 measles cases), progressive, degenerative CNS disease. Measles virus has been isolated from brain tissue in some patients, and all have high titer of measles antibody in the cerebrospinal fluid (CSF). Onset of CNS symptoms is usually years (mean, 7 years) following natural measles infection. The majority of SSPE cases give a history of measles at an early age.

Adults and young infants are more likely to have illness that is prolonged and severe. Prolonged febrile illness is common among malnourished children living in underdeveloped parts of the world, who may also experience gastroenteritis, secondary skin and eye infections, and enhanced severity of their underlying malnutrition. Children with significant cell-mediated immunity deficiency are at high risk of a prolonged, febrile illness with or without the usual rash of measles. Many of these children die of measles virus pneumonia.

Diagnosis

In the past, the diagnosis of measles was always based on clinical findings alone. Because many physicians are now not as familiar with measles, and because of the public health importance of the disease, laboratory confirmation is now considered essential. Determination of acute and convalescent measles hemagglutination inhibition (HI) antibody titers is the easiest and most reliable diagnostic test. HI antibody is detectable with the appearance of the rash and rapidly rises to peak levels in 3 to 4 weeks. Measles virus can be isolated from throat washings during the prodrome and the first 1 or 2 days of the rash.

Prevention of Measles

Passive immunotherapy. Gamma globulin (immune serum globulin [ISG]), in a dose of 0.2 ml/kg, will prevent or modify measles when given at any time during the incubation period. ISG is recommended for all susceptible measles contacts, especially infants 4 to 12 months of age who having waning protection from passive maternal antibody and who are not candidates for measles vaccine.

Measles Vaccines. Live attenuated measles vaccine was first introduced in the United States in 1963, and by 1967 was being widely used. The current "further attenuated" measles vaccines confer lifelong immunity in at least 95% of recipients while causing mild fever or rash 6 to 10 days after immunization in 5% to 15% of recipients. Measles vaccine is now routinely administered beginning at 15 months of age, in combination with mumps and rubella vaccine in a single injection (MMR).

RUBELLA

Rubella virus causes a mild, exanthematous disease (rubella, German measles, 3-day measles) that affects principally children, adolescents and young adults. Rubella is a generally mild illness that rarely causes serious complications. Rubella has clinical and public health importance because of infection of pregnant women and subsequent chronic infection and embryopathy of the fetus and newborn infant. Once a universal disease in the United States, the incidence of rubella has fallen dramatically with the widespread use of rubella vaccine.

Epidemiology

Prior to the availability of rubella vaccine, endemic rubella occurred annually in the late winter and spring. Cyclical epidemics of rubella occurred with a periodicity of 6 to 9 years in which the annual incidence of reported disease increased from 3- to 10-fold over endemic levels. The last epidemic, which occurred worldwide from 1963 to 1965, was the largest observed. Since the introduction of live attenuated rubella vaccine in 1969, the incidence of reported disease has declined to extremely low levels, in part because of national immunization initiatives and the inclusion of rubella vaccine with measles vaccine (MMR). However, serologic surveys carried out in several urban locations in the U.S. indicate that 15% to 25% of persons over 15 years of age remain susceptible, a percentage that has not changed substantially since the introduction of vaccine.

Clinical Features

Rubella virus is highly communicable with person-to-person transmission occurring *via* the respiratory route. The onset of symptoms follows an incubation period of 14 to 18 days with nearly simultaneous onset of rash, fever, and mild upper respiratory tract symptoms. The rubella rash is a salmon-pink, macular exanthem that begins on the face and neck, spreads to the trunk and proximal extremities, and fades within 1 to 3 days of onset. Pruritus during the eruption is often a major complaint. Fever, which is present in only half of cases, is generally low grade. Posterior cervical and occipital adenopathy is a hallmark of rubella which may be present as the only symptom. Node enlargement is present as early as 7 days prior to the rash and peaks with onset of the rash. The occasional presence of generalized adenopathy and splenomegaly may lead to a mistaken diagnosis of infectious mononucleosis. Pharyngitis and conjunctivitis are common.

Approximately 50% of rubella infections are asymptomatic. Children with symptoms experience only mild illness and virtually all recover within 3 to 4 days. The major complication of rubella is acute polyarthralgia involving the proximal interphalangeal joints, metacarpal phalangeal joints, wrists, elbows, or knees. Transient arthralgias occur in 15% to 25% of postpubertal women with rubella, but in a smaller number of children. Joint symptoms usually begin within days of recovery from the rash illness, and they may persist up to several weeks. The pathogenesis of the arthritis may involve immune complexes; rubella virus has been isolated from the joint fluid in acute cases. Rare complications of rubella include thrombocytopenic purpura, pancytopenia, orchitis, and postinfectious meningoencephalitis.

Diagnosis

In practice, the diagnosis of rubella depends on the demonstration of a rise in specific humoral antibody titer. Serum antibody is first detectable within 1 to 3 days of onset of the rash. The HI test remains the standard method for the serologic diagnosis of acute rubella. Titers of less than 1:8 are considered negative, and seroconversion to positive (a four fold rise in antibody titer) is diagnostic of recent rubella. Since the HI test is less sensitive then other, more recently developed serologic methods like enzyme immunoassay (ELISA) and latex agglutination, as many as 10% to 25% of immune persons may have a negative rubella HI titer. None of the newer methods are now sufficiently standardized to make a specific diagnosis of acute rubella, but they are widely used for serologic screening of pregnant women, hospital employees, and so on.

The presence of rubella-specific IgM antibody also indicates recent infection. IgM serology is especially useful in the diagnosis of congenital rubella syndrome in the newborn infant, since, unlike IgG, IgM antibody of maternal origin does not cross the placental barrier.

Both acquired and congenital rubella can also be diagnosed by recovery of rubella virus in cell culture.

Congenital Rubella Syndrome

The risk of fetal infection and the risk of congenital anomaly resulting from infection are both highest when maternal rubella occurs during the first month of gestation and declines thereafter. Laboratory evidence of intrauterine infection is detectable in 60% of infants born to mothers experiencing rubella in the first month of pregnancy. Correspond-

ing estimates for the second and third month are 25% to 40% and 10% to 30%, respectively. Although the risk of congenital anomalies is low when rubella occurs after the first trimester, some second and third trimester infections result in fetal infection and congenital abnormalities that are not detected until later in childhood.

The classic triad of congenital abnormalities due to rubella includes nuclear cataracts, sensorineural deafness, and congenital heart disease. Ocular disease and congenital heart disease result when maternal rubella occurs during the first 60 to 90 days of gestation, while hearing loss results from gestational rubella any time in the first 4 months. Other common findings of congenital rubella noted early in life include low birth weight, thrombocytopenia, purpura, organomegaly, hyperbilirubinemia, hemolytic anemia, osteitis of long bones, meningoencephalitis, and failure to thrive. Most of these phenomena resolve within the first few weeks of life. Many anatomical and physiological abnormalities are detected in some children with congenital rubella as they grow and develop. These include hearing loss, genitourinary tract abnormalities, diabetes mellitus and other endocrinopathies, hypogammaglobulinemia, and mental deficiency. An interesting, but tragic, progressive neurologic disorder that is clinically and pathologically similar to subacute sclerosing panencephalitis has been described in several adolescents with congenital rubella syndrome. This rubella panencephalitis is thought to result from persistence of rubella virus in the CNS.

Live Attenuated Rubella Virus Vaccine

The RA 27/3 virus is now the only rubella vaccine strain distributed in the United States. Rubella vaccine may be administered as a single agent or combined with measles and mumps vaccines in a single IM dose (MMR).

In the United States, the latter preparation is generally used for routine immunization of infants at 15 months of age. Immunization produces seroconversion in 95% of susceptible persons and successfully boosts the antibody titer in previously seropositive persons with low antibody titers.

RA 27/3 vaccine causes fever and rash in 4% and 10% of seronegative recipients, respectively. The most important adverse effects of rubella vaccine are arthralgias and arthritis, which occur in nearly the same frequency as with natural rubella. The rate of adverse joint reactions following vaccination varies with age and sex. The highest risk occurs among postpubertal women, who have a 15% to 25% incidence of arthralgias and a lower incidence of frank arthritis. Males (5%–10%) and prepubertal children of both sexes (2%–10%) have a lower incidence of joint reactions. Immune recipients experience joint symptoms at a frequency that is no greater than controls. The onset of joint symptoms is generally 7 to 21 days after vaccination. The joints most commonly affected are the fingers, wrists, and knees. Although most joint symptoms resolve within a week, persistent and recurrent symptoms for up to 8 years is reported.

Although rubella vaccine virus is shed in the nasopharynx of vaccinees in low titers, studies in school, institutional, and family settings have shown that susceptible contacts of vaccines remain seronegative. Thus, there is no contraindication to immunizing the children of pregnant women according to recommendations. Although rubella vaccine is contraindicated in pregnant women, data indicate that the teratogenic potential of the vaccine virus is low or nonexistent.

Reinfection with Rubella Virus

Persons immune on the basis of both natural disease and as a result of vaccination are frequently reinfected with rubella following exposure to natural disease, or administration of a booster dose of live vaccine virus. Reinfection is almost always asymptomatic and produces an anamnestic humoral antibody response with little or no rubella-specific IgM. Although some cases of reinfection are reported to have occurred during pregnancy with subsequent fetal infection, the paucity of documented cases indicates that reinfection poses very little risk to the fetus.

VARICELLA-ZOSTER VIRUS INFECTIONS

Varicella (chickenpox) is an acute vesicular exanthem that is the manifestation of primary infection with varicella-zoster virus (VZV), a member of the human herpesvirus family. Reactivation of latent VZV infection later in life may result in herpes zoster (shingles), a painful vesicular eruption, which is usually limited to the dermatome innervated by one sensory nerve. The clinical course of both varicella and zoster depends on the patient's age and the presence or absence of underlying cellular immunodeficiency.

Epidemiology

In temperate climates, approximately 50% of children acquire antibody to VZV by 6 years of age, and more than 95% have antibody by 13 years of age. However, in the tropics and some isolated areas, the risk of varicella infection among children is lower, and a significant proportion of adults remain susceptible to infection. An episode of varicella confers lifelong immunity to subsequent disease, although subclinical infections commonly occur upon reexposure to chickenpox. The overall lifetime risk of developing herpes zoster is approximately 4%; the risk increases with advancing age and with the presence of underlying immunodeficiency or chronic illness.

Person-to-person spread of varicella occurs readily among susceptible individuals in household and institutional settings such as day-care centers, schools, and hospital wards. The period of infectivity during varicella is considered to be from 1 to 2 days prior to the onset of the rash until the skin lesions begin to dry and crust over. The mode of virus transmission from persons with varicella is assumed to be *via* the respiratory route, (*e.g.*, airborne spread has been well documented in nosocomial settings). Persons with herpes zoster are also capable of transmitting VZV to susceptible individuals, although they are generally considered somewhat less infectious than persons with varicella.

Clinical Features

As many as 10% to 20% of primary VZV infections are asymptomatic, or mild enough to escape notice. Clinical disease, which is characterized by acute onset of fever and a vesicular eruption, follows an incubation period that is normally 11 to 21 days, but may be as long as 30 days in cases modified by administration of varicella-zoster immune globulin (VZIG). The initial manifestation of low-grade fever is followed by onset of a generalized vesicular exanthem within 12 to 48 hours. Typically, there is a greater concentration of lesions on the trunk than on the face and extremities. The individual lesions appear at first as papules, which rapidly evolve into 1- to 4-mm vesicles on a thin erythematous base. The vesicles evolve into small pustules with infiltration of polymorphonuclear leukocytes into the vesicular fluid, crust over within 2 to 5 days of their appearance, and heal rapidly without scarring. Several crops of lesions may develop over a period of 1 to 5 days. An enanthem with shallow ulcerative lesions on the oropharyngeal mucosa often parallels the appearance of the rash. Varicella causes only mild discomfort and little limita-

tion of normal activity in the overwhelming majority of children. Secondary cases within the same household may be more severe than the index case.

Herpes zoster is characterized by unilateral pain and a vesicular eruption in the dermatomal distribution of a sensory nerve. Thoracic and abdominal dermatomes are more likely to be involved than dermatomes innervated by cranial and sacral nerves. In normal children, the eruption may last from a few days up to several weeks. Children tend to have less postherpetic neuralgia than do adults.

Complications

Secondary bacterial infections of the skin represent the most frequent complication of varicella in healthy children; cellulitis, impetigo, and erysipelas are most common.

A variety of CNS complications are well described with varicella, the most common being acute cerebellitis (cerebellar ataxia), which typically occurs suddenly, 1 to 3 weeks after the rash. Affected children have acute onset of ataxia and dysarthria, and about 30% will have a low-grade CSF leukocytosis. Most children with varicella-associated cerebellar ataxia recover completely in days to weeks. Less common CNS complications include Reye's syndrome, post-infectious encephalitis, aseptic meningitis, Guillain-Barré syndrome, and transverse myelitis. Arthritis, nephritis, nephrotic syndrome, and orchitis are also associated with acute varicella. Hematologic complications include thrombocytopenia and epistaxis. "Hemorrhagic" varicella is a rare but very serious complication characterized by purpura fulminans and diffuse intravascular coagulation.

Children who are immunocompromised, especially children who are receiving chemotherapy or who are organ transplant recipients, can be expected to develop more serious infection with high fever and a more extensive exanthem. Thirty percent or more of immunocompromised children development visceral involvement with varicella, including hepatitis, pneumonia, encephalitis, or myocarditis. Varicella pneumonia is a life-threatening complication that may cause death in as many as 5% to 10% of immunocompromised children with unmodified varicella.

Not only is the rate of herpes zoster higher among children who are immunocompromised, but there is also a risk of visceral dissemination of VZV and death, albeit a lower risk than with varicella.

Intrauterine and Perinatal Varicella

A syndrome of congenital malformations is an unusual but well-documented complication of varicella that affects approximately 10% of infants born to women who develop varicella during the first trimester of pregnancy. Affected infants exhibit circumferential lesions of limbs, limb atrophy, eye defects, or cerebral atrophy.

When maternal varicella develops within the period of 4 days prior to delivery to 2 days after delivery, there is a considerable risk of overwhelming infection occurring in the newborn infant. In such cases, the neonate is exposed to maternal varicella but lacks the protection conferred by passively acquired maternal IgG antibody, which has not yet developed at the time of parturition. Administration of varicella-zoster immune globulin (VZIG) to infants exposed to maternal varicella within this period is strongly recommended, although the efficacy of VZIG in neonates has not been confirmed by clinical trial.

Diagnosis

In most instances, the diagnosis of varicella is based simply on a history of exposure to varicella or herpes zoster and the finding of the typical vesicular exanthem. In many cases, the diagnosis is made by the mother or other lay caretaker of the child who may or may not seek medical attention. Similarly, the diagnosis of zoster is most often based solely on physical findings alone. In the office or clinic, demonstration of multinucleated cells and intranuclear inclusions by Giemsa stain of cells scraped from the base of one or more varicella or zoster skin lesions (Tzank prep) is a simple and rapid technique for diagnosis available to experienced clinicians. VZV may also be recovered from vesicular fluid in cell culture, or acute infection can be demonstrated serologically by demonstration of a fourfold or greater rise in specific VZV antibody titer. While many serologic methods have been described, the fluorescent antimembrane antibody (FAMA) remains the standard method by which other serologic methods are compared.

Treatment and Prevention

Varicella in normal children requires no specific therapy other than symptomatic relief of the pruritus that often accompanies the rash. Either varicella or herpes zoster occurring in immunocompromised children is an indication for specific antiviral therapy. Intravenous acyclovir in a dose of 500 mg/M^2 q8h has been proven to hasten recovery and reduce the risk and severity of visceral complications of varicella and zoster in children with various underlying conditions. Acyclovir has several advantages over adenine arabinoside and alpha interferon which have also been demonstrated to be effective in controlled clinical trials.

Varicella can be prevented by both passive and active immunization. VZIG will prevent or modify infection of susceptible immunocompromised patients when it is administered within 3 days of exposure, but VZIG has no effect when given late in the incubation period or after the onset of symptoms. Recipients of VZIG will either remain seronegative, develop subclinical VZV infection with seroconversion, or develop mild varicella.

Active immunization with an experimental live attenuated varicella virus vaccine will prevent clinical varicella in about 80% of children with acute leukemia and modify illness in the minority that develop symptoms after exposure. VZV vaccine has also been widely tested in normal children and susceptible adults but has not yet been licensed in the United States.

MUMPS

Mumps virus infection is usually classified with the common viral exanthems of childhood, even though mumps is not usually associated with rash illness. Mumps is a self-limited, systemic viral infection of school age children, adolescents, and young adults. Acute parotitis is a common but not universal manifestation of mumps, and clinical disease of the CNS and other organ systems is well known. A live attenuated mumps virus vaccine is now administered routinely combined with measles and rubella vaccines (MMR).

Etiology

The mumps virus is a human paramyxovirus. Some antibodies to mumps virus cross-react with antibodies to the related parainfluenza viruses.

Epidemiology

Except where prevented by immunzation, mumps is a universal disease with a peak age of infection of 5 to 9 years. Ninety percent of the general population will have antibody to mumps by 14 years of age. Outbreaks in institutional settings among children and adolescents are common, especially during the peak transmission season of January to May.

The incidence of mumps has fallen dramatically in developed countries where mumps vaccine is widely used. In 1983 only 3,355 cases were reported in the United States representing an incidence of 1.4 per 100,000 population.

Pathogenesis

Mumps infection is transmitted *via* the respiratory route. Mumps virus is considered less contagious than measles or rubella viruses, and close personal contact is required for transmission to occur. Following replication in the upper respiratory tract, mumps virus spreads *via* the blood to various target organs including the parotid glands. A single attack confers lifelong immunity.

Clinical Features

Infection with mumps virus causes a relatively mild disease in children; about 30% to 40% of cases among children are inapparent. In contrast, adults often have more severe illness with a greater probability of involvement of organs other than the parotid glands.

After an incubation period of 16 to 18 days, the child with mumps experiences onset of fever, headache, and malaise. Acute parotid pain may produce a complaint of earache. Either unlateral or bilateral swelling and tenderness of the parotid is easily observed on examination, with the swollen parotid obscuring the angle of the mandible. The other salivary glands are sometimes involved, and erythema of the buccal opening of Stensen's duct may be seen on examination of the oral cavity.

The parotid swelling and tenderness peak within 2 to 4 days and usually resolve along with the fever and other symptoms within 5 to 7 days after onset.

Complications

CNS. Subclinical CNS infection is thought to be very common during mumps infections. As many as 50% of children with uncomplicated mumps illness have a CSF pleocytosis without symptoms of CNS involvement other than headache.

Meningismus can occur in as many as 5% to 10% of children with clinical mumps, only half of whom will have parotitis. In these cases, the signs and symptoms of mumps meningitis are similar to those of aseptic meningitis caused by other viruses. The CSF findings are also similar, although up to 30% of children with mumps meningitis may have an abnormally low CSF glucose concentration.

Frank encephalitis occurs in only about 1 in 6000 cases of mumps. The pathogenesis of mumps encephalitis includes both the "post-infectious" type, which is probably immunologically mediated, and primary encephalitis, in which mumps virus can be recovered directly from the brain. Symptoms and signs of both types include high fever, altered consciousness, and seizures. Neurologic sequelae and deaths are less likely to occur than following measles encephalitis.

Unilateral, high-frequency hearing loss occurs in as many as 4% of adults with mumps and a smaller percentage of children. Complete deafness occurs very uncommonly. Other well-known CNS complications include cerebellar ataxia, Bell's palsy, transverse myelitis, Guillain-Barré syndrome, and hydrocephalus secondary to stenosis of the aqueduct of Sylvius.

Other complications. In males, orchitis is the most common non-CNS complication of mumps. The rate of testicular involvement is 20% to 30% in postpubertal males; younger boys are rarely affected. About 10% to 20% of cases of mumps orchitis are bilateral. Acute onset of pain, testicular and epididymal swelling, and marked tenderness are the hallmarks that make orchitis difficult to miss clinically. Although testicular atrophy is a common sequela, frank sterility from bilateral mumps orchitis is very rare. Oophoritis complicates about 5% of mumps infections of postpubertal women. Other rare complications of mumps include polyarticular and monoarticular arthritis, pancreatitis, thyroiditis, glomerulonephritis, and myocarditis.

Diagnosis

In most clinical situations, the diagnosis of mumps is made solely on the basis of the history and physical findings. When a laboratory diagnosis is desired, acute and convalescent mumps antibodies can be demonstrated by HI, neutralization, or complement fixation (CF) methods. Virus isolation from oropharyngeal secretions, urine, and CSF is also feasible when there is access to diagnostic laboratory facilities.

The differential diagnosis of parotitis includes infection with other viruses, particularly enteroviruses and parainfluenza viruses, suppurative bacterial parotitis, and a variety of noninfectious causes.

Mumps Vaccine

Live attenuated mumps virus vaccine (Jeryl Lynn strain) was licensed in the United States in 1967, and has been combined with measles and rubella vaccine for routine use since the mid-1970s. Mumps vaccine administration produces seroconversion in more than 95% of susceptible persons and is associated with few adverse reactions.

ERYTHEMA INFECTIOSUM

Erythema infectiosum (fifth disease) is an acute, mild exanthematous disease of school-aged children that recently has been linked to infection with the human parvovirus B19.

Epidemiology

Erythema infectiosum occurs mostly in winter and spring. Outbreaks of disease among children in elementary and secondary schools are well known. As with other childhood exanthems, the clinical illness may be more severe in adults than in children.

Clinical Features

The incubation period has been estimated to be 14 to 18 days (range, 7 to 28). The typical child with erythema infectiosum has abrupt onset of low-grade fever and a characteristic erythematous eruption on the cheeks, which is often described as a "slapped cheek" appearance. In addition, some patients develop an erythematous, macular rash on the upper trunk and proximal extremities, which may evolve into a reticular pattern with central clearing of the erythema. Alternate fading and reappearance of the macular rash occurs in some patients for up to several weeks.

Erythema infectiosum resolves without complication in virtually all children. Rare cases of pneumonia and encephalitis are reported. Children with chronic, compensated hemolytic anemias such as sickle cell disease may suffer an exaggerated drop in hematocrit or hypoplastic crisis during acute parvovirus infection with or without symptoms of erythema infectiosum. Adults have an increased risk of acute, self-limited polyarticular arthritis.

BIBLIOGRAPHY

Anderson LJ: The role of parvovirus B19 in human disease. Pediatr Infect Dis 6:711–718, 1987

Azimi PH, Cramblett HG, Haynes RE: Mumps meningoencephalitis in children. JAMA 207:509–512, 1969

Balfour HH, Balfour CL, Edelman CK, Rierson PA: Evaluation of Wistar RA 27/3 rubella virus vaccine in children. Am J Dis Child 130:1089–1091, 1976

Bart KJ, Orenstein WA, Preblud SR, Hinman AR: Universal immunization to interrupt rubella. Rev Infect Dis 7 (suppl): S177–S184, 1985

Centers for Disease Control: Measles prevention. MMWR 31:217–231, 1982

Centers for Disease Control: Measles—United States, 1986. MMWR 36:301–305, 1987

Centers for Disease Control: Mumps vaccine. MMWR 30:87–94, 1980

Centers for Disease Control: Rubella and congenital rubella syndrome—United States 1984–1985. MMWR 35:129–135, 1986

Centers for Disease Control: Rubella vaccination during pregnancy—United States, 1971–1985. MMWR 35:275–284, 1986

Corba T, Coccia, P, Holman RC et al: The role of parvovirus B19 in aplastic crisis and erythema infectiosum (fifth disease). J Infect Dis 154:383–393, 1986

Cooper LZ, Krugman S: The Rubella Problem. Year Book Medical Publisher, New York, 1969

Feldman S, Hughes WT, Daniel CB: Varicella in children with cancer. Seventy-seven cases. Pediatrics 56:388–397, 1975

Gershon AA, Steinberg SP, Gelb L et al: Live attenuated varicella vaccine. JAMA 252:355–362, 1984

Green RH, Balsamo MR, Giles JP, Krugman S, Mirick G: Studies of the natural history and prevention of rubella. Am J Dis Child 110:348–365, 1965

Johnson RT: Progressive rubella encephalitis (editorial). N Engl J Med 292:1023–1024, 1975

Kleeman KT, Kiefer DJ, Halbert SP: Rubella antibodies detected by several commercial immunoassays in hemagglutination inhibition-negative sera. J Clin Microbiol 18:1131–1137, 1983

Meyers JP: Congenital varicella in term infants: Risk reconsidered. J Infect Dis 129:215–217, 1974

Miller HG, Stanton JB, Gibbons JL: Para-infectious encephalomyelitis and related syndromes: A critical review of the neurological complications of certain specific fevers. Q J Med 25:427–505, 1956

Modlin JF, Jabbour JT, Witte JJ, Halsey NA: Epidemiologic studies of measles, measles vaccine, and subacute sclerosing panencephalitis. Pediatrics 59:505–512, 1977

Nunoue T. Okochi K, Mortimer PP et al: Human parvovirus (B19) and erythema infectiosum. J Pediatr 107:38–40, 1985

Ogra PL, Herd JK: Arthritis associated with induced rubella infection. J Immunol 107:810–813, 1971

Paryani SG, Arvin AM: Intrauterine infection with varicella-zoster virus after maternal varicella. N Engl J Med 314:1542–1546, 1986

Phillip RN, Reinhard KR, Lackman DB: Observations on a mumps epidemic in a "virgin" population. Am J Hyg 69:91–111, 1959

Prober CG, Kirk LE, Keeney RE: Acyclovir therapy of chickenpox in immunosuppressed children—A collaborative study. J Pediatr 101:622–625, 1982

Tardieu M, Grospierre B, Durandy A, Griscelli C: Circulating immune complexes containing rubella antigens in late-onset congenital rubella syndrome. J Pediatr 97:370–373, 1980

Weber DM, Pellecchia JA: Varicella pneumonia, JAMA 192:572, 1965

Weller TH: Varicella and herpes zoster. N Engl Med 309:1362–1367, 1434–1438, 1983

Williamson AP: Varicella-zoster virus in the etiology of severe congenital defects. Clin Pediatr 14:553–559, 1975

32

Acute Diarrhea

Acute gastroenteritis is second only to the common cold as an acute illness and accounts for 3 million pediatric office visits a year in the United States. Worldwide, it affects 500 million children a year and is the major cause of death in children under the age of 4 years. It accounts for 28% of pediatric hospitalizations and is a major factor in malnutrition in the Third World. A number of microbial agents are capable of inducing diarrhea by a number of pathophysiologic mechanisms (Table 32-1).

NORMAL FLORA

The human is born "germ-free" with microflora swallowed later to allow for the development of normal bowel colonization. Local microbial proliferation is favored by available substrate, degree of competition, and oxygen concentration. The proximal small bowel is populated by aerobic flora, primarily streptococci and lactobacilli, in modest numbers of 10^3 to 10^4 organisms. Beyond the ileocecal region, bacterial counts reach 10^{11} organisms

with the low oxygen tensions favoring anaerobic proliferation by bacteroides and enterobacteria as well as coliforms. A normal viral flora has not been demonstrated in the human.

PATHOPHYSIOLOGY OF DIARRHEA

The pathogenicity of enteric bacteria is determined by colonization factors and virulence factors which promote infectivity and overcome the normal host defenses. Colonization factors may include flagellae *(e.g., Vibrio cholerae)*, enzymes such as mucinases or proteases, and pili or fimbriae to allow for bacterial adherence to the mucosal surface. The process of adherence is critical for many bacteria, especially toxin-elaborating or invasive *E. coli*. It requires a specific binding interaction between the bacterial surface and receptor sites on the mucosal epithelial surface. Adherence may be blocked by mucosal mucins or specific host antibodies to bacterial surface antigens.

The virulence of a bacteria may be deter-

Table 32–1. Microbial Etiologies and Frequency of Isolation in Acute Infantile Diarrhea

Etiology	Frequency of Isolation
Unknown	40%
Rotavirus	20%
E. coli, enteropathogenic	10%
Shigella	3%-15%
Campylobacter	3%-15%
Salmonella	4%
Giardia lamblia	4%
Multiple agents	3%
E. coli, enterotoxigenic	2%
Adenovirus	2%-6%

mined by its ability to produce enterotoxins, to invade the epithelial cell directly, or by its resistance to phagocytosis. Diarrhea can thus be induced by a toxin that creates net secretion of fluid from the enterocyte or by invasion and destruction of the enterocyte with release of inflammatory products.

For example, *Escherichia coli* has several potential mechanisms of producing diarrheal disease. First, some strains, termed enteropathogenic, adhere to the mucosal surface and alter the microvillus membrane, inducing leakage and diarrhea. A second group adhere and then invade the mucosal cells and thus are termed enteroinvasive *E. coli*. They elaborate a *Shigella*-like cytotoxin inside the mucosal cell to produce diarrhea. The third group, termed enterotoxigenic *E. coli*, can produce two forms of toxin: one heat-labile, which binds to the mucosal ganglioside GM receptor and activates adenylate cyclose to cause secretory diarrhea, and a second heat-stable toxin, which binds to a glycoprotein receptor and activates guanylate cyclase to induce diarrhea. This third group is of particular relevance, since the enterotoxigenic *E. coli* account for 60% to 70% of "travelers" diarrhea.

The enteroinvasive bacteria produce an inflammatory enteritis, primarily in the ile-um and/or colon, while the enterotoxigenic bacteria have minimal inflammation. In addition to some strains of *E. coli*, the enteroinvasive bacteria include *Shigella, Salmonella, Campylobacter, Aeromonas hydrophilia, Vibrio parahemolyticus, Bacillus cereus,* and *Yersinia enterocolytica.* The common clinical features of enteroinvasive bacteria disease are crampy abdominal pain, fever, bloody diarrhea, and the presence of fecal leukocytes. Some enteroinvasive bacteria can penetrate into the submucosa, especially in the terminal ileum, to produce systemic infection. These include *Salmonella typhi, Yersinia,* and *Campylobacter.*

By definition, enteric viral disease requires enteroinvasion. In contrast to enteroinvasive bacteria, the virus invasion is primarily in the proximal small bowel, producing high-volume diarrheal fluid losses with rare bleeding and minimal inflammatory response. Parasitic disease can run the gamut from proximal infestation with minimal inflammation *(Giardia lamblia)* to raging inflammatory colitis *(Entamoeba).*

VIRAL DIARRHEA

During the past decade, the ability to diagnose viral diarrhea has been greatly enhanced by the application of electron microscopy and ELISA technology. As noted above, following fecal–oral transmission, the viral agents invade the proximal small intestinal epithelium, generally at the villus tip. With cellular lysis and loss of mature villus epithelial cells, there is a resulting compensatory increase in immature crypt epithelium. The net result is reduction in enteric surface area with associated reduction in disaccharidase and dipeptidase activity and impaired absorption of ionic solutes as well as glucose and amino acids. Normally, the virus is shed rapidly with mucosal recovery anticipated over the next 7 to 10 days. This recovery may be delayed in the presence of malnutrition or immune deficiency.

The major viral enteritis in childhood is that caused by rotavirus, a 70-nm RNA virus that is the primary cause of childhood dehydration. The illness is characterized by watery diarrhea, with fever and emesis prominent in the first 48 hours. Isotonic dehydration and compensated metabolic acidosis should be anticipated. Neither stool polys or blood are anticipated. Oral hydration is usually successful unless emesis is protracted. Diagnosis is now available via office kits using ELISA or other specific antibody technology. Immunization studies are also underway with oral attenuated animal strains.

Norwalk-like viruses are a group of 27-nm viruses that are a major cause of epidemic (especially wintertime) viral enteritis, particularly in adolescents and young adults. Symptoms last for 36 to 48 hours with emesis the most prominent followed by fever, cramping abdominal, and moderate diarrhea. Dehydration is uncommon.

Recent studies suggest that adenovirus, a 75-nm DNA virus may account for up to 6% to 8% of infantile diarrhea. Associated respiratory disease is commonly noted. An enterocolitis illness may be seen, and so polys are occasionally noted in the stool. Hospital-acquired rotavirus and adenovirus remain a major pediatric concern. Additional studies are required before the roles of calicivirus, astrovirus, or coronovirus in childhood diarrhea can be determined.

BACTERIAL DIARRHEAS

As noted in the discussion of pathophysiology, a number of mechanisms may be involved in bacterial enteritis. The bacterial disorders are generally classified as either enteroinvasive or enterotoxigenic. The enteroinvasive bacterial enteritis disorders (Table 32-2) will be reviewed first.

Shigella. Worldwide, *Shigella* is the most common cause for clinical dysentery. In the United States, *Shigella sonnei* is the most common species, whereas in Central America and Asia, *Shigella dysenteriae* (Shiga bacillus) is of greater concern. The disease is most common between 1 and 4 years of age, with a predilection for the summer months. The bacteria enter colonic epithelia and elaborate a cytotoxin, producing ulceration and net secretion. The cytotoxin is also a neurotoxin and may produce encephalopathy, seizures, and reduced rectal tone. After an incubation period of 36 to 72 hours, the child develops fever, malaise, cramping abdominal pain, and a large-volume, watery diarrhea that progresses in half the children to mucousy, blood stools. In addition to the presence of stool polys and blood, the peripheral white blood cell count is often markedly elevated, with band forms prevalent. After correction of dehydration, treatment with trimethoprim–sulfamethoxazole is generally advised; this has been shown to shorten the illness, eradicate the organism, and reduce subsequent spread. Untreated

Table 32–2. Clinical Features of Enteroinvasive Bacterial Diarrhea

Feature	Salmonella	Shigella	Campylobactor	Yersinia
Primary age	Infancy	1–4 yr	Infancy–6 yr	2–18 yr
Site of injury	Ileum/colon	Colon	Colon	Ileum/colon
Positive blood culture	Common	Very rare	Rare	Rare
Bloody diarrhea	Rare	Common	Common	Rare
Fecal leukocytes	Variable	Present	Present	Variable
Mucosal ulceration	Variable	Common	Common	Aphthoid

patients may excrete the bacteria for weeks, a major concern in day-care settings. Complications of *Shigella* enteritis include toxic megacolon, cholestatic hepatitis, hemolytic–uremic syndrome, and, in malnourished children, mortality rates approaching 30%.

Salmonella. *Salmonella* is capable of producing a variety of clinical syndromes, ranging from gastroenteritis to bacteremia to typhoid fever to an asymptomatic carrier state. In the United States, *Salmonella enteritidis* and other nontyphoidal forms predominate. Infection is by ingestion of 10^6 to 10^{10} organisms, usually in food. Within 48 hours, the child develops nausea, fever, cramping abdominal pain, and diarrhea that usually progresses to passage of large amounts of mucus, pus, and blood. Multiple stool cultures may be required to confirm the diagnosis. The peripheral white blood cell count is usually normal to low but with a left shift in *Salmonella* gastroenteritis. Because antibiotic therapy does not alter the duration of illness, it is advised only in suspected bacteremia, infants under 1 year of age, and children with hemolytic anemias, immunosuppression, or congenital heart disease. Untreated patients recover over 5 to 10 days, although fecal shedding of salmonellae may last for several months.

Campylobacter. *Campylobacter jejuni* is usually acquired from household pets or contaminated foods. Invasion of both small bowel and colon have been reported. Onset of illness is acute, within a week of exposure, with fever, crampy abdominal pain, and large-volume, usually grossly bloody, diarrhea. Dehydration and bacteremia are rare, but infants may have a relapsing course. Necrosis of the jejunum is a rare complication. Diagnosis is often suspected by noting motile, curved bacilli in the stools. Culture growth requires special media and incubation. While sponta-

neous recovery within 7 to 14 days is the rule, the degree of toxicity and a relapse rate approaching 25% justify treatment with erythromycin in most children.

Yersinia. The diagnosis of *Yersinia* enterocolitica has often been missed because of the culture requirement of cold enrichment. Infection is usually from contaminated food or water. Illness begins with crampy abdominal pain, emesis, and diarrhea, progressing in 25% to bloody stools. Resolution over 3 to 7 days is generally expected. Extraintestinal manifestation may include septic anthritis, erythema nodosum, splenic abscess, myocarditis, nephritis, hepatitis, and, rarely, meningoencephalitis. Sepsis is usually seen only in the immunocompromised child. A chronic form with persistent abdominal pain and protein-losing enteropathy is also encountered. In older children, an acute ileitis syndrome mimicking appendicitis and Crohn's disease is also noted, with marked mesenteric adenitis and a low risk of ileal perforation. Fecal leukocytes are minimally increased, while peripheral leukocytosis may be marked. With suspected sepsis or a course lasting more than 1 week, treatment with tetracycline, chloramphenicol, or trimethoprim–sulfamethoxazole is advised. In the acute ileitis form, radiographic evidence of lymphoid nodular hypertrophy may persist for months after clinical diarrhea has ceased.

Invasive *Escherichia coli*. Enteroinvasive *E. coli* serotypes produce a dysentery-like illness indistinguishable by clinical means from other enteroinvasive bacteria. Stool blood and polys are anticipated. Because invasion beyond the lamina propnea is lacking, perforation of the colon is not seen.

Recently an enterohemorrhagic form of *E. coli* has been reported (*E. coli* 0157:H7). After acquisition from food, most notably cheese or ground beef, severe crampy abdominal pain is followed by watery diarrhea that becomes bloody and persists for up to 10 days. Submucosal edema is striking on barium enema, and hemolytic–uremic syndrome may develop in children. Treatment studies have been limited and inconclusive to date. Diagnosis of *E. coli* disease requires serotyping or DNA probes, and so they are often missed in clinical practice.

***Aeromonas hydrophila* and *Plesiomonas shigelloides*.** *A. hydrophilia* and *P. shigelloides*, natural inhabitants of both fresh and sea water, have recently been implicated in mild-to-moderate watery diarrhea. The duration of illness is less than a week and neither stool polys nor blood is generally noted. *Plesiomonas* is implicated particularly after ingestion of contaminated oysters. The mechanisms of intestinal injury and frequency of toxin elaboration are unknown.

Enterotoxigenic Bacteria. Bacterial toxin elaboration is nearly universal in bacterial enteritis. Even the invasive bacteria produce most of their symptoms from elaboration of toxin. The noninvasive toxigenic bacteria may produce a cytotoxin (as with *Clostridium difficile*) that produces an inflammatory colitis or a toxin with secretory activity but no inflammation (as with cholera of *E. coli*).

Toxigenic *E. coli*. As noted previously, toxigenic *E. coli* (ETEC) may produce either a heat-labile or heat-stable toxin, which enters the intestinal cell by a specific receptor to induce secretory diarrhea. ETEC is now recognized as the cause of nearly 75% of the cases of "traveler's" diarrhea in patients from industrialized countries. An epidemic form is most common in developing nations in children less than 2 years. Infection is from a large inoculum in contaminated water or food.

Clinical presentation is with crampy abdominal pain, urgency, and large-volume diarrhea with neither blood nor polys noted. If more than three stools are passed in less than 8 hours, treatment is usually initiated. The toxin can be bound by use of large doses of bismuth subsalicylate or the bacteria eradicated by trimethoprim–sulfamethoxazole. Other common causes of "traveler's" diarrhea include *Shigella* (15%), rotavirus (10%), and *Salmonella, Giardia lamblia,* or *Camplyobacter* (3% to 5%).

***Clostridium difficile*.** The growth of *Clostridium difficile* is normally limited by the competition of local anaerobic flora. During or after antibiotic therapy, however, the competition is altered and overgrowth of toxin-elaborating clostridia can occur. The cytopathic toxins (termed A and B) induce an inflammatory colitis, beginning with cramping lower abdominal pain and watery diarrhea. Raised yellow-white plaques develop on the mucosal surface, giving a characteristic "pseudo-membrane" appearance on endoscopic evaluation. Fecal leukocytes are prominent, but rectal bleeding is uncommon.

A number of antimicrobial agents have been implicated in the development of this antibiotic-associated syndrome. Ampicillin, clindamycin, or cephalosporins are implicated in more than 80% of patients. Less commonly, penicillin, erythromycin, and trimethoprim–sulfamethoxazole are reported.

There are three treatment options. First, stop the antibiotic and allow the normal flora to assert competitive inhibition of growth of *Clostridium difficile*. In mild cases, this may be effectively employed. Second, bind the toxin with an anion exchange resin, cholestyramine. Third, initiate administration of an antibiotic to directly inhibit growth of *Clostridium difficile*. Two such antibiotics have been successfully employed—vancomycin and metronidazole. Unfortunately, relapse rates of 10% to 25% are reported, with 5% to 10% having multiple relapses. The risks of untreated disease include chronic diarrhea, transmission to other family members, toxic megacolon, and, rarely, colonic perforation.

Food Poisoning from Bacterial Toxins. The ingestion of food containing bacterial toxin is encountered with four distinct bacteria: *Staphylococcus aureus*, *Bacillus cereus*, *Clostridium perfringens* and *Clostridium botulinum*.

S. aureus produces five different heat-resistant enterotoxins. They induce nausea, emesis, and secretory diarrhea within 2 to 6 hours of ingestion, usually from mayonnaise, potato salad, desserts, or meats. High salt and sugar content of the food enhance growth.

B. cereus is an aerobic, spore-forming, gram-positive bacillus that elaborates a heat-resistant toxin, particularly during growth on rice. Following ingestion, acute emesis is noted in 1 to 4 hours or diarrhea in 8 to 22 hours.

C. perfringens, with six exotoxins, rivals staphylococci as the major cause of food poisoning. In contrast to other food-borne toxins, which stimulate net secretion in the absence of cell injury, the heat-labile toxin of *C. perfringens* inhibits oxidative metabolism and is cytotoxic to ileal epithelium. Fever, abdominal pain, and diarrhea ensue within 8 to 14 hours after ingestion.

C. botulinum was long thought to be a risk only with ingestion of the bacterium or spore from improperly prepared foods, such as home-canned vegetables or farm-cured meats. Recently, it has been shown that ingestion of preformed toxin produces a unique syndrome in neonates and young infants up to 6 months of age. Resulting from a neurotoxin, the syndrome is generally one of progressive constipation, hypotonia, hyporeflexia, and cranial nerve dysfunction. The major source of spores and preformed toxin is contaminated honey.

PARASITIC ENTERITIS

While a number of parasites have an enteric component to their life cycle, diarrhea is a feature of only a few. Most significant are *Giardia lamblia*, *Entamoeba histolytica*, *Strongyloides stercoralis*, and *Cryptosporidium*.

Giardia Lamblia. Considered a normal inhabitant of the human small bowel until the 1950s, *Giardia* is now recognized as a significant cause of diarrheal disease. Contact is primarily from contaminated water or person-to-person in day-care settings or other crowded living conditions. Like *Shigella*, infection occurs with low-dose exposure by ingestion of the cyst. In the upper bowel, the organism excysts and divides into trophozoites, which line the mucosal surface and, rarely, invade. The sucking discs of the trophozoite contribute to mucosal injury. Crampy abdominal pain and diarrhea ensue. The degree of injury and duration of symptoms is greatest in infants and patients with deficiency of immunoglobulin A. Bacterial overgrowth may complicate recovery. Stools are loose and moderate in volume, with no fecal leukocytes or blood noted. Carbohydrate malabsorption is common. Eosinophilia is not seen.

The diagnosis is usually established by documenting cysts or trophozoites in the stool. Occasionally, small bowel aspirates or biopsies are required. Intermittent shedding may limit the value of stool studies alone. Treatment is advised for symptomatic children with quinacrine, furazolidone, or metronidazole. Asymptomatic excretors are also treated in day-care settings or in households with recurrence of symptomatic disease in a child.

Entamoeba histolytica. *E. histolytica* is ingested as a cyst, which excysts and divides into trophozoites that infect the colonic mucosa. The trophozoites usually establish a symbiotic relationship with anaerobic bacterial flora to produce a subclinical infection. Rarely, an ulcerative colitis ensues with bloody diarrhea. Invasion beyond the colon can lead to hepatic abscesses or pulmonary infestation. Diagnosis is usually established by examination of a fresh stool or serologically by hemagglutination. Metronidazole remains the treatment of choice.

Strongyloides sterocoralis. *Strongyloides,* or threadworms, live in the proximal small bowel lumen, usually in the absence of symptoms. The ova hatch in the jejunum, with larvae often penetrating intestine to reinfect the host. With heavy infestation, a chronic, recurring mucoid diarrhea and malabsorption may be seen. Diagnosis is by visualization of larvae in the stool, followed by treatment with thiabendazole. Peripheral eosinophilia may be prominent because of a blood-borne larval phase.

Cryptosporidium. *Cryptosporidium,* the newest "player" in the field, is a protozoan parasite usually encountered in sheep and cows. In veterinarians and animal handlers, a mild-to-moderate disease characterized by nausea, emesis, cramping abdominal pain, and up to 1 week of explosive, watery diarrhea has been recognized. Human-to-human transmission in day-care settings is also reported.

In immunocompromised patients, the diarrhea is much more severe and intractable. The most common underlying disease has been acquired immunodeficiency syndrome (AIDS), but post-transplant and lymphoproliferative malignancy patients are also at risk.

Diagnosis is by demonstration of the oocyst in fresh stool. Supportive treatment is the only proven therapy at this time, with gradual spontaneous resolution anticipated.

BIBLIOGRAPHY

Banwell JG, Lake AM: Gut Immunology and Ecology. Unit 17, American Gastroenterology Association Undergraduate Teaching Project, 1984

Barnett BB: Other viruses with etiologic roles in childhood gastroenteritis. J Pediatr Infect Dis 5:575–582, 1986

Dupont HL, Sullivan PS: Giardiasis: The clinical spectrum, diagnosis and therapy. J Pediatr Infect Dis 5:S131–S138, 1986

Giannella RA: Pathogenesis of acute bacterial diarrheal disorders. Ann Rev Med 32:341–357, 1981

Katz M: Parasitic infections. J Pediatr 87:165–178, 1975

Silverman A: Common bacterial causes of bloody diarrhea. Pediatr Ann 14:39–50, 1985

Tallett S, MacKenzie C, Middleten P et al: Clinical, laboratory and epidemiologic features of a viral gastroenteritis in infants and children. Pediatrics 60:217–222, 1977

Viscidi RP, Bartlett JG: Antibiotic-associated pseudomembranous colitis in children. Pediatrics 67:381–386, 1981

33

Tuberculosis

The mycobacteria are a large family of obligately aerobic "higher" bacterial organisms that are widely distributed in nature. Mycobacteria have cell walls with a high lipid content, a property that endows these organisms with the property of acid-fastness, or the ability to hold the color of carbol-fuchsin stain from decoloration by an acid-alcohol solvent. They replicate slowly, requiring 15 to 20 hours to divide *in vitro*, compared with a doubling time of 20 to 30 minutes for coliform bacteria. Many mycobacteria will produce visible colonies on artificial media only after prolonged incubation, so that a definitive diagnosis of mycobacterial disease based on culture of clinical material may take as long as 4 to 6 weeks.

In 1884, Koch demonstrated the human tubercle bacillus, *M. tuberculosis*, to be the cause of tuberculosis. Tuberculosis is known to have afflicted man for centuries, but the disease became widespread during the urban crowding and adverse social conditions that accompanied the industrial revolution in Europe and North America in the 18th and 19th centuries. The marked decline in the incidence of tuberculosis in the past 100 years has been attributed to improved living and

working environments and also to the introduction of effective antimicrobial agents within the past 40 years.

M. bovis, the agent of bovine tuberculosis, is capable of causing human disease that is indistinguishable from disease caused by *M. tuberculosis*. *M. bovis* infection, acquired from ingestion of the milk of infected cattle, is now rarely isolated in developed countries owing to the introduction of bovine tuberculosis control programs.

PATHOPHYSIOLOGY

Untreated tuberculosis is a lifelong infection. Although tuberculosis has the potential to cause disease in virtually every organ of the body, the lungs are the usual portal of entry, the most common site of symptomatic infection, and the source for respiratory spread of the tubercle bacillus from person to person.

Transmission

Transmission occurs *via* the inhalation of droplet nuclei, miniscule droplets of water containing infectious tubercle bacilli that are generated by an individual with active pulmonary tuberculosis *via* coughing, talking, or sneezing. The risk of transmission is directly related to the concentration of tubercle bacilli expelled into the ambiant air and prolonged exposure to contaminated air (the risk diminishes considerably in well-ventilated rooms). Infectious persons are usually elderly or debilitated adults with uncontrolled cavitary or laryngeal tuberculosis, who cough up sputum containing tubercule bacilli identifiable with the AFB (acid-fast bacilli, or Ziehl-Neelsen) stain. Children with active tuberculosis very rarely transmit the disease. Infection *via* ingestion of contaminated milk is virtually nonexistent in the United States but is a common mode of transmission of tuberculosis to children in the developing world.

Primary Infection

Infection begins when the inhaled droplet nuclei reach the terminal bronchioles. An asympmtomatic, small focus of pneumonia develops as the tubercle bacilli replicate at an (usually single) implantation site in a lower or middle lobe lung field. Spread of tubercle bacilli to hilar lymph nodes *via* the pulmonary lymphatics usually occurs, and organisms may also spread hematogeneously to distant organs, especially bone, kidneys, and the apices of the lungs, where replication may occur before the development of tuberculin sensitivity.

At this stage, the infection may follow any of several natural courses. In a small number of children, progression of infection at the original pulmonary implantation site may result in primary tuberculous pneumonia, and enlargement of lymph nodes at the hilum can produce mechanical compression of one or more bronchi with subsequent lobar atelectasis. Ongoing bacillemia and development of tuberculous foci in many organs leads to systemic (miliary) tuberculosis and/or tuberculous meningitis. Either local or systemic progression of primary tuberculosis is most likely to occur in very young children, or in persons of any age with poor nutrition or underlying chronic or immunosuppressive illness.

With the development of tuberculin sensitivity within 6 to 8 weeks after infection, the great majority of primary infections become quiescent and remain clinically unrecognized. The immunologic response to tuberculin protein (defined clinically by the presence of a positive tuberculin skin test) is related to the development of the lymphocyte-mediated immune response and is manifested pathologically by the characteristic granulomatous inflammatory response surrounding tuberculous foci. Healing of the primary lung focus occurs with granuloma formation, which later may become calcified. The presense of a calcified lower or middle lobe focus with ipsilateral hilar adenopathy, the so-called Ghon complex, is an uncommon but highly characteristic radiologic manifestation of healed primary tuberculosis.

Reactivation Tuberculosis

Most people with primary tuberculous infection remain asymptomatic for life, whether or not they receive antituberculous drug therapy. However, 5% to 15% of untreated persons with quiescent tuberculosis will later develop active disease in the lungs, or at another body site such as bone or kidney. Reactivation infection is characterized locally by granuloma formation, central necrosis, and caseation. About half of reactivated lung foci progress to cavity formation. A tuberculous cavity harbors a concentration of organisms that is logs higher than the concentration found in caseous or granulomatous lesions. Drainage of a cavity into an airway leads to endobronchial spread of tuberculosis throughout the lungs. Adolescents and adults with untreated endobronchial cavitary tuberculosis are likely to be highly infectious for close contacts.

Approximately 54% of reactivation disease occurs within the first year of infection and 78% within 2 years. Thus, reactivation is most likely to occur in children within a few years of primary infection. Children under 3 years of age and adolescents are known to have a higher rate of reactivation of tuberculous foci. The risk of reactivation also correlates with the degree of the initial exposure, with systemic viral infections such as measles, and in the presence of underlying malnutrition, steroid therapy, or chronic illness.

DIAGNOSIS

The Tuberculin Skin Test

Two types of skin tests are available for the purpose of determining the presence or absence of tuberculin sensitivity, an indication of current or past infection with *M. tuberculosis*. In both, the test is applied to the volar aspect of the forearm and is read 48 to 72 hours after injection.

The Mantoux test is the definitive test for tuberculin sensitivity. It consists of the intradermal injection of 5 tuberculin units (TU) of either of two well-standardized preparations, old tuberculin (OT) or purified protein derivitive (PPD). A reaction consisting of 10 mm or greater of *induration* is a positive test, 5 to 9 mm of induration is considered a doubtful test, and any reaction less than 5 mm is recorded as a negative. Tuberculin sensitivity is generally maintained for life, but there is probably some loss of reactivity with time in the absence of continue exposure, low-grade infection, or repeat skin testing. Skin testing with OT or PPD does not sensitize tuberculin-negative persons, but repeat testing may produce a booster response in previously positive persons.

The Mantoux test is an important part of the evaluation of any patient in which tuberculosis is part of the differential diagnosis, but careful interpretation means consideration of both false-negative and false-positive reactions. The test may become doubtful or even negative when many years have lapsed since the last test or in the presence of immunosuppressive drug therapy or debilitating disease. False-positive reactions occur in a small number of persons who are infected with nontuberculous mycobacteria, although the majority of such persons have doubtful or negative reactions. Although strengths of PPD other than 5 TU are available, they have little clinical usefulness.

The second method of tuberculin skin testing employs a disposable multiple-puncture device in which the tines are coated with OT or PPD (tine test, Heaf test). The tine test is a convenient method for screening low-risk populations of persons such as school children or college students. Equivocal or positive tine tests must always be confirmed with the standard Mantoux skin test.

Identification of Tubercle Bacilli in Secretions and Tissue Specimens

The high lipid content of the cell walls of all mycobacteria allows the organism to retain the red color of carbol-fuchsin after "decoloration" with a combined acid-alcohol solvent that washs the stain from background tissue and debris and from other microorganisms present in the specimen. When the background material is counterstained with methylene blue, the "acid-fast" mycobacteria are visualized as bright red, slender, slightly beaded organisms with tapered ends against a uniformly blue background. Minor modifications of this time-honored technique have conferred different eponymic labels, such as the Ziehl-Neelsen or the Kinyoun stain. Many microbiology laboratories now employ rhodamine, a fluorochrome stain that appears to enhance the visualization of mycobacteria when compared with the methods using the traditional acid-fast reagents.

PULMONARY TUBERCULOSIS

Primary Lung Disease

As stated above, most children with primary lung foci have clinically inapparent infections that heal spontaneously, but there is a risk of progression of primary infection, particularly in young children. Fever, which occurs with the development of tuberculin sensitivity, tachypnea, cough, and chest pain are characteristic symptoms, which are usually indistinguishable from other bacterial causes of pneumonia. The chest x-ray shows an infiltrate in one or more of the middle or lower lobes of the lung. The presence of hilar adenopathy is highly characteristic of primary tuberculosis; compression of major bronchi may be associated with wheezing and with either hyperexpansion or atelectasis on chest x-ray. Cavity formation may or may not occur with progression of tuberculous pneumonia.

The treatment of primary tuberculous pneumonia is the same as for other types of tuberculosis. In the absence of caseation or cavity formation, tuberculous pneumonia can be treated with 12 months of isoniazid (INH) therapy alone.

A *pleural effusion* may occur suddenly during primary tuberculosis when a subpleural tuberculous lesion ruptures and disseminates tubercle bacilli in the pleural space. This event is accompanied by sudden onset of fever, cough, and pleural pain. AFB stain of the pleural fluid is generally negative, but virtually all children with acute tuberculous pleural effusion will have converted to a positive skin test result. In fact, many authorities suspect that the inflammatory response within the pleural space is largely a result of the recent development of tuberculin sensitivity. Culture of pleural fluid is positive in only 30% of cases. A pleural biopsy will demonstrate the characteristic histology in most cases. Although the natural course of tuberculous pleural effusion is slow, spontaneous resolution, recovery can be hastened by administration of antiinflammatory agents.

Reactivation Tuberculosis

Reactivation of tuberculosis in children and adolescents occurs months to years after an unrecognized primary infection. The apical portion of the upper or lower lobes are the most common sites, and unilateral disease is more common than bilateral disease. Reactivation tuberculosis typically progresses from infiltration of involved lung to caseous necrosis and cavity formation with scarring. In adolescents and adults, there is frequently little or no radiologic evidence of earlier primary tuberculosis (i.e., hilar adenopathy is not apparent). Patients with reactivation tuberculosis may present with fever, productive cough, chest pain, hemoptysis, malaise, and a history of recent weight loss.

Tuberculomas are asymptomatic, smooth-walled "coin" lesions that are usually detected on routine chest x-rays. They represent healed caseous or calcified tuberculous lesions within the lung parenchyma.

The diagnosis of pulmonary tuberculosis is often first suspected on the basis of the history and characteristic findings on chest x-ray. The presence of a positive AFB stain of sputum, bronchial washings, gastric aspirates, or biopsied tissue provides strong presumptive evidence of tuberculosis, but false-positive results sometimes occur because of the presence of mycobacteria other than *M. tuberculosis*. The definitive diagnosis is based on culture of these clinical specimens.

TUBERCULOSIS IN OTHER ORGANS

Extrapulmonary disease occurs in 10% to 15% of reported tuberculosis cases. Virtually any organ can be involved as a result of hematogenous spread of tubercle bacilli during primary infection, a process that is generally contained with the development of tuberculin sensitivity.

Progressive dissemination with disease due to bone marrow, liver, lung, and central nervous system infection is termed *miliary tuberculosis*. Miliary tuberculosis is most often a complication of primary tuberculosis in young children. Affected children experience either abrupt or insidious onset of fever, weight loss, anorexia, and adenopathy for as long as 1 to 4 months before the diagnosis is made and appropriate antituberculous therapy initiated. Anemia, leukopenia, and hyponatremia are commonly present early in the course. The chest x-ray usually shows a reticular, interstitial infiltrate but may be normal early in the course of disseminated tuberculosis. The correct diagnosis is often delayed, in part because of a low index of suspicion on the part of the practitioner. Even when suspected, the diagnosis is often difficult to confirm; approximately 25% of children with miliary tuberculosis will have negative tuberculin skin test results. The most expedient diagnostic procedure is biopsy of lung, liver, or bone marrow, which will demonstrate characteristic granulomas and acid-fast bacilli. Ultimately, cultures of sputum, urine, gastric aspirates, cerebrospinal fluid (CSF), or biopsy material will confirm the diagnosis. Untreated miliary tuberculosis is fatal; otherwise, the prognosis depends on the child's clinical status when therapy is initiated.

Tuberculous meningitis occurs in young children with or without miliary tuberculosis as a result of hematogenous dissemination of tubercle bacilli to the meninges during primary infection. The resulting inflammatory response is greatest at the base of the brain, involving cerebral arteries and cranial nerves, and producing hydrocephalus as a result of obstruction of CSF flow at the ventricular foramina. Affected children present with fever, headache, confusion, lethargy, and signs of meningeal irritation that may progress over days or weeks. With advancing disease, cranial nerve palsies, papilledema, seizures, and increasing obtundation are the rule. As with miliary tuberculosis, the diagnosis of tuberculous meningitis depends on a high index of suspicion on the part of the physician. The tuberculin skin test is positive in about 75% of children, but the chest x-ray may be normal in as many as 50%. Although the CSF is the key to the diagnosis, repeated lumbar punctures may be necessary before the characteristic findings of tuberculous meningitis are reflected in the CSF (*i.e.*, a predominantly lymphocytic pleocytosis with a white blood cell count that is usually less that 1000 per mm^3, increasing protein concentration, and diminishing glucose concentration). AFB stains of the CSF are positive in a minority of cases; examination of the centrifuged CSF pellet and use of rhodamine stain may enhance the chance of finding the organisms microscopically. Early therapy is critical, and the stage of disease at the onset of therapy is the single most important prognostic factor. Both INH and rifampin penetrate into the CSF; corticosteroids are advocated when signs of cerebral edema or hydrocephalus are present. Even with therapy, the overall mortality of tuberculous meningitis is about 20%, and many children have significant neurologic residua.

Tuberculomas are rare, slowly enlarging granulomas of the brain that present as mass lesions. The CSF findings are usually normal, and the diagnosis is most often made at surgery.

Renal infection is the most common form of extrathoracic tuberculosis. Spread to the kidneys during primary infection is thought to be relatively frequent, but reactivation with clinical disease tends to occur years later, and generally only in one kidney. Dysuria, flank pain, hematuria, and sterile pyuria are common presenting manifestations; fever and azotemia are uncommon. By the time the patient presents, the disease is often advanced to the point that intrarenal caseation, cavities, or calcification can be demonstrated by intravenous pyelogram (IVP) or by ultrasound. Development of an obstructive uropathy with healing is an important complication of renal tuberculosis.

About half of cases of tuberculosis involving the skeletal system occur in the spinal column. *Vertebral tuberculosis* (Pott's disease) can occur anywhere in the length of the spinal column but is most frequently found in the thoracic and lumbar vertebrae. Initially, loss of volume of the anterior portion produces the characteristic wedge-shaped vertebral body. Infection then spreads readily across the intervertebral disk space, resulting in obliteration of the disk space and involvement of adjacent vertebrae. With progression of infection, one sees development of an anterior paraspinous abscess, which can extend the length of many vertebrae. The devastating outcome of inadequately treated vertebral tuberculosis is vertebral collapse and paraplegia. The use of antituberculous antibiotics alone is now the standard treatment for vertebral tuberculosis; surgery is reserved for cases in which there is impending spinal cord involvement.

Tuberculous osteoarthritis is infection of contiguous bone and joint space, most frequently in the lower extremities. The earliest clinical manifestation is pain; later there is swelling of the joint due to thickening of the synovium or an effusion of the joint space. Skeletal tuberculosis usually produces extensive destruction of bone and periarticular cartilage. A bone or synovial biopsy is the most expedient means of diagnosis. AFB staining of joint fluid is positive in only 20% of cases, but the culture should be positive in more than 80%.

Tuberculous pericarditis is an uncommon, but life-threatening form of tuberculosis that follows hematogenous spread or rupture of a tuberculous lesion into the pericardial space. The initial pericardial effusion may cause relatively few symptoms until the symptoms and signs of tamponade occur. The later development of constrictive pericarditis is an uncommon complication.

Gastrointestinal tuberculosis, which most often follows swallowing of contaminated food or infected pulmonary secretions, can occur in any portion of the gastrointestinal tract. The ilium and cecum are the most common sites. Replication of tubercle bacilli in lymphoid tissue in these locations produces submucosal granulomatous masses and mucosal ulcerations, which may progress to intestinal obstruction, perforation, or fistula formation. Abdominal pain, diarrhea, constipation, bleeding, and malabsorption are all presenting features. In developed countries, gastrointestinal tuberculosis is frequently mistaken for malignancy until laparotomy. Approximately half of patients will also have active pulmonary tuberculosis.

Tuberculous peritonitis is caused by seeding of the peritoneal space with tubercle bacilli from a caseous abdominal lymph node, from a pelvic site, or from intestinal perforation at a site of intraluminal gastrointestinal tuberculosis. Affected children have insidious onset of fever, abdominal pain, anorexia, weight loss, and increasing abdominal girth (secondary to ascites). Examination may indicate signs of ascites, peritoneal tenderness, multiple masses, or a "doughy" consistency on palpation. The diagnosis of tuberculous peritonitis is most quickly made by peritoneal biopsy.

Tuberculosis can occur in many other organs or organ systems in children, including the lymph nodes, genitalia, skin, larynx, middle ear, and adrenal gland.

CONGENITAL AND NEONATAL TUBERCULOSIS

M. tuberculosis infection has been transmitted to the fetus in rare cases of symptomatic maternal tuberculosis late in gestation. Infants born with *congenital tuberculosis* either are stillborn or have generalized infection at delivery with extensive disease of the liver, lung, bone marrow, and other organs with a mortality that exceeds 90%.

Perinatal or postnatal exposure to tuberculosis also represents a high risk of disseminated or progressive pulmonary disease in immunologically immature newborn infants who typically fail to express tuberculin sensitivity. When the mother has active pulmonary tuberculosis, the risk of transmission to the newborn infant is approximately 50%. The management of these infants is somewhat controversial. Some authorities recommend separation of the infant from the mother at birth until the maternal disease is under control in order to prevent neonatal disease; others consider treatment of the newborn with isoniazid alone to be adequate management. Regardless, all infants returning to households in which a tuberculin-positive person resides should be treated with INH until it can be established with certainty that no contacts have active infection. Follow-up of these infants with regular tuberculin skin testing is mandatory.

TREATMENT

The antibiotic therapy of tuberculosis is based on knowledge of the pathobiology of the organism and the naturally occurring drug resistence observed in populations of *M. tuberculosis* cultivated on artificial media. Effective therapy requires drugs that are active against rapidly dividing tubercle bacilli in the high-oxygen, neutral *p*H environment of pulmonary cavities and also drugs that inhibit the more slowly replicating organisms that inhabit caseous and granulomatous tissues, or exist intracellulary in macrophages, where replication occurs very slowly, if at all.

In addition, mutant tubercle bacilli naturally express resistance to most clinically useful antibiotics at a rate of the order of 1 in 10^5 for INH and 1 in 10^8 for rifampin. In clinical situations where pulmonary cavities may contain more than 10^9 tubercle bacilli, the chance of selecting out a resistant population of organisms is high when only one drug is used, and the rate of treatment failures is substantial. Conversely, clinically inapparent granulomatous foci that contain only 10^3 to 10^4 organisms will be sterilized by a single drug alone. These observations form the rationale for the use of multiple agents to treat clinically advanced disease, while asymptomatic tuberculin converters are usually managed with INH alone.

INH and rifampin now represent the mainstay of antibiotic therapy of children with *M. tuberculosis* infection that is not caused by drug-resistant organisms. Both drugs are bactericidal against both extracellular and intracellular organisms, and both penetrate adequately into the CSF, which is important for the management of CNS tuberculosis. The use of INH and rifampin in combination has allowed the introduction of "short-course" antibiotic therapy of children with most forms of tuberculosis. INH is given orally in a dose of 10 to 15 mg/kg (maximum, 300 mg), and rifampin is given in an oral dose of 15 to 20 mg/kg (maximum, 600 mg) once daily to initiate therapy. Clinical improvement can be expected to occur within 2 weeks, although improvement in the appearance of the chest x-ray may take months. After 2 months of therapy, the dose of both agents can be reduced so that each are administered twice weekly, with the dose of INH doubled. A total of 9 months of therapy is now standard.

If either or both drugs cannot be used for reasons of drug toxicity or recovery of tubercle bacilli that are drug-resistant, then less active agents are added to the regimen, but a longer course is required to ensure complete cure.

These "second-line" antibiotics include streptomycin, ethambutol, para-aminosalicylic acid, and pyrazinamide. Ethambutol, pyrazinamide, or streptomycin (or a combination of the three drugs) should be added to INH and rifampin if the circumstances suggest the possibility of primary drug resistance (infection in a region with a high level of drug resistance such as southeast Asia or Africa, or contact with a person with known drug-resistant tuberculosis) or if there has been previous therapy of the child for tuberculosis. Ethambutol and pyrazinamide may be too toxic for use in young children under certain circumstances, and streptomycin use may also be limited because of potential ototoxicity.

Failure of treatment is manifest by persistence of symptoms, clinical deterioration, or a worsening chest x-ray. These problems raise the specter of primary drug resistance or may indicate that the child is not receiving the prescribed medications.

Problems arising from drug toxicity are rare in children receiving the appropriate dose of INH and rifampin. Approximately 75% will develop an asymptomatic elevation of hepatic transaminases during the first 2 months of treatment, but jaundice and other symptoms occur in fewer than 0.5% of children. Although some authorities advocate regular testing of serum hepatic transaminase levels during the first 2 months of therapy, others consider monitoring unnecessary.

Treatment of Asymtomatic Children with Positive Skin Tests

The term "prophylaxis" is widely used to refer to the treatment of asymptomatic, skin-test–positive persons who have not previously received antituberculous therapy. The standard therapy for skin test "converters" who are under 35 years of age is INH alone for a total of 9 months.

INH treatment for 3 months is also recommended for children under 5 years of age whenever they are exposed to an active case of tuberculosis in the household, regardless of their skin test status. Repeat skin testing is mandatory at the end of the prophylactic regimen; children who convert to a positive test should then receive the full 9 months of INH.

BCG

Bacille Calmette Guérin (BCG) is a live attenuated strain of tubercle bacilli derived from both *M. tuberculosis* and *M. bovis*. BCG is widely administered in the developing world to prevent tuberculosis, and is recommended by the World Health Organization to be given to all infants at birth. However, under controlled conditions, the efficacy of BCG in preventing clinical disease has varied from 0 to 80%, probably because of differences in potency of different BCG preparations.

There is a widely held misbelief that prior BCG administration interferes with the subsequent interpretation of the tuberculin skin test. In fact, tuberculin reactions of 10 mm or greater are rarely caused by BCG infection alone in children when the skin test is applied more than 1 or 2 years after administration of BCG.

INFECTIONS CAUSED BY OTHER MYCOBACTERIA

There are numerous other mycobacteria species that are capable of causing human disease. These organisms are often grouped together under the term "atypical" mycobacteria and they cause a broad spectrum of clinical illness, ranging from pulmonary disease indistinguishable from tuberculosis, to chronic infections limited to the skin and soft tissues. Unlike *M. tuberculosis* and *M. bovis*, the other mycobacteria are ubiquitous inhabitants of soil and water, although many mycobacteria species have limited geographic distributions. Infection is invariably acquired from environmental sources; person-to-person transmission does not occur.

The other mycobacteria are traditionally classified according to their growth characteristics and pigment production into four groups (Runyon classification): photochromagens, scotochromagens, nonchromogens, and rapid-growing mycobacteria. A number of different species, which are identified on the basis of biochemical reactions, are distributed among the four groups.

Nontuberculous Mycobacterial Cervical Lymphadenitis

By far the most common nontuberculous mycobacterial infection of children to come to clinical attention is cervical lymphadenitis. Preschool-aged children are most often infected and *M. avium-intracellulare* or *M. scrofulaceum* are the usual species of mycobacteria recovered. The typical child presents with unilateral, painless, nontender swelling of one or more submandibular or submaxillary nodes in the absence of fever or other systemic symptoms. Ten percent to 15% of children with nontuberculous adenitis will have a draining, open lesion overlying the node.

The management of suspected nontuberculous adenitis is complete surgical excision. Excised nodes show an intense granulomatous reaction, and many will also contain acid-fast bacilli with specific staining. Although the definitive diagnosis rests on culture of the node, as many as 50% to 60% of excised nodes are culture negative, even in the presence of a positive AFB stain.

Since the nontuberculous mycobacteria tend to be resistant to the antibiotics commonly used to treat tuberculosis, their use should be limited to cases in which *M. tuber-culosis* cervical adenitis is part of the differential diagnosis. (In the United States, *M. tuberculosis* causes fewer than 10% of mycobacterial adenitis cases. Furthermore, *M. tuberculosis* adenitis tends to occur in older children in the setting of contact with tuberculosis, bilateral nodal involvement, and a positive chest x-ray.)

BIBLIOGRAPHY

Avery ME, Wolfsdorf J: Diagnosis and treatment: Approaches to newborn infants of tuberculous mothers. Pediatrics 42:519–522, 1968

BCG: Bad news from India (editorial). Lancet 1:73–74, 1980

Committee on Diagnostic Skin Testing: The tuberculin skin test. Am Rev Respir Dis 104:769–775, 1971

Comstock GW, Livesay VT, Woolpert SF: The prognosis of a positive tuberculin reaction in childhood and adolescence. Am J Epidemiol 99:131, 1974

Dutt AK, Stead WW: Present chemotherapy for tuberculosis. J Infect Dis 146:698–704, 1982

Hageman J, Shulman S, Schreiber M et al: Congenital tuberculosis: Critical reappraisal of clinical findings and diagnostic procedures. Pediatrics 66:980–984, 1980

Houk VH, Kent DC, Baker JH et al: The *Byrd* study. In-depth analysis of a micro-outbreak of tuberculosis in a closed environment. Arch Environ Health 16:4, 1968

Jacobs RF, Abernathy RS: The treatment of tuberculosis in children. Pediatr Infect Dis 4:513–517, 1985

Lincoln EM, Sewells EM: Tuberculosis in children. New York, McGraw-Hill, 1963

Nemir RL: Perspective in adolescent tuberculosis: Three decades of experience. Pediatrics 78:399–405, 1986

Nemir RL, Teichner A: Management of tuberculin reactors in children and adolescents previously vaccinated with BCG. Pediatr Infect Dis 2:446–451, 1983

Sahn SA: Miliary tuberculosis. Am J Med 56:495, 1974

Stead WW, Bates J: Evidence of a "silent" bacillemia in primary tuberculosis. Ann Intern Med 74:559, 1971

Strumph IJ, Tsang AY, Schork MA et al: The reliability of gastric smears by auramine-rhodamine staining technique for the diagnosis of tuberculosis. Am Rev Respir Dis 114:971, 1976

Styblo K: Recent advances in epidemiological research in tuberculosis. Adv Tuberc Res 20:1, 1980

Wolinsky E: Nontuberculous mycobacteria and associated diseases. Am Rev Respir Dis 119:107–159, 1979

34

Sexually Transmitted Diseases

GONORRHEA

Neisseria gonorrhoeae is a gram-negative, aerobic diplococci, difficult to grow *in vitro* because it requires a narrow *p*H range (7.2 to 7.6), low CO_2 concentration (2% to 10%), and a temperature of 35°C to 37°C. Nonetheless, *N. gonorrhoeae* causes a number of illnesses in persons of all ages.

Gonorrhea (GC) is the most common reportable infectious disease in the United States. There were 863,677 cases of GC reported in 1984; this averages to more than 428 cases per 100,000 population. Since the majority of GC cases are not reported, approximately 2 million cases of GC are estimated to occur each year. The highest rate per 100,000 population occurs in men 20 to 24 years of age. The highest rates in women occur in women 15 to 24 years of age.

Pathophysiology

N. gonorrhoeae can invade columnar epithelium. Initially, the organisms adhere to mucosal surfaces by means of hair-like projections from the cell wall called pili. These pili have the capacity to protect the organism from antibodies and complement. The risk of developing disease also depends on local factors, such as the thickness of the mucosal wall and its *p*H. Antibody production to GC does not provide solid immunity, and thus reinfection is common. In addition, many strains of *N. gonorrhoeae* have developed mutations that render them penicillin resistant by their production of penicillinases.

Clinical Manifestations

Asymptomatic GC. A person may harbor GC in the pharynx, rectum, vagina, or urethra without demonstrating any symptoms (see below) of the disease. As many as 80% of women and 40% of men may be asymptomatic and serve as reservoirs of infection.

Symptomatic GC.

Gonococcal Ophthalmia Neonatorum. The neonate acquires gonococcal ophthalmia neonatorum after passage through the birth canal of a mother who has GC. After an incubation period of 1½ to 3 days, the infant develops either unilateral or bilateral conjunctivitis with purulent discharge. Untreated, the disease is rapidly progressive, with corneal ulceration, opacification, and blindness resulting. Instillation of 1% $AgNO_3$ into the eyes soon after birth decreases the incidence of this disease. Periodic culturing and treatment, if necessary, of pregnant women eliminates the disease.

Urethritis. After an incubation period of 2 to 5 days, a male who has contracted GC may complain of dysuria or a yellow urethral discharge. The physical examination is usually normal except for the presence of a discharge, the amount of which can be increased by milking the urethra.

Epididymitis. After an incubation period of 2 to 5 days, a male patient with GC-related epididymitis presents with a red, swollen, painful hemiscrotum; bilateral involvement is not as common as unilateral involvement. A urethral discharge may be present. The physical examination reveals a swollen, tender, warm testis and epididymis. The condition must be distinguished from testicular torsion, which is not usually accompanied by a discharge. Lifting the affected testis usually relieves the pain of epididymitis but does not alleviate the pain of torsion (Prehn's sign).

Vaginitis. The prepubertal child may present with a swollen, red vulva. She may have a discharge or dysuria or complain of vaginal itching.

The postpubertal female may present with all the symptoms listed above. She is more likely to have a discharge than is a younger patient.

Cervicitis. Cervicitis is a common GC-associated entity in postpubertal females. It is characterized by a purulent yellow or green discharge accompanied by dysuria. The patient may also complain of pain during intercourse. The endocervix may bleed after swabbing for cultures.

Salpingitis. Salpingitis (also known as pelvic inflammatory disease [PID]) is the inflammation of the fallopian tubes. It is rare in virgins. As with all manifestations of GC, a number of different organisms can cause this entity. The symptoms of salpingitis are those common to all female genital infections (discharge, dysuria, dyspareunia) and lower abdominal pain. The pain may be so severe that the patient walks slightly stooped with a shuffling gait. The diagnosis, however, is confirmed by adnexal tenderness and the elicitation of pain when the cervix is moved on physical examination.

Fitz-Hugh–Curtis Syndrome. Fitz-Hugh–Curtis syndrome is acute perihepatitis and is really a localized peritonitis. It should be suspected in any female with upper right quadrant pain, especially when PID or symptoms of genital infection are present.

Proctitis. GC infection of the rectum is acquired through anal sex. Symptoms include painful defecation, anal discharge, and an inability to sit.

Pharyngitis. The symptoms of GC pharyngitis may be no different from those of pharyngitis caused by other organisms.

Disseminated GC. Disseminated GC results from hematogenous spread of the organism and most commonly manifests itself as arthritis, tenosynovitis, and dermatitis. Septic arthritis in adolescents and young adults is frequently caused by GC. Usually, the arthritis is monarthric, with minimal systemic signs and negative blood cultures. However, the joint fluid may be positive for GC. Occasionally, the arthritis is polyarthric, and there are systemic signs such as fever, chills, dermatitis, and positive blood cultures. The dermatologic lesions may be macular, maculopapular, vesicular, pustular, or purpuric, but the organism is rarely recovered from these lesions.

Endocarditis (with aortic valve involvement) and meningitis may also follow disseminated GC infections.

Diagnosis of GC

The initial suspicion of a GC infection may be verified by demonstration of gram-negative diplococci in polymorphonuclear cells; strictly speaking, there should be at least eight sets of diplococci in each polymorphonuclear cell. Demonstration of gram-negative diplococci from a male patient is usually sufficient to make the diagnosis. However, because the female genital tract contains numerous organisms, some of which are gram-negative diplococci, the criterion of intracellular organisms should be followed.

Cultures of the discharge, affected sites, or associated sites should be obtained. *N. gonorrhoeae* grows best on chocolate agar to which vancomycin, colistimethate sodium, and nystatin have been added. This mixture is known as Thayer-Martin medium. *N. gonorrhoeae* also grows best under conditions of reduced O_2 content so that candle jars of "CO_2 packs" should be used, especially if the sample cannot be transported to the laboratory immediately. If disseminated GC is suspected, a culture of the blood, joint fluid, or skin lesion should be obtained.

Treatment of GC-Related Diseases

The treatment of GC-related diseases is outlined in Table 34-1.

SYPHILIS

Syphilis is caused by *Treponema pallidum*, a slender, coiled, motile spirochete. This organism stains poorly and requires dark-field microscopy or immunofluorescence for detection. It is not easily cultured in vitro.

The rate of syphilis is approximately 14 per 100,000 population. The male rate is between two and three times the female rate. The incidence of congenital syphilis does not show any sex predominance and has been rising since 1978.

Pathophysiology

The organism may be transmitted transplacentally, through blood products, and by mucosal contact.

Clinical Manifestations

Early congenital syphilis. The infected infant may be completely well in his first few weeks of life, may have systemic symptoms, such as weight loss, fever, anemia, and irritability with or without a skin rash, or may have mucocutaneous lesions but is otherwise well. These lesions may be maculopapular, vesicular, or bullous and may initially appear on the distal extremities but later become generalized. Darkening and desquamation of these lesions usually occur. They are highly infectious and may recur before they disappear entirely.

In the first few weeks of life, there may be a purulent, copious nasal discharge, which is blood-tinged. This is the classic "snuffles" of congenital syphilis. The discharge contains live organisms and is highly infectious.

Other findings are hepatosplenomegaly, thrombocytopenia, Coombs-negative hemolytic anemia, leukocytosis, osteochondritis of multiple sites, periostitis, widened epiphyses, and renal dysfunction.

Table 34–1. Treatment of GC-Related Diseases*

Neonatal Gonococcal Ophthalmia
Hospitalization; aqueous crystalline penicillin G, 50,000 units/kg/day IV divided bid × 7 days. Irrigation of eyes with saline solution or buffered ophthalmic solution frequently (as often as qh). Treatment of parents.

Urethritis
Ampicillin, 3.5 g and probenecid, 1 g po
or
Aqueous penicillin G, 4.8 million units IM + probenecid, 1.0 g
plus
Tetracycline HCl, 500 mg po qid × 7 days
or
Doxycycline, 100 mg po bid × 7 days
  (To cover chlamydia, see Table 34-3.)

Epididymitis
Amoxicillin, 500 mg po tid × 10 days
or
Tetracycline HCl, 500 mg po qid × 10 days
or
Doxycycline, 100 mg po bid × 10 days

Vaginitis/Cervicitis
Amoxicillin, 3.0 g or ampicillin, 3.5 g, with probenecid, 1.0 g po
or
Aqueous procaine penicillin G, 4.8 million units IM and probenecid, 1.0 g
or
Tetracycline HCl, 500 mg po qid × 7 days
If prepubertal child, begin evaluation for sexual abuse.

Salpingitis Pelvic Inflammatory Disease
Consider hospitalization if patient is pregnant, a noncompliant adolescent, is experiencing intractable vomiting or is dehydrated, the diagnosis is uncertain, surgical pathology high in the differential, failure to respond to outpatient therapy
Hospitalization therapy
  Doxycycline, 100 mg IV bid
        and
  Cefoxitin, 2.0 g IV qid × 4 days and at least 48 hours after the patient has defervesced

Salpingitis Pelvic Inflammatory Disease *(continued)*
Continue doxycycline, 100 mg po bid to complete 10-day course
Ambulatory therapy
  Cefoxitin, 2.0 g IM *or* amoxicillin, 3.0 g po, *or* ampicillin 3.5 g po *or* aqueous procaine penicillin G, 4.8 million units, each with po probenecid, 1.0 g
        plus
  Tetracycline HCl, 500 mg po qid × 10 to 14 days
        or
  Doxycycline, 100 mg po bid × 10 to 14 days

Fitz-Hugh–Curtis Syndrome
See under salpingitis.

Anorectal GC
Aqueous penicillin, G 4.8 million units IM with probenecid, 1.0 g po; If allergic to penicillin, spectinomycin, 2.0 g IM

Pharyngeal GC
Aqueous penicillin G, 4.8 million units IM with probenecid, 1.0 g po
        or
Tetracycline, 500 mg po qid × 7 days

Disseminated GC
Hospitalization
Aqueous penicillin G, 10 million units IV qd until improvement, followed by amoxicillin/ampicillin, 500 mg po qid × 7 days
        or
Amoxicillin/ampicillin, 3.0 g or 3.5 g, respectively, po each with probenecid, 1.0 g po followed by amoxicillin/ampicillin, 500 mg po qid × 7 days
        or
Tetracycline HCl, 500 mg po qid × 7 days (or longer)— *do not use in pregnancy*
        or
Cefoxitin, 1.0 g/Cefotaxime, 500 mg, either IV qid for at least 7 days (treatment of choice for disseminated infections caused by penicillinase producing *N. gonorrhoeae*)
        or
Erythromycin 500 mg po qid × at least 7 days

*In all GC-related diseases, sexual contacts of the patient should be treated, and the patient should have his syphilis serology determined (see section on syphilis).

Late congenital syphilis. Chronic inflammation produces persistent or recurrent periostitis and bone thickening especially in the skull, clavicles, scapulae, and tibiae. Defective tooth formation may occur, with unusual shapes (peg-shaped upper central incisors, or Hutchinson teeth) or abnormal enamel. A "saddle-nose" is a flattening of the nose due to the destruction of the nasal bone and cartilage by persistent rhinitis.

Other associated features of late congenital syphilis include juvenile aortitis, tabes, paresis, keratitis, and deafness.

Acquired syphilis—primary. At the site of contact (3 to 6 weeks earlier) with *T. pallidum*, a papule appears. It is usually solitary and painless and eventually erodes to form an ulcer with a raised border (a chancre). A chancre may go unrecognized and heals spontaneously in 1 to 2 months, leaving a scar. There may be regional adenopathy accompanying the chancre.

Acquired syphilis—secondary. The secondary form follows the chancre by 1 to 2 months. The patient develops fever, malaise, anorexia, weight loss, myalgias, arthralgias, and lymphadenopathy. A red macular rash begins on the trunk and upper extremities and progresses to a generalized (including palms and soles) copper-colored macular rash. The lesions are very infectious. Erosion of these lesions in moist areas of the body produces plaques called condyloma lata, which are also infectious.

Other associated features of secondary syphilis are meningitis, glomerulonephritis, hepatitis, or periostitis.

Acquired syphilis—latent. Latent syphilis follows untreated secondary syphilis. Early latent syphilis is the first year of latency, while late latent syphilis occurs thereafter. Patients with late latent syphilis are not infectious but have a 40% chance of developing tertiary syphilis. The patient has positive serology with a normal examination, chest x-ray, and cerebrospinal fluid.

Acquired syphilis—tertiary. Late syphilis is slowly progressive and can affect any organ system. It is a disease of adults. Common complications are neurosyphilis and cardiovascular disease.

Diagnosis

Diagnosis can be made by positive dark-field examination. Serum should be obtained for serologic testing. Initially, a nontreponemal test, such as the VDRL, can be used to screen for syphilis. If the VDRL is positive, a treponemal test such as the fluorescent treponemal antibody absorption (FTA-ABS) should be obtained. If the FTA-ABS is positive, the patient is presumed to have syphilis. The VDRL can yield false positive results if the patient has hepatitis, infectious mononucleosis, malaria, varicella, measles, or an autoimmune disease.

All patients with primary, secondary, and congenital syphilis should have repeat nontreponemal tests at 3, 6, and 12 months after treatment; if the patient's disease has been present for more than one year, a repeat test should be done at 24 months since titers decline more slowly if the disease has been present for a longer period of time.

Treatment

The treatment of syphilis is outlined in Table 34-2.

CHLAMYDIA

Chlamydia are intracellular obligate parasites with a cell wall; they contain both DNA and RNA. One type of *Chlamydia trachomatis* causes lymphogranuloma venereum; another type causes genital infections, trachoma, neonatal conjunctivitis, and pneumonia of early infancy.

The prevalence of chlamydia infections of the cervix ranges from 2% to 26%, with the usual reports being 8% to 12%. From 25% to

Table 34–2. Treatment of Syphilis

Congenital syphilis
normal CSF
Benzathine penicillin G, 50,000 units/kg IM
abnormal CSF
Crystalline penicillin G, 50,000 units/kg/day IM or IV × 2 to 3 weeks
or
Procaine penicillin G, 50,000 units/kg/day IM qd × 2 to 3 weeks
acquired syphilis
Early (<1 year's duration)
Benzathine penicillin G, 2.4 million units IM (30,000 units/kg)
or
Tetracycline HCl, 500 mg po qid × 15 days
or
Erythromycin, 500 mg po qid × 15 days
Late (>1 year's duration)
Benzathine penicillin G, 2.4 million units IM weekly × 3 doses
or
Tetracycline HCl, 500 mg po qid × 30 days
or
Erythromycin, 500 mg po qid × 30 days
In Pregnancy
Treat as for early acquired syphilis, except do not use tetracycline (contraindicated in pregnancy) or erythromycin (does not seem to prevent congenital syphilis)
Persistent symptoms
Retreatment should be considered if symptoms of syphilis persist or recur, if there is a four-fold increase in titer with a nontreponemal test, or if a nontreponemal test with an initially high titer fails to show a four-fold decrease within 1 year.

50% of infants born to infected women will develop chlamydia conjunctivitis, and between 5% and 20% of infants will develop pneumonia. Unfortunately, most women with chlamydia are asymptomatic and, therefore, have not been treated.

Pathophysiology

Once introduced to the host, *C. trachomatis* invades cells of the genital tract, conjunctiva, or lower respiratory tract. It multiplies within cells by binary fission; illness is a result of the infected tissues' response to its presence.

Clinical Manifestations

Neonatal conjunctivitis. The form of conjunctivitis caused by chlamydia cannot be distinguished clinically from other forms of conjunctivitis in early infancy. The young infant presents with red conjunctivae and a purulent yellow discharge from his eye(s). Systemic signs of illness may be lacking. There may be no known history of genital infection in the mother.

Pneumonia. The onset of maternally derived chlamydial pneumonia usually occurs in an infant between 1 and 3 months of age. The child presents with a staccato cough and, usually, fever. Eosinophilia ($\geq$400/mm^3) is frequently present. The chest film shows an interstitial pneumonia with hyperaeration.

Cervicitis. The cervicitis caused by chlamydia is indistinguishable, clinically, from that caused by *N. gonorrhoeae* (see section on gonorrhea).

Pelvic Inflammatory Disease. The salpingitis caused by chlamydia is indistinguishable, clinically, from that caused by *N. gonorrhoeae* (see section on gonorrhea).

Fitz-Hugh–Curtis Syndrome. Chlamydia infections have also been associated with Fitz-Hugh–Curtis syndrome (see section on gonorrhea).

Diagnosis

A secure diagnosis is based on cell culture. Rapid presumptive diagnosis may be accomplished by antigen-detection kits using monoclonal antibodies or enzyme-linked immunosorbent assay (ELISA). Giemsa staining of conjunctival scrapings to detect inclusion cells gives a presumptive diagnosis of chlamydia.

Treatment

The treatment of chlamydia is outlined in Table 34-3.

TRICHOMONAS

The trichomonad is a flagellated protozoa that is demonstrated in saline preparations of secretions.

Since *Trichomonas* infection is not routinely reported, its yearly incidence is unknown.

Pathophysiology

The protozoa are introduced to the host usually by intercourse but occasionally by communal bathing or sharing of wet towels. The presence of the protozoae elicits a tissue response of an extremely pruritic vaginal discharge.

Clinical Manifestation—Vaginitis

The patient with *Trichomonas* vaginitis has a foul-smelling vaginal discharge with associated pruritis or dysuria.

Diagnosis

Diagnosis is based on demonstration of the motile protozoa in a fresh saline preparation of secretions.

Treatment

Treatment of *Trichomonas* vaginitis is listed in Table 34-3.

GARDNERELLA VAGINALIS

Gardnerella vaginalis is a short, gram-negative bacillus.

Since *G. vaginalis* infections are not subject to mandatory reporting, the incidence is unknown.

Pathophysiology

The organism interacts with anaerobic vaginal bacteria to produce the characteristic odor of pungent amines.

Clinical Manifestations—Vaginitis

Many women with *G. vaginalis* infections have no vaginal discharge, but the characteris-

Table 34–3. Treatment of *Chlamydia, Trichomonas,* and *Gardnerella vaginalis* Infections

---

Chlamydia
Conjunctivitis
Erythromycin, 50 mg/kg/day po divided into four doses for 10 to 14 days
Topical therapy is unnecessary.
Pneumonia
Erythromycin, 50 mg/kg/day po divided into four doses for 14 days
Cervicitis (or Urethritis in Males)
Tetracycline HCl, 500 mg po qid × 7 days
or
Doxycycline, 100 mg po bid × 7 days
or
Erythromycin, 500 po qid × 7 days (treatment of choice during pregnancy)
Pelvic Inflammatory Disease or Fitz-Hugh–Curtis Syndrome
Same as for GC-related (see Table 34–1)
Trichomonas Vaginitis
Metronidazole, 2.0 g po × 1 day
If patient is pregnant, clotrimazole, 100 mg intravaginally hs × 7 days
Gardnerella vaginalis Vaginitis
Metronidazole, 500 mg po bid × 7 days
or
Ampicillin, 500 mg po qid × 7 days

---

tic odor ("stale fish") is present nonetheless. When a discharge is present, it is generally a thin, white fluid.

Diagnosis

Vaginal epithelial cells studded with bacilli ("clue cells") are present on wet mount or Gram's stain. Gram-positive organisms are rarely present.

Treatment

Treatment of *G. vaginalis* vaginitis is listed in Table 34-3.

HERPES

Herpes is caused by Herpes hominus, a DNA virus. There are two types, herpesvirus I and herpesvirus II. Type I has been associated with nongenital infections of the mouth, lips, eyes, and central nervous system (CNS); it may also cause genital disease. Type II has been associated with genital and neonatal infections but may also cause oral lesions.

The number of new cases of herpes in the United States each year is between 2 and 4 million. The number of cases of neonatal herpes has been estimated to be 1 in 7500 live births.

Pathophysiology

The primary infection of a susceptible host (*i.e.*, one without type-specific antibodies) may be unapparent. Once the primary infection resolves, the virus becomes latent in the ganglion cells of local nerves. Recurrent infections may be precipitated by factors such as fever, trauma, sunlight, or stress.

Clinical Manifestations

Neonatal herpes. Neonates acquire herpes by passage through an infected birth canal; trans-

placental antibodies are not protective. The child becomes ill at the end of the first week of life, but the characteristic skin lesions may be lacking. The infant develops temperature instability, icterus, hepatosplenomegaly, anorexia, vomiting, respiratory distress, and circulatory collapse. The infection is usually fatal.

Genital herpes—First episode/recurrence. The patient may present with dysuria and a painful perineum. The involved genital area is usually erythematous and edematous, with multiple, tiny (2- to 5-mm), shallow ulcers. These ulcers may coalesce into larger ulcers. Occasionally, the patient may present with only one ulcer. Regardless of the number of ulcers present, their common property is their exquisite tenderness.

Disseminated herpes. In malnourished or immunocompromised persons, a herpetic infection may manifest itself as a disseminated disease similar to that described in the section on neonatal herpes.

Diagnosis

When present, the characteristic skin lesions can be diagnostic. Herpesvirus can be cultivated in cell cultures. Sera from acute and convalescent stages can be tested for type-specific neutralizing or complement-fixing antibodies. The antibodies begin to rise at the end of the first week of a primary infection; no rise occurs in recurrent disease. Finally, the diagnosis is suggested by biopsy material that demonstrates acidophilic intranuclear inclusion bodies, multinucleated giant cells, and ballooning degeneration of epithelial cells.

Treatment

The treatment of herpes is outlined in Table 34-4.

HIV (AIDS)

Acquired immunodeficiency syndrome (AIDS) may be acquired sexually in pediatric patients, especially older ones. However, the more common ways for infants and children to acquire the AIDS virus is through blood transfusions or being born to a mother with AIDS. Such a mother would have a high likelihood of being sexually promiscuous or an intravenous drug user. The children have positive serologic tests for the human immunodeficiency virus (HIV) and have no other explanation for their immune deficiency.

Infants with AIDS become ill in early infancy, with failure to thrive, severe intractable oral (and, occasionally, esophageal) candidiasis, and recurrent infections with both common and opportunistic (such as *Pneumocystis carinii*) organisms. These infants have elevated erythrocyte sedimentation rates and progressive reduction in T-lymphocyte helper cells. There is presently no cure.

OTHER SEXUALLY TRANSMITTED CONDITIONS

Treatments of other sexually transmitted conditions are outlined in Table 34-5.

BIBLIOGRAPHY

Bell T: Major sexually transmitted diseases of children and adolescents. Pediatr Infect Dis 2:153–61, 1983

Frau L, Alexander ER: Public health implications of sexually transmitted diseases in pediatric practice. Pediatr Infect Dis 4:453–67, 1985

Neinstein L et al: Nonsexual transmission of sexually transmitted diseases—An infrequent occurrence. Pediatrics 74:67–76, 1984

Sexually Transmitted Diseases—Treatment Guidelines. MMWR 31:#2S, 8/20/82

Table 34–4. Treatment of Herpes

Genital herpes—first episode
Acyclovir ointment, 5%—apply to lesions q3h, 6×/day, × 7 days. Therapy should be started within 6 days of onset of symptoms; it does not prevent recurrences. Sitz baths may also offer relief.

Table 34–5. Treatment of Other Sexually Transmitted Conditions

Pediculosis pubis
   The louse may be killed by lindane 1% lotion, cream, or shampoo (requires prescription)
or
Pyrethrins and piperonyl butoxide (over the counter)
Scabies
The mite may be killed by lindane 1% lotion or cream
or
Crotamiton 10% (treatment of choice for infants and pregnant women)
Condylomata acuminata
This condition is caused by a papova viral infection of the skin or mucous membranes. When the warts occur on the external genitalia, perianal or periurethral areas, treat with podophyllin 10%–25% in compound tincture of benzoin topically, with removal in 1–4 hours.
When the warts occur in the mouth, urethra, or rectum or on the cervix, podophyllin should be avoided.
Cryotherapy, electrosurgery, or surgical removal may be necessary.

35

Mucocutaneous Lymph Node Syndrome (Kawasaki Syndrome)

Mucocutaneous lymph node syndrome (MLNS), an acute exanthematous illness of childhood, was first reported by Kawasaki in 1967 in Japan. Since then it has been reported throughout the world. Victims are usually younger than 5 years, with the peak incidence between 6 months and 2 years of age. However, infants as young as 2 to 3 months of age have demonstrated the clinical syndrome. The male-to-female ratio is approximately 1.5 to 1.6:1. Children of Asian ancestry appear to have the highest risk, followed by black children, whose risk is greater than that of white children. The incidence of MLNS does not vary by season. Secondary cases in the home, school, or neighborhood are rare. There is generally a 1% to 2% mortality rate in the late subacute or early convalescent stage, usually from cardiovascular complications.

ETIOLOGY

The etiology of MLNS is unkown. No bacterial or viral agent has ever been isolated consistently from patients. Since MLNS is similar to leptospirosis clinically, attempts (unsuccessful) have been made to isolate *Leptospira* from patients. Because some investigators have reported "rickettsia-like bodies" in skin and lymph node biopsies, attempts to isolate rickettsia or to discern a rise in antibodies to rickettsial agents have been made. All such attempts have been unsuccessful.

Because the clinical syndrome (see below) includes arthralgia/arthritis, vasculitis, and an elevated IgE level, some investigators have suggested that MLNS represents a new variant of collagen–vascular disease or an immunologic disorder, perhaps mediated by antecedent exposure to a common infectious agent. This line of investigation continues. Since several outbreaks of MLNS have been linked to exposure of victims to shampooed rugs, a hypothetical association of rug shampoo and household carpet mites (which would be airborne after vigorous rug cleaning) has been postulated. These associations have not been verified consistently by other investigators.

CLINICAL MANIFESTATIONS

MLNS is triphasic, with an acute febrile stage (days 1 to 14), a subacute stage (days 15 to 25),

249

and a convalescent stage (days 26 to 60). The clinical manifestations and pathologic processes vary by stage and will be so discussed. The diagnosis of MLNS is based on strict stage specific diagnostic criteria (see Table 35-1).

Acute Febrile Stage

The first phase of MLNS is heralded by a high fever. The fever is an intermittently spiking one, which is only temporarily responsive to intermittent doses of antipyretics. The temperature may be 40° C at its peak; at its trough it may be normal. This type of fever must be present for at least 5 days before a diagnosis of MLNS is entertained. Within 2 to 3 days of the fever's onset, bilateral, nonpurulent, conjunctival injection develops. The injection is particularly marked in the bulbar conjunctivae. Conjunctival involvement is invariable in MLNS and thus constitutes a diagnostic criterion.

Within 1 to 3 days of the fever's onset, another diagnostic manifestation of MLNS in oral mucosa change occurs. These changes are manifested in the lips (erythema and fissuring), in the oropharynx (erythema), and on the tongue (hypertrophy of the tongue's papillae to create a "strawberry" tongue). Lip changes evolve over several weeks, and the fissuring may be so severe that the lips bleed. With the fever's onset comes the rash of MLNS. The rash occurs principally on the face and trunk, is erythematous, and takes several forms. The most common form is erythematous, irregular plaques, which are partially confluent. The next most common form is a morbilliform rash. Eruptions resembling those of scarlet fever, urticaria, or erythema multiforme may also occur. However, the rash of MLNS is never vesicular, bullous, petechial, purpuric, or crusting.

Within several days of the fever's onset, changes in the hands and feet develop. The palms and soles develop a red edema that is indurative. The patient may demonstrate ten-

Table 35–1. Principal Diagnostic Criteria for Mucocutaneous Lymph Node Syndrome

Fever, persisting for more than 5 days
Conjunctival injection
Changes in the mouth consisting of:
   Erythema, fissuring and crusting of the lips
   Diffuse oropharyngeal erythema
   Strawberry tongue
Changes in the peripheral extremities consisting of:
   Induration of hands and feet
   Erythema of palms and soles
   Desquamation of finger and toetips approximately 2
     weeks after onset
   Transverse grooves across fingernails 2 to 3 months after onset
Erythematous rash
Enlarged lymph node mass measuring more than 1.5 cm
  in diameter

(Melish M: Kawasaki syndrome [mucocutaneous lymph node syndrome]. Pediatr Rev 2[4]:107–114, 1980; with permission)

derness of these areas by refusing to hold his bottle or favorite object or refusing to stand. The skin of the dorsum of the hands and feet appears shiny and stretched. Extremity changes are the most distinctive of the diagnostic criteria.

The name of the syndrome suggests widespread lymph node involvement; such is not the case. Only about 50% to 70% of the children have lymphadenopathy, which, when present, is usually only a solitary cervical node (1.5 cm in diameter) that is rarely warm, fluctuant, or tender.

Other reported associated findings in the first stage are irritability, mood lability, lethargy, cerebrospinal fluid (CSF) pleocytosis (predominantly lymphocytes), abdominal pain, diarrhea, liver inflammation, sterile pyuria, urethritis, hematuria, joint involvement (late in the first stage), and the beginnings (clinically undetectable) of cardiovascular involvement. Perivasculitis of the coronary arteries, microvasculitis of the coronary arteries and aorta, and pancarditis with inflammation of the A-V conduction system may be present.

In the acute stage, most patients have an elevated (>20,000) white blood cell (WBC) count with a left shift. The sedimentation rate and levels of C-reactive protein are elevated. Toward the end of this stage, thrombocytosis occurs (see next section). Results of serum IgG, IgM, IgA, rheumatoid factor, and antinuclear antibody assays are generally normal, although IgE levels may be elevated in some patients. Cultures of blood, CSF, and urine are usually sterile.

Subacute Stage

The fever, rash, and lymphadenopathy subside together by day 14, and the subacute stage of MLNS begins. The conjunctivae may still be reddened. The lips are usually still reddened, edematous, fissured, and bleeding. The peripheral extremities begin to desquamate between days 10 and 20, and other parts of the body may desquamate also. The child is still anorexic and irritable. In this stage, joint symptoms (arthralgias or arthritis) may develop in the large joints (knees, hips, elbows). The arthritis may have an associated effusion that persists for several weeks.

The greatest danger to the patient in this stage is due to cardiovascular pathology. Although the pancarditis, which had its onset in the first stage, is improving, the coronary arteries demonstrate a persistent panvasculitis, and may demonstrate areas of thrombosis and occlusion. Some involvement of the coronary arteries probably occurs in all cases of MLNS. Clinically, the child may have sinus tachycardia, a gallop rhythm, muffled heart sounds, or minor electrocardiographic (ECG) abnormalities (prolonged PR interval, ST-T wave changes). Some children develop clinical cardiomyopathy with congestive heart failure, pericardial effusion, and mitral valve insufficiency due to papillary muscle dysfunction. Coronary artery aneurysms occur in approximately 20% of children with MLNS. Sudden death occurs in the subacute stage because of rupture of an aneurysm in a coronary artery or to occlusion of a coronary artery by a thrombus. The risk of death is also increased because of the thrombocytosis which peaks in this stage. Platelet counts of 1.8 million have been reported; counts of 600,000 to 1 million are common.

Laboratory results that were abnormal in the first stage of MLNS usually remain abnormal in the second stage. In children with myocarditis, levels of serum glutamic oxaloacetic transaminase (GOT), creatine phosphokinase (CPK), and lactate dehydrogenase (LDH) are usually elevated. A mild anemia may be present.

Convalescent Stage

In the convalescent phase, the child is returning to normal. His eyes, lips, and extremities are markedly improved; joint symptoms are also resolving. His appetite is increasing, and his irritability is decreasing. Early in this stage, the coronary arteries are still inflamed, and the presence of coronary artery aneurysms are still life-threatening. By the end of this stage, the coronary arteries have developed calcified scars in their walls and recanalization of their lumens; some myocardial fibrosis is still present. One-third of children with coronary artery aneurysms will still have them 1 year later.

Most of the laboratory values, including the platelet count, are normal by the end of this stage.

DIFFERENTIAL DIAGNOSIS OF MLNS

Once MLNS is established, its diagnosis is fairly evident. However, early in the course of the illness, the rash may be confused with that of measles, streptococcal scarlet fever, Epstein-Barr virus infections, or leptospirosis, which can be diagnosed by appropriate cultures or serologic tests. The rash may also be confused with erythema multiforme or drug eruptions. A history of drug use and an improvement in the rash following the cessation of its use is good evidence for a drug eruption. Drug eruption may also be accompanied by eosinophilia, which is not seen in MLNS. Erythema multiforme has a variety of manifestations (vesicles, bullae, crusts) that are not seen in MLNS.

MANAGEMENT OF THE PATIENT

Risk factors have been elucidated to detect the children most likely to develop coronary artery aneurysms or coronary thrombosis:

1. Male gender
2. Age less than 1 year
3. Duration of initial fever of 15 days
4. Recrudescent rash
5. Recrudescent fever
6. WBC count of 30,000
7. Westergren sedimentation rate of 100
8. Presence of cardiomegaly
9. Presence of arrhythmias
10. Evidence of myocardial infarction
11. Prolonged QR interval on EKG
12. Hemoglobin of 10 or less
13. Persistently elevated sedimentation rate for 5 weeks

Children with less than five factors generally do well; children with more than nine are likely to develop an aneurysm or thrombosis. Keeping these risk factors in mind, the management of MLNS by stage is discussed.

Acute Stage

Because of the irritability with which many of these children present, the goal of the initial evaluation is to rule out sepsis. This includes a lumbar puncture in the infant. Cultures of the blood, urine, throat, stool, and CSF (if applicable) are obtained to exclude treatable bacterial diseases. Viral cultures (or ELISAs) and leptospirosis cultures may also be obtained. The complete blood count, sedimentation rate, C-reactive and baseline liver/cardiac enzymes are determined. If MLNS is a serious consideration, a baseline chest film and EKG are also useful.

Many physicians advocate hospitalizing all children with suspected MLNS for a brief period to observe their clinical courses and to assist their families, since the children are often irritable and anorexic. Other physicians use the aforementioned risk factors to select the children who should be hospitalized. If the child with MLNS is not hospitalized, he should be seen as an outpatient two to four times a week.

Hospitalized or not, the child with MLNS should receive aspirin in a dose of 80 to 100 mg/kg/day so that the serum salicylate level is 20 mg/dl. Aspirin has anti-inflammatory and antiplatelet aggregation properties; its use, in high dose, has been associated with a lower incidence of aneurysms. The use of intravenous gammaglobulin at a dose of 400 mg/kg/day for 4 to 5 days early in the illness has also led to a reduced incidence of aneurysms. The use of antibiotics is not indicated. The use of corticosteroids is contraindicated because steroids have been associated with increased development of coronary artery aneurysms. The child with MLNS is frequently anorexic and may require intravenous fluids.

Monitoring of abnormal laboratory results should be done at least weekly with determination of platelet counts, salicylate levels, and sedimentation rates done more frequently, as each case dictates. If an outpatient with MLNS develops any cardiac abnormalities, he should be hospitalized immediately. At the end of this first stage, an echocardiogram is performed to detect subclinical cardiac pathology.

Subacute Stage

After defervescence, the aspirin dose may be halved, with continued monitoring of serum salicylate levels. Supportive therapy is continued. The cardiac examination, complete blood count, erythrocyte sedimentation rate, platelet count, and ECG should be serially monitored. Another echocardiogram should be performed and compared with the first to detect changes in coronary vessels or cardiac size. Any outpatient who develops new risk factors or cardiac decompensation requires hospitalization.

Cardiac failure is managed with standard doses of digoxin. Children with documented coronary vessel anomalies should be continued on high-dose aspirin therapy. A coronary angiogram should be performed on any child presenting with coronary vessel damage or myocardial infarction.

Convalescent Stage

Children with normal echocardiograms should have a repeat study when their platelet count normalizes (in 2 to 3 months). If no abnormalities are found, aspirin therapy may be stopped and the child evaluated every 1 to 3 months.

Children with evidence of coronary artery aneurysms should have serial echocardiograms to assess the progress of aneurysm resolution. A repeat angiogram should be performed in about 1 year.

Children with increasing cardiac symptoms and coronary vessel involvement may require bypass surgery.

BIBLIOGRAPHY

Bell D: Kawasaki update: More answers, fewer questions. Contemp Pediatr 1:20–36, 1985

Crowley D: Cardiovascular complications of mucocutaneous lymph node syndrome. Pediatr Clin North Am 31:1321–1329, 1984

Kawasaki T et al: A new infantile acute febrile mucocutaneous lymph node syndrome (MLNS) prevailing in Japan. Pediatrics 54:271–276, 1974

Melish M: Kawasaki syndrome (mucocutaneous lymph node syndrome). Pediatr Rev 2:107–114, 1980

Melish M et al: Mucocutaneous lymph node syndrome in the United States. Am J Dis Child 130:599-607, 1976

Morens D, Nahmias A: Kawasaki disease: A "new pediatric enigma. Hosp Pract 109–120, 1978

Morens D et al: National surveillance of Kawasaki disease. Pediatrics 65:21–25, 1980

Newburger J et al: The treatment of Kawasaki syndrome with intravenous gammaglobulin. N Engl J Med 315:341, 1986

Part VII:　　　　Gastroenterology

36

Recurrent Vomiting in Childhood

Emesis is one of the most common symptoms in childhood. As indicated in Table 36-1, the potential explanations are legion, some benign and some true emergencies. This is not surprising, since both the normal process of suck, swallow, and gastric emptying and the "pathologic" process of emesis require complex integration of neurologic, muscular, and enteric hormonal systems. Emesis, for example, can be mediated locally by obstruction or centrally by a central nervous system (CNS) "vomiting center" in the reticular formation or a "chemoreceptor trigger zone" in the region of the fourth ventricle near the satiety center.

From the developmental perspective, by 24 weeks' gestation, the fetus is capable of suck and swallow of amniotic fluid, reaching, by term, a rate of 500 ml/24 hours. This rate is equaled by fetal urination to maintain constant amniotic fluid volumes. With intrauterine bowel obstructions (atresias, meconium ileus, etc.), therefore, amniotic fluid volumes would increase, thus producing "polyhydramnios."

While emesis is the clinical focus of this chapter, it is also important to remember that infants and toddlers cannot describe either nausea or dysphagia, two of the prominent early signs of many of the disorders discussed. Anorexia or food refusal, therefore, may be early presenting signs. In infancy, simple regurgitation (mediated primarily by gravity) must be distinguished from the active process of true emesis.

In terms of prevalence, the "functional" disorders listed in Table 36-1 account for the vast majority of children with recurrent emesis. Inappropriate intake occurs in three contexts: overfeeding, hyperosmolar feeding, and aerophagia. Overfeeding is often a conscious or subconscious effort to either "satisfy" a colicky, crying child or meet a cultural demand for a fat (and therefore healthy) baby. Hyperosmolar feedings can result from incorrect formula preparation or efforts to provide calories to fluid-restricted children. While a degree of aerophagia is nearly universal in childhood, a pathologic extreme can be encountered in the severely retarded child (usually in the context of reflux esophagitis) or normal child with excessive gum chewing or carbonated beverage intake.

A hyperactive gag reflex is commonly

encountered early in hypertonic cerebral palsy, producing pharyngeal spasm and secondary emesis. A functional or psychological reaction with nausea is seen in many normal children in response to food appearance or smell.

Gastroesophageal reflux (GER) is one of the most interesting topics in pediatrics today. It is best considered "functional," since we are all born with some reflux due to modest reductions in lower esophageal muscular tone and the short distance over which this "sphincter pressure" is applied to the distal esophagus. Simplistically, if rates of gastric emptying are normal, GER produces benign regurgitation, usually immediately after meals, for up to 6 to 8 months with generally normal growth and development. If gastric emptying is impaired by "pylorospasm" or abnormal gastric peristalsis, the degree of emesis with GER is more severe and often occurs up to several hours after meals, contributing to impaired growth. All forms of GER may be complicated by esophagitis, dysphagia, or aspiration pneumonia. If distal esophageal peristalsis is abnormal on either a primary basis (*e.g.*, tracheo-esophageal fistula) or secondary basis (*e.g.*, sliding hiatal hernia) the duration of reflux symptoms is greatly prolonged. The pressure generated in the lower esophageal sphincter can also be reduced by a number of medications (*e.g.*, theophylline, alcohol, nicotine, caffeine, and progesterone) producing transient alteration in esophageal function.

By definition, anyone with emesis has GER. A difficult clinical dilemma is presented by the child with minimal or no emesis where GER may contribute to esophageal bleeding, reactive airway disease, apnea, impaired growth, or dysphagia. Documentation of GER can be achieved radiographically by barium swallow, but the sensitivity of this test is poor. Even so, the test is usually justified to evaluate gastric emptying and exclude intestinal rotational defects. Monitoring of esophageal *p*H has now become the "gold standard" of documentation of GER. Ideally performed over 24 hours, the frequency and duration of acidification is documented in relation to the symptom potentially attributable to GER. In situations of dysphagia, the sensitivity of the distal esophagus to acidification can also be tested by the Tuttle test of acid perfusion. The documentation of esophagitis in patients with GER occasionally can be made on barium swallow, but the more sensitive test is endoscopic esophageal biopsy.

Pylorospasm is a functional impairment of gastric emptying that is very prevalent in infancy. It may also be the common pathway for emesis with increased intracranial pressure and drug-induced gastritis.

Psychogenic rumination is a rare disorder of impaired maternal–infant interaction. It occurs primarily between 2 and 8 months of age, with voluntary emesis responding dramatically to sensitive nurturing. In older children, bulemia presents as a bing/purge cycle related to anorexia nervosa. This is discussed in greater detail in Chapter 3 (discussed under Anorexia Nervosa).

The enteric obstructions listed in Table 36-1 can occur at any level of the intestine. Most are partial obstructions, often producing intermittent symptoms. Emesis from obstruction beyond the second portion of the duodenum is often bile stained. Abdominal distention is most prominent with distal obstruction. Diagnosis is often confirmed radiographically. If, during barium contrast studies, an area of narrowing is noted, spasm can often be relieved by administration of glucagon, whereas stenosis is not so relieved.

Dysmotility of the intestine is clearly at one end of the spectrum of functional disorders. Any enteritis, especially the viral syndromes of childhood, often is heralded by anorexia and emesis. Chronic enteropathy, as in gluten-sensitive celiac disease, may also

Table 36–1. Disorders Presenting With Recurrent Emesis

Functional
  Inappropriate intake
  Hyperactive gag reflex
  Gastroesophageal reflux
  Pylorospasm
  Psychogenic rumination/bulimia
Enteric Obstruction
  Stenosis, atresia
  Malrotation, volvulus
  Duplication, diverticulum
  Vascular compression
  Annular pancreas, choledochal cyst
  Intussusception
  Ischemia, necrotizing enterocolitis
  Inflammatory
    Antral or channel ulcer
    Eosinophilic gastroenteritis
    Chronic granulomatous disease
    Regional enteritis (Crohn's disease)
    Appendicitis
    Toxic megacolon
Enteric Dysmotility
  Enteropathy (gluten, infectious)
  Pseudo-obstruction
  Peritonitis/pancreatitis
  Emesis gravidarum (pregnancy)
  Pyelonephritis/strep pharyngitis/otitis
Primary Metabolic
  Adrenocortical insufficiency
  Diabetes
  Hypercalcemia/hypocalcemia
  Acidosis syndromes
  Drug-induced/chemotherapeutics
Primary Neurologic
  Cerebral edema
  Subdural hematoma
  Intracranial hemorrhage
  Hydrocephalus
  Meningitis/encephalitis
  Tumor
  Vestibular disorders
  Migraine
  Cyclic emesis
  Familial dysautonomia

present in infancy with emesis. Enteric hormonal factors may also play a role in these situations.

Intestinal pseudo-obstruction is a severe reduction in motility on either a primary or secondary basis. The inherited familial form usually presents in infancy with emesis, distention, obstipation, and impaired growth. Progressive enteric compromise is the rule. In older children, pseudo-obstruction is encountered in many muscular disorders such as dystrophies, amyloidosis, or scleroderma, neurologic disorders such as familial dysautonomia, and endocrine disorders such as diabetes, myxedema, and pheochromocytoma. It may also develop after exposure to pharmacologic agents such as tricyclic antidepressants, botulism, poisonous mushrooms, and phenothiazines. The major complications of pseudo-obstruction are related to stasis with bacterial overgrowth, bile acid deconjugation, steatorrhea, and progressive impairment of intake.

Dysmotility is also prominent, with a number of nonenteric infectious conditions, especially pneumonia, strep pharyngitis, and pyelonephritis, all of which may present with fever and emesis, obscuring the true origin of the illness. Both peritonitis and pancreatitis are frequently associated with profound ileus and emesis.

The metabolic disorders must always be considered in children, especially infants, with dramatic emesis. Diabetes and other acidosis syndromes, while rare, commonly present in this manner. Renal tubular acidosis, organic acid disorders, and aminoacidemia must be excluded. Emesis is also prominent with adrenocortical insufficiency, whether from adrenogenital syndrome or steroid withdrawal. Altered calcium homeostasis, especially hypoparathyroidism, must also be considered. Several medications can induce emesis independent of gastritis. These include theophylline, digitalis, lead, and a host of chemotherapeutic agents employed in cancer therapy, especially *cis*-platinum.

The neurologic disorders of greatest concern are those associated with increased intracranial pressure. Cerebral edema may complicate closed head trauma, Reye's syndrome, urea cycle disorders, and lead poisoning. Cyclic emesis or periodic emesis is rare in childhood. Often seen in the context of family history of migraine, these children present with nausea and variable degrees of emesis at 3-week to 6-month intervals. By definition, the intervals between episodes are marked by normal appetite, growth, and lack of emesis.

As indicated above, the disorders potentially contributing to recurrent emesis in childhood are many. No "cookbook" evaluation with suffice. Clues from the history point to specific studies of exclusion. As a baseline, the investigations listed in Table 36-2 are usually required. The value of a 7-day diary kept when the child is symptomatic cannot be underestimated. It forces prospective assessment on the effects of diet and other activities on the emesis. Radiographic contrast studies are usually required. Sonography, cranial CT

scan, and metabolic studies are more individualized.

There is no simple generic treatment for emesis in childhood. Efforts focus primarily on enhancing gastric emptying by positioning the infant prone with head elevated and somewhat right side down. Feeding consistencies are altered, usually to liquids for enhanced emptying. Medications with "pro-peristaltic" activity, such as metaclopramide, may be employed with some functional and dysmotility conditions. Medications with CNS effects to suppress the vomiting center are also used, especially with motion sickness or chemotherapy-induced emesis. In this category are antihistamines and experimental derivatives of cannabinoids.

Table 36–2. Evaluation of Recurrent Emesis: Baseline studies

1. Seven-day diary of intake, emesis, activities, stools
2. Complete history and physical examination, including thorough neurologic examination
3. Laboratory
    Complete blood count
    Electrolytes, serum urea nitrogen, calcium
    Urinalysis, urine culture
4. Radiographic
    Abdominal flat plate
    Barium swallow, upper gastrointestinal, SBFT
    Abdominal sonography

BIBLIOGRAPHY

Berquist WE, Byrne WJ, Ament ME et al: Achalasia: Diagnosis, management, and clinical course in 16 children. Pediatrics 71:798–805, 1983

Byrne WJ, Cipel L, Euler AR et al: Chronic idiopathic intestinal pseudo-obstruction syndrome in children—Clinical characteristics and prognosis. J Pediatr 90:585–589, 1977

Christie DL, O'Grady LR, Mack DV: Incomplete lower esophageal sphincter and gastroesophageal reflux in recurrent acute pulmonary disease of infancy and childhood. J Pediatr 93:23–27, 1978

Fleisher DR: Infant rumination syndrome. Am J Dis Child 133:266–269, 1979

Herbst JJ, Book LS, Bray PR: Gastroesophageal reflux in the "near miss" sudden infant death syndrome. J Pediatr 92:73–75, 1978

Hilemeier AC, Lange R, McCallum R et al: Delayed gastric emptying in infants with gastroesophageal reflux. J Pediatr 98:190, 1981

37

Abdominal Pain

Acute and chronic abdominal pain remain major diagnostic and therapeutic challenges throughout childhood. While Table 37-1 presents a partial list of contributing conditions to acute abdominal pain, the list is deceiving, not only because of the many conditions omitted, but also owing to the implication that an explanation is usually found. When approaching the problem of abdominal pain in childhood, the emphasis is on the exclusion of significant pathology, the appreciation of the degree of handicap to the child, an understanding of the level of concern of the parents, and close follow-up. Many episodes will go unexplained.

ACUTE ABDOMINAL PAIN

Appendicitis is never an easy diagnosis to make, especially in the nonverbal, early-infancy period. In general, the diagnosis depends on the development of "peritoneal signs" such as rebound pain, localization to the right lower quadrant, and, often, a mass effect on rectal examination. Associated features in infancy include ileus (distention and

Table 37–1. Acute Abdominal Pain in Childhood

Inflammatory
  Appendicitis
  Mesenteric adenitis
  Gastroenteritis
  Pancreatitis
  Peptic gastritis/duodenitis
  Vasculitis
  Cholelithiasis
  Pneumonia
Obstructive
  Intussusception
  Constipation
  Volvulus
  Foreign body
Genitourinary
  Pelvic inflammatory disease
  Cystitis/pyelonephritis
  Testicular torsion

emesis), irritability, and features of either a mass or peritonitis. In older children, a history can be elicited, allowing better appreciation of the progression of disease. Anorexia is nearly universal. In contrast to gastroenteritis, the pain of appendicitis usually precedes the onset of emesis. Fever is less prominent and

261

often mild. The value of blood testing is to exclude other etiologies to the pain. Leukocytosis, while expected, is not universal. Surgical exploration for "probable" appendicitis should be reconsidered if examination reveals significant hematuria, marked pharyngitis, or jaundice. As alluded to above in the reference to peritonitis, the rates of appendiceal perforation are high in childhood, ranging from 25% in adolescence up to 90% in infancy. Of greater concern is the observation that nearly 50% of these children with perforation had been seen by a physician earlier in the course of the illness, but the diagnosis was missed.

Mesenteric adenitis is another major cause of acute lower abdominal pain. Often clinically indistinguishable from the pain of appendicitis, it reflects either a generalized adenopathy (as with streptococcal pharyngitis) or localized adenopathy (as with *Yersinia* enterocolitica). Appetite is often preserved.

Acute infectious gastroenteritis in childhood is frequently accompanied by cramping abdominal pain. In most circumstances, the pain follows nausea or emesis and precedes or accompanies diarrhea. Bacterial, parasitic, and viral etiologies may be implicated. Rapid diagnostic ELISA techniques have been of great value in confirming an infectious etiology.

Pancreatitis is a diagnosis of inclusion in childhood; one must think of it to diagnose it. Clinically, presentation is with acute epigastric or diffuse abdominal pain. Anorexia is severe and emesis prominent because of the degree of associated ileus. Neither is relieved by antacids or meals. Radiation of the pain to the back, a prominent sign in adults, is rare in childhood. Both ascites and pleural effusions (especially left thorax) are common. As noted in Table 37-2, the major etiologies of pancreatitis are infection, blunt abdominal trauma, and medication. Most episodes are moderately severe, but hemorrhagic pancreatitis is truly life-threatening. The diagnosis is confirmed

Table 37–2. Pancreatitis in Childhood: Etiologic Considerations

Genetic
Familial ± aminoaciduria
Cystic fibrosis
Types I, IV, V hyperlipidemia
Familial hyperparathyroidism
Obstruction of Pancreatic Flow
Trauma
Congenital ductular stricture or stenosis
Choledochal cyst, gallstone
Duodenal inflammation (*e.g.*, ulcer, lymphoma)
Pseudocyst
Gastroduodenal duplication cyst
Infection
Viral: mumps, mononucleosis, measles, rubella, coxsackie B
Viral hepatitis, influenza A
Mycoplasma, salmonellosis, ascaris
Drug-Induced
Alcohol
L-Asparaginase
Azothioprine
Furosemide
Thiazides
Estrogens/cortisone
Sulfasalazine
Boric acid poisoning
Miscellaneous
Postoperative
Pregnancy
Reye's syndrome
Graft-versus-host
Post-marasmus
Henoch-Schönlein syndrome
Diabetic ketoacidosis
Vasculitis
Porphyria

by documentation of elevated serum and/or urinary amylase. The sonogram is of particular value in childhood, since swelling of the pancreas is anticipated with acute injury, and the complications of pseudocyst formation and ascites can be excluded. Additional laboratory features include leukocytosis, hyperlipemia, hyperglycemia, and subsequent hypocalcemia. Demonstration of elevated methemalbumin in the serum suggests hemorrhagic pancreatitis. With persistent or recurrent inflammation, complications include pseudocyst formation, endocrine insufficiency (diabetes), and exocrine insufficiency (steatorrhea).

Peptic disorders of the esophagus, stomach, and duodenum can present with acute abdominal pain, usually when complicated by gastric outlet obstruction, perforation, and/or bleeding. More commonly, they contribute to chronic abdominal pain and are thus discussed in more detail later in this chapter.

Abdominal pain may be a cardinal feature of the vasculitic disorders of childhood, primarily Henoch-Schönlein (anaphylactoid) purpura. The pain is usually due to partial or functional small-bowel obstruction by intramural hematomas or the "pseudo-obstruction" of vasculitis-associated ileus. It may then complicate the course of Kawasaki's syndrome, lupus erythematosus, scleroderma, dermatomyositis, or mixed connective tissue disease. In Henoch-Schönlein purpura, the abdominal pain may precede the characteristic rash and edema of the extremities by up to 1 week. Acute enlargement (hydrops) of the gallbladder with right upper quadrant pain is also seen in vasculitic disorders such as Kawasaki's syndrome, polyarteritis, and graft-versus-host disease.

Cholelithiasis is uncommon in childhood, except in the chronic hemolytic disorders such as sickle cell disease or spherocytosis. The diagnostic procedure of choice is sonography.

Pain referred to the abdomen is frequently noted with lower lobe pneumonias. Spinal cord lesions and herpes zoster must also be considered.

In addition to the primary inflammatory disorders presenting with acute abdominal pain, there are a number of primary obstructive conditions in which inflammation is secondary. In the toddler, intussusception is prominent and mandates early recognition and reduction to prevent irreversible ischemia. The triad of abdominal pain, distention, and bilious emesis in infancy should suggest midgut volvulus, usually with malrotation. Constipation, defined as the chronic failure to evacuate the colon completely may present with acute obstruction and severe cramping abdominal pain. Foreign body ingestion should be pursued historically, but rarely contributes to pain by perforation or obstruction. The major site of injury from ingested foreign bodies is the esophagus, with perforation leading to mediastinitis. Chest pain and dysphagia thus mandate exclusion of esophageal injury.

The primary extraintestinal etiologies of acute abdominal pain are in the genitourinary system. Pelvic inflammation from sexually transmitted disease or ectopic pregnancy are, tragically, now major pediatric concerns. Ovarian cyst, endometriosis, and ovulatory pain (mittelschmertz) are more common chronic concerns. Cystitis and pyelonephritis are excluded by careful examination and culture of the urine. In the adolescent male, there is too often a reluctance to admit scrotal pain, so that the embarrassed boy denies abdominal pain even when suffering from severe testicular torsion.

The diagnostic evaluation of the child with acute abdominal pain is summarized in Table 37-3, with additional testing anticipated on an individualized basis. The history focuses on genetic predisposition, the progression of symptoms, and associated signs. The physical examination emphasizes the degree of distention, bowel sounds, localization and referral of pain, and evidence of systemic features of illness. The blood testing is self-explanatory. Radiographic studies should routinely include a chest x-ray and two views of the abdomen, looking for focal alterations, mass effect, free air, obstructive signs, or calcification.

Establishing communication, if not formal

Table 37–3. Diagnostic Approach to Acute Abdominal Pain

Detailed history
Complete physical examination, including rectal and frequently pelvic examination
Urinalysis (+ culture)
Stool: Occult blood, smear for polys
Complete blood count, differential, sedimentation rate
BUN, amylase, glucose
X-ray
   Chest, kidney, ureter, and bladder upright
Surgical consultation
Additional studies as indicated

consultation, with an experienced surgical colleague is a critical phase in the evaluation of acute abdominal pain, independent of obvious concerns such as bleeding or bilious emesis. Surgical training and publications increasingly emphasize a conservative approach to abdominal pain in the child, making communication easier for all involved.

CHRONIC ABDOMINAL PAIN

The approach to chronic abdominal pain does not differ greatly from that outlined above. By definition, all chronic pain has an acute phase, and most acute etiologies can recur; overlap is thus inevitable. Between the ages of 8 and 15 years, nearly 15% of all children seek medical attention for recurring or persistent abdominal pain. Fewer than one in five such children have a significant organic etiology to their pain. The rest have "functional" pain, every bit as real as that from an organic etiology.

Table 37-4 presents those conditions that figure prominently in the differential diagnosis of chronic or recurring in abdominal pain in the child. The list is most impressive for the dozens of explanations not included, especially recurrence of conditions listed in Table 37-1.

As noted above, nearly 80% of children with complaints of chronic abdominal pain will have a functional origin. The features of this condition are specific enough that it is *not* considered a diagnosis of exclusion. Onset is around puberty, persisting into late adolescence. Awareness often follows an acute viral-like syndrome with variable intestinal manifestations. There is a paucity of systemic features such as fever, diarrhea, weight loss, or reduction in rate of growth. Bowel complaints, when present, suggest a colonic dysmotility, with variable constipation and loose stools in the absence of true diarrhea. The associated symptoms are "autonomic," featuring pallor, weakness, flushing, and lethargy. The pain is usually described as periumbilical in origin, prompting Apley to conclude that the further the pain from the umbilicus, the greater the concern of an organic etiology (see Bibliography). The pain is independent of activity, meals, or stool pattern and rarely awakens the child at night. The family history frequently features functional complaints such as spastic colitis or peptic complaints.

To the parent, the greatest frustration from this syndrome lies in the inconsistency with the child's prior behavior. These are primarily "good kids," with histories of excellent school performance and overachieving and with little to gain directly from their incapacity with pain other than the obvious attention. In addressing the psychological issues, the em-

Table 37–4. Causes of Persistent Abdominal Pain

Functional/idiopathic abdominal pain
Irritable bowel syndrome
Inflammatory bowel disease
Carbohydrate intolerance
Peptic esophagitis/gastritis/duodenitis
Constipation
Ovarian cyst/endometriosis
Persistent hepatitis

phasis is on eliciting real or perceived loss, difficulty in handling hostility or sexual feelings, and the degree of parental preoccupation with the child's symptoms. These issues are best addressed in the absence of the parent, emphasizing to the child that you are his advocate, not the parent's advocate.

The diagnostic investigations in the context of probable functional pain are minimized. A 7-day diary of pain, diet, and associated events is mandatory. At least three stool samples are analyzed for occult blood, leukocytes, and reducing sugars. With diarrheal symptoms, routine culture for pathogens and parasite examinations are indicated. A urine sample is analyzed and routinely cultured. The blood studies are limited to a complete blood count and sedimentation rate. A sonogram may be warranted in pubertal girls or with focal pain not adjacent to the umbilicus. If there is a question of relationship to milk products, a breath hydrogen test with lactose is warranted. If results of these screening studies are normal, reassure the child and parent and encourage a resumption of normal diet, normal school attendance, and prior activities.

If the child has depressive features, the family is too oriented to the incapacity, or school attendance cannot be resumed, psychiatric consultation is warranted. Long-term studies suggest that only 2% of children clinically diagnosed with functional pain will eventually prove to have organic illness, usually peptic ulcer or Crohn's disease.

Irritable bowel syndrome is a related "functional" disorder of the colon, most prominent in toddlers and adolescents. In addition to crampy abdominal pain, these children have loose stools and intermittent anorexia and show a more direct relationship of the pain to stressful situations. Because dietary histories in both age-groups often feature low fiber intake, supplementation is often advised and effective.

Inflammatory bowel disease, predominantly Crohn's disease or regional enteritis, is a major concern to the physician and knowledgeable family. These conditions are discussed in more detail in Chapter 41. The features sought in the history include anorexia, reductions in rate of growth or sexual maturity, and extraintestinal manifestations such as episcleritis, synovitis, erythema nodosum, perianal lesions, and anemia. Regrettably, no single laboratory study excludes inflammatory bowel disease.

The peptic disorders of acid-mediated injury to esophagus, stomach, or duodenum vary in clinical presentation largely as a function of age. In infancy, up to about the age of 3 years, presentation is usually as a gastric outlet obstruction. Emesis is prominent, especially with free esophageal reflux. Colicky abdominal pain and reduced rates of growth are prominent. The emesis is usually postprandial, although intervals up to 4 hours are seen. Night arousal is frequent but very nonspecific. Blood in the emesis is more prominent with esophagitis than duodenal ulcer. The response to medical therapy is good, but recurrence rates are high.

In midchildhood, from 3 to 10 years, the pain of peptic disease is often nonspecific and periumbilical rather than epigastric. Night and early morning pain are prominent. The pain is rarely relieved by meals, and anorexia may be severe. Esophagitis may present with dysphagia due to stricture formation, whereas heartburn is rarely described. More than one-third of children with peptic ulcers have a parent with a history of ulcer.

The adolescent with peptic disease will have a more typical peptic history. The pains are usually epigastric and prominent at night, as well as early morning. Stress is not commonly implicated. Bleeding is much more prominent than in the younger children, and duodenal ulcers predominate. Gastric antral gastritis may follow a viral-like illness, presenting with persistent epigastric pain and anorexia in the relative absence of bleeding. The response to medical management is good, but, again, recurrence rates exceed 25%.

Peptic disease complicates a number of childhood illnesses, most prominently pancreatic insufficiency, chronic pulmonary disease, cyanotic heart disease, mastocytosis, and hyperparathyroidism. The minimum screening laboratory assessment includes complete blood count, analysis of three stools for blood, calcium, phosphorus, and fasting gastrin. True Zollinger-Ellison hypergastrinemia is suspected with multiple ulcerations, with frequent recurrence, or in the context of multiple endocrine adenoma. Barium contrast studies and endoscopy are of roughly equivalent value in the diagnosis of duodenal ulcer; however, endoscopy and biopsy greatly increase the ability to diagnose esophagitis and gastritis.

Medical therapy of peptic disease consists of avoidance of binge meals, caffeine, and alcohol. Bland diets are rarely indicated. Antacids are effective, but compliance with the large amounts and frequency of delivery is poor. The new histamine-2 blockers; cimetidine (Tagamet™) and ranitidine (Zantac™) are effective and generally safe for use in school-aged children with documented peptic disease. Dosage and toxicity are not well documented in infancy. Anticholinergics are used rarely to reduce postprandial discomfort. Surgery is indicated for persistent bleeding, perforation, intractable pain, obstruction, or three or more recurrences in 5 years.

The role of chronic constipation in abdominal pain is a greater issue to the primary care physician that the subspecialist. Addressed in more detail in Chapter 44, the critical issue in constipation is the incomplete evacuation of the colon rather than the frequency or consistency of the stool. The pain is crampy in nature, is maximal during or after meals, and clears over a few minutes especially following defecation.

The role of carbohydrate intolerance in recurrent abdominal pain has been clarified greatly over the past decade with the development of noninvasive breath hydrogen testing. Significant lactose malabsorption can clearly contribute to abdominal pain independent of diarrhea. The onset is usually 15 to 60 minutes after meals containing lactose. Thresholds of severity vary with age and antecedent illness. Family histories are usually positive, although often described as "milk allergy" or "dislike" rather than confirmed lactose intolerance.

In the pubertal or postpubertal girl, an ovarian lesion is a frequent concern, and pelvic sonography is usually advised. The demonstration of a small ovarian cyst may, of course, be physiologic and thus independent of the origin of the pain.

Abdominal pain is an uncommon feature of acute hepatitis. If hepatic enzyme elevations are noted, they should be monitored for 3 months to confirm recovery. If they are persistently elevated, hepatitis B, persistent Ebstein-Barr syndrome, Wilson's disease, and alpha 1-antiprotease deficiency should be excluded. Exclusion of chronic active hepatitis requires hepatic biopsy after 3 months of persistent transaminase elevation.

During the past decade, endoscopic evaluation has been available for children of any age with abdominal pain. The resulting data are both helpful and confusing. The value of endoscopic biopsy in the diagnosis of both peptic and chronic inflammatory disease is unquestioned. A "by-product," perhaps, is the frequency with which children with functional-type pain will have mild, nonspecific inflammatory changes in the biopsies of the duodenum and/or colon. Close follow-up of these children is necessary before the significance of these alterations can be understood. Radiographic studies in the child with chronic abdominal pain also are obtained frequently. Any child with indication for an upper gastrointestinal series should have distal views of the small bowel obtained, as well. Flexible colonoscopy has largely replaced the barium enema, except in obstructive circumstances. Meckel's scans, pyelograms, and computerized tomography have limited, individualized applications.

BIBLIOGRAPHY

Apley J: *The Child with Abdominal Pain,* 2nd ed. London, Blackwell Scientific Publication, 1975.

Brender JD, Marcuse EK, Koepsell TD et al: Childhood appendicitis: Factors associated with perforation. Pediatrics 76:301–306, 1985

Christenson MF, Montensen O: Longterm prognosis in children with recurrent abdominal pain. Arch Dis Child 50:110–113, 1975

Galler JR, Neusten S, Walker WA: Clinical aspects of recurrent abdominal pain in children. Adv Pediatr 27:31–42, 1980

Jordon SC, Ament ME: Pancreatitis in children and adolescents. J Pediatr 91:211–215, 1977

Ravitch MM: Appendicitis. Pediatrics 70:414–419, 1982

38

Abdominal Mass

Generalized abdominal distention or palpation of a focal abdominal mass are significant clinical concerns in childhood, with particular prevalence in the neonatal period. While Table 38-1 lists an extensive differential diagnosis, it is important to note that more than 60% of abdominal masses in childhood are renal in origin. The emphasis in physical examination and use of imaging technology is on determining the intraperitoneal or retroperitoneal origin of the mass, the degree of localization, and the relationship to contiguous structures.

GENERALIZED ABDOMINAL DISTENTION

The child with generalized distention usually has an etiology related to hypotonia, ileus, or ascites. Hypotonia of the abdominal muscles, together with increased gaseousness, contributes to the prominent "pot-belly" appearance of the child with celiac syndrome or cystic fibrosis. Prune-belly syndrome is a rare syndrome of congenital hypoplasia of the striated muscles of the anterior abdominal muscles.

An associated deficiency of smooth muscle in the genitourinary collecting system produces obstructive uropathy and hydroureter in more than 90% of cases. Malrotation, phimosis, and imperforate anus may also be seen.

Ileus is the complication of impaired intestinal motility at any level, with distention most pronounced with distal obstruction. Contributing conditions include volvulus, stenosis, Hirschsprung's disease, or chronic constipation.

Intestinal pseudo-obstruction is a progressive or recurring functional ileus in the absence of obstruction. A severe congenital form carries a dismal prognosis. It is more commonly seen secondary to collagen–vascular disease (especially scleroderma or dermatomyositis), primary myopathies such as myotonic or muscular dystrophy, or endocrine disorders, such as hypothyroidism, hypercalcemia, or diabetes. Severe aerophagia may mimic pseudo-obstruction in older children.

Ascites is usually freely demonstrated by eliciting a fluid wave or percussion over the liver. Several potential origins exist, beginning with portal hypertension at any level.

Table 38–1. Abdominal Distention or Mass in Childhood

I. **Generalized distention**
   Hypotonia
      Malabsorption syndromes
      Prune belly syndrome
   Ileus
      Distal bowel obstruction
      Constipation
      Pseudo-obstruction
      Aerophagia
   Ascites
      Portal hypertension
      Pancreatitis
      Protein losing enteropathy
      Chronic renal disease/nephrosis
      Chylous ascites

II. **Focal mass**
   Asymmetric Hepatomegaly
      Hepatoblastoma/hepatocellular carcinoma
      Subcapsular hematoma
      Hemangioma/hamartoma
      Choledochal cyst/hydrops of gallbladder
   Midline mass
      Gastric outlet obstruction
      Pancreatic pseudocyst
      Mesenteric cyst
      Intussusception
      Pregnancy
      Sacrococcygeal teratoma
      Urachal cyst
      Bladder retention
   Lateralizing mass
      Wilms' tumor
      Neuroblastoma
      Hydronephrosis/polycystic kidney
      Renal vein thrombosis
      Ovarian cyst/tumor
      Abscess (appendiceal)
      Splenomegaly
      Crohn's disease
      Hodgkin's/lymphoma
      Constipation

Splenomegaly is anticipated in these children, as well. Hypoalbuminemia contributes to ascites from protein-losing enteropathy, chronic renal disease, nephrotic syndrome, or profound malnutrition (kwashiorkor). Be-

cause pancreatitis should not be overlooked as a cause of ascites, the amylase level should be determined routinely. Chylous ascites usually reflects intestinal lymphangectasia or postoperative lymphatic trauma. Vascular origins include venacaval thrombosis or pericarditis.

FOCAL MASS

A symmetric hepatomegaly may present as a right upper quadrant or epigastric mass. The major concern is exclusion of hepatoblastoma or hepatocellular carcinoma. Subcapsular hematomas, hemangiomas, or even hamartomas may also be noted. Choledochal cyst or hydrops of the gallbladder (the latter prominent in Kawasaki's syndrome and graft-versus-host disease) is often indistinguishable by palpation alone from an enlarged right lobe of the liver. Associated jaundice is anticipated in these children.

The differential diagnosis of a midline mass is more extensive. Gastric atony or distention may reflect outlet obstruction from pylonic stenosis, channel ulcers, or duodenal obstruction. Pancreatic pseudocysts, while arising from the retroperitoneum, are often large enough to palpate in the epigastrium. Blunt abdominal trauma is the major etiology, although any acute pancreatitis may result in the complication of pseudocyst formation.

Mesenteric cyst or intussusception may present as either midline or lateralizing firm masses. Obstructive features may also complicate their presence. Pediatricians cannot overlook pregnancy with uterine enlargement as the cause of a midline abdominal or pelvic mass.

The sacrococcygeal teratoma is most prevalent in early infancy, arising from the retroperitoneum and often most impressively palpated on rectal examination. Urachal cysts and bladder retention syndromes also present as midline pelvic masses.

The most common concern is the lateralizing or flank mass in childhood. Wilms' tumor is the most common retroperitoneal tumor in childhood, accounting for up to 30% of all childhood renal masses. The tumor is firm, is usually nontender, and rarely crosses the midline, although bilateral Wilms' tumor is encountered in 7% of involved children. In the preschool-aged child, presentation is usually asymptomatic but occasionally with hematuria, flank pain, anorexia, emesis, and/or hypertension.

Neuroblastoma, in contrast, is the most common malignant tumor present at birth, and the majority of involved children present before the age of 2 years. The tumor can arise at any level of the sympathetic ganglia, but most involve the adrenal gland and present as a suprarenal mass, often extending across the midline. Symptoms of catecholamine release include hypertension, sweating, tachycardia, or diarrhea. Early metastasis may lead to presentation with proptosis, ecchymosis of eyelids, lymphadenopathy, and bone pain.

With hydronephrosis, hydroureter, or polycystic kidney, bilateral renal masses are frequently noted. Renal vein thrombosis in the neonate presents with unilateral renal enlargement and hematuria.

Ovarian cysts or tumors may present with a mass, even in the absence of significant pain. Pelvic abscess may complicate pelvic inflammatory disease but most commonly is seen as a complication of appendiceal perforation. Fistulas with abscess formation also complicate Crohn's disease with a right lower quadrant fullness or mass palpable. Intestinal lymphomas, especially Hodgkin's or Burkitt's, may present as a localizing abdominal mass.

APPROACH TO DIAGNOSIS

Once distention or a mass is noted, the diagnostic approach begins with a careful physical examination (Table 38–2). The mass is

Table 38–2. Diagnostic Approach to Abdominal Mass

Universal
  Physical examination
  Rectal examination
  Urinalysis
  Flat plate and upright abdominal x-ray
  Abdominal and pelvic sonogram
  Abdominal CT with contrast
Individual
  Specific blood tests
  Nuclear-medicine scans
  Pyelogram
  Anteriogram
  Laparoscopy
  Laparotomy

defined by consistency, mobility, tenderness, and the presence or lack of a bruit. Rectal examination often is critical in confirming the pelvic origin. A fresh urine sample is analyzed routinely. Blood studies are rarely of diagnostic value as "screening" tests but are used to confirm diagnostic suspicions of liver disease, renal failure, pancreatic inflammation, or endocrine function.

The initial radiographic studies remain the kidney, ureter, and bladder (KUB) or flat plate plus an additional view of the abdomen and pelvis. Mass effect, calcification, or fluid is noted. The sonogram is routinely obtained to determine location, consistency, presence of ascites, and relation of the mass to other structures. In many circumstances, a definitive diagnosis is established by sonography. Abdominal CT scans offer greater resolution and the ability to incorporate contrast in the intestinal tract or kidney collecting systems. The added value of nuclear magnetic resonance (NMR) or positron emission tomagraphy (PET) in childhood has yet to be defined.

On an individualized basis, nuclear medicine flow scans (technicium) or avidity scans (gallium) may be needed. Pyelograms may reveal the characteristic renal distortion of Wilms' tumor versus renal displacement of neuroblastoma. Anteriography with venous phase studies may be required to confirm partial venous hypertension or to define vascular flow prior to surgical resection of a mass. Laparoscopy is not employed as often for diagnosis now that improved, less invasive imaging technology is available. Laparatomy is rarely employed diagnostically, although frequently employed therapeutically.

BIBLIOGRAPHY

Aney JB: Abdominal mass in infants and children. Pediatr Clin North Am 10:665–672, 1963

Byrne, WJ, Abel L, Euler AR et al: Chronic idiopathic intestinal pseudo-obstruction in children. J Pediatr 90:585–589, 1977

Goldberg BB, Pollack HM, Capitanio MA et al: Ultrasonography: An aid in the diagnosis of masses in pediatric patients. Pediatrics 56:421–428, 1975

Koop CE: Abdominal mass in the newborn infant. N Eng J Med 289:569–571, 1973

Mollet DL, Ballantine TVN, Grosfeld JL: Mesenteric cysts in infancy and childhood. Surg Gynecol Obstet 147:182–184, 1978

Silverman FN: X-ray diagnosis of intra-abdominal masses in childhood. Postgrad Med 20:545–563, 1956

Tapper D, Lack EE: Teratomas in infancy and childhood. Ann Surg 198:398–410, 1983

39

The first issue in the approach to the evaluation of the child with chronic diarrhea is the definition. Just as "beauty is in the eye of the beholder," diarrhea in an infant is defined by the diaper changer. To the parent, the definition is thus based on frequency and/or consistency, while to the physician, the scientific definition is one of volume (greater than 20 ml/kg/day). It is important to note that teenagers have no idea what normal volume or consistency should be and so they generally underestimate the severity of their diarrhea. The definition is therefore best approached as objectively as possible with the use of a 7-day diet and stool diary kept while the child is fed as normal a diet as possible. The effect of the diarrhea and resultant dietary manipulations on the growth of the child must also be confirmed. Chronicity usually implies persistence beyond 4 weeks or multiple recurrences within 6 months.

Any evaluation begins with the personal examination of a fresh stool sample (Table 39-1). The consistency is recorded, and determination of occult blood, pH, and reducing sugars is routinely performed. In the absence of acids derived from maldigested carbohydrate, the stool pH is generally neutral (6.0 to 7.5).

Analysis for reducing sugars by the Clinitest™ system will confirm the presence of glucose, lactose, fructose, or galactose in the stool. Because sucrose is not a reducing sugar, children on high sucrose diets must have their stools hydrolyzed by acid prior to analysis. A fecal smear can be stained for fat globules, but the interpretation of the stain requires experience, since most infants have some fat globules normally present in the stool. On the other hand, a fecal smear stained with methylene blue is very valuable as a screen for fecal leukocytes or polymorphonuclear leukocytes, a hallmark of colonic inflammation. In ostomy patients or infants with high-volume stool losses, the fecal sample should be submitted for determination of osmolality and electrolyte content to guide fluid replacement and confirm the presence of unabsorbed, osmotically active substances. The stool sample is then submitted to the laboratory for culture of enteric pathogens, analysis for parasites, and exclusion of clostridial toxin (if these tests have not been performed already).

The vast majority of children with persistent or recurring diarrhea have no alteration in the rate of growth, as long as normal caloric intake is sustained. Indeed, in many children,

Table 39–1. The Initial Stool Examination

Consistency
Occult blood
*p*H
Reducing sugars
Qualitative fat stain
Methylene blue stain for polymorphonuclear leukocytes (PMNs)
Osmolality and electrolytes
Culture, parasite analysis, clostridial toxin

Table 39–2. Diarrhea Without Growth Impairment

Inflammatory secretion
Infection/inflammation
Partial obstruction
Ischemia/radiation
Allergy
Primary Secretion
Chloride-losing diarrhea
Neural crest tumor
Functional
Systemic stress
Hyperthyroidism
Dietary indiscretion/medication
Encopresis
Nonspecific diarrhea syndrome

an iatrogenic fall-off weight gain results from the prolonged elimination of high-calorie foods. In Table 39-2, the major conditions contributing to diarrhea in the absence of growth impairment are listed.

The disorders of inflammatory secretion include chronic intestinal infections such as with *Giardia* or enteroinvasive bacteria, or toxin-mediated diarrheas as with *Clostrium difficile* or even cholera. With partial distal intestinal obstruction, diarrhea may result from a prestenotic enteritis independent of the documentation of bacterial overgrowth. Postischemic or radiation enteritis may also be seen in childhood. The role of allergic enteritis in the absence of true enteropathy remains controversial.

Familial chloride-losing diarrhea presents as an intractable diarrhea in infancy. Catecholamine metabolites also induce net secretion in children with neural crest tumors, so that diarrhea is often prominent at the time of diagnosis.

The "functional disorders" imply that stool volume is probably normal, although the consistency is not ideal. Systemic stress or irritable bowel is common in childhood, especially in adolescents. A positive family history is normally anticipated. The intervals of constipation in adults with irritable bowel are less prominent in childhood. Dietary indiscretion refers to excessive intake of poorly absorbed material such as sorbitol, fructose, iced tea, or apple juice. Well water high in sulfates or other salts and chlorinated pool water (swallowed excessively) may contribute. The suspensions used in liquid medications may also lead to diarrhea. When increased frequency of small bowel movements of "loss of control" of liquid stool is reported, one should suspect primary constipation with leakage or encopresis confusing the parent or child as to etiology.

The syndrome of chronic nonspecific diarrhea of childhood accounts for more than 80% of the complaints of diarrhea in the child under 3 years of age. It is not a diagnosis of exclusion. While the pathophysiology remains unclear, it is best considered a disorder of "lazy colon." Digestion and absorption are normal. The clinical features are noted in Table 39-3. The onset may follow an acute enteritis, and interpretation is obscured by the multiple dietary manipulations made in an effort to improve the stool consistency. The syndrome generally presents in the toddler and becomes a source of family concern when the stools escape the diaper and raise the fear that the child will "never be able to be toilet trained." The management consists of addressing the family's concerns and reassuring them of the benign course of the problem. A normal, balanced diet for age is critical, using

Table 39–3. Chronic Nonspecific Diarrhea Syndrome

Onset in first 18 months
Three to six soft to runny stools/day; most formed in the
  morning
Normal growth and absorptive ability
Positive family history of bowel complaints
No sustained response to dietary manipulations
Resolution by age 4 years or at toilet training

Table 39–4. Diarrhea with Growth Impairment: Phases and Disorders of Digestion and Absorption

Intraluminal Phase
  Pancreatic insufficiency
    Cystic fibrosis
    Schwachman-Diamond syndrome
    Hereditary fibrosing pancreatitis
  Enterokinase deficiency
Micellar Phase
  Cholestasis
  Metabolic hepatic disease
  Bile acid malabsorption/deficiency
  Bile acid deconjugation
Brush Border Phase
  Disaccharidase deficiency
  Bacterial overgrowth
Mucosal Phase
  Flat villus lesion (often patchy)
    Gluten-sensitive enteropathy
    Malnutrition
    Acute infectious or prestenotic enteritis
    Milk or soy protein enteropathy
    Giardia lamblia infestation
    "Intractable diarrhea of infancy"
    Eosinophilic gastroenteritis
    Immunodeficiency syndromes
    Bacterial overgrowth
    Dermatitis herpetiformis (? gluten)
    Neomycin and radiation enteropathy
    Chronic enteritis
    Tropical sprue
    Chronic ischemia
  Short-bowel syndrome
    Postresection fistula
  Binding factor deficiency
    Zinc: Acrodermatitis enteropathica
    Copper: Menke's
    B_{12}-binding protein
    Transport deficiencies for amino acids
Delivery Phase
  Abetalipoproteinemia
  Intestinal lymphangiectasia
  Portal hypertension
  Whipple's disease

dairy products unless lactose intolerance is confirmed. Medications to control diarrhea are generally worthless in this setting, although a role for fiber supplements may be appropriate if the diet is deficient in fiber content and the child is near toilet-training age. Once the child is toilet trained, this syndrome ceases to exist, since the child retains the stool longer and the parent no longer has to change dirty diapers.

While diarrhea need not be present in the setting of malabsorption or digestion, reductions of growth rate are generally anticipated. In the assessment of these children, it is critical to recognize the five stages of normal digestion and absorption. The first is the intraluminal phase, relating primarily to pancreatic functions of lipolysis and proteolysis. The second is the micellar phase, relating to normal bile excretion and bile acid function. The brush border phase depends on normal disaccharidase and oligopeptidase activity. The mucosal phase depends on normal villus function and surface area, whereas the delivery phase depends on normal lymphatic and portal venous function. Specific defects can exist at any level in this process, and some, such as bacterial overgrowth, can interfere at a number of levels. Table 39-4, lists a lengthy, but still far from complete, differential diagnosis listed by stage of digestion or absorption.

The classic example of a disorder in the intraluminal phase is pancreatic insufficiency caused by cystic fibrosis. This autosomal recessive disorder is characterized by large, greasy stools in infancy associated with impaired growth and progressive respiratory disease. Fat-soluble vitamin deficiency and severe steatorrhea are the rule; however, up to

20% of children with cystic fibrosis have no significant impairment in pancreatic function. The 72-hour fecal fat analysis will generally reveal more than 40% of undigested long chain fat. The diagnosis is confirmed by the elevation of sweat electrolyte concentration. Schwachman-Diamond syndrome is a condition in which pancreatic insufficiency is noted in the context of bone marrow dysfunction, usually neutropenia and thrombocytopenia. A characteristic metaphyseal dysostosis is noted in older children with osteoporosis prominent in infancy. In contrast to cystic fibrosis, the severity of the pancreatic insufficiency may actually decrease over the years.

The classic example of a disorder of the micellar phase is the infant with chronic cholestasis. The reduction in jejunal levels of bile acids lowers the efficiency of micellar solubilization and subsequent absorption of lipids. Steatorrhea and fat-soluble vitamin deficiency ensue with increased fecal losses of digested, but unabsorbed lipid. Deconjugation of bile acids by enteric bacterial overgrowth will similarly reduce micellar function.

The list of conditions associated with failure of mucosal function is lengthy, but celiac disease remains the preeminent example of these conditions. Celiac disease is now termed gluten-sensitive enteropathy in recognition of the ability of a fragment of gluten to produce the characteristic villus injury.

The presentation is a function of the age and degree of gluten exposure. Classically, the infant presents between 9 and 24 months of age with anorexia, impaired growth, irritability, abnormal stools, abdominal distention, and hypotonia. In younger infants, emesis, severe diarrhea, and edema from a mucosal protein-losing enteropathy are more prominent. In older children, the symptoms are more subtle, with occasional obstipation, anemia rickets, oral ulcerations, delayed puberty, or even infertility. The diagnosis is often suspected by laboratory parameters of malabsorption including hypoproteinemia, hypocalce-

mia, disaccharide intolerance, and a mixed anemia. Modest steatorrhea and reduction in red cell folate may also be noted with any villus injury. The diagnosis is confirmed by biopsy of the jejunum revealing villus epithelial cytotoxicity. Following gluten elimination, a clinical response and histologic recovery on a follow-up biopsy are documented. Challenge with gluten to confirm the lifelong need for gluten restriction is advised prior to the start of school, an age when parents often lose control of the child's diet unless highly motivated.

The mucosal phase is also impaired with other reductions in surface area, as noted with enteric fistulas or following resection of extensive areas of small bowel. Specific epithelial transport deficiencies are also reported for zinc (acrodermatitis enteropathica), copper (Menke's syndrome), vitamin B_{12}, and specific amino acids.

Abetalipoproteinemia is one example of a disorder in the enteric delivery phase. In the absence of betalipoprotein, lipid is digested, is absorbed into the epithelial cell, and is then unable to leave the cell. Severe deficiency of fat-soluble vitamins produces the prominent symptoms of ataxia and hypotonia (vitamin E) and retinal changes (vitamin A). The lack of red cell membrane lipid produces the acanthocyte or spiculated appearance of the erythrocyte.

The evaluation undertaken in the context of suspected maldigestion or malabsorption is listed in Table 39-5. Specific absorptive studies are individualized on the basis of history and screening laboratory data. Regrettably, no single laboratory test either confirms or excludes malabsorption. Three tests are best considered mandatory: the sweat test to exclude cystic fibrosis, the 72-hour fecal fat analysis on a high-fat diet, and the breath hydrogen assay after lactose challenge. The 72-hour fecal fat analysis can provide several valuable pieces of information. First, the parents record all intake for the 3 days of

Table 39–5. The "Malabsorption" Evaluation

History
Physical examination
Growth analysis
Initial stool examination
Bone age determination
"Screening" laboratory tests
   Complete blood count, smear, retic, ESR
   Urinalysis, urine culture
   Sweat test
   Immunoglobulins
   Total protein, albumin, liver function tests
   Red cell folate
Specific absorptive studies (individualize)
   72-hour fecal fat
   Disaccharide tolerance (2 g/kg)
      Breath H_2 excretion
   Duodenal aspirate
      Giardia
      Pancreative enzymes
      Quantitative culture
   Fat-soluble vitamin assays
      Vitamin A, E, D
      Prothrombin time (K)
   Schilling test (vitamin B_{12})
Biopsy of jejunum or colon

the test, allowing review of caloric content and nutrient distribution. To maximize the denominator, the infants are given a diet of at least 25 g/day of long chain lipid, the toddlers a diet of at least 50 g, and the school-aged children a diet of at least 100 g/day.

Breath hydrogen analysis has been one of the major diagnostic advances of the past two decades. Following an oral load of 2 g/kg of a 10% solution of carbohydrate (usually lactose), the breath content of hydrogen is determined. The hydrogen content will be determined by the bacterial fermentation of undigested and unabsorbed sugar, normally in the distal bowel. An early hydrogen peak suggests proximal bowel bacterial overgrowth. An elevation of hydrogen content greater than 20 ppm above baseline is diagnostic of malabsorption of that sugar.

Duodenal aspirates are performed to document jejunal infestation with *Giardia lamblia*, to culture for bacterial overgrowth, or to document pancreatic enzyme response to stimulation. Barium contrast studies are rarely of diagnostic value. Biopsies of the small bowel or colon are indicated for the exclusion of chronic inflammatory enteropathy. The value of serum immunoglobulin levels is greatest in children over 1 year of age. Children with IgA deficiency and transient hypogammaglobulinemia have increased diarrheal symptoms, often due to persistent infection, as with giardiasis. More severe diarrhea is seen with combined immunodeficiency.

If no etiology is apparent, the child is placed on whatever diet is associated with sustained growth while the symptom of diarrhea is minimized, if necessary, with a binding resin such as cholestyramine. In infancy, some of the children develop an intractable diarrhea with net fluid losses regardless of the enteric nutrient provided. The ability to temporarily sustain these infants with parenteral nutrition has revolutionized their care and improved survival from less than 40% to more than 90% during the past 20 years. After an interval on exclusive parenteral nutrition, enteric feeding is resumed with an elemental diet at low levels of caloric demand and slowly advanced. Cholestyramine is often required to bind incompletely absorbed bile acids, one of the many complications of this condition. In the absence of ongoing inflammation, complete recovery is the rule.

BIBLIOGRAPHY

Berg NO, Borulf S, Jakobsson I et al: How to approach the child suspected of malabsorption. Acta Pediatr Scand 67:403, 1978

Gryboski J, Walker WA: Gastrointestinal problems in the infant, 2nd ed. Philadelphia, WB Saunders, 1983

Silverman A, Roy CC: Pediatric Clinical Gastroenterology, 3rd ed. St Louis CV Mosby, 1983

40

Gastrointestinal Bleeding

Recent technological advances allow the same basic approach to the evaluation of intestinal bleeding to be applied to children of all ages. However, the differential diagnosis of likely etiology remains highly age-dependent in childhood. In Table 40-1, the more common etiologies are reviewed in this manner, emphasizing, but not demanding, mutual exclusivity.

NEONATE

In the neonate, the most common explanation of blood in the emesis or stool is maternal blood, either swallowed at delivery or derived during nursing from fissures in the breast. The maternal origin is easily confirmed with the Apt test, which documents the resistance of fetal hemoglobin to denaturation by alkali.

Coagulation defects in the neonate often present with intestinal hemorrhage. Foremost are the failure to provide vitamin K because of oversight in the delivery room and consumption coagulopathies complicating neonatal sepsis or following hypoxic hepatic injury.

Necrotizing enterocolitis is an ischemic

Table 40–1. Common Causes of Intestinal Bleeding in Childhood

| **Neonatal** |
| Maternal blood |
| Coagulopathy |
| Necrotizing enterocolitis |
| Gastric ulcer |
| Malrotation/volvulus |
| Anal fissure |
| Proctocolitis |
| **Infant/Toddler** |
| Polyp |
| Meckel's diverticulum |
| Intussusception |
| Esophagitis |
| Hematoma |
| Hemangioma/telangiectasia |
| Hemolytic–uremic syndrome |
| **Child/Adolescent** |
| Peptic ulcer |
| Portal hypertension |
| Inflammatory colitis |
| Vasculitis |

insult to the intestine that presents with enteric bleeding and pneumatosis or intramural air on radiographic examination of the abdomen. Most common in premature infants after the initiation of feedings, enterocolitis is also heralded by abdominal distention with ileus.

Stress-induced gastric erosions and ulceration can be seen at any age, especially in the context of multisystem disease in the intensive care unit. In the neonate, gastric ulceration and perforation present with catastrophic bleeding and shock.

The cardinal features of neonatal malrotation and volvulus are bilious emesis and small-bowel obstruction; however, intestinal bleeding may also be prominent. Early recognition is the key to minimizing the ischemic infarction of the mid-small bowel.

Bright red streaks of blood on the surface of the stool is a feature of both anal fissures and inflammatory proctitis in the neonate and young infant. While a notorious complication of constipation, anal fissures also develop in the absence of firm stool as a result of the infant's poor relaxation of the external sphincter. Inflammatory proctitis is heralded by the demonstration of polymorphonuclear leukocytes in the stool and is confirmed by proctoscopic visualization and biopsy. Infectious etiologies include *Campylobactor*, *Yersinia*, *Salmonella*, *Shigella*, and enteroinvasive *E. coli*. The role of *Clostridia* toxin in early infancy is obscured by its frequent presence in the stools of normal infants. Dietary protein origins for proctocolitis are also prominent in infancy, especially cow milk, soybean, and even maternal dietary proteins in breast-fed infants.

INFANTS AND TODDLERS

In infancy and young childhood, the three most common causes of intestinal bleeding are polyps, Meckel's diverticulum, and intussusception. The vast majority of polyps are benign juvenile retention polyps, with a peak frequency of bleeding between 2 and 6 years. Most have an acute onset of bleeding, followed by several months of intermittent bleeding. Self-amputation commonly occurs in 4 to 6 months. Familial polyposis of the colon consists of multiple adenomatous polyps with a malignant potential so great as to justify colectomy in childhood. The hamartomatous polyps of Peutz-Jeghers syndrome may occur in either the small or large bowel, with bleeding and/or obstruction as the principal feature. A familial disorder, Peutz-Jeghers syndrome patients may also have pigmented freckles of the oral mucosa. Meckel's diverticulum usually presents with relatively painless but dramatic rectal bleeding. The bleeding is usually ileal in origin, juxtaposed to the ectopic gastric mucosa in the diverticular remnant of the fetal omphalomesenteric duct. While bleeding is the most common feature, obstruction, perforation, and pain are also reported. While occasionally visualized on barium small-bowel follow-through, the major diagnostic technique is a radionucleide scan utilizing technitium 99m pertechnetate concentration in the gastric tissue, especially after potentiation by pentagastrin. The ("Meckel's" scan) may also be positive with gastric duplication, intestinal hemangioma, small-bowel ulceration, ureteral obstruction, and intussusception with severe bowel-wall edema.

Intussusception, usually of the terminal ileum into the colon, is most frequent in the otherwise healthy 18 to 36 month old. The classic presentation is with a "currant-jelly" dark red stool and a palpable abdominal mass. Usually idiopathic in toddlers, a lead-point is more common in older children. Etiologies include Meckel's diverticulum, polyp, lymphoid hyperplasia including lymphoma, and Henoch-Schönlein purpura. When suspected, a barium enema can both diagnose and hydrostatically reduce the intussusception in younger children. Surgical reduction and exclusion of a lead-point is more common in patients over 5 years of age.

Reflux esophagitis is also a common cause of chronic, low-grade intestinal bleeding. In early infancy, streaks of blood are mixed with frequent emesis. In older children, the bleeding is more likely to be occult, and the diagnosis is more difficult prior to the development of substernal pain or dysphagia. A family history of hiatal hernia should be elicited.

Blunt trauma to the abdomen from accidental or nonaccidental (abusive) origin may lead to the development of intramural hematoma and melena. The most common site of the hematoma is near the fixation of the duodenum at the ligament of Treitz, presenting with gastric outlet obstruction and bleeding. Pancreatitis with or without pseudocyst must be also excluded. Intestinal hematomas may also complicate primary coagulopathies such as thrombocytopenia, hemophilia, or vasculitis, as with Henoch-Schönlein purpura.

Hemangiomas or telangiectasia of the bowel may contribute to enteric bleeding. The telangiectasia may be restricted to the stomach or colon or may occur diffusely throughout. Colonic telangiectasia is a feature of Turner's syndrome. Angiodysplasia of the right colon is rare in childhood.

Hemolytic–uremic syndrome usually presents in toddlers and older children with a blood-streaked diarrheal stool and all the features of an acute, often ulcerating, colitis. A microangiopathic hemolytic anemia is present, with acute renal failure anticipated in the next 24 to 72 hours.

CHILD/ADOLESCENT

The peptic disorders of gastric or duodenal ulcer may present at any age. The characteristic relation to meals seen in adults is less common. The pain may be cramping or burning, epigastric or periumbilical, with night pain a prominent feature. Melena or hematemesis will be documented in 20% to 40% of involved children. Gastric ulceration may be secondary to stress or salicylate use. Postprandial acid secretion is often elevated in duodenal ulcer patients but is usually normal with gastric ulcer. With both hiatal hernia and peptic ulcer, a positive family history is anticipated. The syndrome of elevated gastrin-induced hyperacidity (Zollinger-Ellison) is very rare in children but must be excluded with repeated ulcer activity, multiple ulcerations, or evidence of multiple endocrine adenomas. Response rates of peptic disease to treatment with histamine (H_2) antagonists are high, but relapse is common.

Approximately 90% of children with portal hypertension will develop variceal bleeding from esophageal and/or gastric varices. As a rule, in childhood, chronic liver disease produces maximal fibrosis in the portal area, leading to portal hypertension out of proportion to the severity of liver failure. Since hepatic synthetic ability is usually preserved at the time of initial variceal bleeding, the survival rate is high. Approximately 15% of children with portal hypertension have a presinusoidal origin, as with portal vein thrombosis, so that hepatic function is intact.

Rectal bleeding is a nearly universal feature in ulcerative colitis and a more subtle feature of Crohn's disease. With most forms of inflammatory colitis, the diarrheal stools contain leukocytes. Antibiotic-induced or clostridia toxin-mediated colitis may also feature prominent blood loss. A prestenotic inflammatory colitis may complicate colonic strictures after ischemia (as in necrotizing enterocolitis) or with aganglionosis (Hirschsprung's).

Henoch-Schönlein purpura is the most common form of intestinal vasculitis in childhood, and melena will develop during the course of disease in nearly 50% of involved children. Associated features leading to suspicion of the diagnosis include purpura of the buttocks and extremities, edema of the scrotum, ankles, and forehead, and hematuria. Melena is also reported in polyarteritis nodosa but is quite rare in scleroderma or lupus erythematosus.

DIAGNOSTIC EVALUATION

The diagnostic approach to intestinal bleeding begins with an estimate of severity of the bleeding and whether the bleeding is primarily above or below the ligament of Treitz. As the evaluation summarized in Table 40-2 is initiated, surgical colleagues should be apprised of the gravity of the situation in any patient with hemodynamically significant bleeding.

In children with hematemesis, the nasopharynx is first examined as a possible origin and then a nasogastric tube is placed for lavage of the stomach with iced saline solution. The neonate or young infant must be monitored closely for excessive body cooling and salt overload. Neither radiographic or endoscopic evaluation is advised until the child is hemodynamically stabilized. When it is performed in the first 24 to 48 hours, the diagnostic yield of esophagogastroduodenoscopy exceeds that of radiographic contrast studies. Endoscopic sclerosis or laser coagulation may also be available as direct therapeutic intervention. With associated features of obstruction, contrast studies with water-soluble agents are often advised. If the severity of the bleeding interferes with endoscopic evaluation, angiography should reveal the bleeding site and may allow for arterial infusion of clotting agents prior to decisions regarding laparotomy.

In children with melena, a smaller nasogastric tube is passed to lavage the stomach for exclusion of an upper intestinal origin to the bleeding. The abdominal flat plate is reviewed for features of obstruction, as with intussusception. If the bleeding is modest, a limited proctoscopic examination is performed to determine if an inflammatory proctocolitis, internal fissure, or rectal polyp is present. More complete colonoscopy with biopsies should ideally be deferred until results of stool culture are available to mini-

Table 40-2. Evaluation of Significant Intestinal Bleeding

Universal Evaluation
History
Physical examination
Rectal exam
Nasogastric aspirate
Urinalysis
Stool hemoccult, leukocytes
APT test (neonate)
Laboratory studies
   Complete blood count with smear, retic count
   Platelet count, sedimentation rate
   Type and cross-match
   Prothrombin, partial thromboplastin time
   Abdominal flat and upright abdomen
   Alanine aminotransferase, gamma-glulamyl transpeptidase

Individualized Evaluation
Stool culture, clostridia toxin, parasite analysis
Technicium pertechnetate scan
Endoscopy
   Esophagogastroduodenoscopy
   Colonoscopy
Angiography
Barium contrast studies
Exploratory laparotomy

mize the risk of bacteremia. With moderate volume bleeding, especially when recurrent, a technitium 99m pertechnetate "Meckel's" scan is advised prior to the initiation of barium contrast studies. With acute inflammatory colitis, the barium enema is best deferred until flexible colonoscopy and biopsy are performed.

Even when all of the above studies (and more) are performed, an explanation for the bleeding may not be found in up to 30% of children with their first bleeding episode. If the degree of bleeding was modest, bleeding has ceased, and the prior health of the child has been normal, no further studies are warranted other than close follow-up. If, on the other hand, no etiology is established in the midst of active, ongoing bleeding, or if a second episode of dramatic bleeding with a drop in hematocrit has occurred, surgical consultation with exploratory laparotomy is usually warranted. In our last 20 patients under these latter conditions, laparotomy revealed a Meckel's diverticulum in 14 children, hemangiomas in 4, a hamartomatous jejunal polyp in 1, and no explanation in 1 child.

BIBLIOGRAPHY

Bounocore E et al: Massive upper gastrointestinal hemorrhage in children. Am J Roentgenol 115:289–296, 1972

Brayton D: Gastrointestinal bleeding of "unknown origin": A study of cases in infancy and childhood. A.J.D.C. 107:288, 1964

Collins REC: Some problems of gastrointestinal bleeding in children. Arch Dis Child 46:110–112, 1971

Cox K, Ament ME: Upper gastrointestinal bleeding in children and adolescents. Pediatrics 63:408–413, 1979

Nord K: Peptic ulcer disease in children and adolescents: Evolving dilemmas. J Pediatr Gastroenterol Nutr 2:397–399, 1983

Shandling B: Laparotomy for rectal bleeding. Pediatrics 35:787, 1965

Spencer R: Gastrointestinal hemorrhage in infancy and childhood: 476 cases. Surgery 55:718–734, 1964

41

Inflammatory Bowel Disease

Nearly one-third of patients with inflammatory bowel disease (IBD) will have the onset of their symptoms, if not the diagnosis, prior to the age of 20 years. Thus, the burden of early recognition and treatment falls to the pediatrician. The spectrum of symptoms and clinical course are quite broad, often indolent, and defy simple characterization. The two major conditions classified as IBD, ulcerative colitis and Crohn's disease, share many clinical features in childhood and thus, with the exception of treatment, are often considered together. Regretably, the etiology of these conditions remains unknown.

CLINICAL PRESENTATION

For about 60% of children with IBD, the symptoms are obviously intestinal in origin. Such patients present with cramping abdominal pain, tenesmus, weight loss, and diarrhea, which may contain visible blood. More than one-third of the children, however, present with more indolent disease and more prominent extraintestinal or systemic features of IBD. A number of such features are listed in Table 41-1. While this list is not all-inclusive,

Table 41–1 Extraintestinal Manifestations of Childhood IBD

Reduced rate of growth
Persistent anemia
Perianal inflammation
Amenorrhea/delayed puberty
Chronic active hepatitis/cholangitis
Oral aphthous ulcers
Episcleritis/uveitis
Large joint synovitis/arthritis
Erythema nodosum/pyoderma gangrenosum
Renal calculi/obstructive uropathy

the unexplained presence of any two symptoms or the progressive presence of any one feature should lead to the consideration of IBD. The failure to appreciate the significance of these symptoms may lead to a delay in diagnosis and possibly preventable surgery.

The reduced rate of growth with its attendant delay in sexual maturation will complicate the course of more than 80% of children with Crohn's disease and 20% of children with ulcerative colitis. The factors contributing to this reduced rate of growth are summarized in Figure 41-1. The role of corticosteroid therapy after the diagnosis is indicated. Hor-

282

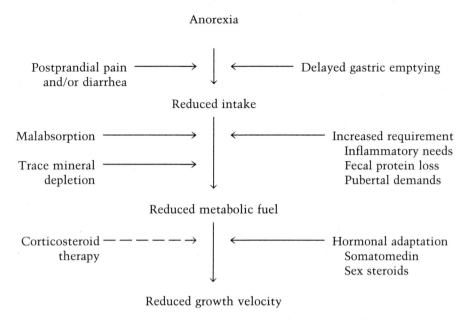

Anorexia

Postprandial pain ⟶ ⟵ Delayed gastric emptying
and/or diarrhea

Reduced intake

Malabsorption ⟶ ⟵ Increased requirement
Inflammatory needs
Trace mineral ⟶ Fecal protein loss
depletion Pubertal demands

Reduced metabolic fuel

Corticosteroid — — — — ⟶ ⟵ Hormonal adaptation
therapy Somatomedin
Sex steroids

Reduced growth velocity

FIGURE 41–1. Interactions in the growth failure of childhood IBD.

monal adaptations, such as reductions in somatomedin, combined with delayed bone ages often lead to confusion with a primary endocrinopathy. Most investigators feel that reduction in net caloric intake is the most important component.

Anemia is commonly noted, often in the absence of significant gastrointestinal GI bleeding. As with other chronic inflammatory diseases, serum iron levels are reduced, but iron therapy fails to correct the anemia. Folate deficiency can complicate treatment with sulfasalazine, and vitamin B_{12} deficiency may develop with extensive ileal disease or resection.

The demonstration of a perianal abscess, fistula, or edematous skin tag should always suggest Crohn's disease. Perianal irritation may also be prominent with ulcerative colitis.

Delayed menstruation or acquired amenorrhea may complicate any chronic nutritional or inflammatory disease in the adolescent female. Similarly, the resumption of a normal menstrual pattern is a valuable marker of disease control.

Chronic hepatitis, with negative viral and metabolic testing, is rare in childhood. When diagnosed in the adolescent, an underlying chronic colitis must be suspected. The liver biopsy may have features of cholangitis, as well as features of chronic active hepatitis. Control of the colitis generally controls the hepatitis.

Aphthous ulcerations of the colonic mucosa are an early feature of Crohn's disease. Recurrent oral aphthous ulcers are also seen, often correlating with disease activity. They are not specific to IBD, since they may occur in any enteropathy or nutritional deficiency. Episcleritis and uveitis are prominent ophthalmologic manifestations of IBD.

Arthritic manifestations complicate the course of more than 25% of children with IBD. Generally the large joints are involved with a nondestructive synovitis that corre-

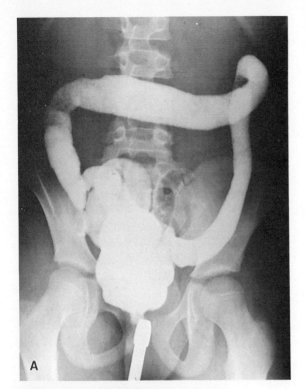

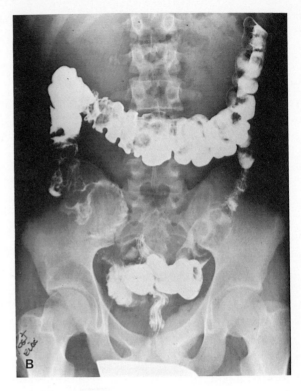

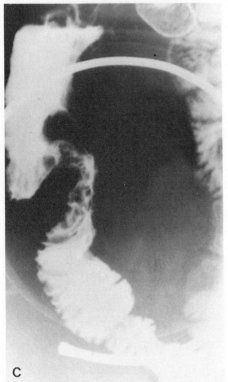

FIGURE 41–2. *(A)* Barium enema: ulcerative colitis. Note the characteristic diffuse "pancolitis" pattern of inflammation with loss of haustral markings throughout the colon. *(B)* Barium enema: Crohn's ileocolitis. Note the severe narrowing or strictures of the cecum and mid-descending colon, with the intervening normal transverse colon. Barium has also refluxed into an inflamed terminal ileum. *(C)* Spot film: Crohn's ileocolitis. Note the fixed narrowing of the terminal ileum with distortion of the cecum and proximal dilatation of the ileum caused by chronic partial obstruction.

lates with intestinal disease activity. Ankylosing spondylitis is also seen with increased frequency in IBD and is progressive independent of intestinal disease activity. Hip or proximal leg weakness may also reflect a fistula or abscess over the psoas muscle.

Of the cutaneous presentations, erythema nodosum is the more frequent and less specific for IBD. While rare, pyoderma gangrenosum may be quite severe. Multiple cutaneous granulomas may also be encountered in Crohn's disease.

Renal manifestations include calcium oxalate stones, obstructive uropathy, and fistulas into the bladder. Renal amyloid may complicate long-term Crohn's disease.

DIFFERENTIAL DIAGNOSIS

With presentation as a chronic enteritis, the initial studies focus on exclusion of infectious bowel diseases. At least two separate stool samples are cultured for the invasive enteric bacteria: *Salmonella, Shigella, Yersinia, Campylobacter,* and enteroinvasive *E. coli.* Even in the absence of a recent history of antibiotic exposure, the stool should also be tested for the toxin of *Clostridium difficile,* the cause of pseudomembranous colitis. Potential parasitic pathogens include *Entamoeba histolytica, Cryptosporidium,* and *Giardia lamblia.* Chronic viral enteritis is entertained only in immunocompromised patients.

An ischemic enteritis mimicking acute IBD may be encountered in the colon of patients with hemolytic–uremic syndrome. Abdominal pain with rectal bleeding is also seen with the small bowel vasculitis of Henoch-Schönlein purpura and may precede the characteristic rash of this condition by several days. Adolescent females on oral contraceptives may also develop an ischemic colitis.

Intestinal lymphoma with involvement of the proximal and distal small bowel may present with fever, weight loss, abdominal pain, and radiographic features of an obstructive nature similar to segmental Crohn's disease. Tubercular involvement of the ileum and cecum is rarely encountered in childhood.

The colitis induced by dietary proteins is restricted to the early infancy period and is rarely a factor in the differential. Eosinophilic enterocolitis is usually obstructive to gastric emptying but may involve the colon.

DIAGNOSTIC PROCEDURES

The history is complicated by the intervals of relative remission that are a feature of IBD in any age-group. Prominent intestinal symptoms include postprandial abdominal pain and diarrhea that can be minimized by reduced intake. A history of nocturnal diarrhea and tenesmus suggests ulcerative colitis. The nutritional history is critical to assessing the influence on growth and the potential sources of caloric supplements in treatment. It is important to realize that a child with a chronic enteropathy (and usually the parents) has no idea what a normal appetite is.

Physical examination must include anthropometric parameters, rectal examination, and complete eye examination in addition to the general examination. Palpation of an abdominal mass or focal abdominal pain will be very critical.

The most important laboratory test is examination of a fresh stool for evidence of occult blood and leukocytes. The complete blood count, reticulocyte count, sedimentation rate, and review of smear should be mandatory. Abnormalities of serum chemistry may include elevations of aminotransferase, reductions in albumin, and low urea nitrogen levels. In well-nourished children with IBD, the sedimentation rate is elevated in approximately 75% of the patients at the time of diagnosis.

Direct visualization of the colon is a mandatory early step in the investigation of IBD and should generally precede contrast studies. Preparation should consist only of a clear liquid diet for 36 hours with mild oral laxatives as needed. Cleansing enemas are avoided because they obscure the interpretation of edema, friability, and mild histologic abnormalities. Using a flexible sigmoidoscope, one can routinely visualize to the mid-transverse colon in children with minimal sedation. Biopsies of the colon and rectum are routinely obtained, even in the absence of apparent disease. In so doing, characteristic features of focal inflammation are found in 75% of patients with Crohn's disease. Diffuse inflammatory ulceration with rectal involvement is a feature of ulcerative colitis, whereas segmental or focal inflammation with aphthoid ulceration is more compatible with Crohn's disease.

Radiographic studies of the intestine are routinely obtained (Fig. 41-2). The barium enema is now generally performed with air contrast to increase mucosal detail. With acute fulminant colitis, the barium enema is relatively contraindicated because of an increased risk for inducing megacolon. The upper intestinal contrast studies should always include visualization of the terminal ileum and cecum with careful observation for fistula formation. Increasing experience with abdominal CT scanning has led to its replacing sonography in the assessment of bowel thickening, mesenteric adenopathy, and possible abscess.

The interpretation of biopsy or resection specimens will focus on distinguishing the pathologic features of Crohn's disease (transmural inflammation, focal ulceration, and prominent granulomas) from those of ulcerative colitis (diffuse inflammation, rectal involvement, and prominent crypt abscess formation) while excluding ischemic disease, graft-versus-host disease, malignancy, and infectious etiologies. Even after radiographic, sigmoidoscopic, and pathologic evaluation, nearly 25% of children with isolated colitis will lack absolute diagnostic features at the time of diagnosis.

CLINICAL COURSE AND THERAPY

Ulcerative colitis in children is usually acute in its presentation. Rarely, the fulminant colitis fails to respond to medical management, necessitating early colectomy. Colectomy under such circumstances should never be performed until hemolytic–uremic syndrome is excluded by urinalysis and review of the peripheral blood smear. Proctitis, with inflammation limited to the rectum, is less common than in the adult.

Medical management of the child with ulcerative colitis begins with a brief interval of relative bowel rest using either clear liquids or brief intravenous hydration to reduce pain, stool frequency, and bleeding. Prolonged parenteral alimentation has never been shown to have significant influence on the course of ulcerative colitis. Long-term nutritional management emphasizes modest increases of caloric intake and a low-residue diet. Antiperistaltic agents to reduce diarrhea are rarely indicated.

Sulfasalazine, soon to be superseded by the active component 5-aminosalicylic acid, is the initial oral medication of choice in ulcerative colitis. An enema form of 5-aminosalicylic acid is now being tested in adults. Gastric upset, rash, headache, and mild hemolytic anemia may complicate therapy with sulfasalazine. All patients on sulfasalazine also require folic acid supplements. Sulfasalazine works best with mild disease and is of proven value in reducing rates of recurrence.

Corticosteroid therapy is eventually required in more than two-thirds of children with ulcerative colitis. Tolerance or compliance with cortisone enemas is maximal in toddlers and motivated adolescents and minimal in 6 to 16 year olds. Chronic corticosteroid use is of limited value in reducing relapse rates.

The vast majority of children will respond well to medical management of their colitis. When surgery is mandated by megacolon, intractable diarrhea, or bleeding, total colectomy with ileostomy or ileorectal pull-through is performed.

Recognizing an extraordinary risk of colonic malignancy in patients with ulcerative colitis as a function of duration of disease (10% per decade of pancolitis), surveillance colonoscopy and biopsies for dysplasia begin at 8 to 10 years after diagnosis, independent of the degree of remission. With our present knowledge, confirmed ulcerative colitis is a premalignant condition with inevitable colectomy.

Due to the indolent nature of their symptoms and the resultant delay in diagnosis, children with Crohn's disease have a greater need for and greater benefit from nutritional management. Residue restrictions are individualized to the obstructive manifestations of the patient. Oral caloric supplements are routinely initiated to increase caloric intake to 125% of the RDA for height and are continued as a function of growth concerns. Multivitamin, mineral, zinc, and iron supplements are routine. Patients on high steroid intakes also require calcium supplements.

The value of sulfasalazine in Crohn's disease is less well established than in ulcerative colitis, but is commonly employed with extensive colonic involvement. Few patients avoid the initiation of corticosteroid therapy.

Prednisone, at doses of 1 to 2 mg/kg, is initiated daily and then tapered to an alternate-day regimen as quickly as possible. With extensive or resistant perianal disease, metronidazole is now employed as an "antibiotic" because of its anti-anaerobic activity. Studies on the value of immunosuppression with 6-mercaptopurine in colonic disease are underway, and preliminary results appear encouraging.

The speed of recovery in patients with Crohn's disease is slower than in ulcerative colitis, a fact attributed to the greater delay in diagnosis and the frequency of obstructive small bowel disease. The value of parenteral alimentation is also well proven when severe malabsorption, fistula formation, or intractable pain preclude oral medication and nutrition. Indeed, dramatic clinical response in Crohn's disease during parenteral alimentation occurs in the absence of anti-inflammatory medication but is not sustained when enteric nutrition is resumed.

Despite responses to medical and nutritional therapy, the majority of patients with Crohn's disease will require surgery within 10 years of diagnosis. Most will be limited resections for strictures, fistulas, or, less commonly, bleeding and perforation. With Crohn's disease, surgery is not undertaken for "cure," since more than 80% of patients will have relapses within a decade of their surgery. While the risk of malignancy is somewhat greater than normal in Crohn's disease, the prophylactic value of surgery is unproven.

The social implications of IBD in children and adolescents cannot be overestimated. Chronic intestinal disease leads to frustrating intervals of active symptoms, absence from school, dietary restriction, medication side effects, overprotective parents, and a too-frequent lack of patient involvement in decisions about diet, medication, and surgery. Intervals of depression and reactive noncompliance should be anticipated and minimized by peer support, education, and a willingness to listen to their concerns.

BIBLIOGRAPHY

Ament ME: Inflammatory disease of the colon: Ulcerative colitis and Crohn's colitis. 86:322–334, 1975

Grand RJ, Homer DR: Approaches to inflammatory bowel disease in childhood and adolescence. Pediatr Clin North Am 22:835–850, 1975

Grand RJ, Kelts DG: Inflammatory bowel disease in childhood and adolescence. Clin Prob Pediatr 10:5–40, 1980

Gryboski JD, Spiro HM: Prognosis in children with Crohn's disease. Gastroenterology 74:807–817, 1978

Hamilton JR, Bruce GA, Abdourhaman M et al: Inflammatory bowel disease in children and adolescents. Adv Pediatr 26:331–341, 1979

Kirsner JB, Shorter RG: Inflammatory Bowel Disease, 2nd ed. Lea & Febiger, Philadelphia, 1980

Whittington PR, Barnes HV, Bayliss TM: Medical management of Chrohn's disease in adolescence. Gastroenterology 72:1338–1344, 1977

42

Infantile Cholestasis

Cholestasis is the result of a reduction in bile flow, at the hepatocellular (intrahepatic) and/or bile ductular (extrahepatic) levels, that leads to increased hepatic and systemic levels of bile components, the most commonly measured of which is bilirubin. Instead of emphasizing disorders of bilirubin production leading to unconjugated hyperbilirubinemia, we will focus on disorders of bile conjugation and excretion that lead to conjugated hyperbilirubinemia. Objectively, these infants present with jaundice and total bilirubins exceeding 1.5 mg/dl with 20% to 70% as the direct reacting or conjugated component. Cholestasis will develop in approximately 1 in 5000 live births.

NORMAL BILE FUNCTION

The formation of bile is an energy-dependent osmotic process of the net movement of water and solutes from hepatocytes into intercellular bile canaliculi. A number of transport systems have been described; one for bile acids, one for organic anions (bilirubin or Bromsulphalein [BSP]), one for organic cations, and one for uncharged organic compounds. Additional systems are proposed for biliary proteins such as secretory IgA and lipids such as lecithin.

Half of the total bile solute is composed of bile acids formed within the hepatocyte from cholesterol and conjugated to either glycine or taurine to increase polarity and facilitate transport into the canaliculus. Bile acids function to clear cholesterol from the liver and to create micelles in the intestine that facilitate long-chain lipid absorption. In fetal life, taurine conjugation predominates, whereas glycine conjugation is greater beyond infancy. After excretion into the intestine, the bile acids may be deconjugated by bacterial dehydroxylases and reabsorbed in the terminal ileum, creating an "enterohepatic" circulation.

Under normal circumstances, 50% of the bile flow in the canaliculus is dependent on bile acids. The other 50% is independent of bile acid secretion and requires integrity of the Na^+-K^+ ATPase pump. This "independent" component of bile flow can be increased by phenobarbital and decreased by estrogens, chlorpromazene, and taurine-conjugated lithocholic acid. Surprisingly, at normal to moderately elevated levels, conjugated bilirubin exerts very little effect on bile flow. The rate-limiting step in the secretion of both conjugated bilirubin and bile acids is at the canalicular membrane.

It is thus not surprising that any insult to the hepatocyte or to the integrity of the canalicular system produces a "generic" cholestasis. Histologically, at the light-microscopic level, the generic components of most of the diseases to be discussed include hepatocellular cholestasis, portal fibrosis, and giant cell transformation. With extrahepatic obstruction, some bile ductular proliferation may also be noted. Giant cells are hepatocytes, containing four or more nuclei, with a pale cytoplasm often containing pigmented granules. In infancy, inflammatory cell infiltrates are rarely noted in any of the disorders.

From the clinical perspective, the major issue when facing a cholestatic infant is the integrity of the extrahepatic biliary system. The categorization of intrahepatic "hepatitis" versus extrahepatic "atresia" is too simple. Thus in Table 42-1, the differential diagnosis is approached in a pathophysiologic basis. An understanding of this differential diagnosis is critical to the organization of the diagnostic evaluation.

DISORDERS OF BILE FORMATION AND SECRETION

The disorders of bile secretion arise when a "normal" hepatocyte is unable to sustain secretion of conjugated bilirubin. Bilirubin "overload" is one possibility, and transient cholestasis will be seen in about 10% of infants with hemolytic anemias. Both Dubin-Johnson and Rotor's syndromes are autosomal-recessive disorders of the specific transport of conjugated bilirubin. Rarely presenting in infancy, these patients have normal transport of bile acids and uncharged compounds. They have minimal hepatomegaly, no pruritis, and normal or minimally elevated hepatic

Table 42–1. Differential Diagnosis of Infantile Cholestasis

Disorders of Bile Formation/Secretion
  Posthemolytic cholestasis
  Dubin-Johnson/Rotor's syndrome
  Benign recurrent cholestasis
  Familial progressive cholestasis (Byler)
  Paucity of interlobular bile ductules (Alagille)
Metabolic/Genetic
  α_1-Antiprotease deficiency
  Cystic fibrosis
  Galactosemia
  Hereditary fructose intolerance
  Tyrosinemia
  Lipid storage disease
Perinatal Infection
  Cytomegalovirus
  Hepatitis B
  Rubella
  Herpes
  Toxoplasmosis
  Syphilis
  Bacterial sepsis/cholangitis
Miscellaneous Hepatocellular
  Parenteral nutrition-associated
  Postischemic hepatitis
  Giant cell (idiopathic) hepatitis
Bile Ductular Obstruction
  Extrahepatic biliary atresia
  Choledochal cyst
  Bile ascites
  Cholelithiasis

enzyme levels. The livers of patients with Dubin-Johnson syndrome are pigmented; those of Rotor's syndrome patients are not.

Benign recurrent cholestasis is characterized by episodic jaundice with pruritis, often precipitated by viral illness, medication, or anesthesia but not progressing to chronic liver disease. Byler syndrome, in contrast, is a progressive hepatic failure disorder involving all transport systems and presenting in infancy with recurrent jaundice and hepatomegaly.

Hypoplasia of the intrahepatic interlobular bile ductules may be seen as part of a distinct clinical syndrome termed Alagille's syndrome. Additional features include a characteristic facies, pulmonary artery hypoplasia or stenosis, vertebral defects, and persistence of the posterior embryotoxin of the eye.

Metabolic/Genetic Disorders

The metabolic and genetic disorders presenting with infantile cholestasis hold specific concern, since early diagnosis and treatment may prevent many of the complications of the disease. In addition to cholestasis, these disorders may present with hepatomegaly, portal hypertension, or growth impairment.

α_1-Antiprotease deficiency, previously termed α_1-antitrypsin deficiency, is discussed in detail in Chapter 43. Only 10% of children with this disorder present with neonatal cholestasis, suggesting that antiprotease deficiency merely predisposes the child to some other hepatic insult.

Cholestasis is a rare complication of cystic fibrosis, usually occurring in association with meconium ileus and coagulopathy secondary to vitamin K deficiency. On liver biopsy, pericholangitis is noted and bile ductules are filled with a viscous inspissated bile.

Galactosemia is frequently characterized by cholestasis, emesis, hepatomegaly, and cataracts. Hypoglycemia, gram-negative sepsis, and growth failure may also be prominent. By definition, the child must have lactose in the diet as a galactose source. Galactose can usually be demonstrated in the urine as a positive reducing sugar (Clinitest) with a negative urine glucose. The disease results from the deficiency of either galactose-1-phosphate uridyl transferase or uridine dephosphate galactose-4-epimerase, both of which can be assayed in peripheral erythrocytes.

Hereditary fructose intolerance usually presents acutely with acidosis, emesis, hypoglycemia, proteinuria, cholestasis, and hepatomegaly. As commonly noted in metabolic errors, laboratory tests reveal moderate prolongation of the prothrombin time with mildly elevated liver enzymes. The spleen is rarely enlarged. Dietary sucrose, fructose, and sorbital must be eliminated from the diet.

Type 1 tyrosinemia results from a deficiency of fumarylacetoacetate hydrolase. Clinically, the majority present in a fashion similar to other metabolic disorders with cholestasis, hepatomegaly, acidosis, and emesis. In contrast to the others, splenomegaly and hematuria are prominent. Hepatic synthetic function is usually severely impaired with hypoalbuminemia, coagulopathy, and reduced cholesterol noted.

Hepatosplenomegaly is anticipated with the lipid storage diseases, especially Niemann-Pick, Gaucher's, and Wolman's diseases. Cholestasis and ascites are prominent associated features in the first several months. Characteristic lipid is routinely found on bone marrow aspirates, precluding the need for diagnostic hepatic biopsy in most patients. A condition of storage of very long chain C-26 lipids, Zellweger syndrome presents with hepatomegaly, hypotonia, cholestasis, and renal cortical cysts. Survival past the first few months is rarely achieved.

Perinatal Infection

Intrauterine infections commonly induce neonatal hepatitis; cholestasis is often anticipated. The most striking exception is the paucity of cholestasis in neonatal hepatitis A infection. Each of these conditions is discussed in detail in Chapter 19. Serologic diagnosis is usually required, with the exception of cytomegalovirus (CMV), which can be cultured. Retinal examination is often critical.

Miscellaneous Hepatocellular Disorders

Cholestasis has recently been identified as a frequent complication of prolonged intravenous alimentation (total parenteral nutrition) in the newborn. As a rule, the infants usually require more than 2 weeks of enteral fasting combined with intravenous administration of aminoacids and carbohydrates. Lipid emulsions appear to have a minimal effect. The development of cholestasis correlates in frequency with degree of prematurity, developing in 50% of neonates less than 1000 g, 20% of those from 1000 to 1500 g, and less than 10% of full-term infants treated with prolonged venous nutrition. The condition is now considered to be a multi-factorial process superimposed on the physiologic cholestasis of prematurity. Risk factors other than degree of prematurity and duration of therapy may include ascending cholangitis or endotoxemia from enteric ischemia.

Postischemic cholestasis is noted after birth asphyxia or neonatal cardiac surgery utilizing hypothermia. Transient but striking increases in aminotransferase levels are noted in the first 48 hours, followed by cholestasis that is minimized by early enteric nutrition and restoration of normal blood flow. The potential patency of the ductus venosus may explain the unique sensitivity of the neonatal liver to ischemic cholestasis.

Despite the space devoted to discussion of differential diagnosis and the implied need for diagnostic tests of exclusion, the majority of infants with cholestasis have either an extrahepatic obstruction of bile flow or an intrahepatic "idiopathic" giant cell hepatitis. As noted above, cholestasis, giant cell transformation of the hepatocytes, and fibrosis are the generic responses of the infantile liver to injuries of many kinds.

Bile Ductular Obstruction

Extrahepatic biliary atresia was originally termed "congenital" atresia, implying an origin from an intrauterine defect in bile duct development. In support of this origin, nearly 10% of infants with extrahepatic biliary atresia have associated anomalies such as polysplenia, preduodenal portal vein, cyanotic congenital heart disease, or malrotation. Against this hypothesis is the observation that few of the infants become clinically cholestatic until 3 to 5 weeks of age. The reigning hypothesis at this time is one of an "infantile obstructive cholangiopathy," originally championed by Landing and associates. This proposes a spectrum from primary intrahepatic giant cell hepatitis to pure extrahepatic biliary atresia as an acquired syndrome. A number of infectious agents have been proposed, most recently reovirus III, as a cholangiopathic infectious disease.

The atresia can occur at all levels of the extrahepatic system, the best prognosis for surgical therapy being with distal ductular atresia with normal bile flow to the gallbladder. Surgical intervention is most successful when attempted prior to 3 months of age. The major procedure employed for the past 20 years is the Kasai procedure, employing a loop of jejunum anastomosed to the porta hepatis after dissection of the portal area in an effort to reach potent bile ducts. Despite surgical intervention, the vast majority of infants progress to biliary cirrhosis, often mandating liver transplant prior to 4 years of age.

Choledochal cysts are saccular dilatations of the distal bile duct, usually lacking both epithelium and smooth muscle. The majority of infants with choledochal cyst present in infancy with jaundice, a right upper quadrant mass, emesis from duodenal obstruction, and/or pancreatitis. Older children may also present with cirrhosis, asymmetric hepatomegaly, portal hypertension, pruritis, or abdominal pain. Ready identification by sonography has revolutionized diagnosis of choledochal cysts.

Bile ascites is a rare complication of bile duct perforation. Presentation is with acholic stools, emesis, mild jaundice, and ascites, the latter often loculated as a cystic mass.

Cholelithiasis is increasingly recognized as a complication of low-flow, lithogenic bile in the context of parenteral alimentation. Hemolytic diseases may also produce bilirubin stones.

DIAGNOSTIC EVALUATION

The evaluation indicated for the infant with cholestatic jaundice is summarized in Table 42-2. The initial assessment is obvious: confirming cholestatic jaundice in contrast to unconjugated hyperbilirubinemia and examining the stool for evidence of bile pigment. The baseline evaluation is a "status" report of the degree of hepatitis, the extent of functional impairment, and the sonogram for screening of liver and spleen size, texture, and extrahepatic structures. The kidneys should be evaluated for the cystic changes in congenital

Table 42–2. Diagnostic Evaluation of Infantile Cholestasis

Initial Assessment
  Complete history/physical examination
  Stool examination for bile pigment
  Bilirubin: total/direct
Baseline Evaluation
  CBC, smear, retic count
  AST, ALT, GGT, Alk Phos
  Total protein, albumin, prothrombin time
  Abdominal sonogram
  Initiation of phenobarbital
Exclusion Studies for Intrahepatic Cholestasis
  Urine/plasma amino acids
  Urine reducing sugars
  Sweat chloride
  α_1-Antitrypsin level
  Hepatitis B serology
  Serology CMV, herpes, rubella, toxoplasmosis, syphilis
  Percutaneous liver biopsy
Bile Flow Investigations
  Duodenal tube drainage
  99mTechnicium iminodiacetic acid scans
  Cholangiogram: operative/transhepatic

hepatic fibrosis or the renal swelling of some storage or infiltrative diseases. Phenobarbital administration is also started at this stage in doses of 2 to 3 mg/kg/day, to maximize bile-acid–independent bile flow. If a decrease in total and direct bilirubin of more than 50% occurs after 10 days on phenobarbital, the likelihood of an atresia is very small.

The exclusion studies are not "cookbook." An emphasis on early exclusion of the treatable metabolic diseases is critical. The urine-reducing sugars sought are galactose with galactosemia (on lactose formulas) and fructose with hereditary intolerance (on sucrose formulas). Interpretation of percutaneous liver biopsies in the age range is not an absolute science. The value of biopsy is greatest in metabolic disorders, especially α_1-antiprotease deficiency and with intrahepatic bile ductular hypoplasia syndromes.

In the infant with acholic stools, especially with failure to respond to phenobarbital, there is a need to confirm bile flow into the small bowel. The simplest test is placement of a small feeding tube into the second portion of the duodenum and aspirating contents hourly for 24 hours while continuing normal feedings to stimulate bile flow. If no definite bile is recovered, nuclear medicine scans are employed. [125]I Rose Bengal scans have been replaced by shorter half-life [99m] technicium iminodiacetic acid (HIDA, PIPIDA) scans. They are ideally performed while the patient is receiving phenobarbital, with repeat scans over 24 hours, because of the slow bile flow of intrahepatic disease even in the absence of atresia.

If the data are inconclusive, an operative cholangiogram is advised for infants younger than 3 months. This should be performed by a surgeon prepared to proceed to a Kasai portoenterostomy if necessary. Thin-needle percutaneous cholangiograms are rarely successful, since proximal ductular dilatation is very rare in extrahepatic atresia.

TREATMENT OF CHOLESTASIS

Obviously, if a specific etiology is established, appropriate dietary or surgical therapy is begun. In far too many circumstances, however, the cholestasis persists. General management principles are outlined in Table 42-3. To maximize bile flow, enteric feeding of protein and long-chain fat are employed. Phenobarbital administration is usually continued, while vitamin D status is monitored for enhanced metabolism in the face of malabsorption. Recognizing that deconjugated bile acids are potentially hepatotoxic, cholestyramine (an anion-binding resin) is often employed to decrease the enterohepatic circulation of bile acids by binding them within the lumen. This is particularly valuable with pruritis. Because cholestyramine acts by exchanging a Cl^- ion, serum chloride levels must be monitored.

Recognizing that poor micelle formation is an inevitable consequence of reduced bile flow, lipid absorption will usually be severely impaired. As medium-chain triglycerides (MCT) do not require micelles for absorption, supplements of MCT oil are advised. Some long-chain lipid is required to meet essential fatty acid requirements. Each of the fat-soluble vitamins will also usually require supplementation. All vitamin levels should be monitored for adequacy, and, in the case of vitamin A, for potential toxicity.

Table 42–3. Medical Therapy of Cholestasis

Treat specific etiology
Promote bile flow
    Enteric nutrient: protein, long-chain lipid
    Phenobarbital
Reduce enterohepatic circulation of bile
    cholestyramine
Compensate for deficiency of micelles
    Medium-chain triglyceride
    Supplemental fat-soluble vitamins: A,D,E,K

BIBLIOGRAPHY

Alagille E et al: Hepatic ductular hypoplasia associated with characteristic facies, vertebral malformations, retarded physical, mental and sexual development and cardiac murmur. J Pediatr 86:63–71, 1975

Green HL, Helinek GL, Moran R et al: A diagnostic approach to prolonged obstructive jaundice by 24-hour collection of duodenal fluid. J. Pediatr 95:412, 1979

Kasai M et al: Surgical treatment of biliary atresia. J Pediatr Surg 3:665–675, 1968

Majd M: Radionuclide studies in the evaluation of neonatal jaundice. In Daum F (ed): Extrahepatic Biliary Atresia, pp 23–32. New York, Marcell Dekker, 1983

Mathis RK, Andres JM, Walker WA: Liver disease in infants. II. Hepatitis disease states. J Pediatr 90:864, 1977

Rosenthal P, Liebman W, Sinatra F et al: String test in evaluation of cholestatic jaundice in infancy. J Pediatr 197:253–255, 1985

Sharp HL: The current status of alpha-1-antitrypsin, a protease inhibitor in gastrointestinal disease. Gastroenterology 70:621, 1976

Thaler MM: Jaundice in the newborn: Algorithmic diagnosis of conjugated and unconjugated hyperbilirubinemia. JAMA 237:58–62, 1977

Watkins JB, Katz AJ, Grand RJ: Neonatal hepatitis: A diagnostic approach. Adv Pediatr 24:399, 1977

43

Hepatitis in Childhood

Hepatitis is a "catch-all" term for any event associated with hepatic inflammation or injury. The definition usually implies serum elevation of the hepatic enzymes released from injured hepatocytes or biliary epithelial cells. The differential diagnosis in childhood is lengthy, including an array of infectious diseases, metabolic errors, drug-induced injury, and vascular compromise.

CLINICAL PRESENTATION

The clinical presentations of hepatitis also are varied, as noted in Table 43-1. It may seem unhelpful to list asymptomatic or subclinical presentations first, but many forms of childhood hepatitis are so mild and self-limited as to escape medical attention. Clinical symptoms of a disease may also vary with age, presenting as jaundice in the infant or as cirrhosis with ascites in the adolescent, a feature of α_1-antiprotease deficiency. Cholestatic jaundice with or without associated pruritus is a common feature, especially with acute disease or drug-induced injury. Hepatosplenomegaly is very prominent in childhood because of the frequency with which Kupffer's cell hyperpla-

sia and/or hepatic fibrosis develop. Storage diseases from metabolic errors commonly include marked organomegaly.

Coagulopathy from impaired vitamin K utilization is especially prevalent when simultaneous impairment in absorption occurs, as with cystic fibrosis or biliary hypoplasia. Abdominal pain, more commonly objective tenderness over the liver edge, is also prominent with acute disease. Anorexia, with or without emesis, is less prevalent in childhood than in the adult. Presentation with ascites, reflecting advanced portal hypertension, is more common in childhood, since portal hypertension secondary to advanced fibrosis usually precedes clinical liver failure. Immune complex mediated rash and/or arthritis may also be noted. Hepatic encephalopathy may be acute in the context of urea cycle disorders or Reye's syndrome or chronic in the setting of advanced hepatic failure.

LIVER FUNCTION TESTS

The liver serves many roles, each of which may or may not be impaired in any given hepatic disease. The specific alterations in bil-

Table 43–1. Clinical Presentations of Hepatitis in Childhood

1. Subclinical or asymptomatic
2. Cholestasis
   Jaundice
   Pruritis
   Fat-soluble vitamin deficiency
      A: night blindness   E: hypotonia, areflexia
      D: rickets   K: bleeding
3. Hepatomegaly
   Symmetric or asymmetric mass
   Pain in right upper abdomen
   Failure to thrive/anorexia
   Rash/arthritis
4. Portal hypertension
   Splenomegaly
   Ascites
   Varices/bleeding
5. Metabolic
   Hyperammonemia (encephalopathy)
   Hypoglycemia
   Hyperaldosteronism
   Androgen excess
6. Elevated liver enzymes
   Parenchymal: alanine aminotransferase (ALT), aspartate aminotransferase (AST)
   Hepatobiliary (microsomal): gamma-glutamyl transpeptidase (GGT)

irubin, lipid, carbohydrate, and protein metabolism must be addressed in each child. Drug metabolism and excretion will be altered, especially for endogenous steroids.

The hepatic "enzymes" are frequently used as markers of disease severity or activity. Thus, is it imperative to understand their significance. The cytoplasmic enzymes are liberated from injured hepatocytes and are thus markers of parenchymal inflammation or injury. The two most commonly measured are the alanine aminotransferase (ALT, previously SGPT) and aspartate aminotransferase (AST, previously SGOT). Both are synthesized in myocardium, skeletal muscle, and kidneys as well as the liver. Whenever ALT and AST elevations are noted, creatinine phosphokinase (CPK) enzyme activity must be measured to guard against the possibility of muscular injury.

Another set of hepatic enzymes are synthesized in the microsomal area. These enzymes (alkaline phosphatase, gamma-glutamyl transferase, and 5 nucleotidase) are elevated in the serum not from cell leakage but in response to stimulated synthesis, especially in the hepatobiliary area from chronic inflammation, cholestasis, or medication. The value of the alkaline phosphatase in childhood is limited by synthesis in growing bone, producing significant elevations in puberty.

True hepatic "function" is not measured by these enzymes; instead, the serum albumin level, prothrombin time, fasting blood sugar level, and cholesterol level are better indications of the synthetic health of the hepatocyte. All are sequentially monitored in the child with hepatitis.

Imaging technology over the past decade has greatly advanced our ability to visualize the liver and biliary system and, to a limited extent, assess function. Advances in sonography allow assessment of hepatic or spleen size, portal vein patency, and biliary structures. Nuclear medicine scans allow determination of hepatic blood flow (technetium 99m), biliary flow (PIPIDA/HIDA), and inflammatory cell mass or lymphoma (gallium). Cholangiograms can now be performed transhepatically with skinny needles or in retrograde fashion by endoscopy (endoscopic retrograde cholangiopancreatography ERCP). Computed tomography (CT) allows estimation of relative consistency of the liver, as well as more detailed analysis of metastatic lesions, cysts, and related structures such as pancreas or lymph nodes.

The value of pencutaneous needle or operative wedge liver biopsy remains high. The major value is in assessment of severity and chronicity of hepatitis, documentation of infiltrative or storage disease, determination of metabolic enzyme activity, and, to a limited degree, estimation of prognosis.

DIFFERENTIAL DIAGNOSIS

The differential diagnosis of childhood hepatitis, as alluded to earlier, is lengthy. Summarized in Table 43-2, the list is categorized as viral, drug-induced, ischemic, metabolic, bacterial, parasitic, and fungal.

Hepatitis A is a single-stranded RNA enterovirus. It is spread by fecal–oral contamination of food or water and in day-care settings. The incubation period is 15 to 45 days, with no carrier state defined. Virus is detectable in blood and stools late in the incubation period but is cleared from both within 1 week of presentation. More than 50% of infected children have subclinical illness. Elevation of ALT is detected with acute symptoms and may remain mildly elevated for several months even though chronic hepatic injury is

Table 43–2. Differential Diagnosis of Childhood Hepatitis

I. Viral hepatitis
    Hepatitis A
    Hepatitis B
      Delta agent
    Non-A, non-B hepatitis
    Ebstein-Barr
    Cytomegalovirus
    Enterovirus
    Herpes simplex virus
    Adenovirus
    Rubella
II. Drug-induced
    Primarily hepatocellular necrosis
      Acetaminophen
      Isoniazid
    Primarily steatosis
      Valproic acid
      Tetracycline
    Primarily cholestasis
      Phenytoin
      Contraceptive steroids
    Primarily fibrosis
      Methotrexate
      Vitamin A
III. Ischemic
    Cardiac failure
    Veno-occlusive disease
    Sickle cell
    Hyperthermia
IV. Metabolic hepatitis
    Reye's syndrome
    α_1-Antiprotease deficiency
    Lipid/glycogen storage disease
    Hemochromatosis
    Wilson's disease
    Urea cycle disorders
    Cystic fibrosis
    Galactosemia/fructose intolerance
    Tyrosinemia
V. Bacterial hepatitis
    Bacterial toxin
    Ascending cholangitis
    Peri-hepatitis (Fitz-Hugh–Curtis)
    Syphilis
    Tuberculosis
    Lipospirosis
    Pyogenic abscess
VI. Parasitic hepatitis
    Visceral larva migrans
    Shistosomiasis
    Amebiasis

(continued)

Table 43–2. Differential Diagnosis of Childhood Hepatitis (continued)

VI. Parasitic hepatitis (*cont.*)
    Liver flukes
    Echinococcosis
    Toxoplasmosis
VII. Fungal hepatitis
    Candida
    Actinomycosis
    Blastomycosis

not seen. The diagnosis of hepatitis A is made by demonstration of hepatitis A antibody IgM, which is present at the time of acute presentation and persists for 3 to 6 months. Hepatitis A antibody IgG persists for many years. Rarely, hepatitis A may lead to fulminant hepatic failure, myocarditis, or bone marrow hypoplasia/aplasia. Prophylaxis is possible by giving immune serum globulin within 14 days of exposure.

Hepatitis B is a spherical DNA hepadnavirus with special relevance in childhood because of its vertical transmission from the mother. Transmission is by contact with infectious body fluids, including blood, saliva, semen, vaginal secretions, and breast milk. The incubation period ranges from 60 to 160 days. As with most forms of viral hepatitis, the majority of children have subclinical disease. Fulminant hepatitis is seen in less than 1%. In contrast to hepatitis A, however, chronic infection develops in 10% of patients, with about one in four of these children having clinically significant chronic hepatitis.

Extrahepatic manifestations are common in hepatitis B, especially immune complex-mediated disorders such as glomerulonephritis, pericarditis, arthritis, and a characteristic rash termed papular acrodermatitis. The chronic hepatitis also is associated with an increased risk for the subsequent development of hepatocellular carcinoma. The diagnosis of hepatitis B is made by documentation of viral antigens and their antibodies in the serum.

Hepatitis B surface antigin (HB$_s$Ag), previously termed Australian antigen, is excess viral coat material that is the first marker of infection. With resolution of infection, surface antigen is cleared from the serum. The antibody to surface antigen (anti-HB$_s$) is protective, and so its presence in the serum, usually 2 months after acute presentation, indicates resolution of infection and immunity. Up to 10% of patients never produce anti-HB$_s$. The hepatitis B core antigen (HB$_c$Ag) is produced universally and persists for years. The hepatitis B e antigens (HBeAg) are a product of the viral core and are present universally for up to 2 months during acute infection. Persistence of HBeAg is a marker of infectivity and persistent liver disease. Antibody to eAg (antiHBeAg) is a marker of relative lack of infectivity.

Prevention of hepatitis B is now possible by passive immunization with high-titer (>1:100,000 anti-HB$_s$) globulin and by active immunization with recombinant DNA vaccine. The latter is advised for at-risk newborns, health care workers, hemodialysis patients, hemophiliacs, and household and sexual contact of HB$_s$Ag carriers. Vaccination requires at least three dose with boosters at 1 and 6 months and, perhaps, 3 years. The value in newborns is unquestioned because if a mother's blood is positive for both HB$_s$Ag and HBeAg, her newborn has an 80% to 90% chance of developing chronic hepatitis B. In contrast, delivery of HB immune globulin at birth followed by active vaccination should prevent 90% of these infections.

Delta hepatitis is a unique, recently described, hybrid RNA virus that requires HB$_s$Ag as an envelope in order to be pathogenic. Delta hepatitis can thus be acquired simultaneously with hepatitis B, producing a biphasic acute hepatitis, or it can complicate established chronic hepatitis B infection, perhaps increasing the risk of fulminant hepatitis or cirrhosis. Delta antigen and IgM antibody serology is now available. The presence of delta agent clearly increases both the morbidity and mortality of hepatitis B. Most prevalent in Italy, South America, and the Middle East, the incidence of delta hepatitis in childhood is small except in hemophiliacs or illicit drug users.

Non-A, non-B hepatitis is a clinical syndrome similar to hepatitis B. A number of viral agents will probably eventually be demonstrated. No serologic markers are available. More than 90% of post-transfusion hepatitis is due to these agents. In addition, up to 50% of sporadic viral hepatitis may be caused by non-A, non-B hepatitis. The majority of infected children are anicteric. Many have a characteristic biphasic pattern of enzyme elevation. Of concern is the chronic hepatitis that develops in up to 40% of infected patients and for which no proven immunoprophylaxis is available.

Epstein-Barr virus induced mononucleosis will be complicated by hepatitis subclinically in 40% of patients and clinically in less than 5%. Modest elevations of aminotransferase with marked elevation of gamma-glutaryl transferase may persist for 6 to 8 weeks. Rarely, acute hepatic failure is seen. Cirrhosis has not been reported. Neither hepatomegaly or hepatitis has been reported with chronic EB virus syndrome.

Cytomegalovirus hepatitis accounts for approximately 15% of post-transfusion hepatitis. Congenital forms are also seen. In older children, the clinical syndrome is similar to Ebstein-Barr mononucleosis with hepatosplenomegaly, adenopathy, and lymphocytosis. Pharyngitis is rare. Elevation of aminotransferase is modest, while jaundice is unusual. Recurrence of symptomatic disease and progression to chronic active hepatitis are rare but reported.

In infancy, hepatitis may complicate systemic viral illness with enterovirus (echovirus, coxsackievirus), adenovirus, herpes simplex, and rubella.

Drug-induced hepatitis is classified by histologic alteration and/or mechanism of injury. Toxic reactions are seen in two forms, those due to direct dose-related toxicity and those due to idiosyncratic host responses. The normal liver contains a number of enzymes and peptides that are the key to detoxification of drugs and their metabolites. These include glutathione transferases and peroxidases, superoxide dismutase and epoxide hydrolase. Genetic predisposition and competitive interaction may determine an individual's susceptibility to drug-induced injury.

As noted in Table 43-2, classification by histologic alteration is easily done, although overlap will occur. For example, phenytoin usually produces a cholestatic process; however, rare children will progress to hepatocellular necrosis. The steatosis induced by valproate may be associated with a mitochondrial dysfunction similar to Reye's syndrome. Fibrosis in the relative absence of "hepatitis" is a feature of methotrexate. Vascular injury is also seen from drug exposure, as with the Budd-Chiari syndrome from estrogens and veno-occlusive disease from doxorubicin. Drug-induced hepatic tumors are rare in childhood but include androgen-induced hepatocellular carcinoma, estrogen-induced adenomas, and anabolic steroid-induced angiosarcoma.

Ischemic hepatitis can develop in the setting of systemic shock, small-vessel occlusion (sickle cell), or veno-occlusive disease. Cardiac failure, especially of the right heart, can lead to hepatomegaly, fibrosis, and, eventually, cirrhosis. Hepatic failure is a feature of acute hyperthermia.

The *metabolic hepatitis syndromes* may present with neonatal cholestasis, childhood cirrhosis, or encephalopathy. Reye's syndrome is discussed in detail in Chapter 72.

α₁-Antiprotease deficiency, previously termed α₁-antitrypsin deficiency, was first described in children in 1969 by Dr. Sharp and his associates. α₁-Antiprotease synthesized in the hepatocyte, is a glycoprotein, that inhibits a number of proteases including trypsin, chromtrypsin, thrombin, elastase, Hageman factor, and collagenase. It thus modulates activation of the complement and coagulation systems while contributing to the tissue or host response to bacterial proteases. Production of α₁-antiprotease is genetically controlled by a series of more than 20 co-dominant alleles that determine electrophoretic mobility and serum concentration. The most common is termed protease inhibitor M (PiMM), while PiZZ and PiSZ are associated with symptomatic liver disease in childhood. These children synthesize anti-protease but appear to be unable to secrete it from the hepatocyte. Since only 10% to 20% of those with increased hepatocellular antiprotease develop liver disease, the deficiency of circulating antiprotease appears to predispose rather than directly induce hepatic injury.

The most common clinical presentation with α₁-antiprotease deficiency is with neonatal jaundice, hepatomegaly, and modest aminotransferase elevations. Up to 50% of these children will progress to significant hepatic cirrhosis. The second clinical presentation is with hepatomegaly and portal hypertension in later childhood. The extra-hepatic manifestations of α₁-antiprotease deficiency include early-onset emphysema and/or membranoproliferative glomerulonephritis.

The diagnosis is made by documenting reduction in serum α₁-antitrypsin level and Pi typing. Histologic analysis of a liver biopsy will reveal the excess α₁-antiprotease as PAS-positive, diastase-resistant cytoplasmic granules, most prominent in the periportal hepatocytes.

The *glycogen storage diseases* of the liver present with hepatomegaly and variable degrees of impaired growth, hypoglycemia, and enzyme elevations. Long-term hepatic complications include fibrosis, cirrhosis, and increased risk for adenoma and hepatoma.

Type I glycogen storage disease (von Gierke's disease) is caused by deficiency of glucose-6-phosphatase and presents in early infancy with failure to thrive, developmental delay, and symptomatic hypoglycemia. Hepatomegaly is pronounced, whereas splenomegaly and jaundice are lacking. Laboratory features include fasting hypoglycemia, lactic acidosis, hyperlipidemia, hyperuricemia, and elevated aminotransferases (ALT, AST). Diagnosis is established by enzyme analysis of hepatic biopsy tissue. Management is usually accomplished by continuous-infusion night feedings and multiple, small daytime meals. Renal enlargement and subsequent renal failure may complicate long-term management.

Type III glycogen storage disease is due to deficiency of the debrancher enzyme amylo-1,6 glucosidase, producing hepatic accumulation of limit dextrins. Massive hepatomegaly, symptomatic hypoglycemia, short stature, and hypotonia are the clinical features. In contrast to type I, the fasting hypoglycemia usually occurs in the absence of acidosis or hyperuricemia. The bilirubin level is again normal, with mild enzyme elevation. Diagnosis is established by enzyme level in leukocytes or muscle in addition to liver. The prognosis is better than for type I.

Type IV glycogenosis results from the lack of the brancher enzyme amylo-1,4-1,6 transglucosidase, producing an accumulation, not of glycogen, but of amylopectin. Presentation is in infancy, with cholestasis, poor feeding, emesis, and impaired growth. Because the hepatomegaly is accompanied by severe fibrosis, splenomegaly secondary to portal hypertension is frequently seen. Enzyme elevations are prominent, often with bilirubin increase as well. Neither hypoglycemia nor acidosis is prominent early in the illness. On liver biopsy, the cytoplasmic amylopectin stains as if it were α_1-antiprotease, and so serum levels of alpha-1-antitrypsin must be documented.

Type VIa is attributed to reductions in hepatic phosphorylase. In this milder disease, the hepatomegaly is maximal when the patient is well, and liver size is reduced with fasting. Hypoglycemia is mild and aminotransferases are normal. Spontaneous resolution in adolescence is the rule. On hepatic biopsy, hepatocytes are enlarged by a structurally normal glycogen. A similar pattern is seen with type IX due to deficiency of phosphorylase kinase.

Disorders of lysosomal function are catagorized as lipid or mucopolysaccharide storage. Because all of the lipid storage disorders of the liver also involve the bone marrow, diagnosis is usually made by bone marrow analysis. The major conditions are Niemann-Pick disease, Gaucher's disease, Wolman's disease, and gangliosidosis. Storage of unbranched C26 lipid is also a feature of hepato–cerebral–renal syndrome (Zelliweger). Of the mucopolysaccharidases, Hurler's syndrome and, less commonly, Hunter's syndrome feature hepatosplenomegaly and progressive hepatic dysfunction.

Iron-overload, *hemachromatosis*, may be congenital (transferrin deficiency) or acquired secondary to transfusion therapy for hemoglobinopathies. Excessive iron intake very rarely contributes to overload in childhood. In both sickle cell disease and β-thalassemia, a combinaton of right-sided heart failure, iron-overload, and non-A, non-B hepatitis may be encountered. Most patients with idiopathic hemachromatosis have minimal hepatic disease until adulthood.

Copper overload, *Wilson's disease,* is due to deficiency of ceruloplasmin and increased hepatic copper binding and is of critical relevance in pediatrics because all of the complications can be avoided by early recognition and management. Hepatic presentations are more common in children, with neurologic presentations more common in the adult. Inherited as an autosomal recessive trait, its presentation may occur between 6 and 20 years as acute hepatitis, chronic active hepatitis, fulminant hepatitis, or portal hypertension. Hemolytic anemia may be an associated feature. More than 90% of involved children have the characteristic copper deposition in the corneal Descemet's membrane, termed Kayser-Fleischer ring, although most are visualized only by slit-lamp examination. Serum ceruloplasmin levels may be normal, and since 24-hour urine copper levels may be elevated in other forms of chronic hepatitis, hepatic biopsy copper content must be used to confirm the diagnosis. D-Penicillamine is the preferred treatment and is required for life. If one family member is diagnosed, all others are screened.

The *urea cycle disorders* present with hyperammonemia and encephalopathy, usually in the neonatal period (see Chapter 71). Those with milder forms and carriers may develop symptoms later in childhood. Modest hepatomegaly and variable aminotransferase enzyme elevation may be seen. In contrast to Reye's syndrome, hypoglycemia is unusual. Neither jaundice nor splenomegaly is anticipated.

The hepatic manifestations of *cystic fibrosis* may include neonatal cholestasis or subsequent focal biliary fibrosis in up to 40% of children with the disease. The neonatal jaundice presentation is usually accompanied by meconium ileus and coagulopathy due to decreased vitamin K absorption. The cholestasis is attributed to inspissated bile and a characteristic pericholangitis. Both are implicated in the subsequent development of the focal biliary fibrosis, which is already established in 10% of patients by 6 months of age. Clinical presentation is usually with nodular hepatomegaly and complicating portal hypertension, splenomegaly, varices, and ascites in adolescence. The elevations of alkaline phosphatase and gamma-glutaryl transferase are often striking.

Galactosemia is the result of the inability to convert galactose to glucose because of deficiency of galactose 1-phosphate uridyl transferase or, rarely, uridine diphosphate galactose-4-epimerase. Galactokinase deficiency is associated with cataracts with no hepatic injury. Presentation is usually in infancy following the introduction of lactose to the diet, with cholestasis, emesis, impaired growth, acidosis, and, frequently, gram-negative sepsis. The diagnosis is first suspected by demonstration of galactose in the urine as a positive reducing sugar (Clinitest™). The confirmation is usually made by enzyme analysis in red cells. Rapidly progressive hepatic failure can by halted, and perhaps reversed in part, by elimination of lactose and galactose from the diet.

Hereditary fructose intolerance presents in infancy following the introduction of foods containing sucrose, fructose, or sorbitol. Cholestasis, hypoglycemia, acidosis, anorexia, and emesis are prominent. Hepatomegaly is prominent, but splenomegaly is not. Laboratory features include hypoglycemia, hypophosphatemia, proteinuria, and prolonged prothrombin time, and moderate aminotransferase elevation. With elimination of fructose sources from the diet, emesis and coagulation defects improve within hours, while the renal tubular dysfunction (proteinuria, hypophosphatemia) resolve within days. Either a standardized fructose tolerance test is performed when the patient is clinically stable or hepatic enzyme determination (usually reduced fructose-1-phosphate aldolase) confirms the diagnosis.

Tyrosinemia type I is due to reduction in hepatic fumarylacetoacetate hydrolase. The majority of involved children present in infancy with hepatomegaly, emesis, fever, and edema. Less commonly, cholestasis, melena, ascites, splenomegaly and hematuria may be encountered. Because hepatic function is severely impaired early in the course of illness, coagulopathy and hypoalbuminemia are prominent. The hepatic histologic features of tyrosinemia, galactosemia, and fructose intolerance are similar, featuring severe architectural disarray, pseudoacinar formation, and minimal inflammation.

Bacterial hepatitis is usually a complication of systemic infection or toxin elaboration. Gram-negative endotoxin, for example, is capable of producing transient cholestasis. Ascending cholangitis may complicate any mesenteric infection, especially inflammatory bowel disease, necrotizing enterocolitis or obstructive biliary disease. An extension of pelvic inflammatory disease into a perihepatitis, usually attributed to *Neisseria gonorrhoeae* or chlamydia, is termed Fitz-Hugh–Curtis syndrome. Both shoulder and pleuritic pain may be reported, and a hepatic friction rub may be heard.

Acquired syphilis is usually a neonatal hepatitis featuring cholestasis, rash, bone change, and hepatomegaly. Nonhemolytic hydrops may be seen with severe infection.

Tuberculosis, presenting as granulomatous hepatitis, has become very rare in childhood. Granulomas in the liver are also reported with sarcoidosis, brucellosis, leprosy, histoplasmosis, tularemia, ascariasis, and schistosomiasis.

Leptospiral hepatic disease is rare but must be excluded in the clinical setting of acute hepatitis with conjunctivitis, rash, hepatomegaly, and meningeal signs. Laboratory features include leukocytosis, elevated sedimentation rate, mild hyperbilirubinemia, and variable aminotransferase elevations. As a systemic vasculitis, elevation of creatinine phosphokinase and cerebrospinal fluid (CSF) pleocytosis may be encountered. The leptospiral organism is present in blood or urine early in the disease, with specific serology positive after 2 weeks.

Less than 10% of pyogenic liver abscesses

occur in childhood. Hepatic reticuloendothelial function is normally so efficient that children at risk include those with immune deficiency (especially leukemia and chronic granulomatous disease), burns, bowel perforation, or hemolytic disease, or following umbilical catheterization. The clinical features are acute hepatomegaly, fever, and abdominal pain. Jaundice is frequently seen. The organism most commonly isolated is *Staphylococcus aureus* with occasional *Enterobacter, Klebsiella,* or anaerobes. The diagnosis is usually pursued by sonography, gallium-67 citrate scintiscan, or CT scan. Needle aspiration under sonographic guidance is used increasingly to obtain cultures.

Parasitic hepatitis can occur in either generalized or cystic form. Visceral larva migrans is a generic term for parasitic disease that includes a circulation through the liver. While *Toxocara canis* is the classic cause, other potential parasites include *Ascaris lumbricoides, Capillaria hepatica,* malaria, *Ascaris suis,* and *Strongyloides.* Worldwide, shistosomiasis remains a major cause of presinusoidal portal hypertension and hepatitis. Amoebic liver abscess complicates about 5% of invasive colitis due to *Entamoeba histolytica.* Following a prodromal course of malaise and respiratory symptoms, the child develops spiking fever, chills, weight loss, and right upper quadrant pain, often made worse by deep inspiration or cough. Jaundice is rare, eosinophilia uncommon, and diarrhea may be mild. Either sonography or technetium liver scans suggest the diagnosis. Serologic testing is now readily available.

Liver flukes, *Clonorchis sinensis* or *Fasciola hepatica,* develop in bile ducts. Clinical features include pruritus, hydrops of the gallbladder, ascending cholangitis, toxic hepatitis, and, eventually cirrhosis or cholangiocarcinoma. Laboratory features include leukocytosis, eosinophilia, and occasional hyperbilirubinemia. Stools or duodenal aspirates often contain ova.

Hydatid disease, due to *Echinococcus granulosus* (dog tapeworm), leads to cystic compression of the biliary system, producing pain, jaundice, and often asymmetric hepatomegaly. On sonography, a fluid-filled cyst is noted. As with amoebic disease, eosinophilia is mild or lacking.

Toxoplasmosis, like syphilis, is of major clinical concern as an intrauterine infection producing neonatal hepatitis. Cholestasis, microcephaly, chorioretinitis, and intracranial calcifications suggest the diagnosis, which is confirmed serologically by specific IgM antibody titer.

Fungal hepatitis is very rare except as a terminal complication of fulminant hepatitis or as an opportunistic infection in immunocompromised children. As such, it presents in the post-transplant child with jaundice and hepatomegaly. In this population, of course, there are multiple potential differential diagnoses, including graft-versus-host, drug-induced hepatitis, veno-occlusive disease, or viral hepatitis.

CHRONIC HEPATITIS

Any process that persists longer than 3 months in a child is termed chronic. Since many of the conditions cited above have specific therapy, and since certain forms of chronic active hepatitis respond to immunosuppression, a major effort is devoted to establishing a diagnosis whenever liver injury has been present for 3 months or longer. As a corollary, more than 90% of uncomplicated viral or drug-induced liver injuries will have resolved clinically within the first 3 months.

An obvious problem, of course, is the question of how long an episode of hepatitis has persisted prior to the original diagnosis. Chronicity is suggested if the liver edge is firm or nodular, splenomegaly is prominent, or cutaneous lesions such as angiomata, telangiectasia, or palmar erythema are present.

The goal is to distinguish the child with a benign chronic "persistent" hepatitis from the child with a more severe chronic "active" hepatitis who is at risk for cirrhosis or significant hepatic failure. The former "persistent" hepatitis is usually viral, whereas the latter "active" hepatitis is more commonly autoimmune, metabolic, or due to hepatitis B or cytomegalovirus. While the major distinguishing features are histologic and thus require hepatic biopsy, exclusion of a few conditions is possible by laboratory means. Thus, any child with chronic hepatitis must have hepatitis B serology performed, ceruloplasmin and slit lamp examination done, and serum level of alpha-1-antitrypsin determined. Autoimmune or "lupoid" hepatitis is a specific chronic active hepatitis with a characteristic immune response. Serologic features include positive anti-nuclear, anti-smooth muscle, and anti-mitochondrial antibodies. The clinical significance lies in an excellent response to immune suppression by corticosteroids with or without azathioprine, but a high relapse rate (up to 50%) when therapy is stopped.

Table 43-3 lists the contrasting features of chronic active versus chronic persistent hepatitis. No biochemical parameters are specific. Both usually have aminotransferase levels greater than 100. The histologic features are most specific. The inflammation in persistent hepatitis is a modest mononuclear infiltrate restricted to the periportal region within a limiting plate. In contrast, in active hepatitis, the infiltrate of lymphocytes and plasma cells extends beyond the limiting plate. In contrast, in active hepatitis, the infiltrate of lymphocytes and plasma cells extends beyond the limiting plate into the surrounding hepatocytes, often producing focal hepatocellular destruction, termed piecemeal necrosis. Usually, the associated fibrosis extends or bridges from one portal area to another, setting the stage for true cirrhosis. If chronic active hepatitis is diagnosed and specific tests for alpha-1-antiprotease deficiency and Wilson's disease are negative, therapy with corticosteroids, 2 mg/kg/day, is usually begun. In the presence of active inflammation and hepatitis B, the weight of present data is against steroid therapy.

The role of liver transplantation in the long-term management of childhood liver disease is now evolving, thanks in no small measure to the greatly enhanced survival with cyclosporine therapy to block rejection. Because matching of donor and recipient is usually limited to size and blood type, rejection remains a perpetual concern. Transplantation has assumed a major role in treatment of end-stage liver disease especially for metabolic liver disease where the transplanted liver corrects the original disease, such as α-1-antipro-

Table 43–3. Characteristics of Chronic Hepatitis

	Form	
	"Persistent"	*"Active"*
Biochemical		
ALT	↑ ↑	↑ ↑
Globulins	NL or ↑	↑
Bilirubin	NL or ↑	↑
Serologic abnormalities	None	Often positive, ANA, AMA, ASMA
Histologic inflammation	Periportal	Periportal, piecemeal necrosis
Fibrosis	Minimal	Bridging portal areas
Limiting plate	Intact	Disrupted
Risk for cirrhosis	Minimal	High

tease deficiency, galactosemia, tyrosinemia, and several of the storage diseases. Infants with biliary atresia and progressive biliary cirrhosis also have been successfully transplanted in large numbers.

BIBLIOGRAPHY

Dubois RS, Silverman A: Chronic active hepatitis in children. Dig Dis Sci 17:575–586, 1972

Hoofnagle JH: Serodiagnosis of acute hepatitis B. Hepatology 3:267–268, 1983

Kaplowitz N: Drug-induced hepatotoxicity. Ann Intern Med 104:826–839, 1986

Krugman S: Viral hepatitis. Pediatr Rev 7:3–10, 1985

Werlin SL, Grand RJ, Perman JA et al: Diagnostic dilemmas of Wilson's disease. Pediatrics 62:47–51, 1978

Zimmerman HJ: Drug-induced liver disease: An overview. Semin Liver Dis 1:93–103, 1981

44

Constipation is best defined as the failure of complete evacuation of the lower colon with defecation. This definition is superior to considerations of stool frequency or consistency as it underscores the pathophysiology and facilitates understanding of the complications of chronic constipation. Normal defecation is a relatively simple process. Stool descends through the colon into the rectal ampulla. Distention of the ampulla produces reflex relaxation of the internal sphincter, allowing stool to enter the upper anal canal. When the child then relaxes the external sphincter and contracts the muscles of the pelvic floor, stool is passed. Valsalva's maneuver assists in this final phase.

In the neonatal period, relaxation of the external sphincter is often poorly coordinated, producing apparent straining by normal newborns with the passage of normal or even soft stools. This is particularly prominent in premature infants.

In early infancy, the major concern is the inability to relax the internal sphincter. This is usually due to congenital lack of ganglion cells of the parasympathetic nervous system, a disorder termed Hirschsprung's disease, which occurs in about 1 in 5000 births. The ganglion cells may be lacking only in the most distal sphincter area (termed short-segment aganglionosis) or for varying lengths of the more proximal bowel. The extent of involvement is limited to the rectosigmoid colon in 75% of cases. Rarely, the entire colon (8%) and even the entire small bowel (1%) may be involved. Presentation is often with failure to pass meconium in the first 24 hours of life, a feature in more than 90% of Hirschsprung's newborns. Abdominal distention, infrequent pencil-thin stools, and acute enterocolitis may be other presenting features. The overall ratio of male to females is about 3.5:1, with positive family histories of the disorder in 8% of patients. The diagnosis of Hirschsprung's disease is suspected by history and by a rectal examination revealing a snug anal canal and empty ampulla. Barium enema may then reveal a characteristic "transition zone" between the dilated proximal intestine and contracted aganglionic segment. A film of the abdomen may reveal increased retention of barium 24 hours after the radiographic study. At university centers, anorectal manometry will reveal characteristic failure of the internal sphincter to relax.

Rectal biopsies are nearly always performed

to confirm absence of the ganglion cells and a characteristic increased acetylcholinesterase activity. As a screening test, rectal suction biopsies have 90% sensitivity, although full-thickness biopsies are subsequently performed. Following diagnosis, a colostomy is performed above the transition zone. At a later time, a definitive "pull-through" procedure is usually performed to restore rectal function.

Beyond the newborn period, there are three major times when constipation develops. The first is in the early months of life, when incomplete evacuation reflects a sensitivity to the changing nature of the infant's diet. This is especially prominent with the transition to whole milk, cheese, and other dairy products.

The second and most common phase begins at 18 to 36 months, when the toddler is first aware of his or her ability to control the passage of the stool, especially if this sensation is deemed unpleasant. When the child senses the entry of stool into the upper anal canal, he or she contracts the external sphincter, tightens the buttocks muscles, and returns the stool to the rectum. When this process becomes the rule, the rectum dilates, the sensation of the need to defecate is reduced, and muscle tone in the lower colon is reduced. All effectively create a vicious cycle guaranteeing incomplete evacuation. The longer the stool is retained, the less water it holds, and the more painful the defecation becomes. Toilet training is thus difficult to achieve. In the parent's eyes, these toddlers seem to expend enormous energy straining to have a bowel movement. In reality, the straining is usually devoted to holding the movement in.

The third most frequent time for the development of constipation in childhood is shortly after the start of school, owing either to ignoring the need to defecate or spending too little time to evacuate completely. Children are often too embarrassed to have bowel movements in school.

In the child from age 3 to 7 years, constipation often develops slowly and may not be apparent to the family until the child begins to leak smears of stool into the underwear, a process termed encopresis. This is generally a leakage around the firm stool in the rectum, and the child is truly unaware of its presence until the soiling has begun. With conscious effort, the soiling is minimized, especially in school. Thus, most "accidents" occur on the way home from school, when playing with friends, or when involved in a family outing. Maximum inconvenience seems to be the rule. Most parents fail to understand that the child is minimally aware of this process, and so punishment is commonly employed. Over time, the child may deny that leakage has occurred or hide the soiled underwear.

The vast majority of children with constipation have this "functional" origin to the process. It is critical to recognize, nonetheless, that the degree of rectal and lower colonic distention creates a truly "physical" incapacity to completely defecate. Other origins of chronic constipation are listed in Table 44-1. The neurologic disorders relate primarily to lack of sensation or impaired motility. Intestinal pseudo-obstruction presents with generalized intestinal and gastric hypomotility. The major endocrine disorder is hypothyroidism. Diabetes in the elderly is commonly associated with hypomotility, although in children, both diabetes mellitus and diabetes insipidus have constipation, primarily due to dehydration. Careful perianal and rectal examination will exclude most anatomic obstructions. Rectal strictures complicating Crohn's disease may present with constipation in adolescents. Anorectal pain due to trauma, fissure, abscess, condylomata, or foreign body must be excluded. The constipating effects of medication in childhood are seen most frequently with codeine, tricyclic antidepressants, and vincristine.

The emotional component to constipation

Table 44–1. Differential Diagnosis of Constipation

1. Functional fecal retention (95%)
2. Neurologic
   Aganglionosis (Hirschsprung's)
   Spina bifida
   Hypotonia/pseudo-obstruction
   Psychomotor retardation
3. Endocrine/metabolic
   Hypothyroidism
   Diabetes (usually due to dehydration)
4. Anatomic obstruction
   Pelvic tumor
   Imperforate anus
   Ectopic anus/anal ring/rectal structure
   Anorectal trauma/fissure/infection
5. Medication
   Narcotics
   Antihistamines
   Antidepressants
   Diuretics
6. Emotional
   Usually secondary

Table 44–2. Complications of Chronic Constipation

Encopresis
Abdominal pain
Anorexia/irritability
Anal fissure
Stercoral ulcer
Enuresis
Obstructive uropathy
  UTI
  Hypertension
  Renal failure

and encopresis is rarely primary. Certainly, some severely emotionally distraught children will have primary incontinence. In the vast majority, the emotional concerns are acquired due to the personal, familial, or peer response to the problem.

Aside from emotional concerns, the complications of chronic constipation are listed in Table 44-2. The issue of soiling or encopresis has already been reviewed. Crampy abdominal pain is a reflection of acquired dysmotility and partial distal bowel obstruction. It contributes to the progressive loss of appetite and, in a few patients, to irritability. Anal fissures are a common complication in the toddler who continues to resist passage of firm stool. Older children are often remarkably free of fissures despite passage of massive stools. On rare occasions, the retention of firm stool creates a rectal ulceration or abrasion, termed stercoral ulcer, which may present with significant bright-red rectal bleeding.

Enuresis coincides with encopresis in nearly 20% of involved 3 to 7 year olds. While this

may reflect common etiologies in control of elimination, the degree of rectal distention may limit bladder capacity, producing secondary enuresis. Similarly, the fecal mass may produce secondary obstruction of ureteral flow, usually from the left kidney. This may lead to bladder or ureteral stasis and infection. Rarely, hydronephrosis may develop, including progression to hypertension and even renal failure.

The treatment of functional constipation (Table 44-3) is to initiate fecal flow and sustain complete evacuation by whatever technique is required for that child. The initial evacuation may require up to 2 to 3 days of enemas or stimulant bisacodyl suppositories. To sustain evacuation, the key is to develop a sense of motivation. In older children, behavioral modification with reward systems ("star-charts") may be all that is necessary to restore the habit of defecation. Biofeedback techniques have also been demonstrated successfully. The majority of children, however, will require some form of laxative. Oral mineral oil will work for many toddlers; however, once encopresis has begun, the oil often aggravates the leakage. Mineral oil is avoided for children under 15 months of age because of fear of aspiration. Products such as senna or milk of magnesia usually work best in the early school-aged children. Parents must be reassured that these medications do *not* create a physical dependence. Once rectal tone is

Table 44–3. Treatment of Functional Constipation

1. Complete evacuation
2. Sustained complete evacuation
3. Motivation to evacuate
   Behavioral modification/biofeedback
   Laxative
4. Dietary
   Elimination of constipating foods
   Encourage fiber
5. Patience

restored, the "motivator" medicine is safely stopped. The role of dietary fiber is greatest in the adolescent or adult who already is motivated. In the young child, it is far more important to decrease the constipating foods, such as dairy products, pasta and related starches, bananas, and pears. Dairy products are usually limited to 12 ounces per day to meet calcium requirements. Once fecal emptying is restored, the fiber agents or stool softeners will be helpful to minimize needs for stimulant medication. The goal of therapy in the first 4 to 8 weeks is to achieve at least two large stools per day, and medication is adjusted to this end. No matter what technique is used, parents and patients must demonstrate patience. Early frustation and, more commonly, too rapid a decrease in medication contribute to most treatment failures. Both children and parents must recognize the frequency of the problem and the need for long-term successful management.

BIBLIOGRAPHY

Davidson M, Kugler MM, Bauer CH: Diagnosis and management in children with severe and protracted constipation and obstipation. J Pediatr 62:263–275, 1963

Ehrenpresis T: Hirschsprung's disease. Dig Dis 16:1032–1051, 1971

Fitzgerald JF: Difficulties with defecation and elimination in children. Clin Gastroenterol 6:283–297, 1977

Kleinhaus S, Boley SJ, Sheran M et al: Hirschsprung's disease. J Pediatr Surg 14:588–597, 1979

Sondheimer JM: Helping the child with chronic constipation. Contemp Pediatr March:12–28, 1985

Part VIII: Renal System

45

Fluid and Electrolyte Management in Childhood

In contrast to the adult, the requirements for fluid and electrolyte in the child are rarely constant. Modifications are required to meet the demands of growth, maturity of renal function, and metabolic activity, and to replace recurring but unanticipated losses. The basic maintenance requirements are quite easily estimated, but compensation for ongoing losses and dehydration can be very complicated.

The total body fluid is divided in two compartments: an extracellular component of plasma and interstitial fluid and an intracellular component. While water passes easily from extracellular to intracellular space, the cell membrane actively restricts sodium chloride to the extracellular compartment. The sodium chloride then draws water out of the cells to balance the osmotic forces generated by intracellular proteins. The extracellular compartment can thus be expanded by increasing plasma sodium chloride, by increasing extracellular protein, or by increasing other extracellular osmotic forces (such as blood glucose concentration).

The requirement for fluid or water, while often expressed as a function of body weight, is actually determined by metabolic activity. Fluid requirements are thus best expressed relative to caloric demand, with estimates made for renal losses, sweating, insensible loss, and enteric fluid loss. Insensible losses are losses through the lung or skin to maintain body temperature and approximate 45 ml/100 kcal under basal condition. Losses due to sweating are minimal (0 to 15 ml/100 kcal) but increase markedly with fever (12%/1° C) and with increased ambient temperature (30 ml/1° C).

Renal water requirements are estimated at 55 ml/100 kcal to allow a renal solute excretion at 220 to 290 mOsm per liter. If extraordinary solute loads are taken in (e.g., concentrated feedings with little free water) or if renal concentrating ability is impaired (e.g., polyuria), these limits must be adjusted. The renal solute load is composed of urea and electrolytes. The solute load generated by dietary lipid or carbohydrate is negligible, since both are metabolized to carbon dioxide and water.

Basic fluid requirements are thus 45 ml/100 kcal of insensible loss plus 55 ml/100 kcal of renal requirement, assuming no significant

RENAL SYSTEM

enteric loss from emesis or diarrhea. To estimate basal fluid need, one must assume 100 ml/100 kcal based on the following kcal requirements of the child. For children weighing from 1 to 10 kg, the caloric requirement is 100 kcal/kg. For children weighing from 10 to 20 kg, the caloric need is 1000 kcal plus 100 kcal for every 2 kg over 10 kg. For children weighing 20 to 70 kg, the demand is 1500 kcal plus 100 kcal for every 5 kg over 20 kg.

SODIUM

As noted above, sodium, primarily coupled with chloride, is critical to the establishment of extracellular fluid volume. Normal children, with renal salt conserving and excretion systems intact, can tolerate dietary intakes of sodium ranging from 10 to 100 mM per day. In children with disorders of salt wasting (*e.g.*, adrenal insufficiency), extreme salt supplementation is mandated. Alternatively, in children with salt retention (*e.g.*, ascites), severe salt restriction may be necessary. In calculating normal sodium requirements, assume a need of 2 to 3 mEq/100 kcal. The regulation of plasma sodium concentration is accomplished by regulation of body water (osmoregulation). Thus, osmoreceptors are stimulated by a 2% rise in plasma osmolality to induce the release of antidiuretic hormone (ADH) from the pituitary to produce the sensation of thirst.

Hyponatremia is defined as a plasma concentration of sodium below 130 mEq/liter. When sodium levels fall below 125 mEq/liter, symptoms such as apathy, anorexia, disorientation, muscle weakness, and, eventually, convulsions can appear. As the normal kidney can excrete almost any fluid load presented to it, it is hard to become hyponatremic in the absence of disorders of the kidney or ADH excretion. As noted in the summary of Table 45-1, it is critical to recognize that hypona-

tremia does not always reflect a reduction in total body sodium.

The syndrome of inappropriate secretion of ADH (SIADH) often complicates pulmonary and neurologic disorders in childhood. With SIADH, there is persistent urinary excretion of sodium in the face of true hyponatremia. Therapy of hyponatremia may thus mandate either salt repletion or water restriction. An artifactual reduction in plasma sodium level will be encountered under conditions of decreased plasma water such as hyperglycemia, hyperlipidemia, or hyperproteinemia.

Hypernatremia, defined as a sodium concentration above 150 mEq/liter, develops when loss of water exceeds solute loss, with failure to replace water loss (hypovolemic) or with administration of excess solute (hypervolemic). In young children, hypernatremia with hypertonic dehydration frequently complicates diarrheal disease or diabetes insipidus. The clinical recognition of the severity of hypernatremia is often delayed by the more subtle signs of intracellular dehydration. The young child presents with irritability, restlessness, a high-pitched cry, "doughy" skin, and fever. The major complications are neurologic. As extracellular sodium increases, water leaves the cell to preserve osmotic balance, thus shrinking the intercellular space. The shrinkage of brain tissue can lead to intracranial hemorrhage. At the renal level, acute tubular necrosis may develop. Replacement of water and salt as needed is done slowly to minimize the risk of acute edema.

POTASSIUM

Potassium is primarily restricted to the intracellular space by the same cell membrane pump that limits sodium uptake. Total body potassium is regulated in the kidney, primarily by aldosterone, which stimulates potassium secretion. As elevated levels of hydrogen

Table 45–1. Differential Features of Hyponatremia and Hypernatremia

	ECF	Total Body Na	Weight	Disease	Therapy
Hyponatremia					
Hypovolemic	↓	↓	↓	Diarrhea, Addison's disease	Salt and water repletion
SIADH	↑	N1/↓	↑	Meningitis, chronic lung	Water restriction
Hypervolemic	↑	↑	↑	Cardiac, renal, or hepatic failure	Water restriction; treat underlying illness
Hypernatremia					
Hypovolemic	↓	N1/↓	↓	Diarrhea, diabetes insipidus	Gradual water and salt repletion
Hypervolemic	↑	↑	↑	Iatrogenic delivery of hypertonic solution	Recognition and gradual water repletion

ion force potassium out of the cell, acidosis reduces available cellular potassium for secretion. Thus, maximal renal potassium losses occur under conditions of elevated aldosterone, high sodium tubular levels, and alkalosis, all common features of diuretic therapy. The normal potassium requirement is 2 to 3 mEq/100 kcal.

Because cell membrane potential is heavily dependent on the ratio of intracellular to extracellular potassium, small reductions in extracellular potassium greatly alter the repolarization of both excitable and secretory cells. Hypokalemia, with plasma concentrations below 2.5 mEq/liter, usually presents with muscle weakness, impaired intestinal motility, anorexia, and cardiac arrhythmias. Potassium losses can be very dramatic in persistent emesis and diarrhea. Therapy consists of gradual repletion of potassium.

Hyperkalemia, defined as a plasma concentration exceeding 6.5 mEq/liter, is usually noted with oliguric renal failure or after massive cellular necrosis. Again, alterations in cellular repolarization lead to severe cardiac rhythm disturbance. To reduce plasma levels, the intravenous delivery of glucose with insulin will enhance cellular uptake of potassium. With severe hyperkalemia, the use of an enteric K^+ trapping exchange resin or emergency dialysis may be required.

RECOGNITION AND MANAGEMENT OF DEHYDRATION

The major disorders of fluid and electrolyte balance are seen in childhood are caused by acute diarrheal dehydration. The first step is to estimate the degree of dehydration, usually expressed as a percentage loss of baseline body weight. As such, a 5% deficit is termed mild, a 5% to 10% deficit is termed moderate, and a 15% deficit is termed severe and approaches shock. The approximate fluid deficits for each category of dehydration are expressed in Table 45-2 for infants and for older children.

The physical signs of dehydration are primarily those of reduced extracellular fluid and thus best reflect true fluid status in isotonic dehydration and underestimate the fluid loss in hypertonic dehydration where intracellular fluid loss predominates. The physical features are summarized in Table 45-3.

Table 45–2. Estimates of Fluid Deficits in Dehydration

Deficit	Severity	Approximate Fluid Deficit	
		Infants	*Older children*
5%	Mild	30–50 ml/kg	10–30 ml/kg
10%	Moderate	70–100 ml/kg	30–50 ml/kg
15%	Severe	120–150 ml/kg	50–75 ml/kg

Table 45–3. Physical Features of Dehydration in Childhood

	Type of Dehydration		
	Isotonic	*Hypertonic*	*Hypotonic*
Skin	Cold, dry	Cold, "doughy"	Cold, clammy
Mucous membranes	Dry	Parched	Clammy
Eyes	Sunken	Sunken	Sunken
Fontanelle	Sunken	Sunken	Sunken
Psyche	Lethargic	Hyperirritable	Lethargic
Pulse	Rapid	Moderately rapid	Rapid
Blood pressure	Low	Moderately low	Very low
Relative frequency	70%	15%	15%

The next phase is to confirm the form of dehydration, based, in large part, on the plasma sodium concentration. Isotonic dehydration, accounting for 70% of childhood dehydration, is defined as a sodium concentration remaining between 130 and 150 mEq/liter. Hypotonic dehydration equates with hyponatremia (below 130 mEq/liter), whereas hypertonic equates roughly with hypernatremia (above 150 mEq/liter). When available, plasma osmolality should be confirmed.

The therapy of severe dehydration consists of two phases. The first is the rapid restoration of blood volume with a bolus of fluid, generally normal saline or lactated Ringer's solutions, given as 10 to 20 ml/kg over 1 to 2 hours. The second phase is a more gradual correction of extracellular fluid and electrolyte deficits over 12 to 24 hours. In hypernatremia, this gradual correction extends over 48 to 72 hours. Knowledge of the composition of fluid lost is of great value in estimating replacement needs. Ongoing losses must be monitored, and, if appropriate, a sample should be submitted to the laboratory for confirmation of electrolyte composition. Table 45-4 summarizes the approximate composition of several fluids that may be lost. With milder dehydration, on an outpatient basis, rehydration is best accomplished with oral electrolyte solutions designed to meet the sodium requirements of diarrhea.

ACIDOSIS

The renal contribution to acid/base homeostasis is primarily by regulation of plasma bicarbonate. Secondary factors include renal hydrogen excretion and renal ammonium formation. The syndrome of renal tubular acidosis (RTA) can arise when either a defect in

Table 45–4. Composition of External Fluid Losses (mEq/liter)

Fluid	Sodium	Potassium	Chloride
Gastric	20–80	5–20	100–150
Jejunal	100–140	5–15	90–130
Bile	120–140	5–15	80–120
Ileostomy	45–135	3–15	20–115
Diarrheal	10–90	10–80	10–110

bicarbonate reabsorption or a defect in hydrogen ion gradient is noted. There are four major forms of RTA encountered in childhood.

Type I RTA is the result of an inability to maintain the normal 800:1 lumen to plasma hydrogen ion gradient in the distal tubule when faced with an acid load. This is thus also referred to as distal RTA. Whereas there is a reduction in renal acid secretion, the renal excretion of sodium, potassium, and especially calcium is markedly increased. The high rate of calcium excretion frequently leads to osteoporosis or nephrocalcinosis and sometimes to rickets. The potassium losses lead to a hypokalemic muscle weakness. The clinical presentation is with acidosis, severe growth failure, and emesis in early infancy. The urine pH is never below 5.8, even after a formal acid load test (75 to 150 mEq/m^2 of ammonium chloride).

Distal RTA can be an isolated genetic defect or can be seen in association with Ehlers-Danlos syndrome, Marfan's syndrome, or nerve deafness. Distal RTA can also complicate acute tubular necrosis, autoimmune disease, vitamin D intoxication, primary hyperparathyroidism, or nephrocalcinosis. There is also a form of distal RTA with bicarbonate wasting, termed type III RTA, in which urine pH rarely falls below 7.0.

Type II RTA is characterized by renal wasting of bicarbonate at the level of the proximal tubule. Following an acid load, the ability to acidify the urine is normal. Potassium excretion is elevated, while calcium excretion is generally normal; therefore nephrocalcinosis is absent. The proximal tubular defect may be isolated but commonly is associated with a generalized tubular transport disorder for amino acids, glucose, phosphate, and uric acid (Fanconi's syndrome). The other name for type II RTA is proximal RTA. Proximal RTA can be induced secondary to vitamin D deficiency, heavy metal intoxication, nephrotic syndrome, secondary hyperparathyroidism, or renal transplant.

Type IV RTA results either from a deficiency of mineralocorticoid or a tubular resistance to aldosterone. Renin levels are decreased. Urine acidification after an acid load is normal. In contrast to the other forms of RTA, the patient has hyperkalemia in addition to the usual features of growth failure, hyperchloremic acidosis, and, occasionally, hypertension. Type IV RTA can complicate Addison's disease, congenital adrenal hyperplasia, obstructive uropathy, pyelonephritis, or interstitial nephritis.

The common features of RTA include reduced plasma bicarbonate, hyperchloremic acidosis, and a high basal urinary pH. Treatment consists of addressing underlying illness, supplementation of bicarbonate or citrate (2 to 15 mEq/kg/day), and increased need for vitamin D and potassium.

BIBLIOGRAPHY

Booth IW, Levine MM, Harris JT: Oral rehydration therapy in acute diarrhea in childhood, J Pediatr Gastroenterol Nutr 3:491–499, 1984

Finberg L: Treatment of dehydration in infancy. Pediatr Rev. 3:113–116, 1981

Maclean WC, Graham GG: Pediatric Nutrition in Clinical Practice. Menlo Park, CA, Addison-Wesley, 1982

Winters RW (ed): The Body Fluids in Pediatrics. Boston, Little, Brown & Co, 1973

Ziegler EE, Fomon SJ: Fluid intake, renal solute load and water balance in infants. J Pediatr 78:561–568, 1971

46

Differential Diagnosis
of Edema

Edema, the hallmark of nephrotic syndrome, may be the presenting or primary symptom in a number of childhood diseases. The edema may be generalized or localized, the latter reflecting local reduction in lymphatic or venous flow. Localized edema is thus encountered with primary lymphedema, thrombophlebitis, ischemia, irradiation, anaphylaxis, or burns, or following surgical disruption of lymphatic or venous circulation.

The major cause of generalized edema in childhood is hypoproteinemia, although cardiovascular compromise is also prominent. As a rule, when the albumin level falls below 2.0 g/dl, edema will be noted. It is of value to note that with hypoproteinemia, the edema often begins in the face, whereas with congestive heart failure, the edema is peripheral, reflecting the influence of gravity. Altered capillary permeability is also a feature of a number of infectious disorders in childhood. For example, periorbital edema is very prominent in Epstein-Barr mononucleosis, roseola, and Rocky Mountain spotted fever.

Hypoproteinemia may result from reduced protein intake or absorption, reduced hepatic protein synthesis, or increased protein loss from the circulation. The first of these, reduced absorption, may reflect inadequate intake (kwashiorkor), impaired digestion (cystic fibrosis), or reduced mucosal uptake due to villus injury (gluten-sensitive enteropathy).

Reduced hepatic protein synthesis may be congenital (analbuminemia). This rare disorder may be minimally symptomatic or severe, as with neonatal hydrops. Acquired reduction in hepatic protein synthesis due to cirrhosis is usually a late feature relative to portal hypertension or ascites. With acute hepatic failure, the long half-life of albumin minimizes the severity of edema for 3 or more weeks.

Increased intestinal protein loss, termed protein-losing enteropathy, can complicate a number of disorders at any level of the intestine (Table 46-1). Acute or chronic enterocolitis is the implicated most frequently. When the half-life of circulating albumin falls below 4 days, hypoalbuminemia and edema ensue. In contrast to renal protein loss, intestinal protein loss is essentially independent of molecular weight, thus loss of immunoglobulins is prominent. The nonselective nature of protein-losing enteropathy is further substantiated by the accompanying loss of lipids, cal-

Table 46–1. Differential Diagnosis of Protein-Losing Enteropathy

Right heart failure/pericarditis
Hypertrophic gastritis (Menetrier's disease)
Gastrocolic fistula
Hypertrophic enteritis (transient exudative)
    Post-viral, eosinophilic
Lymphangiectasia
Protein-induced enteropathy
    Gluten, milk, soy
Enterocolitis
    Microbiologic: parasite, TB, Whipple's disease
    Cow-milk induced
    Obstructive: stricture, Hirschsprung's disease
    Inflammatory bowel disease: Crohn's disease, ulcerative colitis
Graft-versus-host

Table 46–2. Differential Diagnosis of Ascites

Transudates (protein <2.5 g/dl)
    Systemic hypoalbuminemia: decreased synthesis, nephrosis/glomerulonephritis, protein-losing enteropathy
    Portal hypertension: presinusoidal (e.g., venal caval thrombosis), sinusoidal (e.g., metabolic cirrhosis)
    Miscellaneous: beriberi, Gaucher's disease, Meigs' syndrome, pseudomyxoma
Exudates (protein >2.5 g/dl)
    Inflammatory serositis: pancreatitis, tuberculosis, sarcoid, syphilis, vasculitis, bacterial peritonitis
    Primary or metastatic tumor
    Portal hypertension:
        post-sinusoidal (epihepatic vein thrombosis), veno-occlusive disease
Chylous ascites

cium, and trace minerals. Intestinal lymphangiectasia also produces loss of lymphocytes.

Ascites, or the increase in free peritoneal fluid, may be either associated with or independent of generalized edema. The differential diagnosis is summarized in Table 46-2, with categorization by the protein content of the ascitic fluid. Ascitic protein concentrations exceeding 2.5 g/dl are termed exudates, while those below 2.5 g/dl are termed transudates. In general, exudates will also have cell counts in excess of 1000 cells/mm^3, while transudates will have less than 200 cells/mm^3.

Every child suspected of having ascites should have, in addition to a complete history and physical examination, both abdominal and pelvic sonography. Computerized tomography is individualized. Nearly all undiagnosed patients will require sterile abdominal paracentesis, often with sonographic guidance to reduce the risk. The ascitic fluid should be analyzed for color, clarity, total protein, amylase, triglyceride, cell count, cytology, and culture. In chylous ascites, the triglyceride content is at least twice that of the serum and lymphocytes are prominent. A chest x-ray is usually required to exclude associated chylothorax or pleural effusion.

BIBLIOGRAPHY

Fisher DA: Obscure and unusual edema. Pediatrics 37:506–528, 1966

Schussheim A: Protein-losing enteropathies in children. Am J Gastroenterol 58:124–132, 1972

Smeltzer DM, Stickler GB, Schirger A: Primary lymphedema in children and adolescents: A follow-up study and review. Pediatrics 76:206–218, 1985

Waldman TA, Wochner RD, Laster L et al: Allergic gastroenteropathy. N Engl J Med 276:761–769, 1967

47

Acute Renal Failure

Acute renal failure is defined as an acute reduction in renal function, resulting in azotemia or the failure to clear nitrogenous waste products from the circulation. There are three distinct, classical forms, although progression from one to another and overlap exist. Beyond the neonatal period, the frequency of acute renal failure is much lower in childhood than in the adult.

The first form, termed *prerenal* failure, is due to a reduction in renal perfusion. Thus, it may complicate any systemic condition of hypovolemia, hypotension, or hypoxemia. The final common path is inadequate glomerular filtration and inadequate oxygenation for active ion transport. The physiologic response to reduced renal perfusion is secretion of renin and antidiuretic hormone (ADH). The net effect is reduced urine production (oliguria) and increased urine osmolality, even in the face of decreased urinary sodium excretion. The recovery with early restoration of perfusion is rapid. The failure to recognize and reverse the hypoperfusion leads to a transition to intrinsic renal failure and a more permanent suppression of glomerular filtration rate.

The second form, *intrinsic renal failure*, is heralded by acute reduction in glomerular filtration rate (GFR), azotemia, loss of tubular concentrating ability (isosthenuria), and increased urinary sodium excretion. In this form, direct injury to either the glomerulus and/or the tubule is noted. Table 47-1 lists the more common causes of intrinsic acute renal failure. In childhood, hemolytic–uremic syndrome is the most common etiology.

The third form, *postrenal failure*, is the result of hydronephrosis induced by either bladder outlet or bilateral urethral obstruction. The most common time of presentation is in the neonatal period with posterior urethral valves or a neurogenic bladder. Neonates with obstructive uropathy should be suspected of having associated renal dysplasia. Crystalline or uric acid stone uropathy is rare in childhood except in the context of tumor lysis. Prompt recognition of the obstructive component of renal failure is critical, usually mandating surgical decompression.

DIAGNOSIS OF ACUTE RENAL FAILURE

Plasma creatinine and urea are utilized as solute markers that vary inversely with the GFR.

320

TABLE 47–1. Differential Diagnosis of Intrinsic Renal Failure

A. Glomerular disease
   Poststreptococcal nephritis
   Membranoproliferative glomerulonephritis
   Rapidly progressive glomerulonephritis
B. Systemic disease with renal involvement
   Vasculitis: systemic lupus erythematosus (SLE)
   Hemolytic–uremic syndrome
   Henoch-Schönlein purpura
C. Metabolic/drug-induced
   Aminoglycosides/sulfonamides
   Heavy metal intoxication
   Organic solvents
   Hemolysis
   Rhabdomyolysis
D. Pyelonephritis
E. Vascular
   Renal artery thrombosis
   Renal vein thrombosis

Unfortunately, plasma creatinine will be decreased in malnutrition, whereas urea will be disproportionately increased in conditions of increased protein turnover. Beyond infancy, the urine to plasma creatinine ratio will generally exceed 40 with prerenal failure and be less than 20 with intrinsic renal failure.

Even though early reviews defined acute renal failure as oliguria of less than 15 ml/kg/day, urine volume alone is of little diagnostic value, since more than 50% of children with acute renal failure will not have oliguria early in their course. In neonates, oliguria is more specific and acute renal failure should be suspected when urine output falls below 1 ml/kg/hour. In older children, urine osmolality is very valuable as a marker of concentrating ability. In prerenal failure, the urine osmolality usually remains above 500 mOsm, but in intrinsic renal failure, an osmolality greater than 350 is rare. In prerenal failure, the urine sodium concentration will be lower than in intrinsic failure.

Improved renal imaging, especially by real-time sonography, has been a major diagnostic advance in the past decade. Renal size, calyce-al distention, vascular perfusion, and ureteral patency can all be assessed relative to age-matched norms. The radionuclide scans provide critical functional information even at very low GFRs with technitium 99 scans used to measure perfusion. Gallium scans are also advised with inflammatory disease or possible lymphoma. In acute renal failure, the added value of computerized tomography (CT) or magnetic resonance imagery (MRI) scan has yet to be established.

MANAGEMENT OF ACUTE RENAL FAILURE

After exclusion of congestive heart failure or obstructive uropathy, the next step is to exclude prerenal failure and minimize ischemic injury with the use of volume expanders and, occasionally, renal vascular vasodilators. The added value of diuretics has yet to be demonstrated conclusively.

The child is monitored closely with daily weights and strict documentation of intake and output, avoiding catheterization if possible. Blood pressure is monitored closely, and hypertension is managed aggressively. Daily laboratory data should include blood urea nitrogen (BUN), creatinine, electrolytes, osmolality, complete blood cell (CBC) count, and calcium. If hyperkalemia develops, an electrocardiogram (ECG) should be performed and monitored. Transfusion for borderline anemia is discouraged. The hydrational state and cardiac and neurologic status are repeatedly assessed.

In acute renal failure, volume is provided to meet insensible fluid losses plus the documented losses of the previous 24 hours. Within the volume restrictions, maximal calories are provided anticipating a 1% to 2% weight loss.

Protein intake is restricted in the absence of dialysis, seeking around 800 mg/kg/day to maintain positive nitrogen balance. In the uremic child, histidine becomes an essential amino acid. With either peritoneal or hemodialysis, protein losses will increase.

In the absence of ongoing enteric losses, sodium requirements are very low. Potassium intake is also restricted, anticipating hyperkalemia in most forms of acute renal failure. Phosphate levels often increase, mandating use of an oral binding material and calcium supplementation.

Peritoneal dialysis, often by an intermittent technique, frequently is required to manage resistent hypervolemia, pulmonary edema, hyperkalemia, acidosis, or symptomatic uremia, or to allow adequate nutritional intake.

BIBLIOGRAPHY

Anand, SK: Acute renal failure in the neonate. Pediatr Clin North Am 29:791–800, 1982

Feld LG, Springate JE, Fildes RD: Acute renal failure. I: Pathophysiology and diagnosis. J Pediatr 109:401–408, 1986

Fildes RD, Springate JF, Feld LG: Acute renal failure. II: Management of suspected or established disease. J Pediatr 109:567–571, 1986

Hudson EM, Kjellstraud CM, Maugr SM: Acute renal failure in infants and children requiring hemodialysis. J Pediatr 93:756–760, 1976

Kon V, Ichikawa I: Research Seminar: Physiology of acute renal failure. J Pediatr 105:351–357, 1984

48

Chronic Renal Failure

Progressive reduction in renal function can complicate a large number of renal disorders in childhood. As any injury to the renal nephron is associated with a compensating hypertrophy of remaining nephrons, the degree of renal injury must exceed 80% of the nephron mass to produce clinical signs of renal failure. In most circumstances, glomerular and tubular function are equally impaired, except early in the course of rare tubular disorders such as oxalosis.

Children with chronic renal failure usually have a disorder that falls into one of four large groups. First are the children with glomerulonephritis. In this group are the children with hemolytic–uremic syndrome, focal segmental glomerulosclerosis, membranoproliferative glomerulonephritis, Henoch-Schönlein syndrome, and systemic lupus erythematosus. Postinfectious glomerulonephritis rarely leads to chronic renal failure. The second group are the children with congenital renal hypoplasia or polycystic disease. Children in the third group have hereditary nephropathies such as medullary cystic disease, Alport's syndrome, cysteinuria, or oxalosis. The last group are the children with obstructive uropathies with features of outlet obstruction, uretheral reflux, and chronic pyelonephritis. In contrast to the adult, neither vascular nor metabolic renal disease contributes in any major way to chronic renal failure in childhood.

The severity of renal failure is generally classified by the severity of reduction in glomerular filtration as measured by creatinine clearance. The serum level of urea nitrogen is helpful but less specific. When the creatinine clearance exceeds 30 ml/min/1.73m^2, there are few clinical manifestations of the renal impairment other than possible reduction in growth rate. When the clearance is 15 to 30 ml/min/1.73m^2, metabolic complications appear, with terminal renal failure developing below 5 ml/min/1.73m^2.

Since the functions of the kidney are many and complex, the nature of impairment and the adaptation to this must be recognized on a function-by-function basis. From the standpoint of salt excretion, the impaired kidney initially increases the rate of sodium resorption per residual nephron, especially in the context of elevated aldosterone, but the ratio of resorbed sodium to filtered sodium is low, producing an obligatory loss of sodium. Late in renal failure, filtration is also impaired, creating a risk of both salt and water overload or intoxication. Because of hypertrophy of tubular secretion, the renal secretion of potassium is preserved until late in the progression of renal failure except in acute tubular necrosis of the impaired kidney. However, the ability to compensate for increased salt intake or potassium release from ischemic cell injury is greatly limited.

The increase in osmolality of the renal blood flow produces an increased urine flow or polyuria. Renal concentrating ability is initially reduced (hyposthenuria) and subsequently lost (isosthenuria), resulting in a urine specific gravity around 1.010. Hydrogen ion clearance is reduced early in the course of renal impairment with the loss of the tubular ability to produce ammonia. With advanced renal failure comes the loss of ability to excrete titratable acids and a reduction in bicarbonate reabsorption.

The hormonal effects of renal failure are equally significant. Foremost is the inability to complete the hydroxylation of 1,25 dihydroxyvitamin D. The resulting decrease in intestinal absorption and bone mobilization of calcium reduces the serum levels of ionized calcium. This is further aggravated by hyperphosphatemia from increased renal phosphorus retention, a process that correlates in severity with increasing reduction in glomerular filtration. This stimulates the release of parathyroid hormone to mobilize calcium from bone. As a result, osteomalacia develops. If growth has been sustained, true rickets will be seen.

The uremic syndrome has a number of consistent clinical features. Prominent among these is anemia due to contributions from reduced renal synthesis of erythropoitin, shortening of red cell survival, and frequent gastrointestinal (GI) bleeding. The children present with a normocytic, normochromic anemia. Uremic alterations in platelet function also contribute to bruising and bleeding. Additional features of clinical uremia include anorexia, lassitude, recurrent infection, and neurologic symptoms ranging from confusion to tremor to convulsions. Severe pruritus, or itching, also develops, a symptom that improves after parathyroidectomy, suggesting a role of elevated parathormone. Cardiopulmonary manifestations include pulmonary edema and pericarditis.

Growth failure is an early and prominent feature of progressive renal failure. Many factors contribute to this, including anorexia, reduced taste sensation, chronic metabolic acidosis, and electrolyte depletion. Reduction in height velocity will be seen in up to 75% of children. Recognizing that nearly 50% of the entire height is achieved in the first two years of life, the influence of chronic renal disease on height depends more on age of onset than specific disease.

The role of nutrition in responding to the demands of growth has only recently been aggressively addressed. Indeed, in the days before dialysis and transplant, there was little desire to facilitate growth, since excretory needs are proportional to body mass.

It has long been realized that high protein intakes aggravated the nitrogen retention of uremia. It is now recognized that low protein intakes appear to slow the progression of renal failure. Thus protein restriction is advised when the creatinine clearance falls below 25 ml/min/1.73 m^2 or when the serum urea nitrogen exceeds 75 mg/dl. Diets are thus designed to maximize carbohydrate and lipid calories while providing essential amino acids and limited additional protein to meet ongoing losses. In infancy, for example, protein is provided to meet 6% to 8% of total calories, about 40% less than normal intakes for age. Carbohydrate intake may be limited by glucose intolerance, since the action of insulin on a cellular level is impaired in uremia. Lipid calories may aggravate the hypertriglyceridemia of renal failure. Additional dietary factors in the conservative management of renal failure include restricting excessive salt intake, providing alkali to children with acidosis, binding phosphorus to reduce intestinal absorption, and providing vitamin D to minimize osteodystrophy.

Many medications require either renal metabolism or excretion. Their dosage and frequency of delivery must be closely monitored.

The psychological support for these children must be extensive and family based. In addition to the routine depression of chronic illness, these children are often physically weak, self-conscious of their short stature, and usually restricted from many activities and diets of their peers.

While hemodialysis and acute peritoneal dialysis have been the cornerstone of therapy, the major advance in the past decade has been the ability to provide safe, long-term dialysis by the use of continuous ambulatory peritoneal dialysis (CAPD). This technique is slower than hemodialysis, requiring 24 hours to achieve the efficiency of 4 hours of hemodialysis, but carries much less risk and greater ability to sustain a near-normal life-style. The only specific contraindication to CAPD is peritoneal hemorrhage. In the experience to date, CAPD normalizes the uremia, corrects the metabolic complications, and reduces hypertension. It may not reverse osteodystrophy and, because of the high glucose load, may aggravate hypertriglyceridemia. The development of closed dialysate bag technology has reduced the risk of peritonitis to approximately one episode per patient year.

The optimal therapy, of course, is restoration of normal renal function by transplantation. The first successful transplant was performed in 1954 with a donated kidney from an identical twin. While related-donor transplantation remains preferable to nonrelated or cadaveric donors, improved immunosuppression and use of donor-specific transfusion has led to a 10-year kidney survival of 50% to 70%. Graft survival for cadaveric donors increased markedly with the application of a new immunosuppressive drug, cyclosporine. Infection remains a great risk, especially with chronic cytomegalovirus, in the post-transplant patient. Another risk is the recurrence of the original renal disease in the transplanted kidney. This risk is greatest in childhood with oxalosis, membranoproliferative glomerulonephritis, and focal segmental glomerulosclerosis.

BIBLIOGRAPHY

Brouhard BH: The role of dietary protein in progressive renal disease. Am J Dis Child 140:630–640, 1986

Broyer M: Growth in children with renal insufficiency. Pediatr Clin North Am 29:991–1003, 1982

Fine RN: Peritoneal dialysis update. J Pediatr 100:1–7, 1982

Potter D, Feduska N, Melzer J et al: Twenty years of renal transplantation in children. Pediatrics 77:465–470, 1986

49

Nephrotic Syndrome

Since the original description of nephrosis by Bright in 1836, the nephrotic syndrome has remained a major clinical concern in childhood, with an incidence of 2 cases/100,000 children each year. The clinical features are the complications of dramatic proteinuria, usually in excess of 2/g m^2/day (or approximately 50 mg/kg/day). The resulting hypoalbuminemia (usually less then 2.5 mg/dl) leads to fluid leak into interstitial tissues, producing edema and hypovolemia. This is aggravated further by the compensatory hyperaldosteronism that increases renal salt and water resorption. As the liver increases protein synthesis, there is increased synthesis of prebetalipoproteins, elevating the cholesterol level. The associated increase in procoagulant proteins, coupled with reduced fibrinolysins, results in a "hypercoagulable" state, contributing to a clinical risk for thrombosis. The renal leak of protein occurs at the level of the glomerulus, usually as a "selective" proteinuria restricted to lower molecular weight proteins.

Primary nephrotic syndrome is divided into four major clinical conditions: congenital nephrosis, minimal change nephrotic syndrome (MCNS), focal segmental glomerulosclerosis (FSGS), and membranoproliferative glomerulonephritis (MPGN). Secondary nephrotic syndrome accounts for less than 10% of childhood nephrosis; it may be encountered as a complication of amyloidosis, systemic lupus erthematosus, Alport's syndrome, or Henoch-Schönlein anaphylactoid purpura.

Nearly 80% of nephrotic syndrome is caused by an idiopathic condition termed "minimal change" from the paucity of alterations in the glomerulus by light microscopy. On electron microscopy, however, a characteristic fusion of the epithelial cell foot process is noted, a nonspecific lesion noted as a complication, experimentally, of severe proteinuria.

MCNS usually presents between 1 and 6 years of age and has a male-to-female ratios of 3:1. The presenting feature in nearly 80% is edema, often first noted in the face, but easily demonstrated in the extremities. Microscopic hematuria will be seen in about 25%, although gross hematuria is rare (less than 5%). Elevations in blood pressure are encountered in 10% to 20%. The serum level of the third component of complement (C3) is normal. While rare, the prevalence in siblings is 1000-fold greater than in the random population, suggesting a genetic predisposition. A consistent, indeed, nearly diagnostic, feature of MCNS is the excellent response to corticosteroid therapy.

At the time of presentation, the clinical features of FSGS are often indistinguishable from those of MCNS. Again more common in males, the frequency of hematuria (75%) and hypertension (60%) is somewhat greater. The C3 level is normal. The diagnosis requires renal biopsy, in which a segmental sclerosis is noted in some glomeruli. Tubular atrophy may also be seen early in the course of the disease. The mechanism of sclerosis is unknown. Focal glomerulosclerosis can be noted in biopsies from children with Henoch-Schönlein purpura, postinfectious glomerulonephritis, IgA nephropathy, and Alport's syndrome. The presence of focal sclerosis is a poor prognostic sign, since less than 20% of the children will respond to prednisone therapy. The prognosis is felt to be somewhat better if therapy is begun when the proteinuria is asymptomatic, when the sclerotic glomeruli are peripheral, and when less than 20% of the glomeruli are involved. FSGS accounts for about 10% of children with nephrotic syndrome and 40% of those resistent to corticosteroid therapy.

MPGN can also present with the nephrotic syndrome, accounting for 6% to 8% of nephrotic children in most studies. In contrast to both MCNS and FSGS, the children with MPGN are somewhat older, C'3 levels are usually reduced, and the nephritic symptoms of hematuria, hypertension, and azotemia are prominent. It is more common in females. Less than 10% of these children respond to corticosteroid therapy.

The congenital form of nephrosis is rare, but well described, especially in children of Finnish descent. Inherited as an autosomal recessive disorder, the neonates present with proteinuria and ascites. Severe growth failure, psychomotor retardation, and recurrent infection mark early infancy. Renal transplantation is usually required at an early age.

In addition to the vascular thrombosis cited above, all children with nephrotic syndrome are at risk for severe complicating infections, especially cellulitis, peritonitis, and sepsis. While *Streptococcus pneumoniae* is most often implicated, *Pseudomonas*, *Eschericia coli*, and *Haemophilus influenzae* are also prevalent.

When a child presents with edema and a clinical suspicion of nephrotic syndrome, the laboratory evaluation outlined in Table 49-1 is advised. The expected result in children with MCNS is also indicated. The 24-hour urine can also be analyzed for the ratio of urinary IgG to transferrin. A ratio of less than 0.1 is noted with the selective proteinuria of MCNS.

The child is weighed daily with regular blood pressures and strict documentation of urine output. While excessive salt intake is minimized, fluid intake is rarely restricted, except in the child with established renal fail-

Table 49–1. Laboratory Evaluation of Childhood Nephrotic Syndrome

Investigation	Expected Result in MCNS
Urinalysis	Proteinuria, mild hematuria
Complete blood count	Normal
BUN, creatinine	Normal
Total protein, albumin	Reduced
Cholesterol	Greater than 250 mg/dl
C3	Normal
Electrolytes, calcium, phosphorus	Normal
Urine	
Protein, 24-hour	Greater than 40 mg/hr/m²
Creatinine clearance, 24-hour	Normal

ure. While it is tempting to give diuretics routinely, one must remember that the child is already intravascular-volume depleted. When respiratory compromise due to edema or ascites, urethral compression, or skin breakdown demand diuresis, the child is first given intravenous albumin at 1 g/kg over 1 hour, followed by a loop diuretic such as furosemide. Because of the risk of infection, polyvalent pneumococcal vaccine is advised, and the new *Haemophilus influenzae* type B vaccine is given, if not previously received. Fevers are aggressively evaluated with a low threshold for initiation of wide-spectrum antibic therapy.

If the clinical features suggest MCNS (age, 1 to 8 years; normal C3, and minimal hematuria), prednisone therapy is initiated at a dose of 2 mg/kg/day in divided doses. In children with MCNS, 75% will clear their proteinuria within 2 weeks, and 95% will clear in 1 month. The prednisone dose is then tapered over 3 to 4 months. Unfortunately, about 80% of these "responders" will relapse over the next year. Most will respond again and continue in remission when the prednisone is tapered more gradually over 1 year. About 20% will become frequent relapsers, prompting initiation of an alkylating agent such as cyclophosphamide or chlorambucil as well as prednisone.

After 1 month on prednisone, a renal biopsy is generally advised for the "nonresponders" to confirm or exclude FSGS or MPGN. As noted above, the response to medical therapy in both of these conditions is less than 25%, and chronic renal disease is the rule.

BIBLIOGRAPHY

International Study of Kidney Disease in Children, The primary nephrotic syndrome in children. J Pediatr 98:561, 1981

McEnery PT, Strife CF: Nephrotic syndrome in childhood. Pediatr Clin North Am 89:875, 1982

Mahan JD, Mauer SM, Sibley RK et al: Congenital nephrotic syndrome: Evolution of medical management and results of renal transplantation. J Pediatr 105:549, 1984

Oliver W, Kelsch R. Nephrotic syndrome due to primary nephropathies. Pediatr Rev 2:311, 1981

Yoshikawa N, Ito H, Akamatsu R et al: Focal segmental glomerulosclerosis with and without nephrotic syndrome. J Pediatr 109:65, 1986

50

Hematuria and Proteinuria

In the course of childhood, up to 10% of all children will demonstrate at least one episode of documented hematuria or proteinuria. While most have benign, transient origins, either symptom may herald severe chronic renal disease mandating an understanding of the differential diagnosis and the extent of evaluation warranted.

HEMATURIA

Hematuria is defined microscopically as the presence of greater than 5 red blood cells (RBCs) per high-powered field in the spun sediment of 10 ml of freshly voided urine. There are two broad categories of hematuria: that associated with proteinuria, presence of red cell casts in the urine sediment, and acute nephritic symptoms termed "glomerular hematuria"; and that independent of the above, termed "nonglomerular hematuria". Of course, when faced with a reddish urine, the first issue is to confirm true hematuria, as opposed to the clearance of a dietary or medicinal pigment, hemoglobin from hemolysis or myoglobin from rhabdomyolysis. In so doing,

remember that the urine dipstick method will be positive with hemoglobin, myoglobin, or red cells. Thus review of the spun urine sediment to confirm the presence of RBCs is essential. The major pigments or dyes contributing to a reddish urine are from ingested beets, KoolAid, or blackberries, medicinal phenytoin or pyridium, or endogenous bilirubin or porphyrin. Uric acid precipitation in the diaper can also appear pink. *Serratia marscesans* in the stools of infants will also discolor the excreted urine as in the "red diaper syndrome." Regrettably, it has been emphasized recently that the collection of the urine be monitored because disturbed parents or children may add drops of peripheral blood to a normal urine as part of Munchausen's syndrome.

The differential diagnosis of nonglomerular hematuria is listed in Table 50-1. While considered "isolated" hematuria, it is important to look for evidence of pyuria or bacturia. With gross hematuria, the dipstick is also usually trace positive for protein on a plasma-lost basis.

The ability of exercise alone to produce transient hematuria is well documented. This

Table 50–1. Differential Diagnosis of Nonglomerular Hematuria

Renal Origins	Urinary Tract Origins
Exercise-induced	Cystitis
Trauma	Hydronephrosis
Hypercalciuria	Posterior urethral valves
Acute interstitial nephritis	Urolithiasis
Sickle cell disease/	Coagulopathy
hemoglobin S-C disease	Foreign body
Polycystic renal disease	
Renal vein thrombosis	
Wilms' tumor	
Tuberculosis	
Papillary necrosis	

is also called "march" hematuria because of its frequency in the military after long marches. The gross hematuria clears in 24 hours, with microscopic hematuria persisting for up to 1 week. The male-to-female ratio of prevalence approaches 10:1. No specific lesion is demonstrated by the limited biopsy data available. Hematuria is also frequent with blunt trauma to the flanks from sport or vehicular injury.

Hypercalciuria has increasingly been recognized as major cause of recurrent hematuria in childhood. While the mechanism of the hematuria is unknown, these patients have either a defect in tubular reabsorption of calcium or an increase in intestinal calcium absorption. Serum calcium levels, parathormone, and vitamin D metabolism are normal. Suspicion of this condition should lead to screening of the urine from parents and siblings, since it is inherited as an autosomal-dominant disorder. Confirmation is achieved by documenting, in a 24-hour urine specimen, the excretion of more than 4 mg/kg of calcium or greated than 0.25 mg calcium/mg creatinine. Calcium stones are a late feature of this condition, rarely noted in childhood.

Acute interstitial nephritis, usually induced by medications such as penicillin or sulfonamide, is often confused with acute glomerulonephritis because, even in the absence of glomerular injury, proteinuria and red cell casts are commonly seen. Many involved children will have acute renal failure and require dialysis or intensive supportive care. Complete recovery, however, is the rule.

Hematuria may also be a significant feature of sickle cell or hemoglobin S-C disease so a hemoglobin electrophoresis is appropriate in black children with hematuria. Polycystic disease of either the infantile or adult type can present with hematuria in childhood. Either renal vein thrombosis or Wilms' tumor can present as hematuria, usually with an abdominal or flank mass. Although renal tuberculosis is now rare, the classic presentation was as hematuria and sterile pyuria.

Hematuria is a feature of cystitis or acute urinary tract infection and may be the presenting sign. Similarly, hydronephrosis, often the result of posterior urethral valves, can have hematuria, usually in the context of pyelonephritis. Urolithiasis is rare but can be seen with urate stones in tumor patients or as oxalate stones after bowel resection. Coagulopathies such as hemophilia or thrombocytopenia may have complicating hematuria, but rarely as a presenting feature. Both urethral and vaginal foreign bodies must also be considered in the differential diagnosis.

The glomerular forms of hematuria are listed in Table 50-2 and usually present with significant proteinuria, red cell casts, and the additional nephritic features of hypertension, edema, oliguria, and azotemia. Further discrimination of the differential is accomplished by documenting reduction or consumption of the third component of complement (C3). We will first review those glomerular origins of hematuria with normal C3 activity.

The major cause of glomerular hematuria was formerly termed benign recurrent hematuria and is now called Berger's disease or IgA

Table 50–2. Differential Diagnosis of Glomerular Hematuria

Complement Consuming	Normal Complement
Postinfectious glomerulonephritis	IgA nephropathy (Berger's)
Systemic lupus erythematosus	Benign familial hematuria
Membranoproliferative glomerulopathy	Alport's syndrome
Shunt nephritis	Hemolytic–Uremic syndrome
Bacteremia	Henoch–Schönlein purpura
	Polyarteritis/Wegener's
	Rapidly progressive glomerulonephritis
	Hepatitis B

nephropathy. It usually presents acutely with gross hematuria in the context of a viral-like upper respiratory illness. The associated proteinuria is modest, usually 0.5 to 1.0 g/24 hours, and the nephritic features of edema, azotemia, or hypertension are rare. The gross hematuria clears quickly, recurring with subsequent infections. In the interval between significant episodes, microscopic hematuria persists. The persistence of proteinuria or reduced creatinine clearance is a poor prognostic sign, especially when focal scarring is noted on biopsy. Indeed, despite the early benign connotation, up to 30% of these children may progress to chronic renal disease. On renal biopsy, a mild proliferative lesion with focal nephritis is noted with glomerular deposition of immunoglobulin, always IgA and frequently IgG and properdin. Follow-up of asymptomatic children at 6-month intervals is indicated.

Another common cause with normal complement is benign familial or idiopathic hematuria. At first, the hematuria, an autosomal-dominant condition, is isolated. On renal biopsy, a characteristic thin glomerular membrane is noted. Although the hematuria is termed benign, close monitoring of these patients will reveal progression to chronic renal disease in up to 20%.

Alport's syndrome is another autosomal-dominant condition, often presenting with isolated hematuria, although sensorineural hearing loss is an associated feature with age. Up to 20% of involved children represent a gene mutation, since family history is negative. In males, the progression to renal failure is nearly universal, whereas females have a more benign course and often have subclinical hearing loss. On renal biopsy, electron microscopy will reveal a specific fragmentation of the lamina densa and nonspecific foam cells.

Hemolytic–uremic syndrome is a multisystem disorder of thrombosis of microvasculature with renal involvement as an acute glomerular nephritis. As such, it is the most common cause of childhood acute renal failure. Presentation is usually before the age of 5 years, with bloody diarrhea, leukocytosis, and features of acute colitis. Indeed, sigmoidoscopy may reveal diffuse ulceration and pseudomembrane formation. The barium enema will reveal a diffuse colitis, indistinguishable from idiopathic ulcerative colitis. In addition, the stool cultures are often positive for a presumptive pathogen such as *Shigella, Salmonella, Campylobacter, Bartonella,* or enterovirus. More than one family member can be involved, and onset with mononucleosis and with oral contraceptive use has been reported. While enteric features are initially prominent, the child rapidly develops a thrombocytopenia and microangiopathic hemolytic anemia. Other coagulation studies are normal. Both acute rhabdomyolysis and central nervous system (CNS) features such as seizures, hemiparesis, or coma may be encountered. Uremia ensues, usually prompting early dialysis. Although early studies with anticoagulant therapy were unimpressive, more recent studies suggest a value for treatment with fresh frozen plasma. This observation is consistent with recent etiologic investigations suggesting a defect in prostacyclin production or the presence of an inhibitor of fibrinolytic activity. Aggressive supportive therapy is justified by complete recovery in more than 95% of children. The gastrointestinal features generally clear in a week, although colonic stricture has been reported as a long-term complication of the ischemic injury.

Henoch-Schönlein purpura is another multisystem disorder characterized by small vessel vasculitis. Onset is usually with an urticarial then purpuric rash on the lower extremities and buttocks, progressing to swelling of the ankles and knees, colicky abdominal pain, and edema, especially of the extremities, forehead, and scrotum. Intestinal features include ileus, melena, and frequent small bowel intussusception. Hepatomegaly with mild enzyme elevation is common. Although renal biopsies confirm renal involvement in more than 80% of the children, gross hematuria develops in about 60% of reported children, usually within 7 to 10 days of the rash. Significant proteinuria in excess of 2 g/24 hours is seen in more than half of the children. Renal function is usually maintained, however, a rapidly progressive glomerulonephritis will develop in 10% to 15% of children with renal manifestations. The rest can expect a complete recovery, although recurrences and persistent hematuria may be encountered.

Rapidly progressive glomerulonephritis of other etiologies may also be noted, including a form induced by immune complexes in children with chronic hepatitis B. Polyarteritis and, rarely, Wegener's syndrome may present with hematuria.

As noted above, the consumption of C3 is used to distinguish other forms of glomerulonephritis presenting with hematuria. The most common, although less frequent in the past two decades, is postinfectious glomerulonephritis. Previously termed poststreptococcal glomerulonephritis, the new name reflects the development after staphylococcal and pneumococcal disease as well as the nephritogenic strains of *Streptococcus.* Presentation is usually acute, 7 to 10 days after the antecedent infection. Hypertension and oliguria will be prominent, lasting 7 to 10 days. Complement depression and proteinuria may persist for weeks. Persistence of a reduced C3 or proteinuria past 8 weeks suggests a preexisting membranoproliferative glomerulonephropathy, mandating renal biopsy.

Membranoproliferative glomerulonephropathy will also feature hematuria, proteinuria, and C3 depression. Several forms exist, discriminated in part by the presence or lack of immune complexes on biopsy. Although uncommon in childhood, it can develop secondary to conditions such as systemic lupus erythematosus or gold therapy. An immune complex etiology can also be noted with bacteremia as with endocarditis or ventriculoatrial shunts.

The evaluation indicated in a child with hematuria is summarized in Table 50-3. In light of the foregoing discussion, most of the studies are self-explanatory. History focuses on indications of chronic systemic disease such as growth impairment and nephritic features such as edema. Family history is pursued in depth. Physical examination includes growth parameters, blood pressure, and careful abdominal palpation. Many children with gross hematuria will require hospitalization to facilitate the evaluation, support renal function, and relieve the parents' and child's fears. Asymptomatic microscopic hematuria is usually confirmed in three samples over 4 weeks before initiating the work-up as an outpatient.

Renal biopsy indications must be individualized but are generally indicated with the second unexplained episode of gross hematu-

Table 50–3. Evaluation of Hematuria

UNIVERSAL
Complete history, including family
Complete physical examination
Urinalysis (patient and parents)
CBC, platelet count, review of smear
Total protein, albumin, creatinine phosphokinase
Urea nitrogen, creatinine, electrolytes
24-Hour urine for protein, creatinine
   clearance, and calcium
Streptozyme, purified protein derivative (PPD)
C3 complement level
INDIVIDUALIZED
Glomerular
Anti-DNA
Hepatitis B
Prothrombin time/partial prothrombin time
Skin biopsy
Renal biopsy
Nonglomerular
Urine culture
Sonogram
Pyelogram
Hemoglobin electrophoresis
Cystoscopy

Table 50–4. Differential Diagnosis of Asymptomatic Proteinuria

Orthostatic/postural
Benign persistent proteinuria
Subclinical nephrotic syndrome
Membranous glomerulopathy
Chronic pyelonephritis
Congenital renal anomaly
   Renal dysplasia
   Polycystic syndrome

ria and/or persistent microscopic hematuria with reduced renal function or hypertension. Biopsies may even lead to specific therapy with immunosuppression. Each biopsy should be routinely processed for light microscopy, electron microscopy, and immunoflourescence.

PROTEINURIA

Although proteinuria is a feature of glomerular hematuria, it can also be present in an isolated, asymptomatic fashion (Table 50-4). Significant proteinuria is defined as 2+ or greater by dipstick, or greater than 150 mg of protein in a 24-hour urine specimen. It must be remembered that protein is present in everyone's urine, usually 60% derived from plasma leakage and 40% from tubular mucoproteins, termed Tamm-Horsfall protein. Because the urine dipstick method detects only albumin and not globulins, a more precise technique is the sulfosalicylic acid method.

Proteins can be lost either at the level of the tubule or the level of the glomerulus. Tubular proteinuria is usually mild, less then 2 g/24 hours, and is thus rarely accompanied by edema. Tubular proteinuria is seen with heavy metal or analgesic poisonings, cystic disease, Wilson's disease, Lowe's syndrome, or renal tubular acidosis. It is often part of Fanconi's syndrome with glycosuria, phosphaturia, aminoaciduria, and bicarbonaturia.

Glomerular proteinuria is usually more severe, up to 30 g/24 hours. The glomerular leak can be "selective," losing only low molecular weight proteins up to the size of albumin. This is a feature of minimal change nephrotic syndrome. Alternatively, it can be "nonselective," with large molecular weight proteins also lost, as with most forms of glomerulonephritis.

The most common form of isolated proteinuria in childhood is postural or orthostatic proteinuria, often further aggravated by exertion. Seen equally in both sexes, it is mild in severity and renal function, by definition, is normal. It is confirmed by comparing the protein content in urine obtained on arising in the morning with an increased level of proteinuria later in the day. This form is very rare before the age of 5 years, and many of the involved children have resolution of proteinuria by adulthood.

The major goal is to avoid missing subclinical nephrosis or early glomerular disease. With nephrosis, the proteinuria may precede other clinical signs by weeks, but serum abnormalities of reduced albumin and elevated cholesterol should be present. Glomerular lesions are screened by serum complement (C3), while renal anomalies are excluded by sonographic evaluation. Urine culture is routinely suggested. Renal biopsy is rarely required with isolated proteinuria. As with idiopathic hematuria, patients with persistent proteinuria not due to orthrostatic change should be monitored closely for renal status throughout childhood.

BIBLIOGRAPHY

Bergstein JM: Hematuria, proteinuria and urinary tract infection. Pediatr Clin North Am 29:55, 1982

Brenner BM, Hostetter TH, Humes HD: Molecular basis of proteinuria of glomerular origin. N Engl J Med 298:826, 1978

Feld L. Schoeneman M, Kaskel F: Evaluation of the child with asymptomatic proteinuria. Pediatr Rev 5:248, 1984

Habib R: The major syndromes, chap 3, pp 246–257. In Royer P, Habib R, Mathienu H et al (eds): Pediatric Nephrology. Philadelphia, WB Saunders, 1974

Northway J: Hematuria in children. J Pediatr 78:381, 1971

Robinson RR: Isolated proteinuria in asymptomatic patients. Kidney Int 18:395, 1980

West C: Asymptomatic hematuria and proteinuria in children: Causes and appropriate diagnostic studies. J Pediatr 89:173, 1976

51

Enuresis

Enuresis is the involuntary passage of urine. As we all start life happily enuretic from 10 to 20 times a day, it has been difficult to determine precisely when the "normal" becomes cause for concern. A review of the physiology of this process and how it matures is of value here.

The passage of urine from the bladder requires a relaxation of the bladder neck, followed by contraction of the detrusor muscles and relaxation of the internal sphincter. In the infant, the detrusor involuntarily contracts whenever the bladder capacity of 40 to 60 ml is achieved, although no awareness of the degree of bladder fullness occurs until around the age of 2 years. Bladder capacity reaches 90 ml by 2 years and 150 ml by 3 years, the age when a child can void at will from a near-full bladder. By the age of 5 years, the capacity is 200 ml, and the child can first voluntarily stop a urine stream by contraction of the pubococcygeal muscle. Clinically, this translates to 80% of children being dry by day at 2½ years and 80% being dry by night by 3 years. Persistent enuresis, defined as wetting 5 days out of 7, occurs in approximately 10% of children at 5 years, 5% at 10 years, with 2% persisting

into late adolescence. This correlates to a 10% per year spontaneous cure rate. Approximately 80% of enuretics are wet only at night, 15% are wet both day and night, and 5% are wet only by day. In most age-groups, the incidence in males is slightly greater than in females.

In most published studies, nearly 80% of the children with persistent enuresis have an etiology attributed to a maturational delay in attaining adequate bladder capacity and/or bladder sphincter control. The two major "risk" factors in these children are a family history of enuresis and a greater percentage of time spent in the deeper stages of sleep (although wetting itself occurs at all levels or depths of sleep except REM sleep). Because bladder capacity may be a component in this maturational process, the children are encouraged to increase fluid intake and delay urination during the day—so-called "stretching" exercises.

A second group of children, comprising about 10% of childhood enuresis, have an "acquired" form of enuresis, having previously demonstrated the ability to stay dry for several months. Primary emotional problems are usually implicated, some as obvious as the birth of a sibling or death of a family member, and some as subtle as sexual abuse. Individual and family counseling will be required in the more complex or obscure situations.

Less than 5% of enuretic children have an "organic" etiology. A flaccid, neurogenic bladder will be noted in children with a number of spinal cord lesions, especially meningomyelocele. The role of polyuria is demonstrated in diabetes insipidus, diabetes mellitus, or with psychogenic polydipsia. Half of those with an organic etiology have recurrent cystitis, commonly with partial obstruction of the bladder outlet. Constipation may contribute in this manner. On the other hand, urethral stenosis alone is rarely the cause, and routine urethral dilatation is discouraged. Enuresis attributed to seizure equivalents or food allergy has yet to be demonstrated convincingly.

The evaluation of the child begins with a detailed history of enuretic frequency, patterns of wetting, and associated complaints. Both family and social histories are taken in detail. It is important to distinguish independently how the child reacts to the situation and contrast it to the parental response. At some point, all parents convert the "problem" into a "crisis," and the effect on the child can be dramatic. It is thus important to determine the extent that it limits the child's participation in activities such as sleeping at the homes of grandparents or friends.

The physical examination should include growth data, blood pressure, careful abdominal examination including rectal examination, and a thorough neurologic examination. The child should be observed passing the urine stream. The extent of laboratory testing is minimal. A complete urinalysis is performed, recording specific gravity, sugar, protein, and cellular elements. A urine culture is generally advised. Radiographic investigations and urologic consultation are warranted only on an individualized basis to address such specific concerns as constant dribbling, prior cystitis, distended bladder or flank mass, or abnormal urine stream.

THERAPY

The options of therapy fall into four large categories: reassurance alone, bladder-stretching exercises, conditioning alarms, and medication. Certainly, up to the age of 5 years, reassurance alone is advised. This is justified, as well, for a few additional years in light of the spontaneous cure rate, especially with an empathetic parent. Bladder-stretching exercises will take several months of sustained effort. While improvement is noted in 70% of children, cures by stretching alone are rare except in day-only enuresis. In studies over the past decade, conditioning with the use of enuresis alarms has become the most commonly justified course of action. Initially, the child is awakened only when urine passed activates the alarm. Gradually the cortical center is conditioned to sense the bladder fullness that precedes the alarm, awakening the child to void. In children over 7 years of age, cure rates when enuresis alarms of 50% to 90% are reported over 8 to 12 weeks. The relapse rate remains high at 40%. Failure of alarm conditioning will occur with fear of the appliance and sleep so deep that the child does not hear the alarm. The enthusiasm for medication has waned, especially since no recent study has demonstrated superiority to conditioning alarms. The most commonly employed medication is imipramine, a tricyclic antidepressant that is felt to relax the detrusor muscle, tighten the sphincter, and alter depth of sleep. Side effects are common, and severe accidental poisoning is a major risk. Published cure rates with medication over the age of 8 years approach 50%, with an equal relapse rate. Regardless of the type of therapy employed, the critical components for success are the motivation of the child, the support of the family, and the recognition that months of patience will be required for cure.

BIBLIOGRAPHY

Brazelton T: A child-oriented approach to toilet training. Pediatrics 29:121–126, 1962

Foxman B, Valdel RB, Brock RH: Childhood enuresis: Prevalence, perceived impact, and prescribed treatment. Pediatrics 77:482–487, 1986

Oppel WC, Harber PA, Rider RY: The age of attaining bladder control. Pediatrics 42:614–626, 1968

Starfield B: Enuresis: Its pathogenesis and management. Clin Pediatr 11:343–350, 1971

Part IX: Cardiology

52

Childhood Dysrhythmias

All forms of dysrhythmias recognized in adulthood can occur in childhood as well. The majority of these are found in infants or children with underlying structural heart disease, but, with increased awareness and improved technology, they are being diagnosed more frequently in children with structurally normal hearts. Although they are always cause for concern, dysrhythmias in otherwise healthy children are rarely fatal. The presentation of a dysrhythmia can vary greatly, depending on the particular dysrhythmia, the age of the child, the presence or lack of heart disease or other systemic illness, and the duration of the dysrhythmia.

There are a variety of etiologies for dysrhythmias. Some dysrhythmias are congenital and have been diagnosed *in utero*, with complete atrioventricular (AV) block and tachycardia due to reentry pathway (Wolff-Parkinson-White syndrome) being examples. Systemic illnesses such as electrolyte imbalances, hypothyroidism or hyperthyroidism, infectious myocarditis or pericarditis, central nervous system (CNS) trauma or infection, or drug toxicity can result in dysrhythmias. In those children with heart disease, dysrhythmias can arise because of stretching of the right atrium (conditions associated with increased pulmonary venous return or tricuspid insufficiency), or secondary to anesthesia and procedures such as cardiac catheterization or cardiac surgery.

The term *dysrhythmia* is used in preference to the older term, arrhythmia, because the latter implies an absence of rhythm. In all but the case of asystole, rhythm is present but abnormal and more appropriately described as a dysrhythmia. This chapter will address the presentation, electrocardiographic (ECG) findings, and management of some of the more common dysrhythmias. For the sake of simplicity, they have been divided into those with a slow regular rate (bradydysrhythmias), those with a rapid rate (trachydysrhythmias), and those with a rate that is irregular.

To understand dysrhythmias, it is necessary to have a basic knowledge of the conduction pathways within the heart and the normal pattern of conduction. The heartbeat begins in the sinoatrial (SA) node, located in the high right atrium. This node is one of several pacemakers within the heart and has the most rapid rate, varying from 100 to 180 in the newborn to 50 to 100 in the adult. It is modulated by input from both sympathetic and parasympathetic afferents. The impulse arising in the SA node travels through the atria to the AV node. There appear to be three separate areas within the atria, consisting of atrial muscle and Purkinje's fibers arranged in parallel, through which the impulses from the SA node are conducted most rapidly. However, normal conduction does not depend on these, since disruption of these specific areas does not lead to delayed intranodal conduction times. The AV node is located in the lower right atrium, near the septum, coronary sinus, and annulus of the tricuspid valve. Like the SA node, the AV node has sympathetic and parasympathetic innervation. It also has an intrinsic rate that is slower than the SA node (80 to 90 in the newborn; 50 to 70 in the adult). Although the AV node is the only pathway through which impulses are normally conducted from the atria to the ventricles, accessory pathways (such as the bundle of Kent) exist in some people. These allow the atrial impulses to reach the ventricles prematurely, without passing through the AV node. In addition, they can transmit impulses in a retrograde direction from the ventricles to the atria. After passing through the AV node, the impulse is carried into the ventricular septum by the bundle of His. The bundle then branches to form the left and right bundle branches. These branches end as Purkinje's fibers supplying the ventricular endocardium. Depolarization, therefore, begins in the endocardium and spreads outward through the myocardium.

BRADYDYSRHYTHMIAS

Sinus Bradycardia

Sinus bradycardia is a slow heart rate with normal conduction. Congenital sinus brady-

cardia is rare in the absence of other heart disease. However, it occurs commonly in association with a wide variety of disorders. For example, asymptomatic sinus bradycardia can occur with vagal stimulation and in the well-trained athlete. Less benign causes of sinus bradycardia include hypothyroidism, hypopituitarism, hyperkalemia, hypothermia, acidosis, hypoxia, and intracranial hypertension. It is also found following damage to the sinus node, as may occur with the Mustard procedure performed in patients with transposition of the great vessels. A 24-hour ECG is indicated to rule out the presence of a second dysrhythmia, most commonly atrial tachycardia or premature ventricular contractions (PVC) and to document the degree of bradycardia with sleep and activity. In children over 5 years of age, a stress ECG can be used to evaluate the ability of the SA node in raising the heart rate with exercise. Intracardiac electrophysiologic (EP) studies can delineate conduction into and out of the SA node but are rarely indicated in the asymptomatic patient. (These EP studies are done in the cardiac catheterization laboratory. They require the placement of multiple catheters in specific areas of the heart. This allows the propagation of the electrical impulses through the heart to be evaluated.) Patients presenting with sinus bradycardia should be examined for evidence of poor cardiac output (weak pulses, mottling, cool skin, poor capillary refill). In the absence of such signs, no treatment is necessary. Atropine (0.01 to 0.10 mg/kg IV) can be used in patients demonstrating circulatory compromise.

Congenital Complete AV Block

The incidence of congenital complete AV block has been variably reported between 1/15,000 and 1/25,000 liveborn infants. Bradycardia occurs because there is a complete failure of transmission of the atrial impulse to the ventricles. This failure of conduction can occur at the level of the atrium–AV node, the AV node–bundle of His, or within the bundle of His. The ventricular rate is determined by the level of the block and is lower with the more distal lesions. Forty percent of infants with congenital heart block have structural heart disease. The diagnosis is often made *in utero* when fetal bradycardia is detected. Nonetheless, many of these infants have been delivered by emergency Cesarean section when their bradycardia was interpreted as "fetal distress." An echocardiogram can be useful in diagnosing complete AV block by demonstrating the motion of the mitral valve in relation to the ventricles. Assessment for fetal hydrops, evidence of congestive heart failure in the fetus, can be carried out at the same time. ECG shows absence of P waves and QRS complexes that are usually narrow. A wide QRS complex indicates a block below the AV node and is probably an indication for mechanical pacing. The babies most at risk for death in the first year of life are those with a ventricular rate <55 and an atrial rate >140, or those with an associated structural heart disease. Pacemaker therapy should be considered for these infants. Also, infants born with congestive heart failure unresponsive to conventional medical management or another significant medical problem usually require pacing. Many can be treated with diuretics alone or require no treatment at all. Those diagnosed some time after birth carry a better prognosis.

Acquired Complete AV Block

Complete AV block can be a complication of cardiac surgery or may occur in association with a systemic illness. Cardiomyopathies and infections are the most common causes of nonsurgically acquired complete AV block. In the case of the postsurgical patient, the prognosis depends on the site of the block, the ventricular rate and the underlying cardiac disease. With nonsurgical blocks, the outcome depends on the disease process and its reversibility.

TACHYDYSRHYTHMIAS

Supraventricular Tachycardia

The presentation and course of supraventricular tachycardia (SVT) vary with the age of the patient, as does the treatment and the response to treatment. SVT occurs in approximately 1/25,000 newborns. Intrauterine diagnosis has been made. The status of the fetus can range from asymptomatic to fetal hydrops and fetal death *in utero*. While SVT is often benign in the older child, it is frequently life-threatening in newborns. The presentation of newborns and young infants with SVT is similar. They are usually fussy and feed poorly. They often demonstrate hemodynamic compromise with pallor, cool and poorly perfused extremities, cyanosis, and hepatosplenomegaly. ECG usually shows abnormal P waves with a normal QRS complex with a very regular rate. P waves may appear normal or be difficult to discern at all. If a wide QRS complex is present, ventricular tachycardia should be suspected. The very rapid heart rates, as high as 230 to 320 beats per minute, shorten diastole and lead to poor ventricular filling. Chest radiograph may reveal cardiomegaly or pulmonary venous congestion. In infants with evidence of congestive heart failure, vagal maneuvers are very rarely successful in restoring sinus rhythm. The "diving" reflex may be useful in the child who is hemodynamically stable. It is most easily and safely elicited by placing an ice bag on the infant's face. Again, if the child is not critically ill, treatment with digoxin can be started (Table 52-1). This is usually done by administering a total digitalizing dose (TDD) of 25 to 50 µg/kg IV or 40 to

Table 52–1. Drug Therapy in Dysrhythmias

Drug	Indication	Dose	Side Effects
Atropine	Sinus bradycardia	0.01 mg/kg IV	Dry mouth, tachycardia, blurred vision; contraindicated in glaucoma
Digoxin	SVT, atrial flutter or fibrillation	*Load:* 50% stat, 25% q 6–8 hr for 2 doses; premature—20 μg/kg; newborn—30–50 μg/kg; <2 yr—60–80 μg/kg; 2–10 yr—40–60 μg/kg; >10 yr—0.75–1.25 mg *Maintenance:* 5–15 μg/kg/day PO q 12 hr, 0.125–0.25 mg PO q day in adults	Nausea, vomiting, diarrhea, vision disturbances, dizziness, ventricular extrasystole
Lidocaine	Acute ventricular dysrhythmias (PVC, VT)	1 mg/kg/dose slow IV push; can repeat q 5–10 min × 3, follow with continuous infusion of 20–50 μg/kg/min	Hypotension, seizures, asystole; contraindicated in SA, AV or intraventricular block
Phenylephrine	SVT	Children—5–10 μg/kg IV push; adults—0.25–0.5 mg/dose IV push	Tremor, insomnia, tachycardia
Phenytoin	Chronic ventricular dysrhythmias, digoxin-induced dysrhythmias	Children—2–4 mg/kg IV over 5 min, then 2–5 mg/kg/day	Gingival hyperplasia, vertigo, nystagmus, tinnitus, liver damage, hirsutism, blood dyscrasias
Procainamide	SVT, ventricular dysrhythmias	Children—load 3–6 mg/kg over 5 minutes, then 20–80 μg/kg/min IV or 15–50 mg/kg/d PO q 3–6 hr	Prolonged QRS, arrhythmias, GI symptoms, hypotension, lupus-like syndrome; contraindicated in complete heart block and myasthenia gravis
Propranolol	SVT, ventricular dysrhythmias	0.01–0.1 mg/kg/dose IV push *Maintenance:* 0.5–1.0 mg/kg/day PO q 6–8 hr	Hypotension, bradycardia, nausea, vomiting, bronchospasm; contraindicated in asthma or heart block
Quinidine	Ventricular dysrhythmias, SVT, atrial flutter/fibrillation, WPW	Children—15–60 mg/kg/day q 6 hr IV not recommended	Nausea, vomiting, diarrhea, hypotension, AV block, enhanced digoxin effect

70 µg/kg PO over a 24-hour period. One-half of the TDD is usually given initially, followed by one-fourth of the TDD every 8 to 12 hours. Maintenance therapy can then be started in doses of 10 to 15 µg/kg PO divided every 12 hours. Slightly lower doses are used when the drug is given parenterally. When signs of shock are present, synchronized direct current (DC) cardioversion (0.50 watt-sec/kg) is indicated and is a rapid and very effective therapy. While digoxin is effective in more than 75% of cases, there is a delay between drug administration and clinical response. Digoxin therapy should be started following cardioversion. Infants who present before 4 months of age and who are managed with this regimen rarely have a recurrence and can be taken off digoxin by 1 year of age.

Of those infants who do have recurrent SVT, 25% to 50% have Wolff-Parkinson-White (WPW) syndrome. WPW is a frequent underlying cause of SVT in patients of all ages. It is the result of conduction of an impulse from the atria to the ventricles by an accessory pathway, the bundle of Kent, that bypasses the AV node. This impulse reaches the ventricles before that which is conducted along the normal pathway through the AV node. This results in the characteristic ECG findings of a short PR interval followed by a "delta wave," a slurring at the onset of the QRS caused by the fusion of the more rapidly conducted impulse with that conducted normally. Since sudden death has been reported (albeit rarely) in patients with WPW treated with digoxin, electrophysiologic studies have been used to assess potential effects of digoxin on the accessory pathway prior to treatment with this agent. Verapamil, another potentially useful drug in the treatment of SVT and reentrant tachycardia, can also shorten the accessory pathway and worsen the rhythm disturbance in a few patients. If the patient does not demonstrate shortening of the antegrade refractory period through the accessory

pathway (placing the patient at risk for ventricular fibrillation) when given a test dose of ouabain during an EP study, digoxin or verapamil can be safely used. Propranolol and quinidine can be useful in WPW not treated with or not responsive to digoxin. Occasionally, surgical division of the accessory pathway may be necessary.

The older child who presents with SVT is likely to have WPW, although it is not always apparent on the ECG. Older children rarely present with congestive heart failure or shock. Usually, their heart rate is slower than that seen in infants and they present earlier because the child complains of a rapid heart rate or of feeling poorly. The typical findings of a shortened PR interval and delta wave may be present on the ECG. WPW must be suspected in children with recurrent SVT even in the presence of a normal ECG between episodes. Electrophysiologic studies can be used to confirm the diagnosis.

In children with acute SVT without WPW, vagal stimulation is often successful in aborting the episodes. Although digoxin has been the usual therapy, recently verapamil has been used to treat acute episodes of SVT. It is extremely effective in converting SVT to sinus rhythm. However, the incidence of side effects of verapamil is greater than that of digoxin, especially in infants. Verapamil acts primarily at the SA and AV nodes by blocking the transmembrane movement of calcium ions and prolonging nodal conduction times. Advantages of verapamil include very rapid onset of action and little risk of serious dysrhythmias should DC cardioversion be necessary following administration of verapamil. It can be administered intravenously in doses of 0.075 to 0.15 mg/kg IV (maximal dose, 5 mg) and can be repeated once 10 to 30 minutes following the first dose. Potential side effects, although uncommon, include a high degree of AV block, extreme bradycardia, asystole, and hypotension. The patient should be monitored with an ECG in an intensive care setting while the IV dose is slowly being infused. Calcium, isoproterenol and fluids for volume expansion should be available for treatment of the possible side effects before the verapamil is given. Side effects are more common in infants. Care should be taken to check for possible interactions with other medications that the patient is receiving prior to administering the drug. Phenylephrine (5 to 10 μg/kg IV) is another useful agent. If these measures fail, synchronized cardioversion is indicated. Digitalization increases the risk of ventricular fibrillation and should therefore be delayed until after cardioversion or the restoration of sinus rhythm. Long-term management can be accomplished through the use of oral verapamil or digoxin. Digoxin is administered as outlined above. Propranolol and quinidine can be used if these drugs are contraindicated or unsuccessful in preventing recurrences. Surgical ablation of the accessory pathways has been used in chronic, recurrent, disabling SVT.

Ventricular tachycardia

Ventricular tachycardia (VT) is another quite serious tachydysrhythmia. It is rare in children and especially rare in children with structurally normal hearts. Acute episodes of ventricular tachycardia occurring in conjunction with other disturbances are usually poorly tolerated. Some conditions that have been associated with ventricular tachycardia are hypoxia, acidosis, electrolyte disturbances (hypoglycemia, hyperkalemia or hypokalemia), drug toxicity (digoxin, quinidine, caffeine, phenothiazines), inhalational anesthetics, myocarditis, myocardial infarction, and as a result of procedures (due to intracardiac catheters during catheterization or following cardiac surgery). The prognosis of acute VT depends on the etiology, how quickly sinus

rhythm can be restored and whether or not the rhythm disturbance progresses to ventricular fibrillation with circulatory collapse. Chronically, VT can be asymptomatic or can present as syncope. It is rare for ventricular fibrillation to occur in the child with a structurally normal heart and chronic VT.

The characteristic ECG finding of ventricular tachycardia is that of repetitive (>3) contractions arising from the ventricle. The P waves are absent, and the QRS duration is prolonged, causing the QRS complex to widen. It must be distinguished from other dysrhythmias with widening of the QRS complex, including SVT.

Acute ventricular tachycardia almost always requires treatment. In the patient who is hemodynamically stable, the first step is to attempt to remove or reverse the precipitating cause. The first line of drug therapy is lidocaine, given initially as a bolus (1 mg/kg IV). If sinus rhythm is not restored, the lidocaine bolus can be repeated ever 5 to 10 minutes for a total of three doses. Following conversion, the patient can be started on a continuous infusion of lidocaine in a dose of 30 to 50 μg/kg/minute. Procainamide (1 mg/kg IV bolus) is the next line of therapy should lidocaine fail. This can be repeated every 5 minutes for as many as 15 doses. For the patient who is hemodynamically unstable, synchronized DC cardioversion (0.5 to 1.5 watt-sec/kg) is the treatment of choice. Ventricular pacing at a rate more rapid than that of the ventricle is sometimes successful. Propranolol can also be used. Because of the risk of sinus bradycardia following IV administration of propranolol, this therapy should be reserved for those patients with a ventricular pacing catheter in place. Drug levels must be monitored, since pharmacokinetics may be different in the infant and young child than in the older child or adult. Quinidine, procainamide, or phenytoin can be used for long-term suppression of ventricular dysrhythmias. Rarely, there may be a right-ventricular focus for the rhythm disturbance that is amenable to surgical excision.

Ventricular fibrillation

Ventricular fibrillation is truly a life-threatening emergency that rapidly results in death. The ECG shows no complexes, only a wavy tracing. Synchronized DC cardioversion (1 to 2 watt-sec/kg) is the appropriate treatment. This often results in another dysrhythmia, such as ventricular tachycardia, which can be treated accordingly.

IRREGULAR RHYTHMS

Like most of the other rhythm disturbances, dysrhythmias that result in an irregular heart rate are rare in children without heart disease. The most common types of irregular rhythms are premature ventricular contractions and first- and second-degree AV blocks. Bundle branch blocks in children are seen almost exclusively following cardiac surgery for congenital heart lesions.

Premature ventricular contractions (PVCs) are characterized by a widened QRS complex and lack of a preceding P wave. If there is more than one site of origin for the ectopic beats, the shape of the complex may vary. They are relatively uncommon and usually benign in the child with a normal heart. Multifocal beats, couplets (two PVCs occurring in succession), or bigeminy (alternating PVCs and normally conducted beats) rarely require emergency treatment in otherwise healthy children. In the presence of hemodynamic instability, an underlying illness with abnormal ventricular function or prolongation of the QT interval, suppression of the ventricular ectopy is indicated. The treatment is similar to the pharmacologic treatment outlined above for the management of ventricular tachycardia. The mainstay of therapy is lidocaine. Procainamide can also be useful.

First-degree heart block is the result of an abnormality of conduction through the AV node. There is a delay in the conduction of the atrial impulse through the AV node that is manifested on the ECG as a prolonged PR interval. All atrial impulses are conducted to the ventricles. Usually this has no apparent hemodynamic effect. It occasionally occurs as an isolated finding in the otherwise normal child. It can occur in association with infections (e.g, rheumatic fever, diphtheria, and viral myocarditis). It is also seen in association with congenital heart disease and following cardiac surgery. First-degree heart block can also be seen as a drug effect with certain antiarrhythmic agents, including digitalis preparations and propranolol. It is important to realize that this can be a desired effect of the drug and does not necessarily imply drug toxicity. No treatment is required for children with first-degree block. These patients should be followed periodically for progression to more severe forms of heart block.

Second-degree heart block is the result of the intermittent failure of atrial impulses to be transmitted to the ventricles. Two types have been recognized. In the first, Mobitz type I, there is progressive prolongation of the PR interval, eventually resulting in a nonconducted P wave (i.e., a dropped ventricular beat). Usually this block occurs at the AV node. Mobitz type I patterns are most commonly seen in children with congenital heart disease, with or without cardiac surgery. Other etiologies can be infectious or pharmacologic. Patients with type I blocks are rarely symptomatic and do not require treatment. There is a slight risk of progression to complete heart block.

The other type of second-degree heart

block, Mobitz type II, is more serious. With this pattern, the PR interval is constant, but the conduction of the P wave is blocked. When this occurs in isolation, the patient is asymptomatic. However, symptoms develop when several P waves are blocked in succession. The symptoms are usually those of cerebral hypoxia or congestive heart failure, with syncope being one of the most common complaints. The etiology of the type II block is unclear. It is much more likely to progress to complete heart block than is the Mobitz type I block. Acutely, the symptomatic patient can be treated with atropine (0.01 mg/kg IV). Ventricular pacing can be used should pharmacologic therapy fail. In asymptomatic children, further evaluation can be carried out with Holter monitoring or electrophysiologic studies prior to instituting therapy.

While rhythm disturbances are frightening to all concerned, the patient, the parents, and the physicians, they are rarely life-threatening in children. Like other conditions, their successful management depends on a proper diagnosis. A carefully taken history, a thorough physical examination, and an ECG are often sufficient to arrive at the diagnosis and make decisions about treatment. Better diagnostic techniques and pharmacologic agents are improving the understanding and management of the more serious rhythm disturbances, and improving the prognosis, as well.

BIBLIOGRAPHY

Campbell RM, Hammon JW Jr, Echt DS et al: Surgical treatment of pediatric cardiac arrhythmia. J Pediatr 110:501–508, 1987

Davignon A, Rautaharju P, Boiselle E et al: Normal ECG standards for infants and children. Pediatr Cardiol 1:123–131, 1979/80

Garson A Jr: The Electrocardiogram in Infants and Children: A Systematic Approach. Philadelphia, Lea Febiger, 1983

Gillette PC: Cardiac dysrhythmias in children. Pediatr Rev 3:190–198, 1981

Gillette PC, Garson A Jr: Pediatric Cardiac Dysrhythmias. New York, Grune & Stratton, 1981

Porter CJ, Garson A Jr, Gillette PC: Verapamil: An effective calcium blocking agent for pediatric patients. Pediatrics 71:748–755, 1983

Southall DP, Johnston F, Shinebourne EA et al: 24-hour electrocardiographic study of heart rate and rhythm patterns in population of healthy children. Br Heart J 45:281–291, 1981

53

Endocarditis

Inflammation of the endocardium, heart valves, or the adjacent vascular endothelium by bacterial, fungal, or rickettsial agents is termed *infective endocarditis*. About 20% of all cases of endocarditis occur in the first two decades of life. In the past, endocarditis typically complicated acquired rheumatic heart disease, usually in the setting of aortic or mitral valve involvement. Today, because of the more aggressive medical and surgical care offered these patients and the markedly decreased incidence of rheumatic fever, most pediatric cases of endocarditis arise in association with congenital structural heart disease. Patients who undergo cardiac surgery, especially when it entails prosthetic valve or synthetic graft implantation, are at increased risk for endocarditis. Among patients with normal hearts, the presence of intracardiac catheters (central venous lines, ventriculoatrial shunts), significant burns, or overwhelming sepsis with a highly virulent organism are risk factors for endocarditis. Unfortunately, intravenous drug abuse is responsible for an increasing number of cases of endocarditis (in addition to the better publicized cases of AIDS and hepatitis) in the pediatric population.

In the preantibiotic era, endocarditis was uniformly fatal. Antibiotic therapy, however, has not been a panacea; mortality averages 20%, and morbidity is often substantial. For instance, endocarditis can require surgical intervention if severe impairment of myocardial function or development of intractable myopericardial infection result. In addition, other organ systems, notably the central nervous system, kidneys, and lung, may be damaged by a combination of embolic and immune phenomena.

PATHOGENESIS

In most cases, endocarditis results from the seeding of a congenital or acquired heart lesion during a significant bacteremia or sepsis. Patients with tetralogy of Fallot, ventricular septal defect (especially when aortic insufficiency is also present), patent ductus arteriosus, coarctation of the aorta, and valvular aortic stenosis are at highest risk for endocarditis. In each of these defects, an abnormal pressure gradient generates turbulent flow that damages endocardium, valvular tissue, or

349

vascular endothelium. Conversely, endocarditis is rare in children with low pressure gradient defects (isolated atrial septal defect, mild pulmonic stenosis). The initial tissue injury develops distal to the pressure gradient (for instance, on the right ventricular endocardium in association with a ventricular septal defect) except in aortic stenosis, where injury usually occurs on the ventricular sides of the aortic valve leaflets. Tissue damage involves exposure of subendocardial collagen with subsequent deposition of platelet–fibrin aggregates, thrombus formation, and fibrous tissue overgrowth. Further modification of this tissue damage produces the vegetations characteristic of valvular endocarditis; histologically, vegetations consist of a central necrotic core surrounded by a shell of organizing fibrinous tissue coated by a thin layer of fibrin. These vegetations provide an excellent nidus for bacterial growth and replication; up to 10^9 to 10^{10} organisms per gram of tissue may be present. Furthermore, bacteria residing in this relatively avascular and acellular tissue are afforded some protection from natural defenses such as white cell phagocytosis and from circulating antimicrobial agents, making prolonged antibiotic therapy necessary to eradicate infections due to otherwise easily treated organisms.

Children with genetic diseases such as Marfan's or Hurler's syndrome who have structural valve abnormalities are also at increased risk for endocarditis.

The most common acquired heart lesion associated with endocarditis is rheumatic heart disease. In this setting, grossly abnormal aortic and/or mitral valves are prone to colonization during bacteremia.

Endocarditis may develop on prosthetic valves and on artificial grafts (Dacron, Teflon, Gortex) that are slow to endothelialize. The risk of endocarditis is highest in the immediate postoperative period, although late-onset endocarditis can occur.

Endocarditis associated with intravenous drug abuse probably arises in large part because of repetitive injections of particulate matter. In most cases, endocarditis is right-sided involving the tricuspid valve.

CLINICAL FEATURES

In the past, clinicians categorized endocarditis as acute or subacute based on the clinical presentation. Although these terms have now been largely abandoned because treatment and prognosis hinge more on the etiologic agent than the initial clinical setting, it is still important to be aware of the different presentations for diagnostic purposes.

Early symptoms of "subacute" endocarditis are nonspecific and include intermittent fever, malaise, anorexia, myalgias, arthralgias, headache, and backache. This indolent presentation may suggest viral infection, connective tissue disease, or malignancy. Given these symptoms, endocarditis must be highly suspect in patients with known congenital or acquired heart disease or in patients with a previous history of endocarditis. Endocarditis should also be considered in the differential diagnosis of fever of unknown origin in the normal host because 10% to 30% of cases of endocarditis occur without predisposing heart disease.

"Acute" endocarditis, on the other hand, is characterized by a fulminant course with high, spiking fevers, rapid destruction of valvular tissue, onset of congestive failure, and formation of myocardial abscesses.

In either case, cardiac examination is almost always positive for a new or changing murmur. Signs and symptoms of compromised cardiac function, such as congestive failure secondary to valvular disease, suggest that advanced disease is present.

Other signs and symptoms relate to embolic and immune phenomena. In left-sided endocarditis, emboli can occur to the central nervous system (resulting in altered mental status, seizures, focal neurologic deficits, and cerebral abscesses), to the kidneys (infarction with macroscopic or microscopic hematuria), and to the spleen. Cutaneous manifestations include petechiae and splinter hemorrhages of the nail beds. Funduscopic evaluation may reveal Roth's spots (pale areas enclosed by a hemorrhagic halo). Splenomegaly with or without left upper quadrant abdominal pain is often present in long-standing endocarditis.

Cases of right-sided endocarditis are more difficult to diagnose for at least three reasons. First, a right-sided murmur is soft and can easily be overlooked. Second, signs of systemic embolization are rarer in right-sided endocarditis because of the filtering capacity of the lungs (but are present in patients with congenital lesions with right-to-left shunts). Pulmonary emboli are less likely to be symptomatic in the pediatric age-group unless they are large, and multiple septic emboli may be confused with pneumonia. Finally, significant cardiac decompensation is unusual.

Classic signs of endocarditis in adults, such as Osler's nodes (tender intradermal erythematous lesions of the pads of the fingers, toes, hypothenar, and thenar eminences) and Janeway lesions (nontender hemorrhagic lesions on the palms or the soles) are rare in children and are probably immune-mediated.

EPIDEMIOLOGY

Infective endocarditis is most frequently due to bacteria; fungal endocarditis is usually seen only in certain high-risk groups such as critically ill neonates with central venous catheters and immunocompromised patients. Four organisms—*Streptococcus viridans*, *Staphylococcus aureus*, *Staphylococcus epidermidis*, and *Enterococcus*—account for up to 95% of cases of bacterial endocarditis in the pediatric population.

Many other organisms have been reported to cause endocarditis, including *Streptococcus pneumoniae*, group A β-hemolytic streptococcus, *Haemophilus influenzae*, a variety of gram-negative pathogens, *Neisseria gonorrhoeae*, and rickettsiae.

DIAGNOSIS AND TREATMENT

General principles

In view of the possibly nonspecific early presentation of endocarditis, a prompt diagnosis requires a careful history, physical examination, and a high degree of suspicion.

Important historical features besides a history of congenital or acquired heart disease include a preceding upper respiratory tract infection, tonsillectomy or adenoidectomy, dental procedures, urologic instrumentation, cutaneous or systemic staphylococcal infection, drug abuse, or indwelling central vascular catheter. It is notable that no more than one of four patients with heart disease who develop endocarditis have one of these risk factors identified.

When endocarditis is suspected, multiple blood cultures from different sites should be obtained under strict aseptic conditions. It is unnecessary to wait for fever spikes to obtain cultures, because bacteremia is continuous during endocarditis (one to hundreds of organisms per ml blood volume). Blood cultures are positive in 85% to 95% of cases. No further diagnostic benefit is accrued by obtaining more than six blood cultures; indeed, in culture positive cases, the first culture is positive at least 75% of the time. The most common cause of culture negative but surgically or autopsy proven endocarditis is prior antibiotic therapy. When blood cultures are negative, the diagnosis must be made on clinical grounds alone. Patients with culture negative endocarditis, especially those who do not defervesce after a week of antibiotic therapy, have an increased mortality.

Other than the blood culture, laboratory

tests are supportive rather than diagnostic. Typical findings include an elevated erythrocyte sedimentation rate, hematuria, and hematologic abnormalities such as a normochromic, normocytic anemia and a leukocytosis with a left shift. Rheumatoid factor may be present, and the C3 serum complement fraction may be decreased. Echocardiography may reveal valvular vegetations, although a normal study by no means rules out endocarditis.

Initial therapy should be directed at the most likely etiologic agents pending results of cultures and detailed testing of antibiotic sensitivities.

In "acute" endocarditis, the most common pathogen is *Staphylococcus aureus*. Other possible agents include *S. pyogenes*, *S. pneumoniae*, *N. gonorrhoeae*, and *Enterococcus*. Several blood cultures should be obtained over a few hours, and appropriate antibiotic therapy begun promptly.

In "subacute" endocarditis, the usual organism is *S. viridans*. *Enterococcus* or *S. aureus* may also be responsible. Current practice is to obtain six sets of cultures while observing the patient carefully to maximize the chance of recovering an organism to which antibiotic therapy can be best tailored.

Endocarditis following heart surgery can be due to the usual pathogens *(S. viridans, S. aureus, Enterococcus)* as well as indolent *(S. epidermidis,* diphtheroids) and nosocomial organisms (gram-negative bacilli, fungi). Early-onset endocarditis (<2 months) after prosthetic valve replacement is most likely due to *S. epidermidis, S. aureus,* or gram-negative bacilli, whereas late-onset endocarditis is most likely secondary to *S. viridans.*

In the addict, common pathogens include *S. aureus, Pseudomonas aeruginosa, Candida* species, *S. viridans,* and *Enterococcus.* Recently, regional variations of the causative agent have been noted.

The most likely organism to complicate endocarditis secondary to an intracardiac catheter is *S. aureus.* Neonates in particular are at increased risk for complications due to fungal pathogens.

When an organism is recovered, the minimum inhibitory concentration (MIC) and the minimum bactericidal concentration (MBC) of the antibiotic agent(s) in use must be determined, as well as the peak and trough antibiotic serum levels. The peak serum antibiotic level should at least be equivalent to a 1:8 dilution of the MBC. In addition, the trough serum antibiotic level should be equal to or greater than the MIC of the organism. Assuming adequate peak and trough levels can be attained without risking drug toxicity, it is important to follow the levels serially because individual pharmacokinetics can change over a short period of time for a variety of reasons.

Organisms that have high MICs to the usual antibiotics, tolerant organisms (such as *S. aureus* and nutritionally dependent streptococci), and unusual pathogens must have *in vitro* testing performed for antibiotic synergy.

No good data are available for the pediatric population to guide length of antibiotic therapy. In general, therapy has been given intravenously for periods ranging from 4 to 6 weeks up to 8 to 12 weeks for difficult-to-treat organisms. Oral therapy has been administered successfully in certain cases, but more data are required before recommending this mode of treatment.

In some cases, medical therapy alone is insufficient, and surgical intervention becomes necessary. Indications for surgery may include worsening or unmanageable congestive heart failure due to progressive valve destruction/dysfunction, persistent bacteremia despite adequate antibiotic therapy (acceptable antibiotic levels, proven *in vitro* antibiotic synergy), isolation of uncommon organisms with known high mortality (*i.e.,* gram-negative enteric bacilli and fungal pathogens where mortality is greater than 75%), evidence of myocardial abscess formation, purulent pericarditis secondary to valve-ring abscess, and persistent morbid emboli. Some authorities feel that in light of a high mortality in adult patients (>70%), early-onset prosthetic valve endocarditis is also an indication for surgery.

Specific therapeutic guidelines

Recommendations for antibiotic coverage in patients allergic to penicillin and in nonallergic patients are presented in Tables 53-1 and 53-2 for *S. viridans, S. aureus, S. epidermidis,* and *Enterococcus.*

Cleary and Kohl should be consulted for treatment of unusual bacterial pathogens (see the Bibliography).

Fungal pathogens require intravenous administration of amphotericin B for 6 to 12 weeks and, when possible, adjunctive oral 5-flucytosine therapy. Early surgery is advisable when large emboli are obvious.

Therapy of "acute" endocarditis before isolation of an organism should be started with nafcillin and gentamicin or, in the case of patients with a prosthetic valve or penicillin allergy, with vancomycin and gentamicin. It

Table 53–1. Antibiotic Treatment of Common Causes of Endocarditis*

Organism	Treatment No allergy to penicillin		Penicillin allergy	
S. viridans Low MIC (85%)	PEN1 ± STREP or GENT	4 weeks 2 weeks	VANC ± STREP or	4 weeks 2 weeks
High MIC (15%)	PEN2 + GENT	4–6 weeks	VANC + GENT	4–6 weeks
S. aureus Methicillin-sensitive	NAF ± GENT	4–6 weeks 2 weeks	VANC or CEPH	4–6 weeks
Methicillin-tolerant or resistant	VANC	4–6 weeks	VANC	4–6 weeks
S. epidermidis Methicillin-sensitive	NAF ± GENT or RIF	4–6 weeks	VANC ± GENT or RIF	4–6 weeks
Methicillin tolerant or resistant	VANC ± GENT or RIF	4–6 weeks	VANC ± GENT or RIF	4–6 weeks
Enterococcus	AMP OR PEN1 + GENT	4–6 weeks 4–6 weeks 4–6 weeks	VANC + GENT	4–6 weeks 4–6 weeks

*See Table 53-2 for antibiotic dosages.

Table 53–2. Antibiotic Dosages

Abbreviation	Antibiotic	Dose/kg	Maximum dose	Frequency	Route
PEN1	Penicillin G	25,000 units	3.5×10^6 units	q4h	IV
PEN2	Penicillin G	35,000 units	3.5×10^6 units	q4h	IV
STREP	Streptomycin	15 mg	500 mg	q12h	IM
CEPH	Cephalothin	25 mg	2 g	q6h	IV
VANC	Vancomycin	10 mg*	500 mg	q6h	IV
NAF	Nafcillin	25–35 mg	2 g	q4h	IV
GENT	Gentamicin	1.5–2.5 mg*	100 mg	q6–q8h	IV
RIF	Rifampin	7.5–15 mg	300 mg	q12h	PO
AMP	Ampicillin	50–75 mg	2 g	q6h	IV

*Monitor peak and trough serum levels serially.

is recommended that presumed endocarditis that is culture-negative be treated initially with nafcillin and gentamicin pending clinical response. Surgical intervention should be considered if the patient fails to improve.

PROPHYLAXIS

It is recommended that patients with certain congenital structural heart diseases or rheumatic heart disease and patients with a previous history of endocarditis receive antibiotic prophylaxis in situations where bacteremia is likely to occur (prior to dental procedures or instrumentation of the upper airway or genitourinary or gastrointestinal tracts). The most current recommendations for antibiotic prophylaxis as formulated by the American Heart Association can be found in the article by Shulman and associates (see the Bibliography).

BIBLIOGRAPHY

Cleary TG, Kohl S: Anti-infective therapy of infectious endocarditis. Pediatr Clin North Am 30:349–364, 1983

Kaplan EL, Shulman ST: Endocarditis. In Adams FH, Emmanouilides GC (eds): Heart Disease in Infants, Children, and Adolescents, pp 565–575. Baltimore, Williams & Wilkins, 1983

Kavey R-E W, Frank DM, Byrum CJ et al: Two-dimensional echocardiographic assessment of infective endocarditis in children. Am J Dis Child 137:851–856, 1983

Mendelsohn G, Hutchins GM: Infective endocarditis during the first decade of life. Am J Dis Child 133:619–622, 1979

Newburger JW, Nadas AS: Infective endocarditis. Pediatr Rev 3:226–230, 1982

Shulman ST, Amren DP, Bisno AL et al.: Prevention of bacterial endocarditis. Am J Dis Child 139:232–235, 1985, or Pediatrics 75:603–607, 1985

Stanton BF, Baltimore RS, Clemens JD: Changing spectrum of endocarditis in children. Am J Dis Child 138:720–725, 1984

54

Myopericardial Diseases

Diseases of the heart may affect exclusively the endocardium, the myocardium, or the pericardium. Often, however, disease of the myocardium and disease of the pericardium coexist, although symptoms may derive primarily from involvement of only one. The title of this chapter emphasizes this fact even as the discussion, for the sake of simplicity, makes the traditional classification of myocardial and pericardial diseases.

MYOCARDIAL DISEASES

Symptoms of myocardial disease arise for one or more of the following three reasons: (1) inadequate cardiac output (either at rest or during stress); (2) pulmonary and/or systemic congestion; and (3) insufficient myocardial blood flow. The etiologies and symptomatology of pediatric myocardial diseases differ markedly from those of the adult disorders. For instance, although the antecedents of coronary artery disease may originate in the pediatric period, similar disease is rarely observed in pediatric patients (*e.g.*, in association with specific congenital defects in lipid metabolism). A listing of the more common pediatric myocardial diseases is shown in Table 54-1.

Primary cardiomyopathies

Endocardial fibroelastosis. Three-quarters of cases of endocardial fibroelastosis (EFE) occur in association with other congenital heart diseases (coarctation of the aorta, aortic atresia), and symptoms and prognosis are a function of the underlying heart disease. This discussion centers on only the 25% of cases where EFE is an isolated finding (primary EFE). For reasons that are unclear, the incidence of primary EFE appears to be declining.

EFE typically presents in the neonate or young infant but occasionally manifests in adolescence. Although some neonatal cases have been linked to an *in utero* viral infection, the etiology of most cases is unknown. The pathologic hallmark of EFE is a thick whitish-gray plaque of fibroelastic tissue, which invests the endocardium and extends into the underlying myocardium. Histologic examination may demonstrate surrounding inflammation or calcification. Severe disease may involve all chambers of the heart (but rarely the right atrium), as well as the aortic and mitral valves. Symptoms of congestive heart failure (see Chapter 55) predominate when EFE is an isolated finding (25%). In the latter

Table 54–1. PEDIATRIC MYOCARDIAL DISEASES

Primary (idiopathic) cardiomyopathy
    Endocardial fibroelastosis (EFE)
    Dilated (congestive)
    Hypertrophic
    Restrictive
Secondary cardiomyopathy
    Myocarditis
        Viral
        Bacterial
        Other
    Autoimmune disease
        Systemic lupus erythematosus
        Juvenile rheumatoid arthritis
        Dermatomyositis
    Neuromuscular disease
        Duchenne's muscular dystrophy
        Friedreich's ataxia
    Metabolic disease
        Glycogen storage diseases
        Mucopolysaccharidoses
        Lipidoses
    Toxin-related
        Adriamycin
        Heavy metals
        Fluorinated hydrocarbons
    Endocrine disease
        Hyperthyroidism
    Neoplastic disease
        Myocardial tumors
        Pheochromocytoma
    Hematologic disease
        Sickle cell anemia
    Nutritional deficiency
        Protein–calorie malnutrition
        Beriberi (thiamine deficiency)
        Scurvy (vitamin C deficiency)

case, cardiomegaly on chest x-ray corresponds to multichamber cardiac dilatation. Depressed ST segments, inverted T waves, and ventricular hypertrophy on electrocardiogram (ECG) suggest myocardial dysfunction. Presence of complete heart block or Wolff-Parkinson-White syndrome indicates involvement of the conducting system. Echocardiography shows a dilated, poorly contractile heart and, sometimes, mural thrombi. In view of the nonspecific nature of these findings, a definitive diagnosis may require endomyocardial biopsy.

Treatment includes aggressive digitalization and other anticongestive measures. Therapy should be continued for at least 2 or 3 years until clinical, radiologic, and ECG findings return to normal. Earlier withdrawal of support has been associated with a poor outcome. Mortality is somewhat less than 50%. Good prognostic signs include later presentation of disease, clinical stability after initiation of treatment, gradual resolution of x-ray and ECG abnormalities, and survival through 5 years of age.

Dilated cardiomyopathy. Dilated cardiomyopathy is the most common idiopathic cardiomyopathy. Pathologically, it is distinct from EFE; the myocardium may be normal, or patchy areas of fibrosis and necrosis may be evident. Anatomic dilatation represents a compensatory response to diminished myocardial function. The etiology of the myocardial cell dysfunction is unknown. Mitochondrial abnormalities and other nonspecific changes are evident on electron microscopy.

The disease has an insidious onset but an unrelenting course. Symptoms are typical of most cardiomyopathies and arise secondary to congestive heart failure, arrhythmias, and systemic embolization from mural thrombi. Findings on physical examination are consistent with those of congestive heart failure; in addition, a murmur of mitral and/or tricuspid insufficiency and a gallop rhythm may be auscultated. Findings on chest x-ray, ECG, and echocardiogram are similar to those in dilated EFE. Myocardial biopsy may be necessary to confirm the diagnosis.

Treatment is directed at relief of congestive symptoms. Digitalization, when deemed necessary, should be conducted with caution because the injured myocardium is especially arrhythmogenic. Anticoagulation with an agent such as warfarin is used to minimize thromboembolic complications. Afterload-reducing agents are sometimes helpful when acute complications supervene.

Prognosis is poor. Occasionally, even severe disease remits, but this is the exception. Cardiac transplantation is the only definitive therapy.

Hypertrophic cardiomyopathy. Hypertrophic cardiomyopathy generally presents in late childhood or adulthood. Anatomically, myocardial hypertrophy is striking, often with disproportionate involvement of the interventricular septum. Microscopic examination may show a striking disarray of myocardial cell architecture. The etiology is unknown; some cases are familial and suggest autosomal-dominant transmission. Hypertrophic cardiomyopathy also occurs in association with mitral valve prolapse, Friedreich's ataxia, and Noonan's and multiple lentigines syndromes. A similar but transient disease, known as asymmetric septal hypertrophy (ASH), has been described in infants of diabetic mothers.

The disease may be asymptomatic or may cause a host of serious clinical symptoms, including fatigue, dyspnea on exertion, palpitation, angina, and syncope. Myocardial dysfunction may progress to frank congestive heart failure. Symptoms result from a combination of left ventricular outflow obstruction (secondary to the hypertrophied interventricular septum or to anomalous anterior motion of the anterior mitral valve leaflet during systole, both of which encroach upon the left ventricular outflow tract), diminished diastolic filling (secondary to decreased ventricular compliance), and arrhythmias. Symptoms relating to obstruction worsen when preload falls or contractility increases. Conversely, obstructive symptoms abate with an increase in preload or a lessening od contractility.

Cardiovascular examination generally is notable for a palpable thrill and sometimes a double cardiac impulse secondary to a strong atrial contraction. A systolic ejection murmur is characteristically heard at the mid- to lower left sternal border and radiates to the apex. Presence of an S_4 confirms abnormal ventricular compliance. The strength of the pulse varies because of the beat-to-beat variability of the left ventricular obstruction. The underlying pathophysiology has led to the development of helpful diagnostic tests. Thus, auscultation during maneuvers that decrease preload (Valsalva's maneuver), decrease afterload (inhalation of amyl nitrite), or increase contractility (intravenous infusion of isoproterenol) intensify the systolic murmur. Conversely, increasing preload by elevation of the lower extremities diminishes the murmur.

Chest x-ray may show cardiomegaly or a normal-sized heart if hypertrophy occurs at the expense of chamber volume. ECG invariably demonstrates evidence of left ventricular hypertrophy; precordial q waves emphasize hypertrophy of the interventricular septum. Supraventricular tachycardias or Wolff-Parkinson-White syndrome may be noted. Echocardiogram confirms asymmetric septal or generalized cardiac hypertrophy, diminished contractility of the interventricular septum, and often some degree of systolic anterior motion of the anterior mitral valve leaflet.

Therapy includes proscription of exercise and pharmacologic treatment with β-adrenergic blockers (*e.g.*, propranolol) to diminish contractility and lessen left ventricular outflow obstruction. By decreasing heart rate, propanolol may also have the desirable effect of augmenting ventricular filling. Antiarrhythmic therapy may be necessary; in this case, digitalis preparations are usually contraindicated because of their inotropic effects. Calcium channel blockers such as verapamil may improve ventricular compliance. Occasionally, symptomatic relief requires surgical resection of the outflow tract. Unfortunately, surgery does not lesson the risks of myocardial dysfunction, arrhythmia, or sudden death.

Restrictive cardiomyopathy. Restrictive cardiomyopathy is rare in pediatrics. The abnormality is markedly decreased ventricular compliance in the absence of significant myocardial hypertrophy. Symptoms result from pulmonary and systemic venous congestion due to high diastolic filling pressures. In the United States, hemochromatosis and amyloidosis are the usual causes. This disease must be differentiated from constrictive pericarditis, since pericardial resection is curative in the latter case; because of the similarity of hemodynamic and other clinical findings, myocardial biopsy may be required.

In tropical regions, an entity known as endomyocardial fibrosis is common. This disease combines elements of restrictive and hypertrophic cardiomyopathy. The etiology is thought to be due to an autoimmune process. There is sometimes an associated eosinophilia.

Secondary cardiomyopathies

Myocarditis. Infectious myocarditis is the most common cause of cardiomyopathy in the pediatric patient. Nonetheless, a precise incidence has been difficult to establish, in part because many cases are subclinical. In one study from Minnesota, 17% of 90 autopsied children between infancy and 17 years of age who died suddenly and unexpectedly had pathologic evidence of myocarditis. In the same study, myocarditis was present in 2 of 48 (4%) of postmortem examinations of children who died violently. This is consistent with the 2% to 5% incidence found in similar autopsy studies of adults. It has also been estimated that 5% of all viral illnesses are complicated by some degree of myocardial involvement.

Myocarditis was recognized by the late 1800s in association with epidemics of mumps and pleurodynia (now known to be caused by coxsackievirus and echovirus). Since then, the list of etiologic agents has expanded and now includes many viruses, bacteria, rickettsiae, fungi, protozoa, and other parasites.

The pathology of myocarditis depends primarily on the etiologic agent, the age of the patient at the onset of disease, and the duration of myocarditis. Gross examination at autopsy may reveal a normal heart, especially if sudden death occurred early in the course. Usually, the myocardium is soft and pale, and the heart is dilated. Scarring observed on cut section implies a longer duration of disease. Occasionally, there is ventricular hypertrophy. Perinatal coxsackievirus B infection is associated with EFE. Abscesses, petechiae, and hemorrhage usually indicate a bacterial etiology; caseous nodules are a clue to tuberculous myocarditis. Rubella infection during the first trimester has been associated with pulmonic stenosis and persistent patent ductus arteriosus. Microscopically, there is inflammation and necrosis, although necrosis without inflammation is typical of perinatal rubella myocarditis. Initially, the infiltrate is composed of polymorphonuclear cells but is replaced in several days by lymphocytes, histiocytes, and plasma cells. Necrotic areas later are replaced by fibrous tissue and may calcify. Toxins elaborated by bacteria (e.g., diphtheria toxins) induce fatty degeneration. Vasculitis is common in rickettsial infection.

Clinically, there is a spectrum of disease. The incidence of serious disease is highest in neonates, who may acquire the infection transplacentally or postnatally. Coxsackievirus B, an RNA picornavirus, accounts for at least half of the cases in which an etiology is identified. After an incubation period of 2 to 8 days, and usually between 5 and 10 days of age, infants present with nonspecific signs including fever, excessive tachycardia, and lethargy. Symptoms can progress rapidly as respiratory distress, peripheral vascular collapse, and congestive heart failure ensue. Arrhythmias may complicate the cardiac disease. Infants invariably have systemic involvement affecting the brain, liver, adrenal glands, and pancreas; mortality is as high as 50%. Treatment is supportive.

Myocarditis is relatively uncommon in the older infant, but the incidence increases again later in childhood. In this population, the disease is frequently preceded by an upper respiratory infection or gastroenteritis; initial symptoms are again nonspecific, and the course is more insidious. Cardiac involvement may occur suddenly as symptoms of the intercurrent illness resolve. A common symptom is chest pain, which usually indicates concomitant pericarditis. Cardiac examination reveals a diminished S_1 and a gallop rhythm. A pericardial friction rub may be audible. Other signs of congestive heart failure may appear transiently. Chest x-ray reveals cardiomegaly. ECG shows supraventricular tachycardia or possibly atrioventricular dissociation with ectopic beats. Limb and left precordial leads demonstrate ST segment depression and T wave depression or inversion. Voltage is generally diminished. Echocardiogram confirms abnormal contractility and screens for pericardial effusion. Serum myocardial enzymes are elevated early in the course. Prognosis in older patients is very good, although sudden death may occur, presumably secondary to arrhythmias.

Identification of the specific etiologic agent can be difficult. The definitive method is direct isolation or identification of the virus from tissue, preferably from pericardial fluid. This usually is possible only in the first several days of illness. Specific cell lines are inoculated with the sample and later examined for characteristic cytopathic changes. Alternatively, biopsied tissue may be examined for pathognomonic changes by light or electron microscopy or by direct or indirect immunofluorescent techniques. The problem with the latter method is a tendency for myocardium to show nonspecific fluorescence. Finally, paired acute (less than 1 week) and convalescent (at least 2 weeks after onset of symptoms) antibody titers can be assayed by radioimmunoassay (RIA) or enzyme-linked immunoabsorbant assay (ELISA). Greater than a fourfold rise in specific titer is diagnostic.

In all cases, treatment begins with bed rest; clinical and experimental animal studies have linked premature resumption of physical activity to increased mortality. When possible, appropriate antibiotic or antiviral agents should be administered. Development of congestive heart failure demands scrupulous attention to oxygenation and a heightened regard for possible digitalis toxicity as standard therapies (see Chapter 55) are employed. Arrhythmias should be treated aggressively. Some clinicians use a combination of corticosteroid and immunosuppressive (azathioprine) therapy if myocardial disease is severe or prolonged. In this case, it seems prudent to continue azathioprine therapy for a period after steroids are discontinued.

Prognosis after recovery is generally good, although the course may be complicated by subacute and chronic disease, which increase in likelihood in proportion to the degree of initial myocardial involvement.

Myocardial disease associated with connective tissue disease. Among connective tissue diseases that present during childhood, systemic lupus erythematosus (SLE), juvenile rheumatoid arthritis (JRA), and dermatomyositis can be complicated by heart disease.

Some type of cardiac disease occurs in up to 40% of cases of SLE. Most frequently, clinical symptoms (*e.g.*, chest pain) are secondary to pericarditis. Verrucous endocarditis (Libman-Sacks disease) may also develop. Myocardial involvement ranges from subclinical disease to congestive heart failure. Pathologic findings include fibrinoid degeneration of myocardial collagen and focal myocardial necrosis. Myocarditis is less common in JRA and, as a rule, is subclinical in dermatomyositis. ECG and echocardiographic findings are consistent with a dilated cardiomyopathy. Myocardial dysfunction in SLE and JRA usually responds well to steroid therapy.

Kawasaki's disease (see Chapter 35) is discussed briefly here because of its pathologic similarity to infantile polyarteritis nodosa, which is quite rare. The etiology is unknown. Although pancarditis may complicate the initial phase of Kawasaki's disease, the most feared complications result from vasculitis of the major coronary arteries. The vasculitis can cause coronary artery aneurysmal dilatation or thrombosis or can result in arrhythmias. Sudden death occurs in 1% to 2% of patients secondary to severe myocardial dysfunction, arrhythmias, myocardial infarction, or, rarely, coronary artery rupture. Although the risk of sudden death peaks during convalescence, about 3 weeks after the onset of clinical symptoms, sudden death also may occur months or years later. Because most clinically significant disease is limited to the proximal coronary arterial tree, two-dimensional echocardiography has been used to screen for coronary aneurysms. More invasive evaluation with coronary angiography is restricted to patients with positive echocardiograms. Aspirin therapy is commonly employed until all clinical, laboratory, and cardiac abnormalities have resolved.

Myocardial involvement in other diseases.
Myocardial disease characterized by fibrosis, hypertrophy, and, sometimes, infarction, is common in Duchenne's muscular dystrophy, an X-linked recessive disease. Interestingly, there is little correlation between the extent of skeletal muscle and myocardial disease. Symptomatic congestive heart failure is relatively uncommon. Friedreich's ataxia is a less

common neuromuscular disease with autosomal-recessive inheritance that, as a rule, is complicated by cardiac pathology. In addition to hypertrophic cardiomyopathy (see above), pathologic findings include fatty degeneration, fibrosis, and premature coronary atherosclerosis. The clinical cardiac presentation is similar to that of Duchenne's muscular dystrophy. ECG abnormalities (T wave changes, arrhythmias) are sometimes the first clue to the diagnosis. The extent of neurologic disease does not necessarily correlate with myocardial dysfunction.

Nutritional deficiency states that affect myocardial performance include protein–calorie malnutrition, beriberi or thiamine deficiency (especially the infantile form), and scurvy or vitamin C deficiency. Although these disorders are rare in the United States, they are responsible for significant morbidity in many developing nations, where severe dietary deficiencies are common.

A variety of metabolic storage diseases can result in striking myocardial dysfunction. Among the glycogen storage diseases, myocardial pathology is found in types II (Pompe's disease), III, IV (Andersen's disease), and V (McArdle's disease), but clinical cardiac symptoms are significant only in Pompe's disease. Death occurs in infancy secondary to progressive congestive heart failure or to arrhythmias. Many of the mucopolysaccharidoses are complicated by aortic or mitral valve disease. A third category of metabolic disease with cardiac pathology are the lipidoses.

Finally, myocardial disease may accompany hematologic, endocrinologic, or neoplastic disorders or ensue as a side effect of chemotherapy or toxin ingestion.

PERICARDIAL DISEASES

Pericarditis with or without pericardial effusion is the most common type of pericardial disease in the pediatric population. Moreover, the clinical presentation of many of the infectious and inflammatory causes of myocarditis already discussed may be dominated instead by symptoms of pericardial disease. Partial and total congenital defects of the pericardium, pericardial cysts or diverticula, and neoplastic involvement of the pericardium (usually by hematogenous or contiguous spread of a secondary cancer) also occur but are much less common.

Pericarditis. When pericarditis is not complicated by significant effusion, as is often the case during viral pericarditis, the most common cardiac symptom is chest pain that may vary with respiratory effort. Occasionally, the patient experiences palpitations. A friction rub may be audible. Fever, arthralgias, myalgias, and symptoms of upper respiratory or gastrointestinal illness are frequently present. ECG may be unremarkable or may show a characteristic progression of abnormalities. Initially, the ST segment is elevated. As the ST segment returns to baseline, the T wave first lessens in amplitude and then inverts. The latter T wave changes often persist for weeks to months after clinical recovery. In the absence of a large pericardial effusion, other laboratory tests add little information. Although the white blood cell count may be normal, the differential may show a lymphocytosis. Treatment is supportive and consists of bed rest, administration of salicylates (for control of fever, chest pain, and inflammation) or more potent analgesics.

Pericardial effusion. Injury to the pericardium provokes some combination of exudation of fluid, fibrin, and inflammatory cells. Common injuries that produce clinically significant pericardial effusions include viral, bacterial, or other causes of infectious pericarditis; noninfectious inflammatory diseases such as rheumatic fever, SLE, JRA, and uremia; and direct pericardial trauma from accidental (e.g.,

blunt trauma) or surgical (e.g., postpericardiotomy syndrome) events. Pericardial fluid may also accumulate when the local balance of Starling forces is disturbed (increased venous pressure, severe hypoalbuminemia, lymphatic obstruction secondary to tumor) or when leukemic or lymphoma cells "metastasize" to the pericardium.

The symptomatology of a large pericardial effusion depends on its etiology, rate of accumulation, the relative compliances of the pericardium and myocardium, and the filling pressure of the heart as determined principally by the blood volume and degree of venous constriction. The hemodynamic symptoms associated with pericardial effusions of bacterial or noninflammatory etiology may be overshadowed by other symptoms of the underlying disease. A relatively small amount of fluid that accumulates rapidly is more likely to cause circulatory compromise than gradual exudation of an effusion triple or quadruple in volume. Effusions into a fibrotic or constrictive pericardium with reduced compliance result in a steeper rise in pericardial pressure compared to normal. On the other hand, a hypertrophied or stiff myocardium is more resistant to elevations in pericardial pressure. Acute hypovolemia may initiate or markedly exacerbate circulatory insufficiency in the setting of a pericardial effusion; conversely, volume loading may temporally relieve symptoms by increasing the filling pressure of the heart.

Physical signs of pericardial effusion include elevation of venous pressure (distention of jugular veins with increased venous pulsations), tachycardia (a compensation for decreased stroke volume), and, finally, shock (if frank cardiac tamponade supersedes). Pulsus paradoxus (a decrease of more than 10 mm Hg in systolic pressure with quiet inspiration) is a classic sign that aids in the differentiation of a large pericardial effusion from myocardial dysfunction. The physiological explanation of pulsus paradoxus is still debated. On examination, heart sounds are decreased or distant, and the maximal cardiac impulse is reduced. With large effusions, pulsus alternans may be present. Chest x-ray demonstrates globular cardiomegaly (the "leather water-bottle" sign). QRS voltage is diminished, and electrical alternans may be noted on ECG. Echocardiogram provides the best means to document the size of the effusion and may be necessary to rule out myocardial dysfunction.

Treatment of pericardial effusions depends on the etiology and hemodynamic symptoms. Purulent bacterial effusions are best treated initially with antibiotics, barring extreme systemic toxicity or symptoms of tamponade. The latter two circumstances demand immediate drainage. Most clinicians recommend eventual drainage as part of the management for purulent pericarditis.

Although a pericardial tap may be crucial for diagnostic or therapeutic purposes, the procedure may be complicated by laceration of the myocardium or a coronary artery. The patient is placed in the supine position with the head of the bed slightly elevated. Under sterile conditions, an appropriately sized needle is then inserted under the xyphoid toward the spine or the left shoulder at about a 30° angle to the plane of the patient. An alligator clip connected to the V lead of the ECG is attached to the distal end of the needle after it is inserted subcutaneously. The needle is advanced slowly as gentle aspiration is provided continuously. Usually, puncture of the pericardium gives the sensation of a "pop." It is important to monitor the ECG, because inadvertent contact of the needle with the epicardium causes an injury current manifested by ST segment depression. When continuous drainage is desired, a flexible catheter can be threaded through the needle into the pericardial space.

BIBLIOGRAPHY

Feldman W: Bacterial etiology and mortality of purulent pericarditis in pediatric patients. Am J Dis Child 133:641–644, 1979

French JW: Diseases of the myocardium. In Kelley VC (ed): Practice of Pediatrics. Philadelphia, Harper & Row, 1985

Gersony W, Hordof A: Infective endocarditis and diseases of the pericardium. Pediatr Clin North Am 25:831–846, 1978

Guntheroth WG: Diseases of the pericardium. In Kelley VC (ed): Practice of Pediatrics, Philadelphia, Harper & Row, 1985

Harris L, Powell G, Brown O: Primary myocardial disease. Pediatr Clin North Am 25:847–867, 1978

Spodick D: The normal and diseased pericardium: Current concepts of pericardial physiology, diagnosis, and treatment. J Am Coll Cardiol 1:240–251, 1983

Woodruff JF: Viral myocarditis: A review. Am Pathol 101:425–479, 1980

55 Congestive Heart Failure

The function of the heart is to supply sufficient blood flow to meet the metabolic demands of the body for oxygen and other nutrients over time. To accomplish this, the heart must work as an efficient mechanical pump and empty the systemic and pulmonary venous returns into their respective pulmonary and systemic arterial circuits. Congestive heart failure is the clinical syndrome that results from failure of the heart to perform adequately as a pump. In severe heart failure, symptoms relate to engorgement (congestion) of the pulmonary and systemic venous systems, systemic hypoperfusion, and the systemic effects of compensatory mechanisms that attempt to increase cardiac output to match metabolic requirements. Since right-sided or left-sided heart failure or both may be present, symptoms as well as their severity vary from patient to patient.

PHYSIOLOGY

Electrical stimulation of a myocardial cell generates tension and results in cell shortening (contraction) that depends on the resting length of the cell and its load. Within limits, if the cell is stretched at a given load, contraction generates a greater tension and increases cell shortening. In this respect, the heart is analogous to a collection of individual muscle cells. An increase in end-diastolic volume at constant systolic load augments the force of contraction of the heart muscle, which, in turn, increases ejection fraction, stroke volume, and, therefore, cardiac output. This improvement in performance arises because cell elongation aligns the contractile proteins in a more efficient configuration for contraction. The capacity of the heart to increase its output (and perform more work) as its end-diastolic load rises is described by the Starling curve (Fig. 55-1).

It should now be apparent that cardiac output is determined by a complex interplay among four factors: the end-diastolic ventricular load (preload), the resistance against which the heart must pump (afterload), the intrinsic ability of the heart to generate force at a given preload and afterload (contractility), and the heart rate. At a fixed afterload, a decrease in contractility shifts the Starling curve down and to the right, so that an equiv-

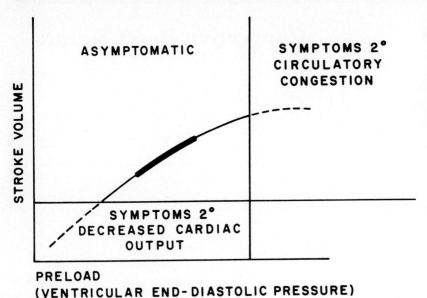

ASYMPTOMATIC

SYMPTOMS 2°
CIRCULATORY
CONGESTION

STROKE VOLUME

SYMPTOMS 2°
DECREASED CARDIAC
OUTPUT

PRELOAD
(VENTRICULAR END-DIASTOLIC PRESSURE)

FIGURE 55–1. Schematization of the Starling curve for the normal heart. Stroke volume as a function of the normal range of preload is indicated by the heavy portion of the curve. Preload can rise or fall outside of the normal range and not produce symptoms. Further increases or decreases in preload, however, cause symptoms related to circulatory congestion and systemic hypoperfusion, respectively.

alent amount of cardiac work requires an increase in preload. A similar shift in the Starling curve can attend an increase in afterload if contractility is unaltered. Conversely, either an increase in contractility or a decrease in afterload moves the Starling curve up and to the left (Fig. 55-2). An isolated increase in heart rate achieved by a pacemaker will raise cardiac output as long as ventricular preload is undiminished. Acute increases in heart rate also improve cardiac contractility when they are mediated by increased levels of circulating catecholamines.

Preload is best assessed by the end-diastolic ventricular pressure, which reflects both the venous return and the pressure–volume characteristics (compliance) of the ventricle. Right ventricular preload is inferred clinically by estimation of the central venous pressure. Accurate determination of left ventricular preload requires the measurement of left ventricular end-diastolic pressure, or of pulmonary capillary wedge pressure in the absence of complicating pulmonary vascular disease. When the compliance of the heart is normal, echocardiographic measurement of ventricular end-diastolic dimensions is a useful measure of preload.

Afterload is easily conceived as the total resistance to ventricular unloading. Clinicians have estimated afterload by using the systolic blood pressure as an indirect measure of peripheral vascular resistance. Blood pressure alone, however, does not reliably mirror changes in afterload; for instance, a decrease in resistance (R) may result in an increase in cardiac output (Q) without a change in pressure $(P = Q \times R)$. In addition, direct measurements of resistance only approximate afterload. A more exact definition of afterload is the arterial impedance, or the instantaneous (rather than the mean) relationship between pulsatile pressure and flow. Unfortunately, this measurement is technically unwieldly. In the clinical arena, the success of pharmacologic efforts to reduce afterload can be judged

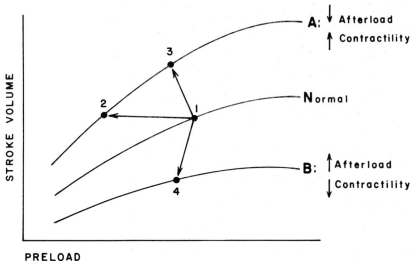

PRELOAD
(VENTRICULAR END-DIASTOLIC PRESSURE)

FIGURE 55–2. Curve N designates the Starling curve for a normal·heart. An increase in contractility or a decrease in afterload shifts the curve up and to the left (curve A). Conversely, a decrease in contractility or an increase in afterload depresses the Starling relationship (curve B). Note that a change in preload can accompany alterations of contractility or afterload. Hence, a shift to curve A could result in no change (1 to 2), a decrease, or an increase (1 to 3) in cardiac output.

from serial assessments of peripheral perfusion and heart rate even if systemic blood pressure does not change.

In the past, simultaneous changes in preload and afterload have precluded confident determination of cardiac contractility. However, the relationship between end-systolic volume and pressure has recently been described as an index of contractility.

DEVELOPMENTAL DIFFERENCES IN MYOCARDIAL RESERVE

The infant heart has a lower reserve capacity to increase its output when confronted with acute stresses than does the more mature heart of an older child, adolescent, or adult. Preload, systolic, and heart rate reserve are each limited.

The infant heart's *preload reserve* is limited for two principal reasons. First, the compliance of the infant heart is less than its adult counterpart; thus, a given increase in diastolic volume in the stiffer infant heart leads to a relatively larger rise in end-diastolic ventricular pressure. Second, the Starling curve of the infant heart plateaus at lower end-diastolic ventricular pressures than does the adult curve. Except when preload is abnormally decreased, only limited increases in cardiac output are achieved acutely by increasing preload.

Isolated contractile elements of the infant

heart generate as much tension as adult elements; however, the infant heart as a whole has fewer myofilaments per unit mass than the adult heart and thus generates less force at the same preload and afterload. Therefore, the Starling curve of the infant heart is depressed compared to the adult's, in part accounting for its decreased *systolic reserve*. In addition, for a variety of reasons, the infant heart does not respond as well as the adult heart to endogenous and exogenous inotropic stimuli. It must also be noted that the oxygen requirement (per unit surface area) of the growing infant exceeds that of the adult. Thus, the young heart at rest is already operating at a very high capacity.

Finally, the *heart rate reserve*, or the ability to increase cardiac output simply by increasing heart rate, is limited in the infant. The resting infant heart rate is already high; marked increases in heart rate shorten diastole and can diminish ventricular filling and compromise myocardial perfusion during diastole.

PATHOPHYSIOLOGY OF HEART FAILURE

The ability of the heart to perform adequately as a pump is a function the metabolic requirements of the body and the prevailing preload, afterload, contractility, and heart rate. The cause of heart failure is always a primary abnormality of one or more of these factors. Symptoms of heart failure arise because of at least one of the following reasons (Fig. 55-2):

1. Depression of cardiac output below a critical level (because of decreased contractility, increased afterload, or markedly increased or decreased preload) causes symptoms secondary to systemic hypoperfusion.

2. Excessive increases in central venous or pulmonary venous pressure (because of an acute volume overload or a more gradual compensatory increase in preload to raise cardiac output *via* the Starling mechanism) produce symptoms referable to systemic or pulmonary venous congestion.

3. Compensatory mechanisms for increasing cardiac output (*i.e.*, high levels of circulating endogenous catecholamines) may have their own systemic effects.

Etiologies

In the adult, congestive heart failure is usually acquired as a physiologic aftermath of coronary artery disease, myocardial infarction, or lung disease. Less commonly, it is a consequence of a congenital defect. The etiology of congestive heart failure in infancy and childhood is fundamentally different (Table 55-1). In infancy, heart failure is frequently due to structural congenital heart disease. In this case, the earlier the onset of heart failure during infancy, the more severe the defect. Heart failure in childhood is more likely to be acquired (*i.e.*, rheumatic heart disease, endocarditis, myocarditis).

A structurally normal heart with intrinsically normal myocardial function may not be able to fulfill its role as a pump in the face of either excessive somatic metabolic requirements and/or an abnormal metabolic or circulatory milieu. Fever, thyrotoxicosis, and other endocrine diseases characterized by high circulating catecholamine levels can precipitate congestive heart failure by increasing systemic oxygen consumption. Pathologic metabolic and circulatory states can precipitate heart failure. These include conditions of increased preload (severe anemia, acute volume overload, cerebral, hepatic or pulmonary arteriovenous shunts), decreased preload (hypovolemia, tachyarrhythmias), increased afterload (systemic hypertension, polycythemia/hyperviscosity), and decreased contractility (hypo-

Table 55–1. Etiologies of Congestive Heart Failure

Structurally normal heart
High output states
  Fever
  Hyperthyroidism
  Increased circulating catecholamines or other drugs
    (theophylline)
  Anemia
  Systemic arteriovenous fistulae
Low output states
  Myocarditis or cardiomyopathy
  Metabolic abnormalities (hypoglycemia,
    hypocalcemia)
  Asphyxia
  Arrhythmias
  Polycythemia
  Systemic hypertension
  Persistent pulmonary hypertension of the newborn
Structurally abnormal heart
Outflow obstruction
  Left heart
    Hypoplastic left heart
    Coarctation of the aorta
    Critical aortic stenosis
  Right heart
    Critical pulmonic stenosis or pulmonic atresia
Obstruction or restriction of venous return
  Left heart
    Hypoplastic left heart
    Mitral stenosis or mitral atresia
    Cor triatriatum
  Right heart
    Hypoplastic right heart
    Tricuspid atresia
    Anomalous pulmonary venous return with
      obstruction
Increased preload
  Left heart
    Ventricular septal defect
    Patent ductus arteriosus
    Truncus arteriosus
    Atrioventricular canal
    Aortic or mitral insufficiency
    Aortopulmonary window
  Right heart
    Ebstein's anomaly
    Pulmonic or tricuspid insufficiency
Other
  Anomalous origin of the left coronary artery

calcemia, hypoglycemia, acute asphyxia, chronic hypoxemia secondary to airway obstruction or cystic fibrosis).

A common cause of heart failure in infancy is structural congenital heart disease. Conversely, up to 90% of all congenital heart defects recognized in the neonatal period include some degree of heart failure. The three most common classes of defects are those that obstruct outflow (especially of the left ventricle) and impose an excessive afterload, those that obstruct venous return and interfere with preload, and those that produce volume overload.

Defects that obstruct ventricular outflow include the hypoplastic left heart syndrome, coarctation of the aorta, and critical aortic stenosis. Early in the course, systemic flow is augmented by a right-to-left shunt across the patent ductus arteriosus. As this fetal vascular channel constricts postnatally, symptoms relating to systemic hypoperfusion become prominent. Pulmonic valvular stenosis or atresia are lesions that obstruct right ventricular outflow.

Left ventricular preload is compromised in hypoplastic left heart syndrome, mitral stenosis or atresia, cor triatriatum and pulmonary vein stenosis. Right ventricular preload is decreased in hypoplastic right heart syndrome, tricuspid atresia, and anomalous pulmonary venous return with obstruction.

Preload is increased in defects characterized by atrioventricular or semilunar valve insufficiency (*i.e.*, atrioventricular canal, Ebstein's anomaly) or in lesions characterized by a large left-to-right intracardiac shunt (ventricular septal defect, patent ductus arteriosus, truncus arteriosus and aortopulmonary window). Symptoms referable to pulmonary edema are especially prominent in these conditions.

A relatively uncommon defect that can produce dramatic heart failure is an anomalous origin of the left coronary from the pulmonary artery. In this case, myocardial contractile function is impaired because of diminished myocardial oxygen delivery.

CLINICAL SIGNS AND SYMPTOMS

The clinical manifestations of congestive heart failure are logical corollaries of its pathophysiology.

In the adult, the earliest manifestation of congestive heart failure is easy fatigability, which can result in an unconscious restriction of physical activity. The infant correlate is feeding difficulty. He may require an hour to finish nursing, instead of the usual 15 to 20 minutes, stopping often for rest between bursts of sucking. Another symptom of congestive heart failure in infancy is failure to thrive. The rate of weight gain is decreased more than the rate of increase in length; head circumference growth is maintained unless failure is severe.

The four cardinal signs of heart failure in children are tachycardia, tachypnea, cardiomegaly, and hepatomegaly.

Tachycardia represents an attempt to maximize cardiac output. When tachycardia is mediated in part by increased catecholamine release, peripheral vasoconstriction with skin pallor and/or mottling, cool extremities, and diaphoresis may also be present.

Cardiomegaly, when due to ventricular dilatation, results from the attempt of a failing heart to increase its output by moving to the right on the Starling curve. Cardiomegaly may not be present when ventricular filling is compromised (for instance, in tachyarrhythmias, obstructed pulmonary venous return, or constrictive pericardial disease). Semilunar valve insufficiency causes ventricular dilatation because a greater end-diastolic volume is required to achieve the same effective stroke volume.

Tachypnea is due to pulmonary venous congestion and may be the first evidence on physical examination of pulmonary interstitial edema. The rapid, shallow respirations characteristic of heart failure maintain alveolar tidal volume and minimize the work of breathing with less compliant, edematous lungs. As failure progresses, transudation of fluid into the alveoli produces rales audible on auscultation. Peribronchial fluid may cause "cardiac" wheezing or a chronic cough. Severe pulmonary edema impairs gas exchange, and the resultant hypoxemia and hypercarbia can provoke anxiety.

Hepatomegaly indicates congestion of the systemic veins. Systemic congestion is often accompanied by systemic hypoperfusion. The consequent decreased renal plasma flow invokes compensatory mechanisms similar to hypovolemia (i.e., stimulation of the renin–angiotensin–aldosterone axis), which increase extracellular fluid volume and exacerbate systemic venous congestion. In contrast to the adult, peripheral edema and jugular venous distention are infrequent indicators of systemic venous congestion.

TREATMENT

General principles

The treatment of acute congestive heart failure begins with minimizing metabolic demands and continues with efforts to improve the performance of the heart as a pump by optimizing preload, afterload, contractility, and heart rate. Ultimately, of course, the underlying etiology of failure must be identified and corrected when possible. Some conditions are amenable to simple medical or surgical treatment; others may require more radical procedures such as heart or heart–lung transplantation.

Supportive measures include antipyresis, institution of a thermoneutral environment, and judicious use of sedation to minimize oxygen consumption. Electrolyte abnormalities, hypoxia, and acidosis should be corrected to increase cardiac contractility and decrease afterload. Precipitating tachyarrhythmias and bradyarrhythmias should also be treated.

Further intervention depends critically on an individualized assessment of preload, afterload, and contractility. For example, reflex diuresis of an infant with a previously well-compensated ventricular septal defect can worsen failure if the infant also presents with dehydration secondary to diarrhea. As suggested by Figure 55-2, use of afterload-reducing agents can be counterproductive in a child with an inadequate preload.

Chronic medical therapy

Traditionally, treatment of mild congestive failure has entailed fluid and salt restriction in conjunction with oral administration of a diuretic (furosemide, chlorothiazide, and/or spironolactone) and possibly a digitalis derivative (i.e., digoxin, a chronic inotrope). Digoxin has a low therapeutic index (ratio of toxic to therapeutic dose) and must be used cautiously. Side effects include tachyarrhythmias and bradyarrhythmias (potentiated by hypokalemia, which can result from concomitant diuretic therapy), increased myocardial oxygen consumption, and gastrointestinal symptoms (nausea, vomiting), which can compromise nutritional status. Current dosage recommendations are based on maturation-dependent bioavailability. Controversy persists whether digoxin is of any value in the special case of a ventricular septal defect; although some clinicians attest to its efficacy, available clinical studies are unconvincing, and many theoretical reasons would suggest that it would not be of significant benefit.

Chronic diuretic therapy with furosemide and the thiazides can result in hyponatremic–hypokalemic metabolic alkalosis. Electrolytes must be monitored periodically; supplemental potassium chloride is often necessary, especially in infants also treated with digoxin. Spironolactone is a potassium-sparing diuretic that competitively inhibits aldosterone (blocks the exchange of sodium for potassium) at the renal collecting tubules.

More recently, some clinicians have employed chronic vasodilator therapy to alter ventricular loading conditions. Some pharmacologic agents can be chosen that dilate primarily resistance arterioles (thus reducing afterload) or capacitance veins (thereby decreasing preload). Other drugs are less selective and dilate both pre- and postcapillary beds (Table 55-2). These agents may be useful in the following situations: (1) conditions in which there is a primary mismatch of afterload to contractility (i.e., systemic hypertension or cardiomyopathy) and (2) conditions that provoke excessive compensatory increases in preload or afterload, thereby producing congestive symptoms and/or decreasing cardiac output. For example, in aortic insufficiency, dilation of the left ventricle compensates via the Starling mechanism for decreased net forward output (up to a point). Thereafter, further dilation may decrease stroke volume (the far right descending limb of the Starling curve).

Acute medical therapy

Congestive heart failure that presents at or near birth usually mandates more sophisticated medical therapy. Infants with severe left ventricular obstructive lesions (critical aortic stenosis, hypoplastic aortic arch) need continuous intravenous administration of prostaglandin E_1 (0.05 to 0.1 μg/kg/min) to maintain ductal patency and thereby achieve adequate

Table 55–2. Vasodilator Therapy of Congestive Heart Failure

Drug/Action	Precapillary arterioles	Postcapillary venules
Hydralazine	+	0
Captopril	+	0
Nitroglycerin	0	+
Nitrates	0	+
Nitroprusside	+	+
Prazosin	+	+

Table 55–3. Relative Adrenergic Activity of Selected Inotropes

Drug	α (Peripheral vasconstriction)	β_1 (Cardiac inotrope)	β_2 (Peripheral vasodilator)	δ
Epinephrine	++++	++++	++	0
Norepinephrine	++++	++++	0	0
Dopamine	++++ (low dose)	++++	++	++++ (high dose)
Dobutamine	0	++++	++	0
Isoproterenol	0	++++	++++	0

systemic perfusion. This drug is also beneficial in infants with ductal-dependent cyanotic congenital heart lesions, which otherwise would be complicated by hypoxic myocardial failure.

Severe congestive heart failure may complicate the course of infants who undergo major cardiac surgery. In these instances, short-term combined therapy with vasodilators and inotropes has proven successful. Certain vasodilators (nitroglycerin, nitrates, nitroprusside) should be used only in intensive care units where continuous hemodynamic monitoring is possible because they are highly potent with a rapid onset of action. In addition, nitroglycerin and nitroprusside are potentially highly toxic because their metabolites include thiocyanate and cyanide. Commonly used inotropes are administered by continuous intravenous infusion. These adrenergic agents vary in their alpha, beta, and delta (dopaminergic) receptor effects (Table 55-3). Thus, although these agents tend to increase myocardial contractility, their side effects include increased myocardial work and oxygen consumption, increased (or decreased for isoproterenol) afterload, tachycardia, and arrhythmias. Accordingly, optimal pharmacologic therapy demands a thorough understanding of the operative hemodynamics in each individual case.

BIBLIOGRAPHY

Alpert BS: Reappraisal of digitalis in infants with left-to-right shunts and heart failure. J Pediatr 106:66–68, 1985

Berman W: Congestive heart failure. In Nelson NM (ed): Current Therapy in Neonatal–Perinatal Medicine. Philadelphia, BC Decker, 1985

Braunwald E: Heart failure: Pathophysiology and treatment. Am Heart J 102:486–490, 1981

Friedman WF, George BL: Treatment of congestive heart failure by altering loading conditions of the heart. J Pediatr 106:697–706, 1985

Green TP: Therapeutic approach to the failing heart. Pediatr Ann 14:304–311, 1985

Rudolph AM: Developmental considerations in neonatal failure. Hosp Pract 20(1):53–70, 1985

56

Hypertension

The measurement of a child's blood pressure is a necessary part of the physical examination. In older children and adolescents, the procedure is fairly simple. Place the blood pressure cuff snugly around the upper arm. The bladder should encircle the upper arm and cover two-thirds its length. The child should be sitting with the arm at heart level and should be as calm as possible. Inflate the cuff until the radial pulse is no longer palpable. Observing the manometer (aneroid or mercury), deflate the cuff at a rate of 2 mm/second. Auscultation over the brachial artery reveals the onset of an audible pulse (the systolic pressure, Korotkoff I sound); further auscultation reveals a muffling of the sound (Korotkoff IV sound) and finally its disappearance (Korotkoff V sound). Because of debate as to which sound truly represents diastole, both Korotkoff sounds IV and V are reported (e.g., 120/80/60). However, because some children have heart sounds audible throughout deflation of the cuff, the Korotkoff IV sound has been used in age- and sex-appropriate blood pressure standards (see below).

Blood pressure measurement in neonates, infants, and some toddlers may be more easily accomplished through ultrasonography. A cuff containing a transducer is placed around the infant's arm or thigh. Ultrasonic waves pass to the underlying artery, the frequency or amplitude of reflected waves is an audible (hissing) sound and is dependent on the velocity of blood in the vessel.

Greatly inaccurate blood pressure measurements result when the cuff size is incorrect (especially, too small), the patient is moving, crying, anxious, or angry, or the equipment is incorrectly calibrated. Errors in determination also occur because of the observer's level of auditory acuity, technique, or preference for particular terminal digits (e.g., 120/80, 106/76, 92/62).

Grids for normal systolic and diastolic blood pressures by age and sex have been developed using data from over 10,000 children and adolescents (see Table 56-1 and Figures 56-1 to 56-6). Using the appropriate grids, the blood pressure (systolic and diastolic) can be compared to that of similarly aged children.

The healthy child who, on one occasion only, has either a systolic or diastolic blood pressure greater than the 95th percentile is said to have high normal blood pressure. If the (otherwise healthy) child's blood pressure

Table 56–1. Classification of Hypertension by Age-Group

Age-Group	Significant Hypertension (mm Hg)	Severe Hypertension (mm Hg)
Newborn		
7 days	Systolic BP ≥ 96	Systolic BP ≥ 106
8–30 days	Systolic BP ≥ 104	Systolic BP ≥ 110
Infant (<2 yr)	Systolic BP ≥ 112	Systolic BP ≥ 118
	Diastolic BP ≥ 74	Diastolic BP ≥ 82
Children (3–5 yr)	Systolic BP ≥ 116	Systolic BP ≥ 124
	Diastolic BP ≥ 76	Diastolic BP ≥ 84
Children (6–9 yr)	Systolic BP ≥ 122	Systolic BP ≥ 130
	Diastolic BP ≥ 78	Diastolic BP ≥ 86
Children (10–12 yr)	Systolic BP ≥ 126	Systolic BP ≥ 134
	Diastolic BP ≥ 82	Diastolic BP ≥ 90
Adolescents (13–15 yr)	Systolic BP ≥ 136	Systolic BP ≥ 144
	Diastolic BP ≥ 86	Diastolic BP ≥ 92
Adolescents (16–18 yr)	Systolic BP ≥ 142	Systolic BP ≥ 150
	Diastolic BP ≥ 92	Diastolic BP ≥ 98

(Report of the Second Task Force on Blood Pressure Control in Children. Pediatrics 79:1–25, 1987).

exceeds the 95th percentile on four separate occasions, he is said to have persistently elevated blood pressure. Measurements should be made on four separate days and not four separate occasions in the same day. Strict attention should be paid to cuff size (especially in obese children), to measurement technique, and to making the child as calm as possible during measurement.

PATHOPHYSIOLOGY

The enzyme renin is located within the renal baroreceptors. Whenever the baroreceptors sense a decreased blood pressure or volume (as in hemorrhage) or whenever there is decreased sodium in the distal tubule of the kidney, renin is secreted. It reacts with its circulating substrate, angiotensinogen, to form the relatively inert peptide angiotensin I, which is converted in the lungs to angiotensin II. Angiotensin II has a very short half-life but is one of the most potent vasoconstrictors known. Its most marked vasoconstrictor activity is in the vessels of the skin, kidney, and splanchnic region, with less effect in the vessels of brain, heart, and skeletal muscle. Angiotensin II also stimulates the adrenal to secrete aldosterone, which leads to sodium retention and, subsequently, an increased blood volume. Thus, through vasoconstriction and increased blood volume, the end result of renin secretion is increased blood pressure. Baseline renin levels show diurnal variation with higher levels in the waking hours and in the upright posture. Hypertension can be associated both with high and low renin levels.

High renin levels are frequently encountered in diseases that compromise the kidneys (renal vessel or renal-associated hypertension)

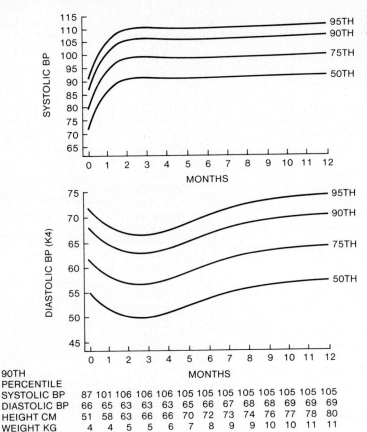

FIGURE 56–1. Age-specific percentiles of BP measurements in boys—birth to 12 months of age; Korotkoff phase IV (K4) used for diastolic BP. (Report of the Second Task Force on Blood Pressure Control in Children. Pediatrics 79:1–25, 1987)

90TH PERCENTILE												
SYSTOLIC BP	87	101	106	106	106	105	105	105	105	105	105	105	105
DIASTOLIC BP	66	65	63	63	63	65	66	67	68	68	69	69	69
HEIGHT CM	51	58	63	66	66	70	72	73	74	76	77	78	80
WEIGHT KG	4	4	5	5	6	7	8	9	9	10	10	11	11

and in hyponatremic states. Low or normal renin levels in the presence of hypertension are associated with primary aldosteronism, pheochromocytoma, aortic coarctation (increased resistance to flow), states of increased cardiac output (thyrotoxicosis, anxiety, exercise), polycythemia (increased blood viscosity), and the use of oral contraceptive agents (increased angiotensinogen activity).

ETIOLOGY

Hypertension may be primary or secondary. In the pediatric age-group, the most common cause of *secondary hypertension* is renal disease.

Acute *renal hypertension* is caused by acute glomerulonephritis (AGN), the hemolytic–uremic syndrome (HUS), nephrosis, and systemic lupus erythematosus (SLE). Because these entities have been discussed in detail elsewhere, they will only be summarized here. In AGN, the patient frequently had nasopharyngitis or impetigo 1 to 3 weeks before becoming ill. The initial process resolved only to be followed by malaise, anorexia, headache, edema, weight gain, decreased urine output, and hematuria. Severely affected children may present with seizures or oliguria/anuria, or in congestive heart failure; if the child is anuric, hyperkalemia and volume overload may be life-threatening. Diagnosis is confirmed by detecting red cell casts

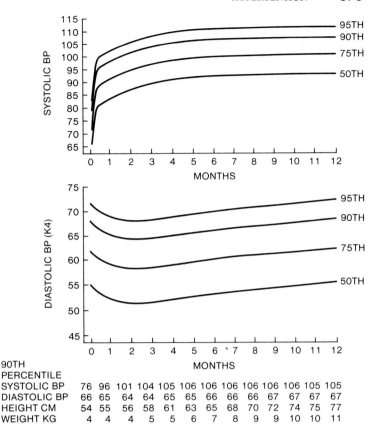

FIGURE 56–2. Age-specific percentiles of BP measurements in girls—birth to 12 months of age; Korotkoff phase IV (K4) used for diastolic BP. (Report of the Second Task Force on Blood Pressure Control in Children. Pediatrics 79:1–25, 1987)

90TH PERCENTILE												
SYSTOLIC BP	76	96	101	104	105	106	106	106	106	106	106	105	105
DIASTOLIC BP	66	65	64	64	65	65	66	66	66	67	67	67	67
HEIGHT CM	54	55	56	58	61	63	65	68	70	72	74	75	77
WEIGHT KG	4	4	4	5	5	6	7	8	9	9	10	10	11

in the urine, elevated serum antistreptococcal titers (ASO), and depressed serum C3 and, occasionally, C4.

The child with HUS is usually younger than 2 to 3 years of age and presents because of diarrhea, usually bloody. He looks ill and may be pale, lethargic or delirious. Urine output may be normal initially but decreases drastically as the disease progresses. Seizures may occur. Diagnosis is confirmed by detecting a microangiopathic hemolytic anemia, thrombocytopenia, fibrin split products, increased creatinine and elevated urea nitrogen. As with AGN, hyperkalemia and volume overload may be fatal.

Nephrotic syndrome is characterized by gradually occurring edema and hypertension.

Diagnosis is confirmed by detecting proteinuria, hypoalbuminemia, hypercholesterolemia, and normal complement levels. Some individuals with nephrotic syndrome have glomerular changes (membranoproliferative glomerulonephritis); they demonstrate hypertension, proteinuria, hypoalbuminemia, hypercholesterolemia, hematuria, and decreased C3.

SLE most commonly affects girls older than 2 years. Its protean manifestations are described elsewhere (see Chapter 96). Diagnosis is confirmed by detecting antinuclear (i.e., anti-DNA) antibodies.

Renal trauma may cause hematuria and hypertension. The trauma may be isolated (as in a blow to the back or abdomen) or multiple

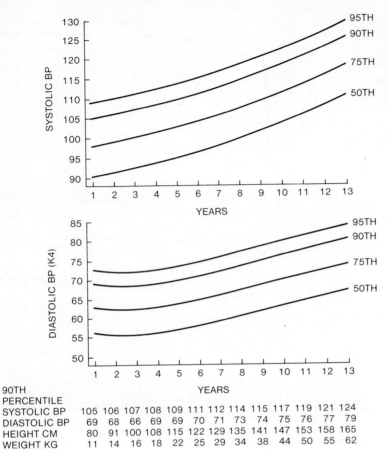

FIGURE 56–3. Age-specific percentiles of BP measurements in boys—1 to 13 years of age; Korotkoff phase IV (K4) used for diastolic BP. (Report of the Second Task Force on Blood Pressure Control in Children. Pediatrics 79:1–25, 1987)

90TH PERCENTILE													
SYSTOLIC BP	105	106	107	108	109	111	112	114	115	117	119	121	124
DIASTOLIC BP	69	68	66	69	69	70	71	73	74	75	76	77	79
HEIGHT CM	80	91	100	108	115	122	129	135	141	147	153	158	165
WEIGHT KG	11	14	16	18	22	25	29	34	38	44	50	55	62

(as in a motor vehicle accident). Intrarenal or subcapsular bleeding may compromise the kidney. Diagnosis is confirmed by intravenous pyelogram (IVP)/radionucleotide scan.

Renal arterial disease is associated with hypertension. Vessels involved are usually the major renal arteries or its branches. Stenotic vessels may be the result of trauma (umbilical artery catheterization), congenital defects, or acquired disease (such as neurofibromatosis, a major cause of renal vessel hypertension). The child may present with failure to thrive, short stature and, in neurofibromatosis, café au lait spots. Although results of urinalysis and renal function tests may be normal, peripheral renin activity may be elevated. A rapid-sequence IVP can detect differences in contrast appearance, disappearance, and volume between the two kidneys and a difference in the sizes of the kidneys. Renal-vein renin ratios (*i.e.*, those exceeding 1.5 or 2 indicate unilateral renal pathology) and selective renal angiograms *via* arteriography solidify the diagnosis of renal vessel disease. A decision is then made whether surgery would be efficacious for the particular patient.

Obstructive uropathy associated with hypertension includes posterior urethral valves, ureterocoeles, ureterovesicular/ureteropelvic obstruction, and bladder diverticula. Gross vesicoureteral reflux (dilatation of the ureter, renal pelvis, or both) leads to renal scarring.

FIGURE 56–4. Age-specific percentiles of BP measurements in girls—1 to 13 years of age; Korotkoff phase IV (K4) used for diastolic BP. (Report of the Second Task Force on Blood Pressure Control in Children. Pediatrics 79:1–25, 1987)

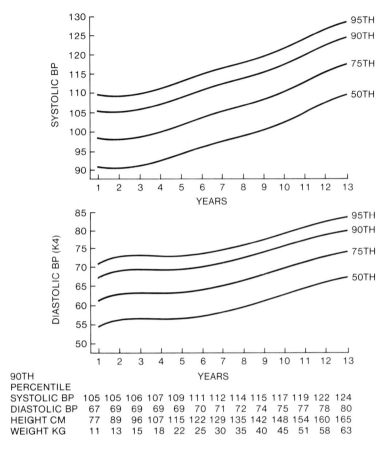

90TH PERCENTILE													
SYSTOLIC BP	105	105	106	107	109	111	112	114	115	117	119	122	124
DIASTOLIC BP	67	69	69	69	69	70	71	72	74	75	77	78	80
HEIGHT CM	77	89	96	107	115	122	129	135	142	148	154	160	165
WEIGHT KG	11	13	15	18	22	25	30	35	40	45	51	58	63

Affected patients may have a history of polyuria, enuresis, multiple urinary tract infections, growth retardation, or fevers of unknown etiology. Diagnosis is suggested by proteinuria, pyuria, and bacteriuria and is confirmed by voiding cystourethrogram which demonstrates the effects of severe, chronic reflux (hydronephrosis, dysplastic or small, scarred kidneys).

Certain congenital renal malformations may also present with hypertension. Polycystic renal disease may present in the neonate as oligohydramnios, a large abdomen containing huge kidneys, respiratory distress, severe hypertension, and dysmorphic facies (low-set ears, underdeveloped chin, flattened nasal

bridge). Cysts are also present in the liver; eventually, portal hypertension develops.

Miscellaneous renal causes of hypertension include renal tumors such as Wilms' tumor, dysplastic kidney(s), hypoplastic kidneys(s), unilateral multicystic kidney, solitary cystic kidney, lead nephropathy, mercury poisoning, radiation nephritis, genitourinary surgery or renal transplant/rejection, renin-secreting tumors, and end-stage renal disease, whatever the cause.

Vascular causes of hypertension include the aforementioned renal vessel abnormalities (stenosis, arteritis, fibromuscular dysplasia, fistula, aneurysm, neurofibromatosis), renal artery thrombosis, aortitis, aortic hypopla-

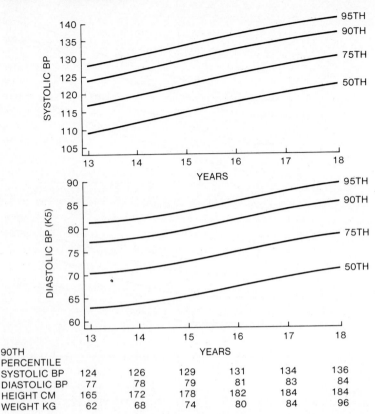

FIGURE 56–5. Age-specific percentiles of BP measurements in boys—13 to 18 years of age; Korotkoff phase V (K5) used for diastolic BP. (Report of the Second Task Force on Blood Pressure Control in Children. Pediatrics 79:1–25, 1987)

90TH PERCENTILE						
SYSTOLIC BP	124	126	129	131	134	136
DIASTOLIC BP	77	78	79	81	83	84
HEIGHT CM	165	172	178	182	184	184
WEIGHT KG	62	68	74	80	84	96

sia, and coarctation of the aorta. Coarctation of the thoracic aorta is frequently associated with cardiac defects (atrial septal defect, ventricular septal defect, patent ductus arteriosus, aortic stenosis, mitral stenosis, mitral insufficiency) and may present in an infant as failure to thrive, respiratory distress, or poor feeding. The infant's examination may reveal a child in cardiac failure with cardiac murmur(s) of left to right shunts, tachycardia, tachypnea, cardiomegaly, a gallop rhythm, rales, and hepatomegaly. The upper extremities have fuller pulses and higher blood pressures than the lower extremities. Diagnosis is confirmed by cardiac catheterization. Unless cardiac failure is intractable and poorly controlled by digitalis, surgery is not performed in infancy; in asymptomatic patients, surgery is postponed until the child is 4 to 8 years of age. Hypertension frequently improves as the infant ages because of the development of collateral arterial circulation; however, sustained hypertension can result in left ventricular hypertrophy. Surgical intervention ideally should take place before hypertrophy occurs. Serial electrocardiograms (ECGs), echocardiograms, and cardiac catheterizations should assist in monitoring cardiac size.

Coarctation of the abdominal aorta is rarer than that of the thoracic aorta. Affected patients present with hypertension, recurrent abdominal pain (secondary to ischemia), fatigue, abdominal bruits, decreased or absent femoral pulses, and blood pressure discrepancy between the upper and lower limbs. Diagnosis is confirmed by arteriography and angiography. Surgical repair may not be feasible.

Endocrine causes of hypertension include primary hyperparathyroidism, primary hyper-

FIGURE 56–6. Age-specific percentiles of BP measurements in girls—13 to 18 years of age; Korotkoff phase V (K5) used for diastolic BP. (Report of the Second Task Force on Blood Pressure Control in Children. Pediatrics 79:1–25, 1987)

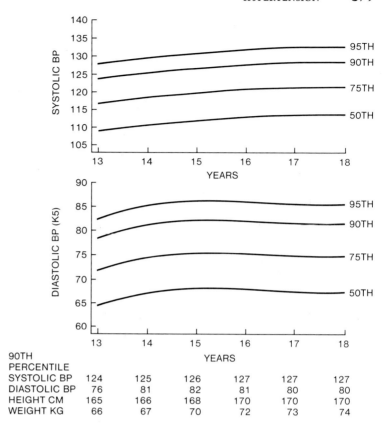

90TH PERCENTILE						
SYSTOLIC BP	124	125	126	127	127	127
DIASTOLIC BP	76	81	82	81	80	80
HEIGHT CM	165	166	168	170	170	170
WEIGHT KG	66	67	70	72	73	74

thyroidism, and adrenal diseases (diseases of both the adrenal cortex and medulla). Adrenal medulla diseases include pheochromocytoma and neuroblastoma. Pheochromocytoma is a tumor affecting individuals of any age but it is more likely after 10 years of age. The tumor may be solitary (one adrenal gland) or in multiple sites (both adrenals, paraspinal sympathetic ganglia in the abdomen, chest, and neck, ovary, testes, kidney, diaphragm, spleen, bladder and aorta). The tumor elaborates dopamine and its byproducts, epinephrine and norepinephrine. If epinephrine constitutes most of the catecholamines, the tumor is in the adrenal medulla. If norepinephrine predominates, extra-adrenal tumor sites must be considered.

Symptoms are related to these products. The patient has hypertension (and, frequently, orthostatic hypotension), headache, nau-

sea, vomiting, diaphoresis, palpitations, and visual disturbances. Polyuria may also be present.

Diagnosis is confirmed by detecting an elevated level of urinary vanillylmandelic acid, a degradation product of norepinephrine and epinephrine. Other diagnostic studies include an IVP (detects adrenal or extra-adrenal mass if it is large and/or displaces the kidney), computed tomography CT scan, arteriography with selective angiography, and adrenal venography with vena caval sampling. Treatment is surgical after the hypertension has been controlled adequately.

Neuroblastoma, a tumor of infancy and early childhood, may also be associated with hypertension (see Chapter 82).

Adrenal cortex abnormalities are also associated with hypertension. Cushing's syndrome (primary or secondary adrenocortical hyperfunction) results in excess cortisol secretion. The syndrome is caused by adrenal tumors, primary adrenal hyperplasia, or adrenal hyperplasia due to adrenocorticotropic hormone (ACTH)-secreting tumors (especially in the pituitary). Tumors are more likely in children, especially girls, younger than 7 years and in those whose cortical production does not decrease with dexamethasone suppression or metyrapone tests. Adrenal hyperplasia is more common in older individuals and in those whose cortisol production is suppressed by high-dose (but not low-dose) dexamethasone and whose urinary 17-OH steroid levels increase when they are given metyrapone.

The patient with Cushing's syndrome has a moon facies, "buffalo hump," short stature, hirsutism, acne, and hypertension. Cutaneous striae, weakness, headaches, amenorrhea, osteoporosis, increased pigmentation, and emotional lability may also be present.

Diagnosis is confirmed by detecting increased plasma cortisol levels and increased urinary cortisol and 17-OH steroids. An IVP with tomography or CT scan is useful to localize the adrenal tumor. Treatment is surgical; pituitary irradiation and an adrenocorticolytic drugs have been used when surgery is not feasible.

Two uncommon forms of the adrenogenital syndrome are associated with hypertension. The adrenogenital syndrome results from the deficiency of enzyme(s) necessary for synthesis of normal steroids. The most common deficiency, 21-hydroxylase, is not associated with hypertension. The two forms associated with hypertension are 11-hydroxylase and 17-hydroxylase deficiencies. The 11-hydroxylase deficiency results in decreased cortisol and aldosterone production, which, in turn, stimulates the pituitary to secrete ACTH. This hormone stimulates the adrenal cortex to form 11-desoxycorticosterone (DOC) and steroids (androgenic and estrogenic). Patients are large and show evidence of virilization. Diag-

nosis is confirmed by detecting a low blood cortisol level, a high blood 11-desoxycortisol level, and DOC, and a decreased urinary aldosterone level. Treatment consists of the administration of corticosteroids, which suppress ACTH secretion, thereby decreasing the levels of DOC and sex hormones. The 17-hydroxylase deficiency is extremely rare. Since corticosteroids, adrenal and sex hormones cannot be synthesized (because of enzyme deficiency), ACTH is increased, leading to excess mineralocorticoid production. The patient lacks secondary sex characteristics and may manifest ambiguous genitalia. Diagnosis is confirmed by detecting decreased blood cortisol level, decreased plasma aldosterone level, decreased urinary 17-ketosteroid and estrogen levels, and increased blood DOC. Treatment includes corticosteroid and sex hormone replacement therapy.

Primary aldosteronism is a very rare cause of hypertension in children. The excess aldosterone results in potassium depletion and decreased plasma renin activity; patients present with failure to thrive, polyuria, and polydipsia. Diagnosis is made by detecting hypokalemia, low plasma renin activity, and increased 24-hour urinary aldosterone. Treatment is surgical.

Miscellaneous causes of hypertension are collagen–vascular diseases, poliomyelitis, Guillian-Barré syndrome, dysautonomia, porphyria, hypercalcemia, Stevens-Johnson syndrome, sympathomimetic therapy, steroid therapy, oral contraceptive therapy, amphetamine use, burns, leukemia, hypernatremia, bacterial endocarditis, and increased intracranial pressure from any cause.

Primary hypertension is hypertension that exists in the absence of any conditions known to elevate blood pressure. There is evidence that both genetic endowment and environmental factors, such as low socioeconomic status and high salt intake, are major factors in the genesis of primary hypertension. Children with primary hypertension may be asymptomatic. When symptoms are present, they include frontal headaches, fatigue, epistaxis, and nervousness. Obesity is present in 50% of patients. Fundoscopic abnormalities are uncommon and, when present, are indicative of hypertension present for at least 1 year.

EVALUATION

When a child with sustained elevated blood pressure presents to medical attention, he deserves a thorough history and complete physical examination. The history should elucidate the child's birth history, presence of chronic conditions or recurrent symptoms, chronic use of medications, growth patterns, urinary tract infections or disorders, dietary history, and family history of hypertension or its complications (renal disease, myocardial infarction, and stroke). The physical examination must be done meticulously, since many of the causes of secondary hypertension have characteristic physical findings. Special emphasis is placed on the fundoscopic and cardiac examinations. The blood pressure is taken in both arms and one leg; in the right arm, the blood pressure is measured with the patient sitting, standing, and supine. The asymptomatic individual with normal findings on physical examination does not merit numerous laboratory studies. However, a routine urinalysis, serum creatinine and urea nitrogen tests, chest x-ray, and electrocardiogram (ECG) are useful screening tests; if results of these are normal, the child is presumed to have primary hypertension and is managed as such, unless new symptoms appear or the hypertension worsens.

MANAGEMENT

The child with sustained hypertension may not require medication to decrease his blood pressure. If he is willing to alter his diet, salt intake, and amount of physical activity, antihypertensive medication may not be necessary.

The hypertensive child who is overweight should attempt to lose enough weight to approach his ideal weight for height and should limit his daily intake of salt (i.e., no salt added at the table). Sympathomimetics such as those present in decongestants should be avoided. Finally, the child should become as physically active as possible. The patient must be motivated to follow his diet; his motivation can be increased if his family supports him emotionally and by action (providing no salt at the table, limiting the amount of high-calorie food in the home, etc.). Parents and child must be patient with the therapy.

If these initial measures are inadequate, a thiazide diuretic is used. The daily starting dose of hydrochlorothiazide is 1 mg/kg, with a maximum of 2 mg/kg (200 mg) per day. Care must be taken to avoid volume depletion and hypokalemia; the latter can be avoided by the provision of a potassium-rich diet. Chronic thiazide use is also associated with hyperglycemia, hypercalcemia, hyperuricemia, and thrombocytopenia.

If the use of a thiazide diuretic does not achieve blood pressure control after 6 to 12 weeks, propranolol or methyldopa is added when diastolic pressures are between 90 and 100 mm Hg. Propranolol is a beta-adrenergic blocking agent; with its use, renin release is blocked and central nervous system vasomotor activity is inhibited. The use of propranolol is contraindicated in the presence of bradycardia (<60 beats/min), heart disease, asthma, gastrointestinal ulcer, or diabetes. Its starting dose is 1 mg/kg/day; increases may be necessary but should be instituted only if the patient is not bradycardic and can increase his heart rate by 20 beats after exercising.

Methyldopa is also used in children. It acts centrally on vasomotor centers and peripherally to decrease arteriolar resistance. Its initial dose is 10 mg/kg/day, and its maximal dose is 65 mg/kg/day. Its significant side effects include lethargy, orthostatic hypotension, and hematologic (hemolytic anemia, thrombocytopenia) and hepatic abnormalities.

If a diuretic plus propranolol or methyldopa does not achieve good blood pressure control, hydralazine is added. Hydralazine vasodilates the peripheral arterioles by relaxing their smooth muscles. Its initial dose is 1 mg/kg/day, and its maximum daily dose is 5 mg/kg (200 mg). Since hydralazine has been reported to induce lupus, antinuclear antibodies should be followed in patients receiving the drug. Side effects of hydralazine include flushing, warmth, and tachycardia; these effects are largely avoided if a beta-adrenergic blocker such as propranolol is used. Hydralazine-associated headaches have also been reported.

HYPERTENSIVE EMERGENCIES

Hypertensive crises (abrupt, marked elevations in blood pressure) occur in renal disease (especially AGN, reflux nephropathy, renal arterial disease, renovascular hypertension, end-stage renal disease), hemolytic uremic syndrome, renin-secreting tumors, and pheochromocytoma, and severe central nervous system pathology. Symptoms include headaches, diplopia, convulsions, congestive heart failure, peripheral edema, facial palsy, and hypertensive retinopathy.

Therapy varies according to etiology. In AGN, furosemide (1 to 2 mg/kg IV) in conjunction with hydralazine (0.15 to 0.2 mg/kg IV or IM) or diazoxide (1.5 to 5 mg/kg IV rapid bolus) are used. In HUS, treatment consists of furosemide and diazoxide (as outlined above); peritoneal dialysis may be required. In renal artery disease, multiple doses of diazoxide or a nitroprusside drip (1 µg/kg/min IV) may be necessary. In end-stage renal disease, intravenous diazoxide (1.5 to 5 mg/kg IV bolus) or a nitroprusside drip is very useful. In pheochromocytoma, diazoxide or nitroprusside therapy is useful to control the blood pressure prior to surgery.

BIBLIOGRAPHY

Bailie M et al: Symposium—Hypertension: Finding a safe and effective therapy. Contemp Pediatr 1:93–106, 1985

Bailie M et al: Symposium—Hypertension: More than ever, a pediatric concern. Contemp Pediatr 1:30–57, 1985

Lieberman E: CIBA Clinical Symposia—Hypertension in Childhood and Adolescence. vol 30, #3, 1978

Londe S: Causes of hypertension in the young. Pediatr Clin North Am 25:55–65, 1978

Report of the Second Task Force On Blood Pressure Control in Children—1987. Pediatrics 79:1–25, 1987

57

Chest Pain

Chest pain is a relatively infrequent presenting complaint in young children but becomes more frequent as children grow older. It is not as common in any pediatric age-group as are headaches or abdominal pain. Like those latter two symptoms, chest pain can be functional, herald serious disease, or have an intermediate significance. Because of parental and, sometimes, patient fear that chest pain is cardiac, the patient usually comes to medical attention promptly.

The properties of the chest pain should be fully elucidated in the history. Because children sometimes have great difficulty in describing the qualities of pain, the historical information may be somewhat imprecise. Regardless, an attempt should be made to answer the following questions: Is the pain sharp (like a knife stab or needle prick) or dull (like someone is sitting on the chest)? Exactly where is the pain located? (Have the patient point to the area.) Does the pain radiate? (Again, have the patient point to the areas of radiation.) Has the child ever had a pain like this before? If so, what made it better and what made it worse? If not, can the child or parent think of anything that brought on this pain? Has the parent or patient tried anything to make the pain better? If so, what was tried, and did it work? What was the child doing when the pain occurred? Does the pain occur with both exercise and rest or with just one of these? Has the child ever awakened from sleep with pain? During the episodes of pain, does the child perspire, become nauseous, vomit, become short of breath, wheeze, or cough? If the chest pain is an initial acute episode, does the child have a fever, respiratory symptoms, or other myalgias? During the pain, can the child feel his heart beating fast or hard? Does skin color change during the pain? How? Has he ever lost consciousness with the pain or without the pain? Does he experience vertigo or light-headedness with the pain? Has the child experienced any trauma prior to the pain's onset? Has the child aspirated a foreign body? Is the child taking any medications or illicit drugs? If so, which ones? when was the child's last meal? Does the pain usually follow a meal? Does the child have symptoms of indigestion?

Does the child have a history of a heart murmur, cardiac surgery, sickle cell anemia, asthma, or other chronic medical conditions or psychosomatic complaints? Is the child under any undue stress? If so, what is it? Does any family member have a history of angina or cardiac disease? Has a family member recently died of cardiac causes?

The patient's physical assessment includes a thorough physical examination. Abnormalities of vital signs should be noted. The color of the skin, mucous membranes, and nail beds should be checked for cyanosis or pallor. The patient's general condition (diaphoretic, apprehensive, in distress due to pain, etc.) is important. Especially informative features of the physical examination are the respiratory, cardiac, and chest examinations. The patient's rate, depth, and symmetry of respiration should be assessed. Is the child splinting or wheezing? On auscultation of the chest is there evidence of rales, decreased breath sounds, wheezing, or other adventitious lung sounds? After determining the point of maximal impulse of the heart, the heart should be auscultated in supine and sitting positions to determine its rate, regularity of rhythm, murmurs, abnormal sounds or splitting of sounds, gallops, or rubs. Palpation for thrills in the chest and neck should be conducted. Pulses should also be palpated for strength and equality of impulses.

The chest wall is inspected and palpated to determine areas of asymmetry, inflammation, or tenderness. The child should be asked to point to the area of greatest pain. When the examiner palpates that area, the child should then be asked if that manuever reproduces the pain. Regardless of the child's answer, bony structures and intercostal spaces should be palpated while observing the child's eyes to detect a response to pain. The vertebral spines should be percussed to determine if pressure on them refers pain to the chest. Finally, the abdomen, especially the midepigastric area, should be carefully palpated for areas of tenderness.

DIFFERENTIAL DIAGNOSES

A cardiac cause for chest pain is suggested by a history of pain precipitated by exercise, palpitations, color changes, syncope, or near-syncope. Although cardiac causes of chest pain are not, as a group, common in pediatrics, they are serious enough to warrant consideration.

Ischemic chest pain results from an imbalance between myocardial oxygen requirements and its oxygen supply. Such an imbalance is caused by a structural lesion or an arrhythmia. Regardless of the cause, ischemic chest pain is described as "squeezing" or "compressing." It can radiate to the back, left arm and jaw, and neck. The young infant with ischemic chest pain may be irritable and diaphoretic, feed poorly, and fail to thrive. During an episode of ischemia or infarction, the patient may demonstrate tachypnea, tachycardia, a gallop rhythm, rales, wheezes, or other signs of heart failure or shock.

Left ventricular outflow tract obstruction causes chest pain precipitated by exercise when the increase in heart rate and the work of the left ventricle creates an oxygen demand–supply imbalance. Left ventricular outflow tract obstruction may result from aortic valve stenosis, subvalvular obstruction, or idiopathic hypertrophic subaortic stenosis (IHSS). The first two entities are associated with loud, harsh systolic ejection murmurs that vary little with manuevers that alter left ventricular filling. IHSS, on the other hand, is associated with a murmur that softens during certain manuevers. IHSS is associated with a pansystolic murmur and an S_4 sound; the electrocardiogram (ECG) may show evidence of a septal Q wave.

Coronary artery anomalies may cause ischemic chest pain. The artery may be compressed because of its anomalous position or, if a fistula is present, may "steal" flow from the remaining coronaries. Chest examination may reveal a systolic or continuous murmur or a gallop rhythm. The ECG may show evidence of infarction or ST-T wave changes.

Mitral valve prolapse (Barlow's syndrome) can be associated with chest pain resulting from ischemia of the papillary muscles and left ventricular endocardium. However, most patients with mitral valve prolapse are asymptomatic. Chest examination may reveal a midsystolic click/late systolic murmur, findings that vary by the position of the patient. The ECG may show evidence of T wave changes, U waves, and tachycardia.

Dissection of an aortic aneurysm produces a sharp, "tearing" pain that radiates to the upper or lower extremities, depending on the site of the dissection. Dissection is usually related to trauma or Marfan's syndrome and is a medical emergency. Depending on the site of dissection, there may be aortic insufficiency. The patient may present in shock.

Arrhythmias can cause an imbalance in myocardial oxygen demand and supply. Prolonged tachycardia is associated with inadequate time for myocardial blood flow. Supraventricular tachycardia over several hours may cause discomfort. If the patient has sensations of palpitations, chest pain, and dizziness, an ECG should be performed at the time of presentation. If the symptoms are chronic, or the initial ECG is normal, continuous Holter monitoring is in order. The same procedure should be followed in patients with ventricular dysrhythmias. Chest pain can also be caused by rhythms that are intermittently too slow to provide the heart with the oxygen that it needs. Such causes of chest pain are unusual in children.

Acquired coronary artery disease, such as that associated with collagen–vascular diseases or mucocutaneous lymph node syndrome, may cause chest pain due to the imbalance of myocardial oxygen demand and supply. Diagnosis is made by echocardiography. Pericardial inflammation due to infectious agents or collagen–vascular diseases, or pericardial infiltration due to tumors may cause pain similar to that of a myocardial infarction. The sharp pain is exacerbated by inspiration, coughing, or movement, and the patient may prefer to sit forward. Radiation of the pain is similar to that of an infarction. A pericardial friction rub is heard on auscultation. The ECG may show ST elevation and low voltage of the QRS complex. Chest x-ray may reveal an enlarged, globular heart.

Noncardiac causes of chest pain are far more common than cardiac causes in the pediatric age-group.

Pulmonary diseases can produce chest pain. Pneumonia or asthma may be associated with tachypnea, cough, wheezing, retractions, or nasal flaring. On auscultation, wheezes, rales, or areas of decreased breath sounds are heard. Pleurisy is associated with a sharp pain aggravated by cough on inspiration. Pneumothorax is associated with a sharp pain peripherally, dyspnea, and areas of decreased breath sounds on auscultation. When pulmonary infarction involves large vessels, there is intense pain, dyspnea, cyanosis, and shock; when smaller vessels are involved, the pain may be transient and variable. Other signs of pulmonary distress may be present. Pulmonary emboli are associated with use of oral contraceptives, debilitation, and hemoglobinopathies.

Gastrointestinal diseases can cause chest pain. Especially notable in this regard are esophageal disorders. Esophageal reflux may produce substernal pain. Patients report that the pain is worse when they are supine and after eating, and is associated with tasting "acid brash" in the mouth. Belching and aerophagia may be common. Esophagitis causes a sharp/burning pain in the lower chest. Other esophageal disorders associated with chest pain are hiatal hernia and esophageal tears (Mallory-Weiss syndrome).

Stomach disorders (spasm, gastritis, gastric ulcers) may produce lower chest and epigastric pain, which can be elicited by palpation of the areas. Other gastrointestinal disorders associated with chest pain include duodenal ulcers, biliary tract and pancreatic diseases.

Mediastinal diseases such as pneumomediastinum, mediastinitis, and tumors can also produce chest pains.

Systemic diseases such as collagen–vascular diseases, malignancies, and hemoglobinopathies can also cause chest pain, as do cervical or thoracic spinal root irritations.

One of the most common causes of chest pain is a disorder of the chest wall. In Tietze's syndrome, or costochondritis, pain is easily reproduced by palpating the enlarged, tender costochondral junctions. The pain may be present for weeks. Another common chest wall disorder causing chest pain is trauma. The patient may not even remember a specific trauma. However, on careful questioning, a history of new exercising or weight lifting may be elicited.

Other chest wall disorders causing chest pain include breast development and herpes zoster. Careful examination of the chest should render these diagnoses readily apparent.

Chest pain may be attributable to emotional disturbances. This pain is vague, sometimes fleeting, localized over the heart with radiation to, or numbness of the left arm. The patient's pain is not brought on by exercise and frequently occurs at rest. The child may have other bodily aches or malaise and may fear that he cannot take in enough air. Consequently, he may panic and shallowly hyperventilate. The child with chest pain of emotional etiology may have a personal history of cardiac disease/surgery or a family member with angina, myocardial infarction, cardiac surgery, or sudden death due to cardiac disease.

Finally, a miscellaneous cause of chest pain in young patients is the precordial catch syndrome. Sharp pain is present along the left sternal border or beneath the left breast; the pain does not radiate. The pain is relieved by change of position, a deep inspiration, or by left chest massage. The pain is short-lived and recurs in no particular pattern. Its cause is unknown and it disappears in time.

MANAGEMENT

Laboratory studies (blood work, chest film, ECG) should be dictated by history and physical findings. Tests should be ordered judiciously; chest films and ECGs are unnecessary for most patients. If a cardiac cause seems likely, an ECG, echocardiogram, and referral to a cardiologist may be in order. If a pulmonary cause is likely, a chest film may be helpful, and appropriate treatment of the underlying disease should relieve the pain. If a gastrointestinal disease is likely, diagnostic studies may not be necessary at all. For example, esophageal reflux and low-grade inflammation may respond to eliminating offending foods, inclining the head of the bed, or the use of antacids or cimetidine. Gastric/duodenal disorders may also respond to a judicious diet and antacids. Chest wall disorders attributable to trauma usually respond to heat, rest, and avoidance of straining chest wall muscles. Other chest wall disorders improve in time (herpes zoster) or with reassurance (breast development, precordial catch syndrome, and emotional disturbances). If, however, severe emotional pathology is suspected, referral to a child psychiatrist or psychologist is indicated.

BIBLIOGRAPHY

Pantell R, Goodman B: Adolescent chest pain: A prospective study. Pediatrics 71:881–887, 1983

Perry L: Pinpointing the cause of pediatric chest pain. Contemp Pediatr 1:71–96, 1985

Brenner J, Berman M: Chest pain in childhood and adolescence. J Adolesc Health Care 3:271–276, 1983

Selbst S: Chest pain in children. Pediatrics 75:1068–1070, 1985

Driscoll D et al: Chest pain in children—A prospective study. Pediatrics 57:648–651, 1976

Part X: Pulmonology

58

Asthma

Asthma is one of the most common chronic diseases encountered in pediatrics. It is a major cause of school absenteeism, pediatric emergency room visits, and hospital admissions. Unfortunately, although significant therapeutic advances have been made in recent years, the overall morbidity and mortality due to asthma remains essentially unchanged. Successful management requires a thorough understanding by both the physician and the patient/family of the pathophysiology and clinical features of the disease.

Although the exact prevalence of asthma is still in question, it is clear that 5% to 10% of children in the United States are at some point afflicted with the disease. Most children with asthma develop signs and symptoms within the first several years of life: about 30% by 1 year of age, 50% by age 2, and 80% by age 5. Prior to puberty, asthma is nearly twice as common in boys as in girls; thereafter, the sex incidence is nearly equal. There is a strong genetic influence on the development of asthma, most likely on a multifactorial basis.

The course and prognosis of childhood asthma may be difficult to predict. Most children will suffer only occasional mild to moderately severe attacks, which are easily controlled. Others will develop severe asthma, which is difficult to control adequately under the best of circumstances and will interfere with daily activities. A significant proportion of children with asthma, probably about 50%, will outgrow their disease by adulthood. Although still somewhat unclear, it appears that those with the mildest disease have the best chance of outgrowing it and that almost all children with severe, persistent wheezing will continue to wheeze into adult life.

Although a strict definition for asthma does not exist, pathophysiologically it is characterized by labile obstruction of both large (>2-mm) and small (<2-mm) airways. The airways are hyperreative to a variety of stimuli and demonstrate a high degree of reversibility of the obstructive process. The elements that contribute to the airway obstruction are smooth muscle spasm (bronchospasm), edema and inflammation of the airway mucous membranes, and intraluminal accumulation of mucus and cellular debris. It is the bronchospastic component that is most readily reversed and hence the target of most of the drugs used in asthma.

Several specific triggers commonly precipitate wheezing in asthmatic children. These include viral respiratory infections, allergen exposure, exercise, atmospheric pollutants, and cold air. Attempts have been made to classify asthma based on the patients' response to these triggers, particularly allergens. In allergic or extrinsic asthma, seen in over 80% of childhood asthmatics, wheezing is precipitated by IgE mediated hypersensitivity reactions to inhaled or ingested allergens. Another group of asthmatics, seen most frequently in the first two years of life and after adolescence, have no evidence of allergic disease, and their asthma has been labeled intrinsic. The exact mechanisms underlying these forms of asthma remain unclear. In both forms, however, it is critical to understand that it is the generalized hyperreactivity of the airway that leads to the pathologic response to these various triggers.

Clinically, asthma is characterized by wheezing, dyspnea, prolonged expiration, use of accessary muscles, and hyperinflation. Cough may also be a prominent feature and, in some cases, may even be the only manifestation of underlying airway hyperreactivity. Although the obstruction is classically expiratory in nature, the child with severe asthma may have significant inspiratory wheezing as well. In the most severe attack, wheezing may even be lacking; only after bronchodilators are given will there be enough air movement to evoke wheezing in such patients.

DIAGNOSIS

The diagnosis of asthma is quite straightforward in most patients. A history of recurrent episodes of wheezing, dyspnea, and cough is obtained in the majority, although some patients present with no history of wheezing but rather a history of recurrent cough, particularly at night. Other patients may present with a history that is entirely consistent with asthma, only to have another diagnosis altogether, such as foreign body aspiration, cystic fibrosis, a congenital malformation of the respiratory or cardiovascular system, or bronchiolitis. A careful history is thus critically important in the evaluation of any patient with recurrent cough or wheezing and should include a complete past medical history, a family history, and a detailed analysis of both specific precipitating factors and the patient's response to previous therapy. It should be emphasized that in some patients, particularly those with less typical asthma, the response to a careful trial of a bronchodilator medication can be a significant diagnostic clue.

Between episodes, the physical examination may be remarkably normal, in stark contrast to the same child with an acute attack who may have wheezing, dyspnea, and markedly prolonged expiration. With more severe disease, chronic changes may include mild growth failure and chest deformities secondary to long-standing hyperinflation. Aside from the examination of the chest, a thorough search for other manifestations of allergic disease should be performed, including allergic shiners, conjunctivitis, and pale, swollen nasal mucosa. In addition, one must look carefully for other clues, such as digital clubbing, that might suggest a diagnosis other than asthma.

Laboratory tests should be used to complement the history and physical in the evaluation of a patient with suspected asthma. In the child with a clear-cut diagnosis and relatively mild disease, no tests may be required. However, in children with more severe disease or in whom the diagnosis may be in question, useful tests include a chest x-ray, eosinophil count, total IgE level, nasal smear for eosinophils, pulmonary function testing, allergy testing, and bronchial provocation testing, using either exercise, cold air, methacholine, or histamine to provoke bronchoconstriction under highly controlled circumstances.

THERAPY

The successful management of asthma requires a carefully balanced program of drug therapy, education, psychological support, and environmental control. It must be individualized for each patient. The goals of therapy are to enable the child and family to lead as normal lives as possible.

As described in Chapter 8, the pharmacologic management of acute asthma relies on a combination of β-adrenergic agents, theophylline, and corticosteroids. In chronic asthma therapy, the same drug classes are used although the approach may be somewhat different.

In the United States, theophylline is generally considered the first-line drug for the chronic management of asthma. It is becoming somewhat less popular because of its narrow therapeutic index, the frequency of adverse side effects, and improvements in available β-adrenergic agents. The usual dose is 20 mg/kg/day, although this may vary considerably in individual patients. Dozens of preparations are available in both long-acting (slowly absorbed) and short-acting (rapidly absorbed) forms. Serum theophylline levels are readily available in most laboratories and may be monitored to prevent toxicity, to maximize the therapeutic effect, and, if necessary, to ensure compliance. It is important to remember, however, that mild side effects, including headaches, stomach aches, and personality changes, are relatively common even without toxic levels and that in occasional patients severe toxicity (usually seizures) may occur without previous milder side effects.

In the last decade, β-adrenergic agonists have assumed a rapidly growing role in the long-term management of asthma. While the effectiveness of epinephrine as a bronchodilator has long been recognized, its short half-life and lack of β2 specificity limited its role in chronic therapy. Now, however, modifications of the catechol nucleus have provided new drugs that are longer acting and far more specific. These include metaproterenol, terbutaline, albuterol, and fenoterol. Each is available both as an oral preparation and metered dose inhaler. All but terbutaline are also available for nebulization, a route of delivery that may be adapted for both chronic and acute use. The inhaled route of delivery offers the distinct advantage of providing a maximum drug concentration to the airway with a minimum of systemic effects. It provides fast, reliable bronchodilation that is particularly useful in the management of exercise-induced asthma, where an inhalation 5 to 10 minutes prior to exercise will prevent most attacks from occurring. Overmedication with a metered dose inhaler is the major concern that must be monitored.

Both theophylline and β-adrenergic agents may be used either on a chronic or intermittent basis. Some children clearly require daily, year-round therapy. More commonly, however, with proper education, a drug may be successfully administered on an intermittent basis. For example, a drug may be started at the onset of a viral respiratory infection or just prior to exercise or allergen exposure. Acute attacks thus may be prevented in many cases with the judicious use of these agents. If they are being used intermittently, β-agonists may be preferable, especially in an inhaled form, because of their more rapid onset of action.

Any child requiring two or more bronchodilators on a regular basis deserves a trial of cromolyn sodium. This agent acts as a mast cell stabilizer and is thus not an effective bronchodilator but rather acts as a prophylactic agent.

It appears to be highly effective in a majority of patients while some patients appear to have no response at all. It is used solely as an inhaled agent and comes in three forms: a metered dose inhaler, a nebulizable solution, and a powder form delivered in a spinhaler. It is extremely safe and has very few side effects. Its major disadvantages are its cost and the need for daily use.

If a child's asthma remains poorly controlled even after bronchodilator therapy has been maximized, corticosteroids may be necessary. In many cases, they may be used in short, 5- to 7-day courses in an acute attack; these brief courses are extremely safe and have been shown to reduce morbidity significantly when an acute attack is otherwise difficult to control. The most severe asthmatics, however, will require steroid therapy on a more regular basis. If possible, an inhaled preparation should be used to minimize systemic side effects. When this is not successful, every attempt should be made to use the minimum possible dose, preferably on an every-other-day schedule, and to monitor for side effects, including growth failure, adrenal suppression, and cataracts.

In addition to drug therapy, the effective management of childhood asthma requires extensive education, self-help skills, psychological support, and environmental control, including both allergen avoidance and elimination of pollutants like cigarette smoke. This approach is time-consuming and for many patients, particularly those with more severe disease, will be greatly facilitated by referral to a pediatric allergist. These adjuncts to pharmacologic therapy are extremely worthwhile, however, since they allow the great majority of asthmatics to lead normal, active lives.

Asthma is a common, chronic disease in childhood. Successful management requires a thorough understanding of the disease and a carefully planned program combining pharmacotherapy with patient education and environmental manipulation. Few diseases in pediatrics are as challenging or as rewarding to manage.

BIBLIOGRAPHY

Eggleston PA, Banks JR: Asthma in children. In Lichtenstein L, Fauci A (eds): Current Therapy in Allergy, Immunology and Rheumatology, p 23. St. Louis, CV Mosby, 1985

Hen J: Office evaluation and management of pediatric asthma. Pediatr Ann 15:111, 1986

Isles A, Levison H: Treatment of childhood asthma. J Respir Dis (suppl) August 1982, pp 60–71

Leffert F: The management of chronic asthma. J Pediatr 97:875, 1980

McFadden ER: Pathogenesis of asthma. J Allergy Clin Immunol 73:413, 1984

Rachelefsky GS, Siegel SC: Asthma in infants and children—Treatment of childhood asthma: Part II. J Allergy Clin Immunol 76:409, 1985

Siegel SC, Rachelefsky GS: Asthma in infants and children: Part I. J Allergy Clin Immunol 76:1, 1985

59

Bronchiolitis

Bronchiolitis is the most common lower respiratory tract infection among infants and young children. At least 75% of cases are caused by infection with respiratory syncytial virus (RSV). Other etiologic agents include adenovirus, parainfluenza virus, and influenza virus. Bronchiolitis occurs in yearly epidemics with a peak incidence between November and March, corresponding to the presence of RSV in the community. Most cases occur in infants less than 6 months of age.

Clinically, the typical infant has coryza and cough for a few days, followed by the development of wheezing, tachypnea, retractions, and variable degrees of dyspnea. Widespread rales and rhonchi are frequently present. Constitutional symptoms include irritability, poor feeding, and fever in about half of patients. Apnea is also frequently encountered, particularly in infants under 2 months of age.

Radiographic findings include hyperinflation, increased peribronchial markings, and, in some cases, areas of segmental atelectasis or consolidation. Hypoxemia and CO_2 retention are also common complications. The diagnosis of bronchiolitis has traditionally depended on these laboratory features in com-

bination with a consistent clinical and epidemiologic picture. Today, however, advances in viral diagnostic techniques frequently allow one to define a specific etiologic agent as well. Fluorescent antibody and ELISA techniques using nasopharyngeal secretions are available in most hospitals and provide for the rapid identification of RSV and other viral pathogens.

The physiologic basis for the wheezing and tachypnea in bronchiolitis is related primarily to obstruction of small airways. The hypoxemia and hypercarbia are the result of ventilation–perfusion mismatch. Pathologically, there is necrosis of the mucosal epithelium with loss of ciliary function. This, combined with increased mucus production and submucosal edema, leads to obstruction in the small bronchi and bronchioles.

Although most cases of bronchiolitis have been considered to be benign and self-limited, it remains a significant disease in terms of both morbidity and mortality. Among patients hospitalized with bronchiolitis, approximately 1% will die and 2% to 5% will develop respiratory failure. Preexisting cardiopulmonary disease, particularly congenital heart disease and bronchopulmonary dysplasia, imparts significantly greater risk for progressing to respiratory failure with at least 25% of deaths attributable to bronchiolitis occurring in such infants. While absolute indications for mechanical ventilation do not exist, a pCO_2 greater than 60 is certainly an ominous sign, especially if associated with apnea, increasing respiratory effort, or altered consciousness.

Most infants with bronchiolitis can be successfully managed at home with careful monitoring of hydration and evidence of increased respiratory distress, fatigue, or feeding difficulties. When the respiratory rate exceeds 60 breaths per minute, hospitalization is generally required, since that degree of tachypnea is commonly associated with hypoxia (pO_2 <60 mm Hg) and with an increased risk of aspiration during feeding. In the hospital, management generally consists of oxygen, hydration, nutritional support and close observation for evidence of respiratory failure. No convincing data exist supporting the use of β-adrenergic agents, theophylline, corticosteroids, or antibiotics in the treatment of bronchiolitis, although a trial of one or more might be indicated in the severely ill patient.

Recently, a new antiviral agent, ribavirin, has been licensed for the treatment of RSV-associated bronchiolitis. Ribavirin is delivered as a nebulized aerosol and has been shown to lead to more rapid clinical improvement and improved arterial blood gas values in several small trials. While the indications for the use of this agent are not entirely clear, it should certainly be strongly considered in any infant with RSV bronchiolitis who has underlying cardiopulmonary disease or impending respiratory failure.

The final and possibly most important aspect of acute bronchiolitis is its relationship to subsequent episodes of wheezing. The incidence of childhood asthma in patients who had bronchiolitis is between 40% and 50%.

The critical question has been whether the damage incurred by an episode of bronchiolitis leads to asthma or, rather, whether bronchiolitis represents the response to an RSV infection in an infant predisposed to reactive airway disease. Long-term studies have shown that there are residual pulmonary function abnormalities in a high percentage of asymptomatic patients who had had bronchiolitis, and it has been estimated in a carefully controlled study that wheezing in 9.4% of the population of children who currently wheeze could be attributed to bronchiolitis. Thus, although the acute illness may appear benign in most cases, significant long-term consequences appear very real.

In summary, bronchiolitis is a common viral respiratory infection affecting infants and very young children. RSV is the major pathogen. Supportive care and observation are all that are generally required with careful monitoring for evidence of respiratory failure. In view of the substantial long-term consequences, however, it is clear that more is needed, either in terms of vaccination programs or more widespread use of antiviral agents, both of which are being studied aggressively.

BIBLIOGRAPHY

Hall CE, McBride JT, Walsh EE et al: Aerosolized ribavirin treatment of infants with respiratory syncytial viral infection. N Engl J Med 308:1443, 1983

McConnochie KM, Roghmann KJ: Bronchiolitis as a possible cause of wheezing in childhood: New evidence. Pediatrics 74:1, 1984

Welliver RC: Viral infections and obstructive airway disease in early life. Pediatr Clin North Am 30:819, 1983

Wohl ME: Bronchiolitis. Pediatr Ann 15:307, 1986

Wright PF: Bronchiolitis. Pediatr Rev 7:219, 1986

60

Cystic Fibrosis

Cystic fibrosis (CF) is the most common lethal inherited disease in the United States. It has an incidence of approximatley 1:2,000 in whites and 1:17,000 in American blacks. The disease is characterized by chronic obstructive pulmonary disease, exocrine pancreatic insufficiency, and excess loss of electrolytes in the sweat. The basic biochemical defect is as yet undefined, and the diagnosis is made by collecting sweat by pilocarpine iontophoresis and analyzing for chloride content. Most of the clinical manifestations of CF are related to obstruction of organ passages by unusually viscous mucous secretions. The life expectancy for patients with CF is currently about 21 years.

Although CF may present with a variety of symptoms (Table 60-1), pulmonary disease remains the most common presenting feature, as well as the most common cause of morbidity and mortality. Wheezing, chronic cough, and recurrent pneumonia are the most common pulmonary presentations of CF. There is marked variation in the onset of these symptoms, ranging from severe wheezing or recurrent pneumonia in infancy to chronic cough as an adolescent or young adult. Then, over a period of months to years,

bronchiectasis and air trapping usually develop, with diffuse mucus plugging of bronchi. Flare-ups of bronchitis are generally characterized by increased cough, dyspnea on exertion, weight loss, and fatigue; there may be no fever, leukocytosis, or acute x-ray changes.

Early in the disease, the major pulmonary pathogens are *Staphylococcus aureus* and *Haemophilus influenzae*. Over time, however, virtually all patients become colonized with mucoid strains of *Pseudomonas aeruginosa*, a problem that is quite unique to CF and generally impossible to eradicate. A variety of treatment regimens are used for these pulmonary infections; although it may not be possible to sterilize the mucus, treatment is generally thought to improve quality of life and survival. While no single protocol has been proven most effective, postural drainage is routinely used, along with some combination of oral or inhaled "prophylactic" antibiotics and intermittent courses of IV antibiotics.

In addition to chronic bronchitis and mucous plugging, pulmonary complications in CF include recurrent pneumothoraces, reactive airway disease, and hemoptysis. Over time, there is increasingly severe ventilation–perfusion mismatch with resultant hypoxia,

Table 60–1. Common Manifestations of Cystic Fibrosis

Respiratory Tract
- Recurrent wheezing in infancy
- Chronic cough
- Recurrent bronchitis/pneumonia
  Colonization with mucoid *Pseudomonas aeruginosa*
  Nasal polyps
Gastrointestinal System
  Meconium ileus
  Meconium plug
  Ileal/jejunal atresia
  Cholestatic jaundice
  Rectal prolapse
  Steatorrhea
  Failure to thrive
  Vitamin deficiency
  Hypoproteinemia/edema
Metabolic
  Hypotonic dehydration
  Hypokalemia/alkalosis

digital clubbing, pulmonary hypertension, and cor pulmonale. Once cor pulmonale develops, the prognosis is very poor, with most patients dying of cardiopulmonary failure within 2 years.

After pulmonary disease, gastrointestinal (GI) complications of CF are the most common presenting features and causes of morbidity. Approximately 10% of patients with CF present with neonatal intestinal obstruction secondary to meconium ileus, in which large amounts of unusually viscous meconium obstruct the terminal ileum. Meconium ileus is frequently associated with a poorly developed large bowel (microcolon), ileal atresia, and meconium peritonitis secondary to perforation of the bowel. At least 99% of infants with meconium ileus will be found to have CF. The meconium plug syndrome is a similar condition that is less severe and less frequently associated with CF. Beyond the neonatal period, patients with CF may develop a "meconium ileus equivalent," in which tenacious mucus becomes impacted in the terminal ileum.

About 90% of patients with CF have evidence of exocrine pancreatic insufficiency. This leads to malabsorption with resultant steatorrhea, hypoproteinemia, fat-soluble vitamin deficiency, and, frequently, failure to thrive. Rectal prolapse is commonly seen, presumably due to excessively bulky stools. Fortunately, pancreatic enzyme replacement therapy, with careful attention to adequate nutrition and vitamin supplementation, will usually alleviate these problems.

The final major GI manifestation of CF is hepatobiliary disease. Cholestatic jaundice is commonly encountered in the neonatal period. As adolescents and young adults, about 5% of CF patients develop biliary cirrhosis with hepatosplenomegaly and esophageal varices.

Metabolic complications of CF result from excess loss of sodium, potassium, and chloride in the sweat. Hypotonic dehydration, hypokalemic alkalosis, and heat stroke are commonly encountered in warmer climates. In addition, endocrine pancreatic insufficiency with diabetes mellitus is occasionally seen, as is recurrent pancreatitis.

As noted, the diagnosis of CF is made by detection of an abnormally high sweat chloride level, generally considered to be over 60 mEq/L. It is extremely important that the sweat test be done in a reference laboratory using the pilocarpine iontophoresis method. As can be ascertained from the above discussion, there is a multitude of indications for performing a sweat test. It is becoming increasingly clear that early diagnosis is linked to improved survival, and, hence, an early sweat test is warranted for any infant or child manifesting a symptom consistent with the diagnosis of CF. An early diagnosis also may be critically important for genetic counseling. For these reasons, neonatal screening programs for CF have been instituted in some areas using dried blood spots for the assay of immunoreactive trypsin.

Rapid advances have been made in recent years in defining the genetics of CF. It has long been known that the disorder is inherited as an autosomal-recessive trait and that about 5% of whites in the United States are heterozygous carriers of the CF gene. Until recently, however, details of the CF gene itself were entirely lacking. If the gene responsible for CF could be identified, it would not only enable prenatal diagnosis, but might also allow for the definition of the basic biochemical defect responsible for this heterogeneous disorder. Researchers have now located the gene on the long arm of chromosome 7 by means of linkage studies, and the gene itself will soon be identified.

In summary, cystic fibrosis is a relatively common disorder that may present in a variety of ways. Although the outlook is improving, most patients still die of the disease's pulmonary complications by the third decade of life. Most encouraging are the rapid advances that have been made in defining the CF gene, the result of which could be a cure of the disease through an alteration of the underlying biochemical defect.

BIBLIOGRAPHY

Dolan TF: Update: Cystic fibrosis. Pediatr Ann 15:196, 1986

Park RW, Grand RJ: Gastrointestinal manifestations of cystic fibrosis: A review. Gastroenterology 81:1143, 1981

Rosenstein BJ, Langbaum, T.S., Metz, S.J.: Cystic fibrosis: Diagnostic considerations. The Johns Hopkins Med J 150:113, 1982.

Stern RC: Cystic fibrosis: Recent developments in diagnosis and treatment. Pediatr Rev 7:276, 1986

Wood RE, Boat FF, Doershuk CF: State of the art: Cystic fibrosis. Am Rev Respir Dis 113:833, 1976

61

Acute Respiratory Failure

Acute respiratory failure may be defined as the development of significantly altered arterial oxygen and/or carbon dioxide tensions during an acute illness. While no strict guidelines exist, an arterial Po_2 <60 mm Hg and a Pco_2 >45 mm Hg are generally considered consistent with the diagnosis. Functionally, the diagnosis is most often made based on an elevated Pco_2, although there are some cases in which the Pco_2 remains normal as the Po_2 falls.

Respiratory failure is not a specific diagnosis but rather the result of a wide variety of underlying conditions. Any disease complicated by significant alveolar hypoventilation may result in respiratory failure. Thus, it may occur in cases of pneumonia, asthma, bronchiolitis, cystic fibrosis, pulmonary edema, epiglottitis, or any other condition with impaired air movement and/or gas exchange. It may also occur, however, in patients in whom the airways and pulmonary parenchyma are completely normal; that is, ventilation may be inadequate because of abnormalities in respiratory control (e.g., central nervous system disease), weakness of the respiratory muscles (e.g., Guillain-Barré syndrome), or structural abnormalities of the thoracic cage

(e.g., scoliosis). It is these patients in whom respiratory failure is most commonly missed.

In some children, respiratory failure results from a failure of the lungs to deliver sufficient oxygen to the pulmonary capillary blood, leading to arterial hypoxia. Carbon dioxide elimination is frequently normal or even increased in these patients. This normocapnic form of respiratory failure occurs in a variety of situations, including a group of disorders labeled the adult respiratory distress syndrome. In this syndrome, diffuse pulmonary infiltrates develop as the result of an infectious or toxic insult to the lung, and severe hypoxia may follow as a consequence of ventilation–perfusion imbalance.

The diagnosis of acute respiratory failure is made by arterial blood gas determination, using the guidelines noted above. The clinical manifestations are generally those of the underlying disease, although restlessness is frequently present early in the course and is often replaced by central nervous system depression, with impaired consciousness and confusion as more pronounced hypercapnia develops.

The treatment of respiratory failure must

400

aim to quickly restore adequate gas exchange and ensure that hypoxia, hypercapnia, and acidosis do not reach hazardous, life-threatening levels. Aggressive therapy should be aimed at relieving the underlying disease whenever possible, and supplemental oxygen should be provided as needed. If the P_{CO_2} continues to rise in spite of the initial therapy, or if the P_{O_2} remains below 60 mm Hg on 60% O_2, intubation and mechanical ventilation will be required. It is highly advantageous to predict the need for intubation before dire circumstances arise and thus to perform it in a controlled, semi-elective fashion.

The goals of therapy are to restore the P_{CO_2} to normal and maintain adequate oxygen saturation while using the minimum ventilatory pressures and the lowest possible inspired oxygen concentrations. Close monitoring in an intensive care unit is essential, following the clinical status, arterial blood gas values, and, ideally, continuous oxygen saturations by pulse oximetry. The patient should be weaned from mechanical ventilation as quickly as possible because of the hazards of both the oxygen and the ventilatory pressures. It is critical that close attention to the underlying disease process and general supportive care be maintained throughout.

Fortunately, advances in pediatric intensive care in recent years provide the means for the successful management of the great majority of children developing respiratory failure during an acute illness. For those children with respiratory failure superimposed on a chronic illness (e.g., cystic fibrosis), the prognosis depends on the nature of the specific chronic illness and may vary widely. Whatever the cause, however, the prognosis will always be improved by making the diagnosis as early in the course as possible.

BIBLIOGRAPHY

Anas NG, Perkin RM: Resuscitation and stabilization of the child with respiratory disease. Pediatr Ann 15:43, 1986

Newth CJL: Recognition and management of respiratory failure. Pediatr Clin North Am 26:617, 1979

Pagtakhan RD, Chernick V: Respiratory failure in the pediatric patient. Pediatr Rev 3:247, 1982

Pfenninger J, Gerber A, Tschappeler H et al: Adult respiratory distress syndrome in children. Pediatrics 101:352, 1982

Raphaely RC: Acute respiratory failure in infants and children. Pediatr Ann 15:315, 1986

Part XI:

Endocrinology and Metabolism

62

Diabetes Mellitus

Diabetes is a chronic metabolic disorder. Because of a lack of or antagonism to insulin, the diabetic is hyperglycemic. Insulin, a polypeptide synthesized in the beta cells of the pancreatic islets, exerts many actions through its binding to outer cell surface membrane receptors in the liver and adipose tissues. When insulin binds to a receptor, there is a lowering of intracellular cyclic adenosine monophosphate (cAMP) and, subsequently, decreased activity of cAMP-dependent hormones. Receptor-bound insulin also suppresses glucagon secretion, facilitates glucose and amino acid entry into adipose and muscle cells, and participates in the adipose cell transport of fatty acids.

There are two major types of diabetes: insulin-dependent (juvenile) and non-insulin dependent (maturity). In juvenile diabetes, the pancreas' insulin-producing capacity is severely limited because of beta cell depletion or exhaustion. Several mechanisms have been postulated to explain this destruction: (1) abnormal stimulation of beta cells with their eventual exhaustion, (2) destruction of beta cells by an immune mechanism, (3) a genetically determined low insulin response, and (4) abnormal activity of both alpha and beta cells in which high levels of glucagon stimulates gluconeogenesis and ketogenesis.

Maturity-onset diabetes may also occur in children, although it is more common in adults. Such children have abnormal insulin responses rather than lack of insulin. If the children are obese, they may respond to insulin stimulation with abnormally high levels of insulin, and consequently, hypoglycemia. The mechanism by which obesity increases the need for insulin and stimulates its production is unclear.

Other rare forms of primary diabetes include transient diabetes of the neonate, lipodystrophic diabetes, in which there is insulin resistance, and diabetes in long-term survivors with cystic fibrosis.

Secondary diabetes occurs when insulin is antagonized, as in hyperadrenocorticism, hyperthyroidism, growth hormone excess, or pheochromocytoma. If glucose is unavailable, as in starvation or glycogen storage diseases, secondary impaired glucose tolerance may occur. Secondary diabetes also may occur with certain drugs, most notably thiazide diuretics.

PATHOPHYSIOLOGY OF ACUTE DIABETES

Reduced entry of glucose into cells raises the blood glucose. Since the cells require glucose, gluconeogenesis is stimulated in an attempt to supply the sugar, which, in fact, only further increases the hyperglycemia and the catabolism of proteins. As amino acids accumulate, the uncontrolled diabetic develops negative nitrogen balance. As the absolute or functional insulin deficiency continues, further metabolic derangements lead to diabetic ketoacidosis (DKA; see Chapter 63).

CLINICAL FINDINGS

In the asymptomatic child, diabetes may present as transient hyperglycemia or glucosuria postprandially or in times of stress or illness. The child may have had symptoms of hypoglycemia in the past; however, findings of the child's physical examination are usually normal.

In the classic presentation of juvenile diabetes, the child may come to medical attention because of weight loss, polydipsia, polyphagia, or polyuria (especially nocturnal enuresis). Other than the demonstration of recent weight loss, the physical examination may be unrevealing.

The presentation and physical findings of the child presenting with DKA are presented in Chapter 63.

Regardless of the presentation of the child, the physician should ask about any signs and symptoms (with their duration) accompanying hyperglycemic episodes, precipitating factors of these episodes, a history of recent change in weight, general health, school performance, moods, a history of recent illnesses, and a past history of symptoms of hypoglycemia (see below). A family history of diabetes is important information that should be elicited.

DIAGNOSIS

The child presenting in diabetic ketoacidosis usually leaves no doubt about his diagnosis as there are characteristically abnormal laboratory values (see Chapter 63).

Children with fasting whole blood glucose concentrations of ≥120 mg/dL or a 2-hour postprandial (or random) whole blood glucose concentration of 180 mg/dl are hyperglycemic. These blood glucose determinations should be made on at least two different occasions when the child is free of infection and stress and is not fasting. Abnormal glucose metabolism may be verified during a glucose tolerance test. The child is given 1.75 g/kg (maximum, 100 g) of glucose delivered in an oral solution. The glucose and insulin concentrations are assayed at the onset and at 30, 60, 90, 120, 180, 240, and 300 minutes.

TREATMENT

The new diabetic generally requires 0.5 to 1.0 unit/kg/day of insulin. If the child can be maintained on a single daily injection, two-thirds of the insulin should be an intermediate-acting type (neutral protein Hagedorn [NPH] or Lente) and the other one-third a rapid-acting type (regular insulin). The single daily dose (both types of insulin) should be given 30 to 45 minutes before breakfast, drawn up in the same syringe, and injected into the arm, thigh, buttock, or abdomen. An older child can give his own insulin injection. The dosage of insulin is then dictated by clinical response. If the child spills much more glucose in the morning than afternoon, the amount of regular insulin is increased; if the opposite is true, the amount of intermediate-acting insulin is increased. Increases are on the order of 10% at a time.

If nighttime hyperglycemia with morning glucosuria occurs, if the patient is a preschooler or is undergoing rapid growth (as in adolescence), two daily injections of insulin are helpful to maintain control. Two-thirds of the daily dose is given before breakfast and one-third in the late afternoon. Both injections contain intermediate- and rapid-acting insulin in a 2 to 3:1 proportion. According to response, adjustments are made as described above.

The diabetic child's nutritional requirements are similar to those of a nondiabetic child. Total caloric intake should approximate 1000 calories plus 100 calories/year of life and should be composed of 15% protein, 30% fat, and 55% carbohydrate. Most of the fat should be polyunsaturated and from vegetable sources (margarine, vegetable oil, lean meats, poultry, and fish) rather than saturated fats from animal sources. Cholesterol intake should also be limited. Carbohydrates should be complex (starches) rather than simple sugars (candy, cookies, carbonated beverages). If carbonated beverages must be consumed, they should be of the diet variety, sweetened with saccharin rather than sorbitol.

Meals should be taken regularly. Occasional excesses are permissible, and the diet should not be so rigid as to be unpleasant. In general, 20% of the calories are provided at breakfast, 20% at lunch, 30% at dinner, and 30% at midmorning, midafternoon, and evening snacks. A proper diet goes hand-in-hand with adequate exercise. The diabetic child needs exercise to remain physically and psychologically well. If he becomes hypoglycemic during exercise, he may need to ingest a simple sugar (juice, candy) during or immediately after exercise or to decrease his daily dose of insulin by 10%.

The diabetic child or his parent should monitor glucosuria and ketonuria before meals and in the evening using a second-voided specimen (first void is discarded; second void, 30 to 60 minutes later, is tested). Compliance is a problem because of inconvenience, embarrassment, or denial. When performed appropriately, however, urine screening is quite useful. If the child spills ≥2% glucose for 48 hours, his insulin dose should be increased by 10%; if he spills no glucose and has symptoms of hypoglycemia, his insulin dose should be decreased by 10%. Failure to spill glucose in the absence of symptomatology is not an indication to reduce insulin.

The symptoms of hypoglycemia are due to catecholamine release (trembling, sweating, anxiety, tachycardia) and to cerebral glucopenia (hunger, sleepiness, mood changes, confusion, seizures, or coma). Causes of hypoglycemia include excess insulin, decreased oral intake, and exercise without increasing caloric intake. Treatment includes the ingestion of a carbohydrate snack or 0.5 mg glucagon IM if the child cannot take oral fluids or food (intractable vomiting, stupor, seizures, coma). Early morning or nocturnal hypoglycemic episodes can alternate with hyperglycemic episodes 4 to 6 hours later especially when >2 units/kg/day of insulin is taken (Somogyi phenomenon). This phenomenon is felt to be secondary to the body's reaction to the (excess) insulin-induced hypoglycemia. Gradual reduction (10% over 3 days) of the insulin dosage, instituting twice daily (rather than once daily) insulin doses, and changing from beef–pork insulin to pure beef or pure pork have all been effective in diabetics with the Somogyi phenomenon.

In times of illness, surgery, or undue stress, the diabetic may require additional insulin. However, if he is vomiting, his insulin requirements may decrease.

Children with diabetes may develop antibodies to thyroid tissue, adrenal tissue, gastric parietal cells, and intrinsic factor (with subsequent malabsorption of vitamin B_{12}). Long-term diabetics also suffer diabetic retinopathy and nephropathy in as few as 10 years of disease if adequate disease control is not attained.

Children with diabetes feel alienation, resentment, denial, anger, and fear of the consequences of the disease. Their parents may feel guilty and helpless and may overprotect the child or impose a rigid diet on him. The child may rebel and "forget" to take his insulin or to eat properly. The physician should counsel both patient and parent. Psychotherapy may be necessary in severe cases. Peer groups and diabetic summer camps are also helpful.

BIBLIOGRAPHY

See Chapter 63.

63

Diabetic Ketoacidosis

Diabetic ketoacidosis (DKA) is the most important cause of acute morbidity and mortality in the diabetic child. It is characterized by high levels of blood glucose and serum ketones, glucosuria, and a state of acidosis.

PATHOPHYSIOLOGY

With insulin lack, there is hyperglycemia with glucosuria occurring at plasma glucose levels above 160 mg/dL. Insulin lack is associated with lipolysis; free fatty acids accumulate because lipid synthesis is severely limited. Fatty acids are oxidized to acetyl CoA, which accumulates because of citric acid cycle malfunctioning. To decrease the amount of acetyl CoA, acetoacetic acid and beta-hydroxybutyric acid are formed. Small amounts of these ketone bodies can be used as sources of energy by peripheral tissues. However, the large amounts produced in DKA exceed the tissues' capacity to oxidize them. Since the renal threshold for ketones is limited, ketonuria results. Excretion of the anion moiety of the ketone body requires a cation; thus, electrolytes are depleted in DKA. Water is lost with these solutes so that dehydration occurs. Finally, carbonic acid accumulates because of the body's attempts to decrease its load of hydrogen ions. Carbonic acid dissociates into H_2O and CO_2, the latter of which stimulates hyperpnea with a lowering of P_{CO_2}. However, if the basic pathology of DKA is not managed aggressively, renal and pulmonary compensations are inadequate and the acidosis worsens.

CLINICAL PRESENTATION

The patient with DKA presents with dehydration (dry skin and mucous membranes, flushed cheeks, sunken eyes), abdominal pain, vomiting, Kussmaul's respirations, hyperpnea, somnolence, and, sometimes, coma. If the state of DKA was precipitated by an illness, signs of that illness may be present. The patient may have a fruity odor to his breath.

Laboratory abnormalities include hyperglycemia, glucosuria, ketonemia, ketonuria, metabolic acidosis (decreased pH, P_{CO_2}, and $HCO_3{}^-$), elevated blood lipids, total body depletion of sodium and potassium, and leukocytosis.

MANAGEMENT

Laboratory measurements. Serum electrolytes, glucose, blood urea nitrogen (BUN), calcium, phosphorus, ketones, osmolality and acid–base parameters should be determined at presentation and every 2 to 4 hours thereafter until the child is stable. Testing with Dextrostixs is done every 1 to 2 hours until the patient is stable. The urine is examined microscopically for evidence of infection and is serially examined for the presence of glucose and ketones.

Fluids. The degree of dehydration in DKA is usually on the order of 10%. Normal saline solution can be used as the initial hydrating solution, since it is hypotonic relative to the patient's hyperosmolar serum. Too rapid a correction of dehydration causes too rapid a correction of hyperosmolarity, which can precipitate cerebral edema. Usually, the saline solution is infused at 20 to 30 ml/kg during the first 2 hours. Thereafter, one should correct half of the calculated deficit in the next 7 to 8 hours and the other half of the deficit in the following 16 hours.

When the serum glucose is 250 to 300 mg/dL, the infused solution should contain glucose (5%).

Electrolytes. After the first bolus of fluid has been given and the patient has voided, potassium should be administered. Total body potassium is invariably depleted during DKA even if serum potassium is normal, since intracellular potassium moves to the extracellular compartment with acidosis. Abnormalities of serum potassium have cardiac effects, which can be followed by electrocardiogram (*i.e.*, hypokalemia is associated with low T waves and U waves; hyperkalemia is associated with high-peaked T waves). Provision of potassium must take into account both maintenance and losses. Therefore, potassium replacement should be on the order of 5 to 6 mEq/kg/day. Potassium should be delivered as KCl alternating with KPO_4 in the first 8 hours because (1) the use of normal saline solution usually causes excess chloride delivery to the body, which aggravates the acidosis, and (2) the body is phosphate-depleted. Phosphate is necessary for the formation of 2,3-diphosphoglycerate (2,3-DPG), which affects the oxygen dissociation curve. If there is a deficiency of 2,3-DPG, the curve shifts to the left, which may lead to impaired oxygen delivery, tissue hypoxia, and a worsening of the acidosis. Since excess infusion of phosphate may precipitate hypocalcemia, serum calcium should be measured periodically during therapy for DKA.

Bicarbonate. Administration of appropriate fluids and insulin usually is sufficient to correct the acidosis. However, when the patient's pH is below 7.1 or his HCO_3^- is <5 mEq/L, 2 mEq $NaHCO_3$/kg should be infused slowly over 30 to 60 minutes, with measurement of the pH at the end of the infusion. Aklalosis is to be avoided because it shifts the oxygen dissociation curve to the left, facilitates potassium's exodus from the extracellular to the intracellular space, leading to hypokalemia, and worsens cerebral acidosis because of the passage and action of CO_2 in the brain.

Insulin. The patient in DKA should receive a bolus insulin dose (0.1 unit/kg), followed by a steady infusion of 0.1 unit/kg/hour. Such a steady delivery avoids the fluctuations of serum insulin concentration that accompany intermittent insulin therapy and is associated with a fairly linear decline in serum glucose (ideally, 80 to 100 mg/dL/hour). Insulin sufficient for 6 to 8 hours may be added directly to the saline infusion or may be given in a separate intravenous line.

When the serum glucose approaches 300 mg/dL, the patient should be given a glucose-containing solution intravenously. The insulin drip can be halved (0.05 units/kg/hour) or subcutaneous insulin (0.25-0.5 u/kg) can be given q6–8 hours. After DKA is controlled, short- and intermediate-acting insulin is used (see Chapter 62).

Ketones. Acetoacetate and beta-hydroxybutyrate are present in DKA, with the concentration of the latter exceeding that of the former by a ratio of 3 to 8:1. However, the nitroprusside reaction that measures serum ketones measures only acetoacetate. Beta-hydroxybutyrate dissociates to acetoacetate as acidosis is corrected. Hence, ketonemia and ketonuria may persist even as the patient improves, and this does not imply failure of therapy.

BIBLIOGRAPHY FOR DIABETES MELLITUS AND DIABETIC KETACIDOSIS

Behrman R, Vaughan V: Nelson Textbook of Pediatrics, 13th ed, pp 1248–1264, Chapter 20: Metabolic Disorders—Diabetes Mellitus. Philadelphia, WB Saunders, 1987

Golden M et al: Management of diabetes mellitis in children younger than 5 years of age. Am J Dis Child 139:448–452, 1985

Kreisberg R: Diabetic ketoacidosis: New concepts and trends in pathogenesis and treatment. Ann Intern Med 88:681–695, 1978

Kaye R: Research and practice in the treatment of insulin-dependent diabetes: A survey of 53 pediatric diabetologists, Pediatrics 74:1079–1085, 1984

Rosenbloom A et al: Classification and diagnosis of diabetes mellitis in children and adolescents. J Pediatr 98:320–323, 1981

64 Hypoglycemia

Hypoglycemia is the pathophysiologic state in which there is an abnormally low concentration of glucose in the blood. The numerical definition of hypoglycemia varies by age:

In the premature infant, <20 mg/dL
In the full-term infant younger than 3 days, <30 mg/dL
In the full-term infant older than 3 days, <40 mg/dL
In infants and children, <50 mg/dL

GLUCOSE HOMEOSTASIS

After a meal, the level of blood glucose rises, stimulating insulin secretion. Insulin promotes glucose entry into tissue and inhibits gluconeogenesis. As the blood glucose level falls, insulin secretion is reduced. If insulin secretion is excessive or prolonged, the result is hypoglycemia.

During fasting, insulin secretion is inhibited so that glucose uptake by tissues is limited. In addition, glucose is released from glycogen (glycogenolysis) in the liver, and glucose is formed in the liver from amino acids and lactate (gluconeogenesis). Hormones released during fasting augment these processes. Adrenal glucocorticoids and glucagon promote gluconeogenesis. Catecholamines and glucagon promote glycogenolysis. The cellular effects of insulin and insulin secretion are antagonized by these substances. Inadequate secretion of any of these hormones or the inability of the liver to respond to them will result in hypoglycemia.

CLINICAL PRESENTATION

The symptoms of hypoglycemia are due to the compensatory secretion of epinephrine. These effects include palpitations or tachycardia, sweating, flushing, weakness, nervousness, and hunger. If the hypoglycemia remains unresolved, the patient may demonstrate cerebral effects such as headaches, confusion, and irritability. If the hypoglycemia is severe and prolonged, seizures, coma, and irreversible brain damage may ensue. Severe, prolonged hypoglycemia may be fatal.

Typically, symptoms of hypoglycemia occur 2 to 6 hours after meals (postprandial hypoglycemia). Symptoms occurring before breakfast are typical of fasting hypoglycemia.

In the neonate, hypoglycemia can be manifested by jitteriness, cyanosis, pallor, diaphoresis, hypothermia, apathy, apnea or tachypnea, weak or high-pitched cry, hypotonia, difficulty in feeding, and seizures. These symptoms also may occur with sepsis, meningitis, asphyxia, mineral abnormalities, and central nervous system (CNS) anomalies. Therefore, the infant with such symptoms deserves a thorough evaluation.

ETIOLOGY

Neonatal Hypoglycemia

Hypoglycemia may occur in the neonate because hepatic enzymes necessary for gluconeogenesis are not fully operative until several hours or days after birth. Thus, if the infant is given nothing by mouth (kept NPO) after birth and the enzyme activities are subnormal, hypoglycemia can result. Hypoglycemia may result in infants of diabetic mothers and infants with erythroblastosis fetalis due to hyperinsulinism. At autopsy, these infants demonstrate hyperplasia of their pancreatic beta cells. Infants who have been malnourished *in utero* (for any reason) and are of low birth weight may have reduced hepatic glycogen stores, thus curtailing glycogenolysis. Septic infants or infants who are severely ill with respiratory, cardiac, or CNS diseases may be hypoglycemic because of their increased metabolic needs. Other infants who are at risk include those whose intravenous infusions are interrupted and those with metabolic disorders (see below).

Postprandial Hypoglycemia

Postprandial hypoglycemia may be functional, as with hypersecretion of insulin after a meal or increased tissue response to normal insulin secretion. It may also occur in early stages of diabetes mellitus, when insulin secretion may be erratic.

Leucine stimulates beta cells to secrete insulin; a patient with this variant demonstrates increased beta cells in the pancreas. Leucine-sensitive hypoglycemia may be familial. Finally, hypoglycemia may occur after pylorus-bypass surgery because glucose absorption is so rapid that the resultant hyperglycemia leads to enhanced insulin secretion, which causes hypoglycemia several hours after eating.

Fasting Hypoglycemia

Patients with fasting hypoglycemia may have a variety of serious conditions. Beta cell hyperplasia, adenoma, and nesidioblastosis (islet cell hyperplasia) all cause excessive insulin secretion. Hyperinsulinism is also seen in association with panhypopituitarism.

Hypoglycemia may also occur when there is a deficiency of hormones or agents that maintain blood glucose level. These include growth hormone, adrenocorticotropic hormone (ACTH), catecholamines, thyroid hormones, and glucagon. Any defect in the liver enzymes that control glycogenolysis or gluconeogenesis will predispose the affected individual to hypoglycemia. Thus, glycogen storage diseases, fructose metabolism disorders, galactosemia, and maple syrup urine disease are associated with hypoglycemia.

Hypoglycemia can result from a number of adrenal and hepatic disorders, such as adrenal insufficiency, congenital adrenal hypoplasia, and hepatic damage due to toxins, tumors, leukemic infiltrates, and hepatitis.

Another type of hypoglycemia is ketotic hypoglycemia. This variant is the most common cause of hypoglycemia in children. The exact cause of the episodic attacks is unknown, but a deficiency of endogenous gluconeogenic amino acids, notably alanine, has been noted in affected children. The attacks occur in the morning and are associated with periods of stress, infection, or fasting. Ketonuria is also present. Affected children are otherwise well and have normal insulin levels and glucose tolerance test results between attacks. Episodes respond briskly to glucose administration.

Miscellaneous causes of hypoglycemia include ingestion of drugs or toxins (insulin, alcohol, salicylate, and propranolol), kwashiorkor, sarcomas, impaired intestinal glucose absorption, and Reye's syndrome (see Chapter 72).

EVALUATION

The patient presenting with hypoglycemia merits a thorough history and physical examination. Information on the timing, frequency, and description of the attacks (with associated symptoms) should be elicited. A history of drug or toxin ingestion should be investigated, and a family history of similar episodes or food intolerances (such as fruits) should be sought. The patient's growth and usual state of health are assessed. Evidence of hormonal dysfunction and abdominal masses are investigated during the physical examination.

Laboratory tests are indicated by the child's history and physical findings. In addition to appropriate assays of hormone function, a glucose tolerance test should be performed to assess both glucose and insulin levels in the fed and fasting states. The glucagon tolerance test challenges the liver's ability to form glucose from stored glycogen; the alanine tolerance test challenges the liver's ability in gluconeogenesis. Other tolerance tests (galactose, fructose, leucine, tolbutamide) are dictated by history and physical findings.

MANAGEMENT

The hypoglycemic patient should immediately be given glucose orally or intravenously (10 to 25 ml of a 50% dextrose solution). A dextrostix glucose test should be done, and a blood glucose and insulin evaluation should be obtained at the same time. Because the glucose administration may cause a rebound insulin secretion, the blood sugar level may quickly fall. The patient should be carefully monitored and, when awake, receive frequent carbohydrate feedings or, if incapable of taking oral feedings, receive intravenous glucose. An intramuscular injection of glucagon may also terminate the attack in some individuals.

The long-term management of these patients is as varied as the causes of their hypoglycemia. Children with ketotic hypoglycemia should be fed frequently, especially during times of illness or stress. Children with hormonal deficiencies respond to their exogenous replacement. Children with hyperinsulinism may improve with diazoxide (10 mg/kg/day divided bid). Children with tumors may improve when the tumors are removed. Children with hepatic enzyme deficiencies improve when appropriate dietary restrictions are imposed. Regardless of the etiology of the hypoglycemia, affected patients and their families benefit from ongoing psychological support.

BIBLIOGRAPHY

Behrman R, Vaughan V: Nelson textbook of Pediatrics, 13th ed, pp 1264–1273, Chapter 20: Metabolic Disorders—Hypoglycemia. Philadelphia, WB Saunders, 1987

Cornblath M: Hypoglycemia in infancy and childhood. Pediatr Ann 10:356–363, 1981

Pagliara A et al: Hypoglycemia in infancy and childhood I and II. Pediatrics 82:365–379, 558–577, 1973

65

Sexual Development

PRECOCIOUS PUBERTY

Precocious puberty is present when secondary sex characteristics appear before age 8 in girls and age 9 in boys. Isosexual precocious puberty refers to development appropriate to one's own sex, whereas heterosexual precociousness refers to development appropriate to the opposite sex.

Premature thelarche denotes bilateral breast development without other signs of puberty. The usual patient is a 2- to 4-year-old girl with breast buds of 2 to 3 cm with no changes in the areola or nipple. One breast may be developing faster than the other. Growth and bone age are normal. Puberty is usually attained at the normal age. Premature thelarche may represent increased sensitivity to low levels of endogenous estrogens, use of exogenous estrogens (creams, oral contraceptive pills), or the first sign of precocious puberty. Treatment includes reassurance and close follow-up.

Premature adrenarche denotes the isolated appearance of pubic, and sometimes axillary, hair before age 8 without other signs of puber-

ty. The usual patient is 6 to 8 years old with an elevated urinary 17-ketosteroid level for age (but not elevated for the amount of pubic hair present) and a normal bone age. Puberty usually occurs normally. Evidence of marked virilization or estrogenization suggests an adrenal disorder or certain gonadal tumors. Treatment is reassurance and close follow-up, unless physical signs suggest a tumor.

Both premature thelarche and adrenarche may herald the first signs of precocious puberty or be isolated events.

True precocious puberty has its genesis in the pituitary or hypothalamus and is associated with increased gonadotropin levels relative to age. It may be idiopathic or due to a pituitary/hypothalamic insult (tumor, injury, infection, hydrocephalus), neurofibromatosis, tuberous sclerosis, the McCune-Albright syndrome (café au lait spots, fibrous dysplasia, bone cysts), and rare gonadotropin-secreting tumors (teratoma, hepatoblastoma, chorioepithelioma). Ovarian tumors (granulosa cell tumors, arrhenoblastomas, lipid cell tumors, thecomas, dysgerminomas, and cysts), testicular tumors (Leydig cell tumors, seminomas),

415

adrenal tumors, adrenal hyperplasia, exoge-nous estrogens, anabolic steroids, or andro-gens, and, rarely, hypothyroidism, can cause incomplete puberty, an infrapituitary disorder with stimulation of testosterone or estrogen production independent of gonadotropin lev-els.

More than 80% of girls with precocious puberty have the idiopathic variety, compared with only 50% of boys; the hypothalamic–pituitary axis is prematurely activated for unknown reasons. Since 50% of the boys and 20% of the girls have an organic cause of their precocious puberty, the evaluation of this condition must be thorough.

The history should include details of the patient's birth, growth patterns, and the long-term use of medications. A history of enceph-alitis, seizures, headaches, behavior changes, visual symptoms, abdominal pain, and geni-tourinary symptoms should be sought. A family history of age of menarche of siblings, mother, and grandmothers, neurofibromato-sis, Mc-Cune Albright syndrome, or tuberous sclerosis is also important. The physical examination should be complete, with special emphasis on the neurologic examination, ophthalmoscopic (fundoscopic and visual fields evaluation), and genital examinations, including Tanner staging of genitalia, pubic hair, and breasts. Evidence of feminization in boys and virilization in girls may indicate het-erosexual precocious puberty, which is usual-ly adrenal or gonadal in origin. A rectal exam-ination should be performed.

Initial laboratory tests that are useful to determine the etiology of the puberty are dis-cussed below. Skull x-rays may demonstrate a lesion in the area of the sella. Hand and wrist films generally demonstrate an advanced bone age; a retarded bone age suggests hypo-thyroidism. Since there is variation in follicle-stimulating hormone (FSH) and luteinizing hormone (LH) levels during a 24-hour period, single determinations are not always useful.

High LH levels suggest a gonadotropin-secret-ing tumor or choriocarcinoma, the latter of which can be diagnosed by a positive urine pregnancy test result, since human chorionic gonadotropin cross-reacts with LH. A 24-hour urine sample for 17-ketosteroids is also obtained to determine levels of androgen pro-duction.

In girls, ovarian tumors cause only 5% of precocious puberty. If an ovarian tumor is strongly suspected, its presence frequently can be verified by the rectal examination and confirmed by a computed tomography (CT) scan. Serum estradiol levels are commonly elevated with ovarian granulosa cell tumors. Serum progesterone and urinary pregnanediol are increased in ovarian thecomas. Some endocrinologists recommend obtaining a vag-inal smear to ascertain the degree of estrogen-ization of vaginal cells; certain ovarian tumors produce excesses of estrogen or pro-gesterone and will affect the type of cells seen on smear. An electroencephalogram (EEG) is also recommended by some, since as many as 80% of children with idiopathic precocious puberty have abnormal EEGs.

If an adrenal cause for precocious puberty is suspected (*i.e.*, if evidence of heterosexual pre-cocious puberty is present), laboratory tests should include the aforementioned ones and a 24-hour urine sample for 17-ketosteroids and pregnanediol. If a girl has a normal 24-hour urinary 17-ketosteroid level but elevated serum testosterone, an adrenal cause is unlikely and an ovarian tumor is probable. If a child has an elevated 17-ketosteroid level sup-pressed by dexamethasone, congenital adrenal hyperplasia is likely; a level not suppressed by dexamethasone indicates an adrenal or gonad-al tumor.

Treatment varies according to the cause. Tumors and cysts should be removed, if pos-sible. Congenital adrenal hyperplasia is treated by glucocorticoid therapy. Idiopathic and severe variants of cerebral precocious puberty can be treated in girls, with medroxy-progesterone acetate IM every other week for several years or until age 8. Because of its extensive side effects related to glucocorticoid excess, its use should be weighed carefully.

The child with precocious puberty requires reassurance that he is not a "freak." Parents must be supportive and should treat the child in an age-appropriate fashion, since intellectual and emotional growth are not usually accelerated.

DELAYED PUBERTY

Delayed puberty is present if secondary sex characteristics have not begun to appear by age 14 to 15 in girls and age 15 to 16 in boys, although some normal adolescents do not begin puberty until 14 to 15 years of age.

The causes of delayed puberty are the same as those of short stature and also primary and secondary hypogonadism. Primary hypogonadism includes Turner's syndrome (female XO or XX/XO mosaic), Klinefelter's syndrome, inflammation, torsion, or tumor of the ovary or testis, certain drugs (i.e., cyclophosphamide, high-dose steroids), and miscellaneous causes. Secondary hypogonadism includes anorexia nervosa (see Chapter 3), pituitary lesions, and certain syndromes (Prader-Willi, Kallman, Laurence-Moon-Biedl).

The evaluation of adolescents with delayed puberty should include a complete history and physical examination and assessments of serum gonadotropins, which are elevated in primary hypogonadism and are decreased in pituitary-associated secondary hypogonadisms. Determination of karyotype may also be useful.

The treatment of delayed puberty depends on its cause. Constitutionally delayed adolescents can be reassured. If there are no signs of puberty by age 16 in males or 15 in females, referral to an endocrinologist for evaluation and possible hormonal therapy is indicated.

MENSTRUATION AND ITS DISORDERS

Physiology

Menstruation occurs as the adolescent growth spurt is slowing; this is not usually before at least a Tanner 4 breast stage is achieved and the body composition is at least 24% fat. These changes generally occur in American girls at approximately 12.5 years. Menstrual periods are often irregular in timing, amount, and duration in early adolescence because of hypothalamic–pituitary–gonadal immaturity. Cycles are frequently anovulatory. Once mature menstrual periods are established, they generally last 3 to 7 days and occur consistently every 21 to 45 days. Each individual's cycle is fairly consistent in length and is measured from the beginning of one menstrual period to the beginning of the next. Blood loss is 35 to 55 ml or an average of 4 to 5 well-soaked pads or tampons each day.

The menstrual cycle is divided into a follicular stage and luteal stage. Low serum level of FSH (and later LH) stimulates an ovarian follicle to produce estrogen during days 5 to 14 (of a hypothetical 28-day cycle). Under the effect of estrogen, the endometrium proliferates. A certain critical level of estrogen triggers an LH surge (which in turn, triggers ovulation 8 to 12 hours later). Ovulation occurs at approximately day 14. Subsequent luteinization of the graafian follicle gives rise to the progesterone-producing corpus luteum. Estrogen is also produced but to a lesser degree than progesterone; both hormones inhibit FSH and LH secretion. The endometrium develops coiled glands, increased vascularity and increased glycogen content of cells. If pregnancy does not occur, the corpus luteum atrophies, estrogen and progesterone production fall, and FSH secretion begins to rise in preparation for the next cycle. Further degradation of the endometrium is associated with menstrual bleeding (days 1 to 5 of cycle).

Amenorrhea

The absence of menstrual flow can be primary or secondary. Primary amenorrhea is also known as delayed menarche. *Primary amenorrhea* may be of three types: (1) delayed sexual development, (2) delayed menarche with some development of secondary sex characteristics, and (3) delayed menarche with evidence of virilization.

Delayed sexual development is present when there is no evidence of pubic hair or breast buds by age 14 to 15. There has usually been no growth spurt. Knowledge of the FSH and LH levels will assist in diagnosis. If FSH and LH levels are high, ovarian failure is usually the etiology (most commonly, Turner's syndrome (XO) or its mosaic, other forms of gonadal dysgenesis, or ovarian damage due to irradiation or chemotherapy). If FSH and LH levels are normal or low, a central nervous system (CNS) disorder or systemic disease is usually the cause (most commonly, hypogonadotropic hypogonadism, deficiencies of LH-releasing factor, panhypopituitarism, Prader-Willi syndrome, CNS tumors, regional enteritis, or anorexia nervosa). If FSH and LH levels are low or normal and the evaluation is negative, true idiopathic delayed puberty is the cause.

An adolescent with *delayed menarche with some development of secondary sex characteristics* may show evidence of normal estrogen (breast and genitalia development) and androgen (axillary and pubic hair) effects. Careful attention must be paid to the presence of external or internal genital anomalies, such as vaginal/uterine cervical agenesis or imperforate hymen. When the uterus and cervix are absent, the girl may have testicular feminization syndrome (*i.e.*, the genotype is XY, ovaries are absent, the testes are insensitive to androgens, and there is age-inappropriate estrogen effect).

If the girl's examination is normal, her vaginal cells demonstrate estrogen effect, and she demonstrates withdrawal bleeding after intramuscular progesterone, her diagnosis is delayed menarche. If the girl's examination is normal but she does not bleed after intramuscular progesterone (with low or normal FSH and LH levels), her diagnosis may be hypogonadism, especially due to hypothalamic causes (stress, weight changes), a CNS tumor, or chronic disease. If she does not bleed and FSH/LH are elevated, gonadal dysgenesis or ovarian failure should be suspected.

Delayed menarche with evidence of virilization is uncommon; it is associated with congenital adrenocortical hyperplasia, ovarian tumors, adrenal tumors, polycystic ovaries, gonadal dysgenesis, incomplete testicular feminization (*i.e.*, no excess estrogen effect), and hermaphroditism (*i.e.*, both ovarian and testicular tissue present). Most of these conditions are diagnosed by karyotype (buccal smear) or measurement of serum testosterone, FSH, and LH in conjunction with urinary 17-ketosteroids (an indicator of adrenal androgen production).

Secondary amenorrhea is the abrupt cessation of menses for 3 to 4 months after previously regular cycles. Sometimes, oligomenorrhea precedes the amenorrhea. The adolescent with secondary amenorrhea deserves a complete history (stresses, weight changes, medications, drugs, chronic illnesses, pregnancy) and physical examination, including a pelvic examination. A pregnancy test should be done because conception is one of the most common causes of amenorrhea.

If the pregnancy test result is negative, a vaginal smear can be examined for estrogen effect, or intramuscular progesterone can be given. If withdrawal bleeding occurs, the diagnosis is usually hypothalamic amenorrhea due to physical or emotional stresses (very common), weight changes, or illness. Other, less common causes include diabetes mellitus, thyroid disease, ovarian tumors, and polycystic ovaries (Stein-Leventhal syndrome). In the last entity, hirsutism is frequently present, and frank virilization may be present. It is believed that the hypothalamic–ovarian feedback mechanism is deranged. LH levels are elevated throughout the cycle without a midcycle surge. FSH levels are low to normal. Excess LH induces excessive ovarian estrogen and androgen production. Ovulation cannot occur, and the ovaries enlarge with multiple cysts. Serum testosterone and urinary 17-ketosteroids are usually elevated; the latter, being deprived from gonads, is not generally suppressed by dexamethasone.

If no withdrawal bleeding occurs after intramuscular progesterone, and FSH and LH levels are high, suspect gonadal dysgenesis or ovarian disease; if FSH and LH levels are low to normal, suspect hypothalamic amenorrhea, CNS tumor, chronic disease, or pituitary infarction.

The girl with secondary amenorrhea and hirsutism/virilization may have ovarian pathology (polycystic ovaries, tumors) or adrenal disease (adrenocortical hyperplasia, tumors, Cushing's syndrome). Diagnostic tests include serum FSH, LH, testosterone, 17-hydroxy-progesterone, urinary 17-hydroxy-corticosteroids, and 17-ketosteroids with a dexamethasone suppression test if the latter is elevated.

Dysfunctional Uterine Bleeding

Dysfunctional uterine bleeding includes any increase or decrease in the amount of timing of menstrual bleeding and is usually due to anovulatory cycles. In adolescents, the genesis of these cycles is generally hypothalamic. An excess of FSH (due to hypothalamic–pituitary–gonadal immaturity) fosters unchanging estrogen levels, which cause endometrial proliferation. If such proliferation is not opposed by progesterone, menstrual bleeding, when it occurs, is due to a proliferative, not a normal secretory, endometrium.

The girl with dysfunctional uterine bleeding deserves a complete history (especially menstrual), physical (including pelvic) examination, a pregnancy test, and a complete blood count (with particular attention paid to the hematocrit and platelet count). The differential diagnosis of dysfunctional uterine bleeding includes pregnancy, a spontaneous abortion, tubal pregnancy, blood dyscrasias, thyroid disorders, adrenal disease, diabetes, tumors of the uterus, vagina, or ovary, oral contraceptive problems (missed pills, breakthrough bleeding), side effects of intrauterine devices, endometritis (irregular bleeding with pelvic pain, fever, discharge), and nongenital tract bleeding (urinary, rectal, colonic).

In addition to the minimal work-up described above, other tests are ordered, according to the findings of the history or physical examination. If a girl presents with severe bleeding, marked anemia, or unstable vital signs, she should be admitted to the hospital. If no other cause for the severe menstrual bleeding is obvious, the patient should be given progestins every 4 hours until the bleeding stops, and then twice daily for 10 to 14 days. A normal withdrawal flow will follow 2 to 4 days after the last dose. The patient should then be cycled with Ortho-Novum or Enovid-E for the next 3 to 4 months. Any patient with severe bleeding that does not respond to progestins within 1-2 days requires an endocervical dilation and curettage.

If bleeding is mild or moderate in dysfunctional uterine bleeding, Enovid-E (2.5 mg bid) or Ortho-Novum (2 mg bid) for 10 days should be used; alternatively, Provera 10 mg/day for 7 days, can be used. Cessation of bleeding is expected within several days, and a normal withdrawal flow will follow 2 to 4 days after the last tablet. The patient can then be cycled for several months with either Enovid-E or Ortho-Novum.

Dysmenorrhea

Painful menstruation is a common adolescent complaint. Approximately 50% of adolescent girls experience menstrual pain within 3 to 5 years of their menarche. Typically, crampy, lower abdominal pain develops within hours of the onset of the period and lasts for approximately 24 hours. Nausea, vomiting, diarrhea, or constipation may accompany the cramps. Other associated symptoms include headaches, breast tenderness, backache, abdominal bloating, pain in the medial thighs, and mood swings. The pain is believed to be mediated by unusually high levels of prostaglandins, which increase uterine contractions and irritate endometrial nerves. Dysmenorrhea may be primary or secondary; the majority (95%) of adolescents with dysmenorrhea have the primary variant with completely normal examinations. The rare adolescent with secondary dysmenorrhea may have endometriosis, ovarian cysts, chronic pelvic inflammatory disease, or anatomic defects of the uterus or vagina.

Some girls with dysmenorrhea can continue their daily activities during the day(s) of pain; for these patients, acetaminophen or aspirin may be the only therapy needed, since either medication inhibits prostaglandin synthetase. For girls whose pain causes them to miss school or social activities, aspirin may be tried (q 4 h as long as the pain persists) for severe periods, or a more potent prostaglandin inhibitor, such as naproxen, may be used. Finally, for girls whose pain is so severe that they must remain in bed, naproxen is used as needed; relaxation or biofeedback techniques are also helpful. In some older teenagers, induction of anovulatory cycles (which are not associated with prostaglandin rise) for several months by use of cyclic hormones (birth control pills) permits the patient to have several pain-free months.

All girls with dysmenorrhea deserve reassurance that the pain does not imply that they are abnormal. They should be encouraged to rest properly, to exercise, and to eat a nutritious diet. The physician should also discuss the cultural meaning of the pain for that patient's family, and counsel both patient and mother, if necessary. The use of intrauterine devices should be avoided in girls with dysmenorrhea, since such devices are associated with menstrual cramps.

Mittelschmerz (Ovulatory Pain)

A unilateral lower abdominal crampy pain occurring at midcycle each month for several minutes to several hours is mittelschmerz (literally, "middle pain"). Usually the pain occurs on alternating lower abdominal quadrants, from month to month, and is believed to be due to peritoneal irritation by the contents of the ruptured ovarian follicle. If the patient presents with her first episode or in severe pain, a surgical etiology may be initially considered. However, in girls whose pain is chronic, cyclical, and self-limited, the diagnosis is fairly straightforward: The patient should be reassured.

BIBLIOGRAPHY

Precocious puberty

Emans SJ, Goldstein DP: Pediatric and Adolescent Gynecology, pp 59–69. Boston, Little, Brown Co, 1977

Hofmann A: Adolescent Medicine. Reading, Mass: Addison-Wesley Publishing Co., 1983; 160–80.

Shen JTY: The Clinical Practice of Adolescent Medicine, pp 267–83. New York, Appleton-Century-Crofts, 1980

Pubertal delay

Emans S, Goldstein D: Pediatric and Adolescent Gynecology, pp 72–88. Boston, Little, Brown, and Co, 1977

Frawley T: Pituitary and Adrenal Disease. In Shen JTY: The Clinical Practice of Adolescent Medicine, pp 269-270. New York, Appleton-Century-Crofts, 1980

Hofmann A: Adolescent Medicine, pp 174–176. Reading, MA, Addison-Wesley, 1983

Menstruation and its disorders

Emans SJ, Goldstein DP: Pediatric and Adolescent Gynecology, pp 71–99, 101–104. Boston, Little, Brown Co, 1977

Hofmann A: Adolescent Medicine, pp 253–262. Reading, MA, Addison-Wesley, 1983

Kreutner AK, Hollingsworth DR (eds): Adolescent Obstetrics and Gynecology, pp 25–45. Chicago, Year Book Medical Pub, 1978

Shen JTY: The Clinical Practice of Adolescent Medicine, pp 349–361. New York, Appleton-Century-Crofts, 1980

66

Diabetes Insipidus

Diabetes insipidus (DI) is a metabolic condition in which antidiuretic hormone (vasopressin) is either lacking or, if present, has little effect on its end organ, the kidney. In the nonrenal form, disease or injury to neurohypophysial structures may result in DI. Such etiologies include tumors in the sella or optic chiasm area, surgery in the region of the pituitary or hypothalamus, head trauma, encephalitis, and leukemia. There is also a hereditary form in which there is a congenital lack of neurosecretory cells of the supraoptic and paraventricular nuclei.

The renal form of the disease (nephrogenic diabetes insipidus, or NDI) is a hereditary (probably X-linked recessive) disorder. The distal tubule and collecting duct, through a biochemical or enzymatic derangement, are unresponsive to vasopressin. Normally, vasopressin increases the permeability of these structures to water and causes it to be reabsorbed into the hypertonic medullary interstitium. In NDI the urine cannot be concentrated even in response to an elevated plasma solute load. If the patient does not drink a large amount of water, in the face of high urine losses, he becomes dehydrated.

Clinically, the patient has polyuria and polydipsia. The urine volumes are large (4 to 12 liters/day) and very hypotonic. The child's thirst is unquenchable. He may have a history of repeated episodes of vomiting and dehydration, constipation, hyperthermia, weight loss, failure to thrive, or developmental delay. Children with inherited DI will demonstrate their symptoms in early infancy. Older children may present with enuresis, lack of perspiration, and bizarre efforts to obtain more water, such as drinking from toilet bowls. Children with central nervous system (CNS) disorders may also present with symptoms attributable to their underlying diseases.

The urine of a patient with DI has a specific gravity of 1.001 to 1.005 and an osmolality of 50 to 200 mOsm/kg water (usually 80 to 120 mOsm/kg). Even with marked dehydration, the specific gravity may not rise above 1.010. Levels of serum and urinary arginine vasopressin can be determined by radioimmunoassay. In patients with DI, water deprivation of 6 to 12 hours leads to dehydration, with an increased serum osmolality and low urine osmolality. If exogenous vasopressin is given, the patient with central DI responds with a rise in urine osmolality, while the patient with NDI shows no response.

Treatment of central DI includes allowing the patient free access to water, correction, if possible, of the CNS lesion, intranasal administration of desmopressin (initial dose, 2.5 to 5.0 μg bid), or intranasal administration of lysine-8-vasopressin, and administration of chlorpropamide. Intramuscular vasopressin (Pitressin) lasts longer than that delivered intranasally, but its injection is painful. Chlorpropamide potentiates the action of vasopressin but is associated with hypoglycemia.

Treatment of NDI includes provision of adequate water for the patient, adequate caloric intake, and a diet rich in carbohydrates and fats and poorer in protein, salt, and phosphorus. Decreasing the body's solute load by decreasing protein intake is important, since more water is required to excrete a high solute load. Finally, thiazide diuretics paradoxically reduce urine volume and increase urine specific gravity in NDI, especially in conjunction with low sodium intake. If thiazides are used, potassium may be lost in the urine, and its supplementation may be required.

BIBLIOGRAPHY

Behrman R, Vaughan V: Nelson Textbook of Pediatrics, pp 1181–1183. Chapter 19—the endocrine system—Disorders of the hypothalamus and pituitary. Philadelphia, WB Saunders, 1987

Greger N, Kirkland R, Clayton G et al: Central diabetes insipidus—22 years' experience. Am J Dis Child 140:551–554, 1986

67 Syndrome of Inappropriate Antidiuretic Hormone Secretion

In the syndrome of inappropriate antidiuretic hormone secretion (SIADH), the level of arginine vasopressin is inappropriately high for the blood's osmolality and is not suppressed by dilution of body fluids. SIADH is associated with central nervous system (CNS) disease (meningitis, encephalitis, brain tumors and abscesses, intracranial bleeding, head trauma, and Guillian-Barré syndrome), certain malignancies (pancreas, duodenum, lung), and miscellaneous causes (pneumonia, tuberculosis, porphyria, certain drugs). The mechanism of injury in CNS disease is probably hypothalamic; in certain malignancies, the tumors may secrete vasopressin.

Clinically, the patient may be asymptomatic if his serum sodium level is at least 120 mEq/L, or he may be nauseated and irritable or confused. If the serum sodium is lower than 110 mEq/L, he may be stuporous, comatose, or seizing.

Serum sodium and chloride are low. The serum is hypotonic, and the urine's osmolality is greater than it should be for the degree of serum hypotonicity present. Renal excretion of sodium continues despite hyponatremia.

SIADH responds to treatment of the underlying disorder, restriction of fluids, and hypertonic saline infusion if severe hyponatremia and neurologic symptoms are present.

BIBLIOGRAPHY

Behrman R, Vaughan V: Nelson Textbook of Pediatrics, 13th ed, pp 1183–1184. Chapter 19—The endocrine system—Disorders of the hypothalamus and pituitary. Philadelphia, WB Saunders, 1987

424

68

Hypothyroidism

Hypothyroidism results from deficient production of thyroid hormone and may be congenital or acquired. The thyroid gland may be enlarged, small, or absent.

The etiologies of hypothyroidism are multiple. Since the thyroid is under the control of the pituitary and hypothalamus, disease in these structures (hypopituitarism, tumors, hemorrhages, etc.) can limit the amount of thyroid-stimulating hormone (TSH) and thyroid-releasing hormone (TRH) produced and secreted. TRH stimulates the synthesis and release of TSH, which, in turn, activates the thyroid to release its hormones. There may be isolated deficiencies of TRH or TSH, and the thyroid may be unresponsive to TSH; all of these conditions will also lead to hypothyroidism.

The thyroid gland itself may be the cause of hormonal deficiency. The gland may be aplastic, hypoplastic, or ectopic because of dysgenesis or maternal radioiodine treatment (for thyroid cancer) during pregnancy. The gland may be incapable of producing its hormones because of defects in iodide trapping, in iodide incorporation into active organic compounds, and in thyroglobulin (TG) synthesis. The active thyroid hormones thyroxine (T_4) and triiodothyronine (T_3) are stored in the gland as T_3 and T_4 and are released from TG by the action of enzymes. Failure of the enzymes to release T_3 and T_4 from TG also leads to a deficiency in circulating hormones.

Hypothyroidism may be secondary to severe lack of dietary iodine (endemic goiter), subtotal thyroidectomy, maternal ingestion of iodides or antihyperthyroid drugs taken during pregnancy, overdosage of antihyperthyroid medications, and damage to the thyroid gland (infections, autoimmune disease). Of these, an autoimmune disease (lymphocytic thyroiditis) is the most common cause of acquired hypothyroidism in pediatrics.

Lymphocytic thyroiditis (Hashimoto's thyroiditis) is characterized by lymphocytic and plasma cell infiltration of the gland. Fifty percent of the patients have antibodies to their thyroid tissue. There is a male-to-female ratio of 1:4 to 7. Familial clusters of cases occur, and other family members may have antithyroid antibodies. The disease may coexist (in the same gland) with Graves' disease and may be associated with other autoimmune disorders, such as diabetes mellitus.

CLINICAL CHARACTERISTICS

Clinically, the infant with congenital hypothyroidism (cretinism) presents in the first few weeks of life. The male-to-female ratio is 1:3. There may be a history of prolonged physiologic jaundice in the immediate neonatal period. The infant is lethargic, sleeps a great deal, cries infrequently, and has a poor appetite. Because of his large tongue, he may suck poorly, choke, and become dyspneic during feeding. He has noisy respirations and is likely to be constipated. Hypothermia is common, and his skin is cold and mottled.

If he has not been treated by 3 to 6 months of age, he will demonstrate growth delay, large fontanelles, hypertelorism, a flattened nose, a gaping mouth from which his large tongue protrudes, a short, thick neck, dry skin, sparse hair, a raspy cry, and generalized hypotonia. He appears dull. If the condition persists, his development will be delayed and his mental development will be retarded.

The patient with acquired hypothyroidism will also have dry skin, constipation, and dullness. His previously normal pattern of growth may cease. Depending on his age, his development may be relatively unaffected. A goiter (thyroid gland enlargement) may or may not be present. The child with lymphocytic thyroiditis may have a variable-sized, sometimes nodular thyroid that is firm and nontender. Clinically, the child may be euthyroid. A child with suppurative thyroiditis (usually secondary to infection or trauma) presents with a markedly tender, swollen, warm, erythematous gland, the size of which may limit neck movements and swallowing.

EVALUATION

In hypothyroidism, serum T_3 and T_4 levels are low or borderline. Such levels are measured by radioimmunoassay, as is the TSH level. If the defect is in the thyroid, TSH levels are high; if the defect is in the pituitary or hypothalamus, TSH is low. When the patient's TSH is low, a TRH challenge test can determine whether the defect is hypothalamic (TRH deficiency) or pituitary (TSH deficiency). Normally, TSH peaks in ½ to 1½ hours after administration of TRH. If the patient responds to TRH, his defect is localized to the hypothalamus. If there is no TSH rise in response to the challenge, there may be pituitary failure.

Serum thyroxine-binding globulin (TBG) measurement may be useful. It is measured by the T_3 uptake resin test. The product of the serum T_4 concentration and the T_3 uptake is the T_4-T_3 index, which is elevated in hyperthyroidism and decreased in hypothyroidism. The index gives a measure of free serum T_4.

Technetium 99m (as pertechnetate) scanning of the thyroid is useful to detect a lack of functioning thyroid tissue, ectopic thyroid tissue, or thyroid masses. It has a lower half-life and is associated with lower radiation exposure than radioactive iodine.

A child with suppurative thyroiditis usually has normal thyroid function study results and merits incision and drainage of the gland with appropriate antibiotic administration. A child with lymphocytic thyroiditis may also have normal thyroid function tests, although the TSH may be slightly elevated. A thyroid scan reveals irregular distribution of the isotope. Fifty percent of the patients have antithyroid antibodies in titers greater than 1:16.

MANAGEMENT

Prompt treatment of congenital hypothyroidism is necessary to avoid permanent mental retardation. If treatment is instituted past 3 months of age, the child's growth may normalize, but he has only a 10% chance of normal mental development.

Since 30% to 50% of T_3 is derived from deiodination of T_4, treatment of hypothyroidism with oral sodium-L-thyroxine will provide adequate levels of T_4 and T_3. Normal levels of T_4 ensure normal levels of T_3; therefore, monitoring of T_4/T_3 levels assesses adequacy of therapy. In infants, the initial dose of sodium-L-thyroxine is 6 to 10 µg/kg/day. The dose for older children and adolescents is 4 µg/kg/day. If a goiter is present, it slowly decreases in size with therapy. However, therapy will not alter antithyroid antibody levels in lymphocytic thyroiditis.

BIBLIOGRAPHY

Behrman R, Vaughan V: Nelson Textbook of Pediatrics, 13th ed, pp 1195–1199. Chapter 19: The endocrine system—Disorders of the thyroid gland. Philadelphia, WB Saunders, 1987

Fisher D: Hypothyroidism in childhood. Pediatr Rev 2:67–74, 1980

Foley TP: Goiter in children. Pediatr Rev 5:259–272, 1984

69

Hyperthyroidism

Hyperthyroidism results from excessive secretion of thyroid hormone. Although there are several causes for this disorder, the most common cause, by far, is a diffuse toxic goiter (Graves' disease). Such a goiter may be congenital if the mother has or recently had Graves' disease. An IgG immunoglobulin long-acting thyroid stimulator (LATS) crosses the placenta and stimulates the infant's thyroid. More commonly, however, Graves' disease is acquired. LATS is present in at least 50% of patients with Graves' disease. Toxic goiter is felt to be an autoimmune disease, since the gland is infiltrated with lymphocytes and plasma cells and it is associated with other autoimmune disorders such as pernicious anemia and myasthenia gravis. Antithyroglobulin antibodies may also be present.

Although young children may present with Graves' disease, the usual pediatric patient is an adolescent. The male-to-female ratio in congenital hyperthyroidism is $1:1$ and in acquired hyperthyroidism, $1:5$. There may be a gap between onset of symptoms and diagnosis on the order of several months.

CLINICAL PRESENTATION

The patient is irritable, restless, and hyperactive, and emotionally labile. He appears anxious and alert and demonstrates tremors. His appetite is ravenous, yet he gains no weight or even loses weight. His eyes are exophthalmic. The thyroid gland may be palpable and visible; it may have an associated bruit. Bone age is advanced, and infants may demonstrate cranial synostosis. The patient sweats excessively, is tachycardic and tachypneic, and has an elevated blood pressure. Older patients may complain of palpitations. Patients, particularly neonates, may develop life-threatening cardiac decompensation. Congenital hyperthyroidism usually remits in early infancy but may persist for several years. Thyroid "storm" is an acute form of hyperthyroidism in which there is severe hyperthermia and tachycardia; delirium, coma, and death may follow.

The patient with Graves' disease usually demonstrates elevated thyroxine (T_4) and triiodothyronine (T_3) with low thyrotropin levels. LATS is found in 50% of the patients.

MANAGEMENT

Treatment of Graves' disease may include subtotal thyroidectomy, medical therapy, or use of radioactive iodine; iodine is generally not used in children, and surgery is performed only if medical therapy is unsuccessful or unfeasible.

Medical therapy of congenital hyperthyroidism consists of Lugol's solution (1 drop q 8 h) and propylthiouracil (10 mg q 8 h); if the infant is quite ill, parenteral fluids, digoxin, and propranolol may be necessary.

Medical therapy of acquired Graves' disease consists of propylthiouracil (100 to 150 mg tid) or methimazole (10 to 15 mg tid); both drugs inhibit iodine incorporation, thus leading to a reduction in thyroid hormones. The dose is adjusted according to the child's response; overdosage can cause hypothyroidism. Clinical response is evident in 2 to 3 weeks and adequate control occurs in 4 to 14 weeks. Treatment should continue for several years and should be tapered slowly before complete discontinuation. Relapses occur in 25% of patients, usually in the first 6 months after therapy is stopped. Therapy may be resumed in such patients.

BIBLIOGRAPHY

Behrman R, Vaughan V: Nelson Textbook of Pediatrics, 13th ed, pp 1199–1204. Chapter 19: The endocrine system—Disorders of the Thyroid Gland. Philadelphia, WB Saunders, 1987

Foley TP: Goiter in Children. Pediatr Rev 5:259-272, 1984

70

Short Stature

When an infant or toddler presents with short stature, it is frequently in association with failure to gain adequate weight (see Chapter 3). Although this association may also exist in older children and adolescents, they are more likely to present with short stature alone. Short stature may be due to growth failure or to marked deceleration of growth so that the child's growth drops from its usual percentile.

The causes of short stature include familial, constitutional delay, prematurity, malnutrition, emotional depression, hypothyroidism, chronic debilitating illnesses, endogenous or exogenous cortisol excess, inflammatory bowel disease, growth hormone deficiency, skeletal dysplasia, Turner's syndrome, and miscellaneous causes. Most cases of short stature are due to genetic (familial) or constitutional delay. In constitutional growth delay, the child's height and weight are normal at birth and in early infancy, but growth falls below the mean in late infancy or early toddlerhood. Although puberty's onset may be delayed, the adult height is usually normal.

The child with a history of prematurity or being small for gestational age may continue to be small. Malnutrition, malabsorption, or chronic debilitating illness causes growth retardation through the lack of adequate calories. Emotionally deprived children fail to grow for reasons not completely understood, but felt to be related to hypothalamic suppression. Hypothyroidism has been discussed in Chapter 68. Chronic high-dose exogenous steroid therapy (for chronic disease) frequently results in growth retardation. Endogenous cortisol excess (Cushing's syndrome) results in a constellation of signs (moon facies, "buffalo hump," hirsutism, hypertension, fatigue, striae, voice deepening, clitoral hypertrophy, and amenorrhea) in addition to growth delay. Growth hormone deficiency results from pituitary dysgenesis. Growth is normal in the first year or two of life but is retarded after age 2, and the child appears infantile in body habitus. Other signs of pituitary dysfunction may be present. Skeletal dysplasia (such as achondroplasia) is characterized by short extremities with a normal sized (or nearly so) trunk and head. Turner's syndrome (genotype XO) is characterized by a webbed neck, low posterior hairline, small mandible, prominent ears, epicanthal folds, and a broad chest. Miscellaneous causes of growth failure include rickets (vitamin D deficiency) and hypoparathyroidism.

The child with short stature deserves a thorough history (pattern of growth, birth and prenatal history, presence of chronic disease, medication usage, developmental milestones, and the growth patterns of parents and siblings) and a complete physical examination, upon which many of the conditions listed above will be obvious. Usually, however, the child with short stature appears normal. An adolescent with short stature may also have delayed puberty, for which he should be evaluated (see Chapter 65). Evaluation is dictated by the results of the history and physical examination. A bone age determination may be useful.

The short individual needs reassurance and, occasionally, counseling. If growth hormone deficiency is diagnosed, replacement therapy is recommended and is frequently very successful.

BIBLIOGRAPHY

Frasier S: Short stature in children. Pediatr Rev 3:171-178, 1981

Frawley T: Pituitary and adrenal disease. In Shen JTY (ed): The Clinical Practice of Adolescent Medicine, pp 273–274. New York, Appleton-Century-Crofts, 1980

Hofmann A: Adolescent Medicine, pp 170–172. Reading, MA, Addison-Wesley, 1983

Root A, Diamond F, Bercu B: Short stature—When is growth hormone indicated? Contemp Pediatr 4:26–56, 1987

71

Inborn Errors of Metabolism

INTRODUCTION

In 1908, Garrod first advanced the concept of an inborn error of metabolism. He proposed that the clinical findings in alkaptonuria (urine that darkens on standing, bluish-brown pigmentation of the sclerae and ears, and arthritis) were due to the absence of the hepatic enzyme that metabolized homogentisic acid. This suggestion eventually evolved into the one gene–one enzyme hypothesis that united the fields of biochemistry and genetics.

New inborn errors are constantly being identified, adding rapidly to the hundreds of metabolic diseases already described. Conceptually, it is helpful to divide inborn errors of metabolism into the following three groups based on the time and mode of presentation:

1. Diseases which have an acute onset in the neonatal period. These disorders are fatal or highly morbid if incorrectly diagnosed or untreated.
2. Diseases which have an insidious onset during infancy or early childhood. Some of the diseases in this category are fatal and currently have no treatment (*e.g.*, Tay-Sachs disease), whereas others are not lethal but are morbid without diagnosis and treatment (*e.g.*, phenylketonuria).
3. Diseases in which clinical manifestations are not apparent until late childhood, adolescence, or adulthood.

Obviously, phenotypic variability of some diseases does not always allow them to fit unambigously into one category. This chapter, however, addresses the recognition and laboratory diagnosis of, and outlines current therapy for, the relatively few diseases in the first group. Although, individually, these inborn errors of metabolism are rare, together they contribute significantly to neonatal morbidity and mortality. Therefore, metabolic disease should be considered in the differential diagnosis of every sick neonate. Today, laboratory tests can make a rapid and specific diagnosis and allow early institution of appropriate therapy if available. Early diagnosis and treatment is essential for survival and optimal long-term neurologic outcome.

PATHOPHYSIOLOGY

Symptoms of metabolic disease in the newborn usually are due to the abnormal accumulation of one or more toxic metabolites (*e.g.,* ammonium in the urea cycle disorders, organic acids in the organic acidemias). Occasionally, symptoms occur secondary to the underproduction of essential metabolites (*e.g.,* glucose in glycogen storage diseases I and III, ATP in the disorders of pyruvate metabolism). In addition, signs and symptoms may arise from both mechanisms: in congenital adrenal hyperplasia, for example, hyponatremia, hyperkalemia, and vomiting arise from a deficiency of cortisol synthesis, while excessive production of adrenal androgens causes the characteristic physical stigmata (ambiguous genitalia) in the female infant.

CLINICAL PRESENTATION

Inborn errors of metabolism usually present in the newborn period after a symptom-free interval of from one to several days after birth. The onset and progression of symptoms often correlate with the introduction and advancement of protein-containing feedings (breast milk, infant formulas). Disorders of pyruvate metabolism and the electron transport chain and the poorly understood transient hyperammonemia of the newborn, on the other hand, typically present on the first day of life with respiratory distress and metabolic (lactic) acidosis.

Undoubtedly, many cases of metabolic disease have been mistakenly diagnosed as sepsis, sudden infant death syndrome, or other disorders. There are at least two lines of evidence which indicate that the incidence of many newborn metabolic diseases has been underestimated. First, the diagnosis of metabolic disease has often been made in a proband whose family history is notable either for one or more siblings who died mysteriously in the neonatal period, or for unexplained male neonatal deaths on the maternal side of the family. Second, newborn screening tests have

demonstrated that certain diseases have a greater incidence than clinical experience had suggested.

Most metabolic disease occurs in full-term rather than in preterm infants (except for transient hyperammonemia of the newborn). Moreover, because preterm infants are at greater risk for other illnesses, a sick full-term infant is much more likely to have a metabolic disease than his preterm counterpart.

The signs and symptoms of metabolic disease (Table 71-1) are protean and usually nonspecific; thus, metabolic disease can masquerade as several other more common neonatal emergencies (Table 71-2). Almost without exception, infants are lethargic, feed poorly, and/or fail to thrive. Acute life-threatening symptoms may also develop, such as unrelenting vomiting, coma, seizures, apnea, or respiratory distress. The presence of other symptoms, including jaundice, hepatomegaly and/or hepatic dysfunction, hypoglycemia,

Table 71-1. Signs and Symptoms of Metabolic Disease in the Newborn

Central Nervous System
  Lethargy, poor suck
  Irritability
  Hypotonicity or hypertonicity
  Seizures
  Coma
Gastrointestinal
  Poor feeding
  Vomiting
  Diarrhea
Cardiopulmonary
  Apnea
  Tachypnea
  Respiratory distress
Hepatic
  Jaundice
  Hypocoagulability
  Hepatomegaly
Miscellaneous
  Culture-positive sepsis
  Abnormal odor of skin or urine
  Coarse or dysmorphic facies
  Cataracts
  Infentile "Reye's" Syndrome

Table 71-2. Masqueraders of Metabolic Disease in the Newborn

Sepsis
Asphyxia
Central nervous system catastrophe
Gastrointestinal tract obstruction
Nonstructural cardiopulmonary abnormalities
Hepatic failure

diarrhea, unusual skin or urine odor, and coarse or dysmorphic facial features are somewhat more specific and allow the clinician to focus on a smaller number of diagnoses.

An acute life-threatening illness, in addition to disorders of pyruvate metabolism and the electron transport chain, suggests the urea cycle enzyme deficiencies, the organic acidemias, certain disorders of amino acid metabolism, galactosemia, and congenital adrenal hyperplasia.

Jaundice is the presenting symptom in deficiencies of the glucose-6-phosphate dehydrogenase and pyruvate kinase enzymes secondary to hemolysis. In Crigler-Najjar syndrome, jaundice is probably due to a deficiency of the hepatic enzyme that conjugates bilirubin. Indirect hyperbilirubinemia is the rule for these disorders. Other disorders present with a mixed indirect and direct hyperbilirubinemia. These include galactosemia, α_1-antitrypsin deficiency, and hereditary tyrosinemia. Hereditary fructose intolerance only presents with mixed jaundice when fructose is introduced into the diet (as a sucrose-containing formula or as fruit feedings).

In addition to the above disorders characterized by mixed hyperbilirubinemia, a diverse group of storage diseases present with hepatomegaly and/or liver dysfunction. Storage diseases, however, tend to present later in the neonatal period or early in infancy. Some of these disorders may be heralded by coarse facial features noted at birth (GM_1 gangliosidosis, β-glucuronidase deficiency, I cell disease, and infantile sialidosis).

Hypoglycemia may occur because of an inability to liberate glucose from hepatic glycogen stores during periods of fasting (glycogen storage diseases I and III) or secondary to defective gluconeogenesis (fructose-1, 6-diphosphatase deficiency). Recently, deficiencies of medium and long-chain fatty acyl CoA dehydrogenases have been described which present with recurrent nonketotic hypoglycemia and a clinical course suggestive of Reye's syndrome.

Relatively recent discoveries have blurred the traditional distinction between inborn errors of metabolism and genetic syndromes characterized by a host of dysmorphic features. For instance, the primary abnormality in cerebrohepatorenal (or Zellweger syndrome) is now thought to be defective fatty acid oxidation within the peroxisomes. Neonatal adrenoleukodystrophy and possibly glutaric acidemia type II are other disorders associated with a characteristic phenotype.

DIAGNOSIS

Prenatal diagnosis

Prenatal diagnosis is possible for an ever-expanding number of metabolic diseases. Early tests used amniocentesis to obtain amniotic fluid or amniocytes for chemical or enzyme activity analysis, respectively. Not all disorders have been amenable to these techniques. For example, in ornithine transcarbamylase (OTC) deficiency (a urea cycle disorder) there are no abnormal metabolites in the amniotic fluid, and the OTC enzyme is not expressed in amniocytes. Diagnosis has been established by analysis of OTC activity in fetal liver biopsy specimens. More recently, biopsy of chorionic villi with linkage analysis of restriction fragment length polymorphisms has made prenatal diagnosis possible when DNA of the mother and a known proband can be similarly analyzed. It is the application of newer genetic techniques which is rapidly increasing the number of disorders for which prenatal diagnosis is possible.

Postnatal diagnosis

Prenatal diagnosis can be attempted when a particular disease has been unequivocably identified in a family member. Occasionally, a mother at risk for a similarly affected fetus may decline prenatal diagnosis. In this case, the neonate should be treated prophylactical-

ly while appropriate diagnostic tests are undertaken. A diagnosis can sometimes be made by analysis of cord blood.

An inborn error of metabolism should be strongly suspected when any of the following five scenarios exist:

1. A positive family history of unexplained or suspicious neonatal deaths (previous siblings, males on the maternal side of the family).
2. The presence of a constellation of the signs and symptoms in Table 71-1.
3. Entertainment of any of the diagnoses

Table 71-3. Laboratory Findings Suggestive of Metabolic Disease

	Galactosemia	Glycogen storage disease	Fructose-1,6-diphosphatase	Maple syrup urine disease	Nonketotic hyperglycinemia	Glutaric acidemia type II	Pyroglutamic acidemia	Organic acidemias	Diseases of pyruvate metabolism	Disorders of ureagenesis	Transient hyperammonemia of the newborn
Hypoglycemia	±	+	+	±	−	±	−	−	±	−	−
Metabolic acidosis ± elevated anion gap	+	+	+	+	−	±	+	+	+	−	±
Respiratory alkalosis	−	−	−	−	−	−	−	−	−	+	−
Hyperammonemia	−	−	−	N−1+	−	N−1+	−	N−3+	N−1+	1+−3+	2+−4+
Direct hyperbilirubinemia	+	−	−	−	−	−	−	−	−	−	−
Urine Clinitest+	+	−	−	−	−	−	−	−	−	−	−
Acetest+ or Ketostix+	−	+	+	+	−	−	−	+	±	−	−
DNPH	−	±	±	+	−	−	−	±	±	−	−
Abnormal odor/color	−	−	−	+a	−	+b	−	+cd	−	−	−
Neutropenia/thrombocytopenia	−	−	−	−	±	−	−	±	−	−	−
Vacuolated lymphocytes	−	−	+	−	−	−	−	−	−	−	−

a maple syrup or burnt sugar
b sweaty feet
c sweaty feet—isovaleric acidemia
d cat urine—multiple carboxylase deficiency

listed in Table 71-2 at any time, but especially when available evidence does not support the given diagnosis. It is important to remember that culture-positive sepsis frequently complicates some of the metabolic diseases (*e.g.*, galactosemia).

4. Failure of infants to improve with the usual therapy.
5. Identification of any of the laboratory abnormalities listed in Table 71-3.

If metabolic disease is suspected, a basic "metabolic battery" should be obtained, including urine non-glucose reducing substances, plasma ammonium, qualitative urine ketones, serum electrolytes and glucose, pH, complete blood count, and serum lactate (if a metabolic acidosis and/or elevated anion gap are not accounted for by ketonemia). Simple diagnostic algorithms are presented in Figures 71-1 and 71-2. If metabolic disease is strongly suspected yet the metabolic battery is completely negative, analysis of plasma and urine for amino and organic acids should be performed using quantitative column chromatography and gas chromatography-mass spectrometry. It may be necessary to send plasma and urine samples to regional metabolic/genetic centers.

In two circumstances, hepatocytes and skin fibroblasts must be harvested immediately postmortem for enzyme studies or storage: (1) the fulminant course of the disease did not allow an unambiguous determination of metabolic disease or (2) despite strong suspicion of metabolic disease, all antemortem tests could not define a specific defect (as might well be the case in disorders of pyruvate metabolism or the electron transport chain).

TREATMENT

It cannot be overemphasized that early consideration of metabolic disease and institution of appropriate therapy is crucial for the

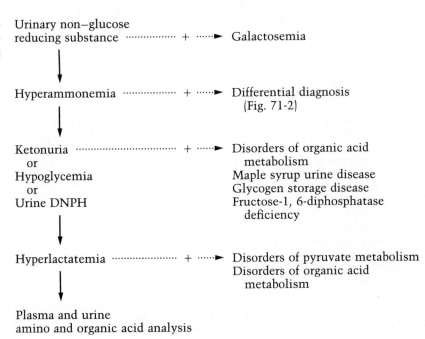

FIGURE 71-1. Initial algorithm for diagnosis of metabolic disease with acute neonatal onset.

Urinary non–glucose reducing substance ·········· + ······► Galactosemia

Hyperammonemia ·········· + ······► Differential diagnosis (Fig. 71-2)

Ketonuria ·········· + ······► Disorders of organic acid metabolism
or
Hypoglycemia   Maple syrup urine disease
or   Glycogen storage disease
Urine DNPH   Fructose-1, 6-diphosphatase deficiency

Hyperlactatemia ·········· + ······► Disorders of pyruvate metabolism
Disorders of organic acid metabolism

Plasma and urine amino and organic acid analysis

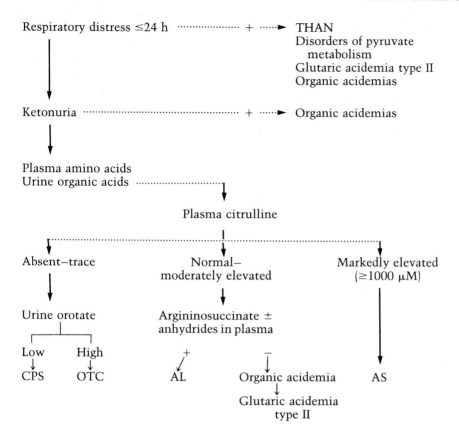

Respiratory distress ≤24 h ·················· + ·······▶ THAN
Disorders of pyruvate
metabolism
Glutaric acidemia type II
Organic acidemias

Ketonuria ·································· + ·······▶ Organic acidemias

Plasma amino acids
Urine organic acids ·······················

Plasma citrulline

Absent–trace

Normal–
moderately elevated

Markedly elevated
(≥1000 μM)

Urine orotate

Argininosuccinate ±
anhydrides in plasma

Low   High
CPS   OTC

+
AL

−
Organic acidemia

AS

Glutaric acidemia
type II

CPS = carbamyl phosphate synthetase deficiency; OTC = ornithine transcarbamylase deficiency; AL = argininosuccinate lyase deficiency; AS = argininosuccinate synthetase deficiency; THAN = transient hyperammonemia of the newborn.

FIGURE 71-2. Algorithm for differential diagnosis of hyperammonemia.

optimal outcome for those disorders amenable to treatment. In urea enzyme deficiencies, for example, both the intelligence quotient and the severity of defined abnormalities on cranial CT scans significantly correlate with the duration of hyperammonemic coma.

The acute life-threatening disorders demand intensive general supportive care measures including correction of dehydration, restoration of normal acid–base and electrolyte status, assisted ventilation, and antibiotic therapy. Nutritional therapy is important for many metabolic disorders. Toxic products accumulate in certain disorders (ammonium: urea cycle enzyme deficiencies; branched chain amino acids: maple syrup urine disease; organic acids: organic acidemias) because of excessive protein intake. Metabolites of galactose are toxic in galactosemia; these infants require complete elimination of dietary lactose (glucose–galactose). In all disorders, aggressive intravenous nutrition with dextrose and lipid should provide sufficent calories (70–120 calories/kg) to prevent tissue catabolism.

Toxic metabolites must be removed as

quickly and efficiently as possible. Hemodialysis is most effective and removes metabolites distributed through total body water. Peritoneal dialysis is the second best and exchange transfusion a distant third alternative. Therefore, optimal acute therapy may necessitate transport to a center with infant hemodialysis capabilities.

Various metabolic therapies, many of which are still investigational, have been used to activate alternate excretory pathways and/or provide missing compounds to facilitate normal metabolism. A state-of-the-art review of this therapeutic modality for disorders or ureagenesis can be found in the second work listed in this chapter's bibliography.

After resolution of the acute abnormalities, long-term dietary therapy may dictate use of special formulas (*e.g.*, a non–galactose-containing formula for galactosemia, other special products for maple syrup urine disease and the organic acidemias). Occasionally, certain disorders respond to megavitamin therapy. A classic example is vitamin B_{12}-responsive methylmalonic acidemia.

Even with the best care, normal long-term nutrition and growth are a challenge to maintain. Metabolic disorders characterized by protein intolerance tend to become symptomatic during intercurrent infections. Strict enforcement of dietary therapy is often difficult. It is important to provide sources of family counseling and support as early as possible.

BIBLIOGRAPHY

Batshaw ML: Hyperammonemia. Curr Prob Pediatr 14(11):1–69, 1984

Brusilow SW, Dunney M, Waber LJ et al: Treatment of episodic hyperammonemia in children with inborn errors of urea synthesis. N Engl J Med 310:1630–1634, 1984

Brusilow SW, Valle DL: Symptomatic inborn errors of metabolism in the neonate. In, Current Therapy in Neonatal–Perinatal Medicine 1985–1986, Nelson NM (ed): Philadelphia, BC Decker, 1985

Burton BK: Inborn errors of metabolism: The clinical diagnosis in early infancy. Pediatrics 79:359–369, 1987

Komrower GM: Inborn errors of metabolism. Pediatr Rev 2:175–182, 1980

Stanley JB, Wyngaarden JB, Fredrickson DS, Goldstein JL, Brown MS (eds): The Metabolic Basis of Inherited Disease. New York, McGraw-Hill, 1983

72

Reye's Syndrome

In 1963, Reye and associates described a clinical entity of acute encephalopathy with fatty degeneration of the viscera. Early studies reported fatality rates in excess of 80%. During the past decade, however, the mortality rate has been reduced to below 40% by early recognition and aggressive supportive care. The syndrome is defined clinically, with the etiology still unknown.

CLINICAL PRESENTATION

The majority of involved children are between 3 and 12 years of age. However, presentations are seen in infancy and even adulthood. The incidence in males and females is about equal with a somewhat greater prevalence in rural environments. The characteristic clinical criteria for diagnosis are summarized in Table 72-1. A prodromal viral upper respiratory illness is nearly universal. Epidemic influenza B and episodic varicella are the most commonly implicated viral disorders, but onset following influenza A, mononucleosis, enterovirus, adenovirus, and herpes simplex are all reported. An interval of clinical improvement is followed within 7 to 10 days by the development

Table 72–1. Diagnostic Criteria for Reye's Syndrome

Historical:
  Prodromal viral illness
  Interval of recovery
  Persistent emesis
  Lethargy, confusion
Laboratory
  ALT/AST increased more than 3 times normal
  Ammonia normal or elevated
  Cerebrospinal fluid (CSF) cell count normal
  Mitochondrial injury: histologic, biochemical

of persistent emesis over 12 to 24 hours. Neither fever nor diarrhea is prominent. Neurologic manifestations ensue with a metabolic encephalopathy that may progress with variable speed through the clinical stages outlined in Table 72-2. Milder disease is defined as remaining in grades 1 and 2, generally persisting over 48 to 96 hours, with complete recovery the rule. Independent of the encephalopathy, the neurologic examination reveals no focal abnormalities. The liver is usually slightly enlarged with a normal spleen.

Early laboratory features include moderate elevation of ALT (serum glutamic pyruvic transaminase [SGPT]) and AST (serum glu-

Table 72–2. Clinical Staging of Reye's Syndrome

Grade	Clinical Features
I	Quiet, lethargic but responsive
II	Confusion, delirium, combativeness
III	Obtunded, decorticate
IV	Coma, decerebrate, hyperpnea
V	Coma, flaccid paralysis, seizures

tamic oxaloacetic transaminase [SGOT]) to levels of 200 to 2500 IU with a normal bilirubin. The creatine phosphokinase (CPK) level is also usually increased, while the prothrombin time is variably prolonged. In infancy, both hypoglycemia and hepatomegaly are more prominent. Ammonia levels are high-normal to elevated, with striking elevations coinciding with advanced encephalopathy. Analysis of the spinal fluid reveals few cells, mild reduction in glucose, and advancing increases in CSF pressure. Additional laboratory features may include elevated amylase, reduction in serum lipids, and elevations in lactate and pyruvate.

On biopsy of the liver, light microscopy will reveal an increase in microvascular fat, a reflection of an increase in hepatic triglyceride to more than 30%. In contrast to usual hepatitis, neither inflammation nor cholestasis is prominent. With electron microscopy, severe distortion of the mitochondira is seen. The significance of the mitochondrial injury is confirmed with hepatic enzyme analysis. The activities of mitochondrial enzymes (ornithine transcarbamylase, carbamyl phosphate synthetase, pyruvate dehydrogenase, and monoamine oxidase) are uniformly reduced, contributing to the hyperammonemia and hypercatecholaminemia of Reye's syndrome. In contrast, the activities of hepatic cytosolic enzymes (glucokinase, pyruvate kinase) are normal.

Efforts to identify the etiology of the injury to the mitochondria have been inconclusive. Toxin studies remain appealing, with special interest in the role of salicylates. In 1984, a pilot Federal Drug Administration (FDA) study revealed that 97% of Reye's patients compared, to less than 50% of age-matched controls, had ingested salicylate during the acute phase of the illness. It is known that, *in vitro*, salicylate is capable of uncoupling mitochondrial oxidative phosphorylation and inhibiting ADP-ATP translocase activity, thus reducing mitochondrial matrix ATP. Coincident with reduction in salicylate use, the incidence of influenza-associated Reye's syndrome appears to have been reduced.

DIFFERENTIAL DIAGNOSIS

The differential diagnosis of encephalopathy in early childhood is limited. Primary disorders of urea cycle enzyme activity must be excluded, especially partial deficiency of ornithine transcarbamylase (OTC) and carbamyl phosphate synthetase (CPS). In these conditions, hepatomegaly is modest, and hyperammonemia is prominent, while increases in AST and ALT values are generally modest. Isovaleric and related organic acidemias may also present with acidosis and encephalopathy. Carnitine deficiency may present as a Reye's-like syndrome with progressive muscle weakness. Hypoglycemia, hepatomegaly, and encephalopathy will also be encountered in infantile galactosemia and fructose intolerance. Hyperammonemia may also be noted with medication toxicity as with valproic acid. In viral encephalitis, greater CSF alterations and focal neurologic signs are anticipated. With fulminant or ischemic hepatitis, hyperbilirubinemia is anticipated, although hepatic biopsy may be required to distinguish fulminant hepatitis from Reye's syndrome.

The treatment of clinical Reye's syndrome is early and aggressive, recognizing that uncomplicated recovery depends on minimizing the complications. On first suspicion of the disorder on grounds of historic or physical examination, the minimal evaluation is ALT, glucose, prothrombin time, and ammonia determination.

MANAGEMENT

The initial management is initiation of intravenous 10% or 15% glucose with electrolytes to correct for the emesis-induced dehydration. Vitamin K supplementation is routinely given. If the child is comatose (higher than Grade 2), he is admitted to the intensive care unit. Analysis of spinal fluid is mandatory, and studies to exclude urea cycle disorders (amino, organic, and orotic acids) are begun. Intracranial pressure is monitored directly *via* placement of a subarachnoid bolt, intraventricular catheter, or epidural transducer. Cerebral edema is managed aggressively; this includes intubation and hyperventilation to reduce the P_{CO_2} to 20 to 25 mm Hg. Arterial pressures are monitored. Cooling blankets are used to prevent fever. Fluids are restricted to 1200 to 1500 ml/m^2/day.

Osmotic diuretics to reduce cerebral hydration are initiated to maintain an intracranial pressure of less than 20 mm Hg while maintaining a cerebral perfusion pressure above 50 mm Hg and serum osmolality from 290 to 320 mOsm/L. Persistent intracranial hypertension often requires initiation of pentobarbital therapy. Agents to reduce ammonia directly, such as arginine or benzoate, remain investigational.

PROGNOSIS

The prognosis is closely tied to the clinical staging of the disease on admission. If the patient is admitted and stable with grade 1 signs, complete recovery is the rule. With grade 3 manifestations, 5% mortality is anticipated, increasing to 25% when the patient is admitted in grade 4 and close to 100% in grade 5. Long-term neuropsychiatric complications are common, with school problems, for example, reported in 80% of survivors of grade 3 disease. Mortality and morbidity are both worse in infantile Reye's syndrome.

BIBLIOGRAPHY

Brunner RL, O'Grady DJ, Pantin JC et al: Neuropsychologic consequences of Reye's syndrome. J Pediatr 95:706–711, 1979

Pantin JC: Reye's syndrome, diagnosis and management. Gastroenterology 69:511–518, 1975

Reye RDK, Morgan G, Baral J: Encephalepathy and fatty degeneration of the viscera: A disease entity in childhood. Lancet 2:749–752, 1963

Stanko KM, Ray G, Dominquez LB et al: Reye's syndrome and salicylate use. Pediatrics 66:859–864, 1980

Part XII: Hematology

73

Transfusion Therapy

INDICATIONS FOR TRANSFUSION

There are three primary situations in which transfusion therapy is indicated:

1. Maintenance or restoration of an adequate circulating blood volume to treat or prevent shock
2. Replacement of a specific blood component such as a plasma protein (*e.g.*, Factor VIII) or formed blood element (*e.g.*, platelets) because its deficiency has produced or is likely to produce adverse symptoms
3. Removal of harmful substances by exchange transfusion

There is only one indication for a transfusion of red blood cells. The sole indication is to provide the patient with sufficient oxygen-carrying capacity to prevent or correct tissue hypoxia.

TREATMENT OF ACUTE HEMORRHAGE

The acute loss of 10% of the circulating blood volume generally is not associated with any significant alterations in the circulation. A hemorrhage resulting in a 20% decrease in the blood volume will not produce a decrease in blood pressure in the supine patient. When the blood volume has been reduced by 30% to 40% clinical evidence of shock will be observable in most patients. This is reflected by a fall in right auricular pressure (central venous pressure), decreased cardiac output, a fall in arterial pressure, an increase in heart rate, and constriction of the veins and venules primarily in the skin, muscles, kidneys, and gastrointestinal tract. Symptoms and signs include pallor, sweating, thirst, light-headedness, restlessness, and air hunger. One of the more reliable signs of peripheral vasoconstriction is the temperature of the nose; if a patient lying in a reasonably warm room has a cold nose, circulatory failure should be strongly suspected.

A useful guide to the volume of blood loss in acute hemorrhage is the systolic blood pressure. In an adult, if this is below 100 mm Hg, the blood volume is probably less than 70% of normal. Other standards must be applied in infants and children. A guide for suspecting a hemorrhage of 30% or more of the blood volume for children under 4 years of age is a systolic blood pressure of less than 65 mm Hg; for children 5 to 8 years of age, 75 mm Hg; for children 9 to 12 years of age, 85 mm Hg; and for children 13 to 16 years of age, a systolic pressure of less than 90 mm Hg.

The blood volume of premature infants is approximately 105 ml/kg, whereas in the full-term infant, the blood volume is close to 85 ml/kg. By 3 months of age, the blood volume is similar to that of the normal adult, 70 to 75 ml/kg.

The pulse rate is a less reliable guide than the blood pressure as an indicator of the magnitude of a hemorrhage. In general, a persistent pulse rate of over 100 beats per minute in an adult is associated with a 20% reduction in blood volume. Standards for infants and children are close to the following: newborn, greater than 170 beats per minute; 1 to 11 months, greater than 160 beats per minute; 1 to 2 years, greater than 130 beats per minute; 2 to 6 years, greater than 120 beats per minute; and 6 to 10 years, greater than 110 beats per minute.

Estimation of the hemoglobin level is not a reliable indication of the extent of hemorrhage. A period of 24 to 36 hours may elapse before the plasma volume is restored to normal and sufficient hemodilution has occurred to reflect the extent of blood loss. Even after the loss of 10% of the blood volume, only half the decrease has been replaced at the end of 24 hours. A reduced hemoglobin or hematocrit level within 3 to 6 hours of hemorrhage suggests a blood loss of greater than 20% to 25% of the blood volume, whereas a normal hemoglobin level 6 hours after a hemorrhage suggests that the blood loss has not been substantial. In patients in shock or preshock, hemoglobin determinations must be performed on central venous blood. Capillary samples from vasoconstricted extremities will result in falsely elevated hemoglobin or hematocrit determinations as a consequence of stasis and hemoconcentration.

TREATMENT OF ACUTE BLOOD LOSS

When the history and physical examination indicate that the patient has sustained a significant acute loss of blood, replacement therapy with whole blood, colloid, or saline solution is indicated. Transfusion is also justified when the loss of blood is less than 20% of the blood volume but may recur. In such circumstances, blood of any storage age is suitable. When the amount of blood to be transfused in a period of 24 hours is equal to or greater than the patient's blood volume, the age of the transfused blood becomes important in terms of the alterations in coagulation factors, platelets, and oxygen transport mechanisms that it may produce. Blood stored for periods in excess of 48 hours lacks adequate numbers of functional platelets and has insufficient quantities of Factor VIII. The use of specific component therapy rather than reliance on fresh whole blood is an effective means of managing coagulation disturbances produced by massive transfusions of whole blood.

When whole blood is not immediately available, plasma, "plasma protein solutions" or saline solution may be used to restore the blood volume. The infusion of a volume of saline solution equal to the volume of blood lost will not restore the blood volume, but infusions of much greater quantities can effectively restore the circulation to normal.

Transfusions following hemorrhage should be administered until the central venous pressure has been restored to normal or, if such information is not available, until the blood pressure and pulse have returned to a satisfactory level and the signs of peripheral vascular insufficiency have disappeared. The infusions initially may be administered rapidly. In adults in shock, the acute infusion of 500 ml in a period of 3 to 4 minutes produces no difficulty.

TREATMENT OF ANEMIA

Packed red cells should be used in all situations in which only a red cell mass deficit exists. This is the usual situation in most patients with chronic anemia. Whole blood should be reserved for those clinical situations characterized by hypovolemia that is accompanied by signs of circulatory insufficiency. The adverse effects of whole blood include the unnecessary increase in the intravascular volume, the presence of potentially antigenic plasma proteins, and the administration of large quantities of potassium, sodium, ammonia, and citrate. It has been estimated that 80% to 90% of all transfusions administered in the United States should be in the form of packed red blood cells.

The rapid correction of red cell mass deficits, (*i.e.*, anemia) is rarely necessary at hemoglobin levels about 6 g/dl. Increases in cardiac output or elevations in the blood-lactate-to-pyruvate ratio rarely are observed in adults at rest until the hemoglobin concentration falls below 6g/dl. In the absence of physical stress or associated pulmonary or cardiac disease, most patients can tolerate hemoglobin values of 3 to 6 g/dl. without developing signs of congestive heart failure.

The decision to transfuse an anemic patient should not be made on the basis of the hemoglobin concentration alone but should include an assessment of the patient's cardiac and pulmonary status, level of physical activity, and the prospects of correcting the anemia with hematinic agents, such as iron, folic acid, or vitamin B_{12}. Patients with iron deficiency, the most common form of severe anemia in childhood, rarely will require a transfusion.

When, in the judgment of the physician, a transfusion is required, the amount of packed red cells to be administered can be determined by formula No. 1 (see below). This formula can be further simplified by assuming that the patient's blood volume is approximately 75 ml/kg and that the concentration of hemoglobin within the packed cells is 22 and 24 g/dl. The simplified formula will be formula No. 2. Another popular formula (formula No. 3), based on the same principles, employs the hematocrit.

1. $\text{Volume of cells} = \dfrac{\begin{array}{c}\text{patient's weight (kg)} \times \\ \text{blood volume (ml/kg)} \times \\ \text{(Hb desired} - \text{Hb observed)}\end{array}}{\begin{array}{c}\text{hemoglobin concentration} \\ \text{of packed cells (g/dl)}\end{array}}$

2. $\text{Volume of cells} = \dfrac{\begin{array}{c}\text{patient's weight (kg)} \times 75 \times \\ \text{(Hb desired} - \text{Hb observed)}\end{array}}{24}$

3. Volume of cells = patient's weight (kg) × increment in Hct desired

When packed red cells are administered to an anemic patient in incipient heart failure, their rate of administration should not exceed 2 ml/kg/hour. The administration of ethacrynic acid or furosemide, which are rapid-acting diuretic agents, prior to the transfusion is a valuable means of decreasing the chances of producing circulatory overload. Ethacrynic acid should never be added to the red cell suspension, since it is a potentially hemolytic agent.

In severely anemic patients in frank congestive heart failure, partial or complete exchange transfusion with packed red cell suspensions has been demonstrated to be an effective means of both correcting the anemia and improving the cardiac status. The use of ethacrynic acid followed by packed red cell transfusion has been shown to be equally effective. The choice of exchange transfusion or diuretic plus simple transfusion is generally determined by the urgency of the situation. In patients requiring emergency surgery, the use of exchange transfusion will decrease the waiting time to operation.

CHOICE OF RED CELL PRODUCT

Whole blood may be modified in order to remove some of its non-red cell components. In Table 73-1 are listed the currently available red cell products and the chances of the product producing one of the more common transfusion-related side effects. A brief description of the usual indication for each product is as follows:

Whole Blood (<21 days' storage). There are limited indications for whole blood in pediatric patients. It may be used in cases of acute blood loss if more suitable products are not immediately available.

Fresh Whole Blood (<72 hours' storage). Fresh whole blood has higher levels of coagulation factors and 2, 3-DPG; and lower ammonia and potassium levels than does blood stored for longer periods, thus making it more suitable for exchange transfusion in neonates and to replace blood lost in acute hemorrhage.

Fresh Whole Blood (<4 hours' storage at room temperature). Leukocyte transfusions have been shown to improve the chances for survival in septic, neutropenic neonates. Leukocytes may be obtained by pheresis or harvested from whole blood. Alternately, if fresh blood is administered *via* exchange transfusion within 4 hours of drawing, it can deliver the same number of viable leukocytes with considerably less preparation time and morbidity.

Packed Cells (<35 days' storage). A unit of packed cells is similar in its cellular constituents to whole blood but with about 40% of the plasma and citrate removed. It is the component of choice in cases of red cell loss or underproduction.

Washed Packed Cells. The washing process removes about 90% of the white cells and more than 99% of the plasma. Its main use is in patients with a history of nonhemolytic transfusion reactions and in other circumstances in which transfusion of leukocytes and plasma is contraindicated.

Table 73–1. Currently Available Red Blood Cell Products

| Product | Percentage of Nonred Cell Components Remaining in Each Red Cell Product | | | | |
	Plasma	*PMNs*	*Lymphocytes*	*Coagulation Factors*	*Platelets*
Whole Blood (<21 days)	100%	100%	100%	Decreased V,VIII, II,VII,IX,X	<1%
Whole Blood(<48 hrs)	100%	100%	100%	Decreased V,VIII	<1%
Whole Blood (<4 hr)	100%	100%	100%	100%	>90%
Packed Cells	20–50%	100%	100%	20–50%	<1%
Leukofiltered cells	10%	<5%	<5%	10%	<1%
Washed packed cells	<1%	10%	10%	<1%	<1%
Frozen deglycerolized cells	<1%	<5%	<5%	<1%	<1%

(Nathan & Oski: Hematology of Infancy and Childhood, 3rd ed. Philadelphia, WB Saunders, 1987)

Frozen Deglycerolized Packed Cells. The processes of freezing and thawing red cells involve extensive washing with solutions of differing osmolalities, a process that removes over 95% of the white cells. Only 1/106 of the original plasma is retained. This is the red cell product most nearly free of non-red cell components and therefore is the product of choice for chronic transfusion.

Leukofiltered Blood. Passing blood diluted with saline through cotton wool fiber containing filters removes approximately as many white cells as does freezing or washing. Alternatively, passing citrated whole blood stored longer than 7 days through microaggregate blood filters removes much of the leukocyte and platelet debris. Either technique may be used to prepare leukocyte-poor blood when frozen blood is not available.

Irradiation of Red Cell Products. Irradiation of any blood product serves one purpose: to prevent lymphocytes in that product from proliferating when transfused into a host with congenital or acquired deficiency in cell-mediated immunity, an event that could cause transfusion-associated graft-versus-host disease (TAGVHD). TAGVHD may occur from 4 to 30 days after transfusion of blood products containing viable lymphocytes. Once it is acquired, there is no effective therapy. The mortality rate in TAGVHD is greater than 90%. All blood products except fresh frozen plasma can cause TAGVHD. The minimum dose of lymphocytes needed to cause TAGVHD is about 1×10^7 per kg.

Lymphocytes in blood products may be inactivated by irradiation; either cesium 137 irradiators or cobalt 60 therapy machines may be used. Radiation in doses of up to 10,000 rad has little or no effect on red cells; and up to 5000 rad may be used without affecting granulocyte or platelet function and survival. The most commonly recommended dose is 1500 rad, although 5000 rad is used in the author's laboratory.

HAZARDS OF TRANSFUSION THERAPY

The use of blood or blood products carries a significant risk to the recipient. The adverse effects may be immediate and include hemolytic transfusion reactions, febrile reaction, allergic reactions, infections from bacterial contamination, pulmonary insufficiency from microaggregates, air embolism, circulatory overload, and the potential hazards of the plasticizers used in the polyvinyl chloride plastic bags. The adverse effects that are delayed in their appearance include the delayed hemolytic reaction, isoimmunization to both cellular and plasma antigens, hemosiderosis, the development of graft-versus-host disease in the immunocompromised blood transfusion recipient, and the transmission of diseases such as hepatitis, cytomegalovirus disease, Epstein-Barr virus, syphilis, malaria, Chagas' disease, and human immunodeficiency virus. Because of these multiple risks, blood and blood products should be regarded as drugs and never administered without a precise indication.

BIBLIOGRAPHY

Conley CL: Anemia: Accurate diagnosis and appropriate therapy. Hosp Pract 19:57, 1984

Fosburg MT, Kevy SV: Red cell transfusion. In Nathan DG, Oski FA (eds): Hematology of Infancy and Childhood, 3rd ed, p 1562. Philadelphia, WB Saunders, 1987

Stockman JA III: Red cell transfusion in the newborn. Indications and unique blood banking needs. Am J Pediatr Hematol Oncol 3:205, 1981

74

Anemia

THE DIFFERENTIAL DIAGNOSIS OF ANEMIA

Anemia is generally defined as a reduction in red cell mass or blood hemoglobin concentration. The limit for differentiating anemia from normal states is generally set at two standard deviations below the mean for the normal population. This definition will result in 2.5% of the normal population being classified an anemic. Conversely, the values for hemoglobin-deficient individuals will be distributed in such a fashion that some will be placed within the normal range. These individuals, who have the potential for a hemoglobin concentration in the upper part of the normal range, may be recognized only after a response to treatment.

Since the primary function of the red cell is to deliver and release adequate quantities of oxygen to the tissues in order to meet their metabolic demands, it is apparent that some measures of both body oxygen metabolism and accompanying cardiovascular compensations are required to complement the current laboratory definition of anemia. The fact that

hemoglobin concentration alone is insufficient to judge whether a patient is "functionally anemic" is best illustrated in patients with cyanotic congenital heart disease or chronic respiratory insufficiency or in patients with mutant hemoglobins that alter hemoglobin's affinity for oxygen.

With these caveats in mind, a useful statistical definition of anemia is provided in Table 74-1 that recognizes the effect of age and sex on the designation of anemia.

CLASSIFICATION OF ANEMIAS

Anemias may be classified on a physiologic or a morphologic basis. As will be illustrated, a combination of both approaches is often employed in the initial differential diagnosis.

The best approach for providing an understanding of the multiple disorders capable of producing anemia is to separate the causes of anemia into three categories of functional disturbances:

450

Table 74–1. Values (Normal Mean and Lower Limits of Normal.) For Hemoglobin, Hematocrit, and MCV Determinations

Age (yr)	Hemoglobin (g/dl)		Hematocrit (%)		MCV (μ)	
	Mean	Lower Limit	Mean	Lower Limit	Mean	Lower Limit
0.5–1.9	12.5	11.0	37	33	77	70
2–4	12.5	11.0	38	34	79	73
5–7	13.0	11.5	39	35	81	75
8–11	13.5	12.0	40	36	83	76
12–14:						
Female	13.5	12.0	41	36	85	78
Male	14.0	12.5	43	37	84	77
15–17:						
Female	14.0	12.0	41	36	87	79
Male	15.0	13.0	46	38	86	78
18–49:						
Female	14.0	12.0	42	37	90	80
Male	16.0	14.0	47	40	90	80

(Nathan DG, Oski FA: Hematology of Infancy and Childhood, 2nd ed. Philadelphia, WB Saunders, 1981; with permission)

1. Disorders of cell proliferation, in which the rate of red cell production is less than expected for the degree of anemia
2. Disorders in erythrocyte maturation, in which erythropoiesis is largely ineffectual
3. Disorders in which erythrocyte destruction or red cell loss is primarily responsible for the anemia.

It will immediately be recognized that these three categories are not mutually exclusive. More than one mechanism may be present in some anemias, but one functional disorder is generally the major reason for the patient's anemia. Table 74-2 classifies the anemias most commonly encountered in infancy and childhood into these three categories of functional disturbance.

Anemias may also be classified on the basis of red cell size and then further subdivided according to red cell morphology. In this type of classification, anemias are subdivided into microcytic anemias, normocytic anemias, and macrocytic anemias. This classification is also arbitrary, and categories are not mutually exclusive. During the course of a disease, classification of the patient's anemia may change from one category to another as a result of other clinical or pathologic variables. In Table 74-3, the more common anemias of infancy and childhood are classified on the basis of their characteristic cell size.

EVALUATION OF THE ANEMIC PATIENT

The initial diagnostic approach to the anemic patient includes a detailed history and physical examination and a minimum of essential laboratory tests. Tables 74-4 and 74-5 list those features of the history and physical examination that are most helpful in providing clues to the etiology of anemia. The initial laboratory tests should include determination

Table 74–2. Physiologic Classification of Anemia

A. **Disorders of red cell production in which the rate of red cell production is less than expected for the degree of anemia**
  1. Marrow failure:
     a. Aplastic anemia:
        Congenital
        Acquired
     b. Pure red cell aplasia:
        Congenital:
          Diamond-Blackfan syndrome
          Asse's syndrome
        Acquired:
          Transient erythroblastopenia of childhood
          Other
     c. Marrow replacement:
        Malignancies
        Osteopetrosis
        Myelofibrosis:
          Chronic renal disease
          Vitamin D deficiency
     d. Pancreatic insufficiency-marrow hypoplasia syndrome
  2. Impaired erythropoietin production:
     a. Chronic renal disease
     b. Hypothyroidism, hypopituitarism
     c. Chronic inflammation
     d. Protein malnutrition
     e. Hemoglobin mutants with decreased affinity for oxygen
B. **Disorders of erythroid maturation and ineffective erythropoiesis**
  1. Abnormalities of cytoplasmic maturation:
     a. Iron deficiency
     b. Thalassemia syndromes
     c. Sideroblastic anemias
     d. Lead poisoning
  2. Abnormalities of nuclear maturation:
     a. Vitamin B_{12} deficiency
     b. Folic acid deficiency
     c. Thiamine-responsive megaloblastic anemia
     d. Hereditary abnormalities in folate metabolism
     e. Orotic aciduria
  3. Primary dyserythropoietic anemias (types I, II, III, IV)
  4. Erythropoietic protoporphyria
  5. Refractory sideroblastic anemia with vacuolization of marrow precursors and pancreatic dysfunction
C. **Hemolytic anemias**
  1. Defects of hemoglobin:
     a. Structural mutants
     b. Synthetic mutants (thalassemia syndromes)
  2. Defects of the red cell membrane
  3. Defects of red cell metabolism
  4. Antibody-mediated
  5. Mechanical injury to the erythrocyte
  6. Thermal injury to the erythrocyte
  7. Oxidant-induced red cell injury
  8. Infectious-agent-induced red cell injury
  9. Paroxysmal nocturnal hemoglobinuria
  10. Plasma-lipid-induced abnormalities of the red cell membrane

(Nathan DG, Oski FA: Hematology of Infancy and Childhood, 2nd ed. Philadelphia, WB Saunders, 1981)

Table 74–3. Classification of Anemias Based on Red Cell Size

A. **Microcytic anemias:**
  1. Iron deficiency (nutritional, chronic blood loss)
  2. Chronic lead poisoning
  3. Thalassemia syndromes
  4. Sideroblastic anemias
  5. Chronic inflammation
  6. Some congenital hemolytic anemias
B. **Macrocytic anemias:**
  1. With megaloblastic bone marrow:
     Vitamin B_{12} deficiency
     Folic acid deficiency
     Hereditary orotic aciduria
     Thiamine-responsive anemia
  2. Without megaloblastic bone marrow:
     Aplastic anemia
     Diamond-Blackfan syndrome
     Hypothyroidism
     Liver disease
     Bone marrow infiltration
     Dyserythropoietic anemias
C. **Normocytic Anemias:**
  1. Congenital hemolytic anemias:
     Hemoglobin mutants
     Red cell enzyme defects
     Disorders of the red cell membrane
  2. Acquired hemolytic anemias:
     Antibody-mediated
     Microangiopathic hemolytic anemias
     Secondary to acute infections
  3. Acute blood loss
  4. Splenic pooling
  5. Chronic renal disease (usually)

(Nathan DG, Oski FA: Hematology of Infancy and Childhood, 2nd ed. Philadelphia, WB Saunders, 1981)

Table 74–6. Sources of Error in Blood Cell Counts Specific for Electronic Counters

1. *Incorrect diluent or lysis agent* for particular instrument
2. *Extraneous particles in diluting fluid* (or containers, at any step)
3. *Presence of cell type that was not to be counted*
4. *Destruction of cell type that was to be counted*
5. *Error in metered delivery of cells after dilution:* pump, valves, tubing, connections, cut-off switch
6. *Partial obstruction of aperture* (impedance type instrument)
7. *Coincidence loss*
8. *Threshold setting:* sensitivity or potentiometer setting not determined by proper calibration
9. *Carry-over* from one specimen to the next
10. *Spurious pulses from sensing region* of equipment, owing to air bubbles
11. *Spurious signals* from electrical or RF interference
12. *Instability,* or intermittent failure of electronic components

(Nathan DG, Oski FA: Hematology in Infancy and Childhood, 2nd ed. Philadelphia, WB Saunders, 1981)

Table 74–7. The Relationship of RDW and MCV in a Variety of Disease States

RDW	MCV		
	Low	*Normal*	*High*
Normal	Heterozygous α or β thalassemia		Aplastic anemia
High	Iron deficiency Hemoglobin H	Chronic disease	Folate deficiency
	S-β-thalassemia	Liver disease Myelotoxic chemotherapy	Vitamin B_{12} deficiency
		Chronic lymphocytic or myelogenous leukemia Mixed deficiencies Sideroblastic hemoglobin SS of SC Myelofibrosis	Immune hemolytic anemia

(Bessman JD, Gilmer PR Jr, Gardner FH: Improved classification of anemias by MCV and RDW. Am J Clin Pathol 80:322, 1983)

pany, Ardsley, NY) and the Fisher Autocytometer (Fisher Scientific Company, Pittsburgh, PA). In this technique, cells passing through a flow chamber cause deflections in a beam of light that are converted to electric pulses by a photomultiplier tube.

Readers are encouraged to consult other references for details of operation of electronic counters and to familiarize themselves with potential sources of error. Some of these potential errors are listed in Table 74-6. Of concern in the evaluation of anemia is the recognition of the fact that increased white cell counts (generally in excess of 25,000 cells/mm³), as a result of turbidity, produce a slight but significant false elevation in the hemoglobin measurement. A very high white cell count can also elevate the hematocrit and the MCV because the white cells are counted and sized with the red cells. Cold agglutinins in high titer tend to cause spurious macrocytosis with low red cell counts and very high mean corpuscular hemoglobin concentrations (MCHCs). Warming either the blood or the dilutent will eliminate this problem.

Electronic cell sizing has provided another useful means of categorizing anemias based on the red cell distribution (RDW), which is derived from the red blood cell histogram that accompanies each analysis. The RDW is an

Table 74–8. Classification of Red Cell Hemolytic Disorders by Predominant Morphology (Nonhemolytic Disorders of Similar Morphology Are Enclosed in Parentheses for Reference)

SPHEROCYTES
  Hereditary spherocytosis
  ABO incompatibility in neonates
  Immunohemolytic anemias with IgG- or C3-coated red cells*
  Acute oxidant injury (hexose monophosphate shunt defects dur-
      ing hemolytic crisis, oxidant drugs and chemicals)
  Hemolytic transfusion reactions*
  Clostridium urelchii septicemia
  Severe burns, other red cell thermal injury
  Spider, bee, and snake venoms
  Severe hypophosphatemia
  Hypersplenism[†]
BIZARRE POIKILOCYTES
  Red cell fragmentation syndromes (micro- and macroangiopathic hemolytic anemias)
  Acute oxidant injury[†]
  Hereditary elliptocytosis in neonates
  Hereditary pyropoikilocytosis
ELLIPTOCYTES
  Hereditary elliptocytosis
  Thalassemias
  (Other hypochromic-microcytic anemias)
  (Megaloblastic anemias)
STOMATOCYTES
  Hereditary stomatocytosis
  RH$_{null}$ blood group
  Stomatocytosis with cold hemolysis
  (Liver disease, especially acute alcoholism)
  (Mediterranean stomatocytosis)
IRREVERSIBLY SICKLED CELLS
  Sickle cell anemia
  Symptomatic sickle syndromes
INTRAERYTHROCYTIC PARASITES
  Malaria
  Babesiosis
  Bartonellosis
SPICULATED OR CRENATED RED CELLS
  Acute hepatic necrosis (spur cell anemia)
  Uremia
  Red cell fragmentation syndromes[†]
  Infantile Pyknocytosis
  Emixien-Meyerhof pathway defects[†]
  Vitamin E deficiency[†]
  Abetalipoproteinemia
  Heat stroke[†]
  McLeod blood group
  (Postsplenectomy)
  (Transiently after massive transfusion of stored blood)
  (Anorexia nervosa)[†]

*Usually associated with positive Coombs' test.

(Continued)

Table 74–8 (Continued). Classification of Red Cell Hemolytic Disorders by Predominant Morphology (Nonhemolytic Disorders of Similar Morphology Are Enclosed in Parentheses for Reference)

TARGET CELLS
  Hemoglobins S, C, D, and E
  Hereditary xerocytosis
  Thalassemias
  (Other hypochromic-microcytic anemias)
  (Obstructive liver disease)
  (Postsplenectomy)
  (Lecithin: cholesterol acyltransferase deficiency)
PROMINENT BASOPHILIC STIPPLING:
  Thalassemias
  Unstable hemoglobins
  Lead poisoning[†]
  Pyrimidine 5′-nucleotidase deficiency
NONSPECIFIC OR NORMAL MORPHOLOGY
  Emixien-Meyerhof pathway defects
  Hexose monophosphate shunt defects
  Unstable hemoglobins
  Paroxysmal nocturnal hemoglobinuria
  Dyserythropoietic anemias
  Copper toxicity (Wilson's disease)
  Cation permeability defects
  Erythropoietic porphyria
  Vitamin E deficiency
  Hemolysis with infections[†]
  Rh hemolytic disease in neonates[*]
  Paroxysmal cold hemoglobinuria[*†]
  Cold hemagglutinin disease[*]
  Hypersplenism
  Immunohemolytic anemia[*†]

[†]Disease sometimes associated with this morphology.
(Nathan DG, Oski FA: Hematology of Infancy and Childhood, 2nd ed. Philadelphia. WB Saunders, 1981)

index of the variation in red cell size, and thus can be used to detect anisocytosis. In the normal patient, the histogram is virtually symmetrical. The RDW is computed directly from the histogram; it is calculated as a standard statistical value, the coefficient of variation of the red cell volume distribution. The formula can be expressed as follows:

$$RDW = \frac{SD}{MCV} \times 100$$

Because RDW reflects the ratio of SD (standard deviation) and MCV, a wide red cell distribution curve in a patient with a markedly increased MCV may still generate a normal RDW number. The RDW in normal individuals ranges from 11.5% to 14.5%, but it may vary as a function of the model of the electronic cell counter employed. The top normal value for infants appears to range from 15.5% to 16.0%

Bessman and associates (see Bibliography) have provided a classification of anemias based on MCV and RDW that appears in Table 74-7.

The Blood Film

Films made on coverglasses are preferable to those made on glass slides because a greater proportion of the blood on the film is technically suitable for microscopic examination. The proper processing of blood films on coverslips is fast becoming a lost art. The details of preparation and examination can be found in manuals of laboratory hematology, but the lucid and succinct instructions of Wintrobe (3) deserve reproduction here (see Bibliography). Wintrobe states:

(1) Use a small drop of blood, only 2 to 3 mm in diameter, taken either from a stylet wound, as described earlier, or from a syringe or needle tip used in venipuncture immediately after the venipuncture has been performed (anticoagulants are not to be used as they will alter the morphologic appearance); (2) hold the coverglasses only by their edges, placing one crosswise over the other, and allow the blood to spread between them for about two seconds; (3) quickly but gently separate the coverglasses by pulling them laterally, in opposite directions to one another but in the plane of the spreading film, just before the film reaches the edges (do not squeeze or lift the coverglasses from one another); (4) quickly air-dry the films, either by placing them face up on a clean surface if the humidity is low, or by moving them through the air while holding them by their edges with your fingertips.

If the procedure has been carried out successfully, the blood will be spread evenly and there will be neither holes nor thick areas in the preparation. A multicolored sheen will be seen on the surface of the dried, unstained film if light glances off from it at the proper

Table 74–9. Diagnostic Significance of Red Cell Inclusions

Inclusion	Staining Agent	Diagnostic Significance
Basophilic stippling	Wright's stain	Represent aggregated ribosomes. May be observed in thalassemia syndromes, lead poisoning, iron deficiency, syndromes accompanied by ineffective erythropoiesis and pyrimidine 5'-nucleotidase deficiency.
Howell-Jolly bodies	Wright's stain	Represent nuclear remnants. Observed in asplenic and hyposplenic states, pernicious anemias, and severe iron deficiency anemia.
Cabot rings	Wright's stain	Appear as basophilic rings, circular, or twisted figure eights. Considered to be nuclear remnants or artifacts. Observed in lead poisoning, pernicious anemia, and hemolytic anemias.
Heinz bodies	Brilliant cresyl blue, methyl violet	Represent denatured or aggregated hemoglobin. Observed in patients with thalassemia syndromes or unstable hemoglobins, following oxidant stress in patients with enzyme deficiencies of the pentose phosphate pathway and in patients with asplenia or chronic liver disease.
Siderocytes	Prussian blue counterstained with Safrinin	Represent nonhemoglobin iron within erythrocytes. Seen in increased numbers in peripheral circulation following splenectomy. Observed in increased numbers in patients with chronic infection, aplastic anemias, or hemolytic anemias.

(Nathan DG, Oski FA: Hematology in Infancy and Childhood, 2nd ed. Philadelphia, WB Saunders, 1981)

angle, for the thin layer of closely fitting cells acts like a diffraction grating. Later, under the microscope, after staining, the red cells will be seen next to each other, but neither overlapping, nor in rouleau formation, and central pallor will be visible; lymphocytes will have a readily distinguished cytoplasm, rather than a minimal zone bearing closely on the nucleus as occurs in thick films or those which dry too slowly.

The examination of the peripheral blood film is the single most useful procedure in the initial evaluation of the patient with anemia. The blood film should first be examined under low power in order to determine the adequacy of cell distribution and staining. Signs of poor blood film preparation include loss of central pallor in red blood cells, polygonal shapes, and artifactual spherocytes. Artifactual spherocytes, in contrast to true spherocytes, show no variation in central pallor and are larger, rather than smaller, than normal red cells. Never attempt to interpret a poorly prepared blood film.

Once the adequacy of the blood film is determined by low power examination, the blood film should be examined under $1000\times$ magnification.

Cells should be graded as to size, staining intensity, variation in color, and abnormalities of shape. A classification of red cell hemolytic disorders can be made based on their predominant morphology. Such a classification is presented in Table 74-8.

The blood film should also be examined for the presence of basophilic stippling and red cell inclusions. The significance of some of these findings is described in Table 74-9.

BIBLIOGRAPHY

Bessman JD, Gilmer PR Jr, Gardner FH: Improved classification of anemias by MCV and RDW. Am J Clin Pathol 80:322, 1983

Conley CL: Anemia: Accurate diagnosis and appropriate therapy. Hosp Pract 19:57, 1984

Oski FA: Differential diagnosis of anemia. In Nathan DG, Oski KFA (eds): Hematology of Infancy and Childhood, 2nd ed, p 289. Philadelphia, WB Saunders, 1981

Sickle cell anemia is a genetic disorder in which a single codon mutation on chromosome 11, involving the beta globin gene, results in a substitution of valine for glutamic acid in the sixth position of the beta chain. This amino acid substitution alters the physical properties of the hemoglobin molecule so that it polymerizes upon deoxygenation, converting the cell from a biconcave disc into a sickle-shaped cell.

Sickle cells are less deformable than normal erythrocytes in the circulation and tend to fragment. This fragmentation contributes to their shortened red cell life span and the presence of anemia. These abnormal cells also occlude the microcirculation and result in ischemia and organ injury.

Children with sickle cell anemia are frequently admitted to the hospital as a consequence of one of four major complication or "crises": (1) vaso-occlusive crisis, (2) splenic sequestration crisis, (3) aplastic crisis, and (4) infection.

The *vaso-occlusive,* or painful, crisis is the most common reason for hospitalization of patients with sickle hemoglobinopathies. During this event it appears that sickle cells obstruct the flow of blood in the microcircu-

lation resulting in tissue hypoxia and infarction. Pain, although most common initially in the extremities, can occur anywhere in the body and quickly become generalized. The vaso-occlusive crisis is managed with the liberal administration of oral or intravenous fluids and the provision of analgesics. A minimum of twice the maintenance volume of fluids should be provided using 0.3 normal saline solution with potassium in a 5% dextrose solution. Patient weight should be monitored frequently. Urine specific gravity measurements are of no help in assessing the patient's state of hydration, since most patients with sickle cell anemia will have developed hyposthenuria by 2 years of age. Intravenous fluids should be continued until the patient's oral intake is sufficient to provide adequate hydration.

The most dreaded and serious form of vaso-occlusive episode is the occlusion of large vessels in the central nervous system. This complication occurs in approximately 5% of patients and may result in hemiplegia and extensive and permanent neurologic deficits.

Table 75-1 describes the analgesic agents available for sickle cell anemia patients, dosages, and routes of administration (see Bibli-

Table 75–1. Recommended Initial Dose and Interval of Analgesics Necessary to Obtain Adequate Pain Control in Sickle Cell Disease*

	Maximum Dose	Route	Interval	Comments
Severe Pain				
Morphine	0.15 mg/kg/dose (max, 10 mg)	SC, IM	q2½h	Drug of choice
Meperidine	1.5 mg/kg/dose (max, 100 mg)	IM	q2h	Increased incidence of seizures; avoid in patients with renal or neurologic disease
Moderate Pain				
Oxycodone (Percocet, Percodan)	1–2 tabs/dose (1 tab = 5 mg)	PO	4h	
Methadone	0.15 mg/kg/dose	PO	Q6H	Effective in patients usually requiring parenteral narcotics; *not for routine use*
Meperidine	1.5 mg/kg/dose (max, 100 mg/dose)	PO	q3½h	
Mild Pain				
Codeine	0.75 mg/kg/dose	PO/SQ	q4h	May be effective up to 6 hours
Aspirin	1.5 g/m²/24 hours divided into six doses	PO	q4h	May be given with a narcotic for added analgesia
Acetaminophen	1.5 g/m²/24 hours divided into six doses	PO	q4h	May be given with a narcotic for added analgesia
Ibuprofen (Motrin)	300–600 mg/dose	PO	q6h	

*Continuous intravenous infusion of narcotic provides excellent pain control but should be performed only by institutions familiar with its use.
(Lubin B: Hematology/Oncology Clinics of North America. Philadelphia WB Saunders [in press])

ography). Depending on the severity of the pain, an appropriate drug can be chosen.

The acute *splenic sequestration crisis* is the second most common cause of death, after infection, in sickle cell anemia patients under 5 years of age. Although the etiology of this complication is unknown, it often appears to follow or be associated with a viral infection. This splenic sequestration "crisis" can occur rapidly, with acute and massive enlargement of the spleen. The patient literally bleeds into himself and this pooling of blood in the spleen produces profound anemia and signs of hypovolemic shock. Prompt intervention using red cell transfusions and plasma volume expanders is required. Following transfusion, the spleen often returns to its previous size. Splenic sequestration crises tend to recur. Because of the danger of death with these episodes, most physicians recommend that splenectomy be performed in patients over 2 years of age who have experienced this problem. If the first sequestration event occurs prior to age 2 years, patients should receive periodic transfusions to avoid a second sequestration episode and then have their spleens removed after their second birthday.

The *aplastic crisis* is usually precipitated by infection with a human parvovirus and is associated with the rapid development of profound anemia. In patients with sickle cell anemia, red blood cell survival is in the range of only 10 to 20 days, compared with 120 days in a normal individual. Patients maintain a hemoglobin of 5.5 to 9.5 g/100 ml by increasing the rate of red cell production by five- to sixfold. When this compensatory response is dampened by the presence of infection, the hemoglobin concentration plunges precipitously. These aplastic crises may simultaneously occur in multiple family members with sickle cell anemia. During an aplastic crisis, the patients demonstrate reticulocytopenia and markedly reduced numbers of erythroid precursors in the bone marrow. The white cell count and the platelet count generally remain normal. At the nadir of an aplastic crisis, the hemoglobin may reach 1 g/100 ml, and death may occur as a result of severe heart failure. Erythroid aplasia usually terminates spontaneously in about 10 days, accompanied by a shower of nucleated red blood cells followed by a brisk reticulocytosis. Management during the acute episode in the presence of severe anemia and reticulocytopenia is with red cell transfusions.

Overwhelming *infection*, particularly during the first 3 to 5 years of life, is another serious complication of sickle cell anemia. Patients begin to become functionally asplenic by as young as 4 months of age. This hyposplenism or asplenism makes the patient with sickle cell anemia particularly vulnerable to infections with encapsulated organisms such as *Streptoccoccus pneumoniae* and *Haemophilus influenzae*. Children with functional hyposplenia are 300 to 600 times more likely than normal children to develop overwhelming pneumococcal and *Haemophilus influenzae* sepsis and meningitis.

Patients should receive penicillin prophylaxis from 4 months of age until 5 years of age. Patients who present with fever, a temperature of 102° F or 39° C, without an obvious source should be promptly cultured and begun on antibiotic therapy. Cefuroxime appears to be an appropriate initial antibiotic.

Patients with sickle cell anemia are also at increased risk for the development of pneumonia. It is often difficult to distinguish infection from infarction in patients with chest disease; they may even coexist. Some features that may help to distinguish these two entities are described in Table 75-2.

Table 75–2. Differentiation of Pneumonia versus Pulmonary Infarction

Common Clinical Features	Features Favoring Pneumonia	Features Favoring Pulmonary Infarction
Chest pain	Age <5 years	Age >5 years
Infiltration	Chills	Associated painful crisis
Fever	Upper lobe involvement	Clear x-ray at onset
Leukocytosis	Elevated bands (>1000/mm³)	Positive V-Q scan
Rub or effusion	Erythrocyte sedimentation rate	Lower lobe disease
Hypoxia	>20 mm/hr	Negative cultures
	Bacteriology: positive blood, sputum cultures or cold agglutinins and mycoplasma titers	

(Adapted from Nathan DG, Oski FA: Hematology of Infancy and Childhood, 2nd ed. Philadelphia, WB Saunders, 1981)

BIBLIOGRAPHY

Mills ML: Life-threatening complications of sickle cell disease in children. JAMA 254:1187, 1985

Poncz M, Kane E, Gill FM: Acute chest syndrome in sickle cell disease: Etiology and clinical correlates J Pediatr 107:861, 1985

Brown AK: Sickle cell anemia in children: Life threatening complications. AM J Pediatr Hematol Oncol 4:385, 1982

Castro OL, Lubin BH, Pearson HA: Managing sickle cell emergencies. Patient Care 19:92, 1985

76

Bruising and Bleeding

Excessive bruising and bleeding can be the result of (1) a deficiency of one of the coagulation factors, (2) a quantitative deficiency of platelets, (3) a qualitative abnormality of platelets, or (4) an abnormality of the vessels—either excessive capillary fragility or the presence of vasculitis.

Some features of the history and physical examination allow for the categorization of the suspected bleeding disturbance into either a defect of the fluid phase of coagulation or an abnormality of platelets or vessel wall. The distinguishing characteristics are described in Table 76-1. The steps in the coagulation pathway are illustrated in Figure 76-1.

When one suspects a bleeding disorder, initial laboratory studies should include a partial thromboplastin time, a prothrombin time, a

Table 76–1. Clinical Features that Serve to Distinguish Bleeding as a Result of a Defect in the Fluid Phase of Coagulation from a Platelet or Capillary Defect

Clinical Features	Coagulation Defects	Platelet and Capillary Defects
Bleeding from superficial cuts and abrasions	Usually not excessive	Often profuse and prolonged
Spontaneous bruises and hematomas	Often deep and spreading hematoma Only a few at any one time	Usually small, superficial, and multiple
Hemarthroses	Common in severe cases	Very rare
Bleeding from deep cuts and tooth extractions	Onset often delayed for minutes or hours; not permanently controlled by local pressure	Onset usually immediate; frequently permanently arrested by local pressure
Most common bleeding manifestations	Deep tissue hemorrhages, often involving joints and muscle; prolonged bleeding after injury	Epistaxis, menorrhagia, and gastrointestinal bleeding
Petechiae	Rare	Common

464

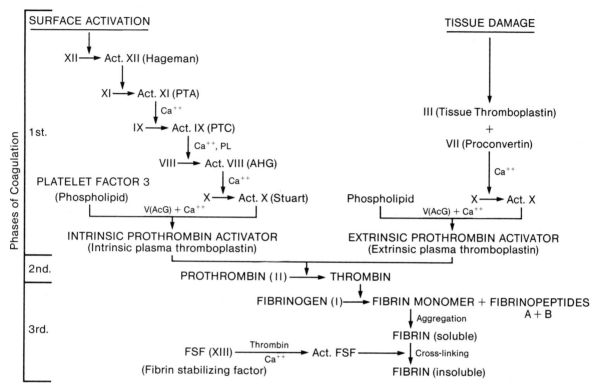

FIGURE 76–1. The coagulation scheme.

platelet count, a smear to examine platelet morphology, and a standardized Ivy bleeding time. This battery of tests allows a presumptive diagnosis of a bleeding disturbance. The only defect not detected by one of these procedures in an inherited deficiency of Factor XIII (fibrin-stabilizing factor). The use of such tests in arriving at a presumptive diagnosis is illustrated in Table 76–2. Once a provisional diagnosis has been made, it can be confirmed by assay of specific clotting factors. The mode of transmission of the inherited defects of coagulation is listed below:

> Sex-linked recessive (disorders primarily of males)
> > Factor VIII (AHF) deficiency
> > Factor IX (PTC) deficiency

Autosomal dominant (disorders of both sexes; one parent affected)
> Factor XI (PTA) deficiency
> von Willebrand's disease

Autosomal recessive (disorders of both sexes; parents appear normal)
> Prothrombin deficiency
> Factor V (proaccelerin) deficiency
> Factor VII (proconvertin) deficiency
> Factor X (Stuart-Prower deficiency
> Factor XII (Hageman) deficiency—no bleeding associated with this disorder
> Factor XIII (fibrin-stabilizing factor) deficiency

Afibrinogenemia, congenital
von Willebrand's disease (severe form)

Table 76–2. A Diagnostic Approach to the Bleeding Patient

Platelets decreased, PT prolonged, PTT prolonged	Platelets normal, PT prolonged, PTT prolonged	Platelets normal, PT normal, PTT prolonged	Platelets normal, PT prolonged, PTT normal	Platelets normal, PT normal, PTT normal	Platelets decreased, PT and PTT normal
Consider: Disseminated intravascular coagulation, particularly in patients with sepsis or hypoxia	*Consider:* Vitamin K deficiency.	*Consider:* Congenital Factor VIII deficiency Congenital Factor IX deficiency Congenital Factor XI deficiency Congenital Factor XII deficiency von Willebrand's disease Heparin treatment	*Consider:* Congenital Factor II deficiency Congenital Factor VII deficiency	*Consider:* Factor XIII deficiency Platelet dysfunction von Willebrand's disease	Determine cause of thrombocytopenia
Tests to confirm: Thrombin time Fibrin split products Factor V assay Red cell fragmentation	If vitamin K has not been given, administer vitamin K, 2.0 mg IV Repeat PT and PTT in 4 hours	*Tests to confirm:* Factor VIII, IX, XI, XII assay Bleeding time (prolonged in von Willebrand's disease)	*Tests to confirm:* Factor II assay Factor VII assay	*Tests to confirm:* Factor XIII assay Bleeding time Platelet adhesiveness Maternal and infant drug history	
	Bleeding stops PT normal PTT normal → *Diagnosis:* Vitamin K deficiency		Bleeding continues PT abnormal PTT abnormal → *Consider:* Congenital Factor V deficiency Congenital Factor X deficiency Congenital fibrinogen deficiency Severe liver disease → *Tests to confirm:* Factor V assay Factor X assay Fibrinogen assay		

466

If the patient is found to be thrombocytopenic, it must be determined whether the low platelet count is the result of inadequate platelet production or accelerated platelet destruction. Simple studies that assist the physician in this determination include a bone marrow examination to determine the adequacy of megakaryocyte number, and an examination of the peripheral smear. Young platelets tend to be large (>2.5 μ in diameter). In patients with destructive thrombocytopenias, young platelets are usually evident on the blood film. If the results of the bone marrow examination and peripheral smear are indecisive, the patient can be administered platelets and their survival determined.

77

Hereditary Coagulation Disorders

THE HEMOPHILIAS

Hemophilia A (factor VIII deficiency) and hemophilia B (factor IX deficiency) are bleeding disorders that are inherited as X-linked recessive traits. The two disorders are clinically indistinguishable but can easily be differentiated by factor assays. In general, the severity of the bleeding manifestations correlates well with the level of factor activity as determined in the laboratory. For example, patients with factor VIIIC values of less than 0.03 units per ml (3% activity) are termed severe hemophiliacs and experience spontaneous hemorrhage into joints and soft tissues. Patients with 3% to 10% activity are termed moderate hemophiliacs and bleed excessively from moderate trauma, whereas mild hemophiliacs, patients with 10% to 15% of normal activity bleed excessively only from major trauma or at the time of surgery.

Both hemophilia A and B are heterogeneous conditions, but the degree of severity of the disease tends to be uniform within families. factor VIII deficiency (hemophilia A) is four to five times more common than factor IX deficiency. It is estimated that 1 in 10,000 males in the United States has factor VIII deficiency.

In both forms of hemophilia, patients require replacement therapy most commonly for treatment of acute hemarthroses and muscle hemorrhage. Bleeding from the genitourinary and gastrointestinal tracts and bleeding within the central nervous system are, fortunately, far less common.

Treatment is based on the replacement of the necessary factor either in the form of factor concentrates or fresh frozen plasma. Recommended doses for the treatment of these two conditions are listed in Tables 77-1 and 77-2. Mild factor VIII deficient patients also may benefit from the administration of DDAVP (desmopressin) which produces a transient increase in factor VIII C activity.

VON WILLEBRAND'S DISEASE

Von Willebrand's disease is believed to be the second most common inherited hemostatic defect after hemophilia A. It is a very heterogenous disease, with the majority of cases inherited in an autosomal-dominant fashion. Patients may experience severe mucous membrane bleeding, particularly nosebleeds, or merely easy bruisability. Women frequently manifest menorrhagia. The bleeding ten-

468

Table 77–1. Recommended Dosages of Factor VIII for Hemophilia A*

Type of Bleeding	Initial Dosage (U/kg)	Repeat Dosage (U/kg)	Other Treatment
Acute hemarthrosis†			
Early	10	Seldom necessary	Ice packs, non-weight bearing; sling or light-weight splint may be helpful; rarely, joint aspiration (see text)
Late	20	20q12h	
Intramuscular hemorrhage†	20–30	20q12h; often several days of treatment required for extensive hemorrhages	Non-weight bearing; complete bed rest for iliopsoas hemorrhage
Life-threatening situations‡	50	25–30q8–12h *or* Preferably, bolus dose of 25 U/kg followed by continuous infusion, 3–4 U/kg/hour	
Intracranial hemorrhage			
Major surgery			
Major trauma			
Tongue or neck bleeding with potential airway obstruction			
Severe abdominal pain‡	20–40	20–25q12h	
Tongue and mouth lacerations‡	20	20q12h	An antifibrinolytic agent (tranexamic acid or EACA), sedation, NPO in small child; local application of orahesive gauze may be beneficial for gum bleeding
Extractions of permanent teeth‡	20	20q12h; however, often not necessary in uncomplicated extractions	Antifibrinolytic agent beginning 1 day preop; continue 7–10 days
Painless spontaneous gross hematuria	None		Increased PO fluids; corticosteroids and/or Factor VIII are used by some

*Refers to heat-treated or otherwise virus-attenuated Factor VIII.

†In infants and children under 4 years of age, some still prefer to use cryoprecipitates rather than virus-attenuated lyophilized Factor VIII concentrates. In individuals who have mild hemophilia A, it is preferable to use desmopressin rather than lyophilized Factor VIII concentrates.

‡These cases should be treated in a comprehensive hemophilia center. If a case is first seen in another hospital, the hemophilia center should be contacted and the patient transferred after emergency treatment is given at the local hospital.

(Reprinted with permission from Lusher JM: Hemophilia. Hematol Rev 1985.)

Table 77–2. Recommended Dosages of Factor IX for Hemophilia B

Type of Bleeding	Initial Dosage and Source of Factor IX (U/kg)*	Repeat Dosage and Source of Factor IX (U/kg)*	Other Treatment
Acute hemarthrosis†			
In individual with mild hemophilia B	15 (FFP)	None	Seldom necessary
Early, in severe hemophilia B	20 (PCC)	None	Ice packs; non–weight bearing; a sling may be useful; rarely, joint aspiration
Late (pain, swelling, limitation of motion) in severe hemophilia B	30 (PCC)	20–25 (PCC) q12h	
Intramuscular hemorrhage†			
In individual with mild hemophilia B	15 (FFP)	10–15 (FFP) q12h	Non–weight bearing; complete bed rest for iliopsoas hemorrhage
In severe hemophilia B	30–40 (PCC)	30 (PCC) q12h; several days of treatment may be required for extensive intramuscular hemorrhage	
Life-threatening situations‡			
Intracranial hemorrhage			
Major trauma	50 (PCC)	20–25 (PCC) q12h _or_ Bolus dose followed by continuous infusion	AT III concentrate or 300 ml FFP as a source of AT III; add heparin to reconstituted PCC
Tongue or neck bleeding with potential airway obstruction			
Severe abdominal pain‡			
In mild hemophilia B	15 (FFP)	10 (FPP) q12h	
In severe hemophilia B	40 (PCC)	20 (PCC) q12h	
Tongue and mouth laceration‡			
Extraction of permanent teeth			
In mild hemophilia B	15 (FFP)	10 (FFP) q12h	An antifibrinolytic agent (EACA or tranexamic acid)
In severe hemophilia B	30 (PCC)	20 (PCC) q12h; however, may not be necessary in uncomplicated extractions	An antifibrinolytic agent begun day after PCC is stopped; orahesive gauze may be helpful for gum bleeding
Painless spontaneous gross hematuria	None		Increased PO fluids; corticosteroids and/or PCC used by some

*FFP = fresh frozen plasma; PCC = heat-treated or otherwise virus-attenuated prothrombin complex concentrate. As soon as a nonthrombogenic Factor IX concentrate is licensed and available, it would become the preferred product for most of the above situations.
†In infants and children under 4 years of age, some physicians still prefer to use FFP rather than PCC, even in those patients with moderately severe hemophilia B.
‡These cases should be treated in a comprehensive hemophilia center. If a case is first seen in another hospital, the hemophilia center should be contacted and the patient transferred after emergency treatment is given at the local hospital.
(Reprinted with permission from Lusher JM: Hematol Rev 1985)

dency is usually more severe in childhood and adolescence and improves in adulthood.

The disease can be traced to either the lack of a protein complex termed von Willebrand's factor or the presence of an abnormal protein complex. Von Willebrand's factor is a multi-formed glycoprotein complex that associates with Factor VIII procoagulant.

Laboratory testing reveals a number of abnormalities, and the diagnostic picture may be clouded by the existence of patients who satisfy only some of the laboratory criteria for diagnosis. Fluctuation in the levels of von Willebrand's factor (*e.g.,* in conditions such as pregnancy and liver disease, which raise its level in the serum) also contribute to the diagnostic difficulties.

In general, patients have evidence of both abnormal platelet function (a prolonged bleeding time) and a deficiency of clotting factor VIII. Platelet dysfunction in von Willebrand's disease can be measured by the ristocetin aggregation test, which measures the ability of the ristocetin protein to aggregate cells. Platelet counts are normal. All of these abnormalities are corrected by infusions of factor VIII-containing preparations. The platelet activity is not abnormal in hemophilia, and hemophiliac plasma will correct the platelet defect in von Willebrand's disease. Cryoprecipitates of plasma fractions rich in factor VIII are the current therapy of choice.

DISSEMINATED INTRAVASCULAR COAGULATION

Disseminated intravasular coagulation (DIC) is an acquired pathophysiologic process characterized by the intravascular consumption of platelets and plasma clotting factors, factors II, V, VIII, and XIII and fibrinogen. This widespread coagulation within the circulation results in the deposition of fibrin thrombi in small vessels and the production of a hemorrhagic state. The accumulation of fibrin deposits in the microcirculation produces mechanical injury to the red cells, leading to erythrocyte fragmentation and a hemolytic anemia.

The most common causes of DIC are infection, shock, tissue injury, endothelial damage, hypoxia, and acidosis. The clinical manifestations of DIC are variable and are determined in part by the associated disease process and in part by the severity of the coagulation deficiency.

Laboratory abnormalities include the presence of a hemolytic anemia with red cell fragmentation visible on the peripheral blood film, variable degrees of thrombocytopenia, and a prolongation of the prothrombin time, the partial thromboplastin time, and the thrombin time, and the presence of fibrin degradation products in the plasma.

Treatment must be directed primarily at the underlying condition rather than the coagulation disturbance. Platelets and plasma may be given to control major bleeding, but success, in general, depends on the ability to correct the primary condition rather than the coagulation abnormalities.

THROMBOCYTOPENIA

The thrombocytopenic patient most frequently displays petechiae and purpura. It is rare for such signs to be present in patients in whom the platelet count exceeds $50,000/mm^3$ unless the patient has intrinsically defective platelets or has taken exogenous agents that have modified platelet function.

In the thrombocytopenic patient, a prompt decision must be made regarding its etiology. The three general categories of thrombocytopenia are; 1. Destructive thrombocytopenia—the increased rate of platelet destruction surpasses the ability of the bone marrow to produce platelets 2. Aregenerative thrombo-

cytopenia—the production of platelets is compromised and is unable to keep up with the normal physiologic demands for platelets
3. Sequestration thrombocytopenia—platelets are trapped within a vascular bed, usually an enlarged spleen. Examples of these various forms of thrombocytopenia are listed in Table 77-3.

Table 77–3. Differential Diagnosis of Thrombocytopenia in Children

DESTRUCTIVE
Primary Platelet Consumption Syndromes
  Immunologic
    Idiopathic thrombocytopenic purpura
    Drug-induced thrombocytopenic purpura
    Infection-induced thrombocytopenic purpura
    Post-transfusion purpura
    Autoimmune or lymphoproliferative disorders
    Neonatal immune thrombocytopenias
    Allergy and anaphylaxis
    Post-transplant purpura
  Nonimmunologic
    Chronic microangiopathic hemolytic anemia and
      thrombocytopenia
    Hemolytic uremic syndrome
    Thrombotic thrombocytopenic purpura
    Catheters, prostheses, or cardiopulmonary bypass
    Congenital or acquired heart disease
Combined Platelet and Fibrinogen Consumption Syndromes
  Disseminated intravascular coagulation
  Kasabach-Merritt syndrome
  Other causes of local consumption coagulopathy
  Miscellaneous causes
  Specific to the neonate
    Phototherapy
    Perinatal aspiration syndromes
    Persistent pulmonary hypertension
    Rhesus alloimmunization
    Post-exchange transfusion
    Polycythemia
    Metabolic disorders
  Glomerular disease
  Preeclampsia
  Fatty-acid–induced thrombocytopenia
IMPAIRED OR INEFFECTIVE PRODUCTION
Congenital and Hereditary Disorders
  Primary hematologic processes
    TAR syndrome
    Other congenital thrombocytopenias with megakaryo-
      cytic hypoplasia
    Fanconi's aplastic anemia
    Bernard-Soulier syndrome*
    May-Hegglin anomaly*
    Wiskott-Aldrich syndrome*
    Miscellaneous hereditary
    Thrombocytopenias (X-Linked or autosomal)*
    Mediterranean thrombocytopenia
  Associated with Trisomy 13 or 18
  Metabolic Disorders
    Methylmalonic acidemia
    Ketotic glycinemia
    Holocarboxylase synthetase deficiency
    Isovaleric acidemia
Acquired Disorders
  Aplastic anemia
  Marrow infiltrative Processes
  Drug- or radiation-induced
  Nutritional deficiency states (iron, folate, or vitamin B_{12})
SEQUESTRATION
  Hypersplenism
  Hypothermia

*These hereditary thrombocytopenias can be associated with normal or increased bone marrow megakaryocytes.
(Nathan DG, Oski FA: Hematology of Infancy and Childhood 2nd ed. Philadelphia WB Saunders, 1981)

IDIOPATHIC THROMBOCYTOPENIC PURPURA IN CHILDHOOD

Idiopathic thrombocytopenic purpura (ITP) is a relatively common cause of petechiae and purpura in children. It is usually an acute, self-limited disorder often precipitated by an antecedent viral illness (Table 77-4). From a review of almost 1400 patients, the clinical manifestations at the time of presentation include skin bleeding (100%), epistaxis (25%), minimal splenomegaly (10%), oral bleeding (7%), gastrointestinal bleeding (5%), hematuria (5%), and intracranial hemorrhage (1%).

The platelet count is less than 40,000/mm^3 in most patients. Large platelets and atypical lymphocytes are often present in the peripheral smear. Since leukemia is commonly associated with thrombocytopenia, a bone marrow examination should be performed in most

Table 77–4. Differential Features of ITP in Childhood

Acute	Chronic
Onset at under 10 years of age	Over 10 years
Onset acute with preceding viral illness	Insidious
Male: female equal	More common in females
Platelet count less than 20,000/mm³	20,000 to 75,000/mm³
Immunoglobulins normal	IgA often decreased
No other immunologic abnormalities	Other immunologic abnormalities present in both propositus and other family members
Platelet-associated IgG antibody markedly elevated	Modestly increased
No common pattern in HLA typing	Increase in A3, B7, or A26,W16 haplotypes

(Nathan DG, Oski FA: Hematology of Infancy and Childhood, 2nd ed. WB Saunders, Philadelphia, 1981)

patients to confirm the diagnosis and to reassure the parents.

In 80% to 90% of children who develop ITP, uneventful recovery will ensue within 3 weeks to 6 months. Listed below are those features that help to distinguish the acute, self-limited disorder from that which is more likely to result in chronic disease.

It seems reasonable to use corticosteroids in the treatment of children with ITP when the platelet count is less than 20,000/mm³. They should be given initially for a period of no longer than 3 weeks. Steroid therapy does not improve the eventual outcome but can produce a more rapid return to normal in the platelet count. Platelet transfusions are generally of no benefit because the transfused platelets are rapidly destroyed. In children who develop chronic ITP, removal of the spleen will produce a return of the platelet count to normal in approximately 75% of instances.

Recently it has been demonstrated that the intravenous administration of gamma globulin will rapidly raise the platelet count in patients with ITP. This form of therapy, while not curative, may often be of clinical benefit in the bleeding patient and may serve to defer the need for splenectomy in the patient with chronic ITP.

BIBLIOGRAPHY

Aledort LM: Current concepts in diagnosis and management of hemophilia. Hosp Pract 17:77, 1982

Hathaway WE: Use of antiplatelet agents in pediatric hypercoagulable states. Am J Dis Child 138:301, 1984

Kelton JG, Gibbons S: Autoimmune platelet destruction: Idiopathic thrombocytopenic purpura. Semin Thromb Hemost 8:83, 1982

Lusher JM: Diseases of coagulation: The fluid phase. In Nathan DG, Oski FA (eds): Hematology of Infancy and Childhood, 3rd ed, p 1293. Philadelphia, WB Saunders, 1985

Walker RW, Walker W: Idiopathic thrombocytopenia: Initial illness and long-term follow-up. Arch Dis Child 59:316, 1984

78

Splenomegaly

The spleen is one of the major components of the reticuloendothelial system. It is comprised of two distinct but closely related elements: the white pulp and the red pulp. The white pulp comprises histiocytic macrophages, lymphocytes, and plasma cells, whereas the red pulp is composed of the Billroth's cords and splenic sinuses. As a consequence of its dual anatomic construction, the spleen serves dual functions. The two primary functions are the filtration of particulate matter and formed elements from the blood and the production of humoral factors required for the opsonization of infectious organisms. Splenic enlargement can be observed in disease states in which either the clearing function of the spleen is excessive or in circumstances in which antigenic stimulation is either massive or prolonged. During fetal life and early infancy, the spleen is also the site of erythropoiesis. In response to needs for augmented red cell production, the spleen may continue to serve as a site for erythrocyte production, and this also is reflected by the presence of splenomegaly.

The spleen is normally palpable as a soft organ in most infants born prior to 40 weeks' gestation. In this circumstance, the spleen can be felt 1 to 2 cm below the left costal margin in the midclavicular line. The spleen can be palpated in approximately 30% of normal full-term infants and in 10% of healthy infants at 1 year of age. By age 12, about 1% of normal children still have a spleen that is palpable approximately 1 cm below the left costal margin. In healthy infants and children, the spleen, when palpable, is soft and nontender and feels much like a normal lymph node.

Occasionally, it is difficult to distinguish a spleen from a renal mass. On physical examination, the spleen descends with inspiration, whereas the kidney remains relatively immobile. The superior margin of the spleen cannot be felt while it is usually possible to define the upper pole of a kidney. When a spleen enlarges, it usually descends downward and medially whereas the enlarged kidney is felt anteriolaterally. If careful physical examination cannot distinguish the two organs, then imaging techniques such as sonography or liver–spleen scans with technitium sulfur colloid should be used.

The causes of splenic enlargement can be conveniently grouped by the use of the mnemonic *SPLEEN: S*equestration, *P*roliferation, *L*ipid, *E*ngorgement, *E*ndowment, and i*N*vasion.

SEQUESTRATION

The spleen sequesters effete red cells at the end of their normal 120-day life span. Abnormal red cells are also retained within the red pulp of this organ. Two main mechanisms are operative under conditions that result in splenic sequestration of erythrocytes. The first is an alteration in the surface properties of the red cell. The presence of immunoglobulins or complement on the surface of the red cell results in their recognition, detention, and ultimate phagocytosis by the monocytes and macrophages within the endothelial lining of the spleen. Diseases accompanied by antibody coating of red cells are generally associated with some degree of splenomegaly. Examples of such diseases include Rh and ABO isoimmunization during the newborn period and "autoimmune" hemolytic anemias later in life.

Splenic sequestration causes a loss of the normal deformability of the erythrocyte. Red cells may lose their normal deformability as a result of alterations in membrane proteins, intracellular deposition of precipitated or aggregated hemoglobin, or as a result of alterations in cell water, cations, or metabolic intermediates such as adenosine triphosphate.

Hereditary hemolytic anemias that are accompanied by alterations in red cell deformability include sickle cell anemia, hemoglobin C disease, thalassemia major, many of the unstable hemoglobins, some of the enzyme deficiencies such as pyruvate kinase deficiency, hereditary spherocytosis, hereditary elliptocytosis, and hereditary stomatocytosis.

The enlargement of the spleen should not be accompanied by generalized lymphadenopathy in patients in whom splenomegaly is produced by sequestration of red cells. A history of anemia or jaundice may be present in the patient or in other family members. Examination of the well-prepared peripheral blood smear and a determination of the patient's hemoglobin, red cell indices, and reticulocyte count should enable the physician to make a preliminary decision that the patient's splenomegaly is primarily a result of an alteration of the red cell.

PROLIFERATION

Many viral and bacterial infections result in a proliferation of the white pulp of the spleen. Chronic immunologic stimulation from any cause can also result in splenomegaly.

Examples of viral infections that commonly result in splenic enlargement in pediatric patients include infectious mononucleosis (Epstein-Barr virus) and cytomegalovirus infections. Splenic enlargement in these diseases is usually accompanied by lymphaenopathy, a history of fever and sore throat, a nonspecific rash in some instances, laboratory evidence of hepatic dysfunction, and the presence of atypical lymphocytes in the peripheral blood smear (see Chapter 29).

Bacterial infections frequently accompanied by splenic enlargement include severe pneumonias, typhoid fever, bacterial endocarditis, and indolent septicemias. The other manifestations of the disease usually dominate the clinical picture, and isolated splenomegaly is rarely present as a diagnostic enigma.

LIPID

The large and heterogeneous group of disorders in which "foam cells" or lipid-laden macrophages accumulate within the spleen and bone marrow result in splenomegaly. Lipids appear to accumulate in the spleen in these disorders because of defects in catabolism of sphingolipids or other related metabolic intermediates. Many of these disturbances have sufficiently distinct clinical manifestations, which may lead to a presumptive diagnosis.

ENGORGEMENT

Engorgement of the spleen may produce splenomegaly; leukopenia and thrombocytopenia are also common findings in patients with splenic engorgement. Localized engorgement can result from splenic trauma and the accumulation of blood within the splenic capsule. Splenic engorgement can be observed in children with portal hypertension that is a consequence of hepatic disease, with primary disease in the portal vein or splenic vein, or with congestive heart failure.

Portal hypertension secondary to liver disease has many causes in pediatric patients. Diseases to consider in such circumstances include chronic hepatitis, cystic fibrosis, Wilson's disease, cirrhosis secondary to intrahepatic biliary atresia, and the consequences of ascending infection via the umbilical vein following catheterization in the neonatal period. In patients with portal hypertension, hepatomegaly, ascites, esophageal varices, internal hemorrhoids, and historical features of liver disease may be found. In patients with congestive splenomegaly as a result of portal vein thrombosis or obstruction to the splenic vein, diagnosis often may be made only with contrast studies of the portal circulation.

Acute splenic engorgement, the so-called "sequestration crisis" may also be observed in patients with sickle-cell anemia. In this circumstance, for unknown reasons, the spleen rapidly fills with blood, and the patient literally bleeds within himself. These patients, usually under the age of 5 years, may present with signs of profound hypovolemia and anemia. This complication of sickle cell anemia is one of the primary causes of early death.

ENDOWMENT

Abnormalities in the category of endowment are rare causes of splenomegaly. Among congenital causes of splenomegaly may be included splenic hemangiomas, splenic cysts, and splenic cystic hygromas.

INVASION

Splenomegaly may accompany a variety of malignant processes. Fifty percent to 60% of children with leukemia may have splenomegaly at the time of diagnosis. Splenomegaly tends to be more common and of greater size in patients with myelogenous rather than lymphatic leukemia. Other manifestations of the disease tend to dominate the clinical picture, and it is extremely rare for isolated splenomegaly to be the sole historical or physical finding in a child with leukemia.

Lymphomas may also be associated with splenomegaly. In this circumstance, isolated splenomegaly may prove to be a source of real diagnostic confusion.

Splenomegaly is generally present in patients with histiocytosis, but this is rarely an isolated finding.

The spleen may be the site of metastatic disease. The most common pediatric tumor associated with metastases to the spleen is neuroblastoma.

The spleen may be the site of granuloma formation in diseases such as sarcoidosis, tuberculosis, and some of the systemic fungal infections.

DIAGNOSTIC TESTS

Investigation of a patient with splenomegaly should begin with a careful history and physical examination and a complete blood count.

Additional studies that may be indicated include a bone marrow examination, a lymph node biopsy, a computed tomogram of the abdomen and a study to exclude the presence of portal hypertension and esophageal varices. Specific etiologic tests should be deferred until a correct general categorial assignment can be made for the cause of the splenic enlargement.

BIBLIOGRAPHY

Boles ET Jr, Baxter CF, Newton WA Jr: Evaluation of splenomegaly in childhood. Clin Pediat 2:161, 1963

Tunnessen WW Jr: Splenomegaly, In Signs and Symptoms in Pediatrics, p 340. Philadelphia, JB Lippincott, 1983

79 Lymphadenopathy

It must be appreciated that the lymphatic tissue forms a larger percentage of the total body weight during infancy and childhood than in adult life, and as a result lymphoid tissue is easily palpable in many areas of the body. The relative abundance of lymphoid tissue is reflected by the size of the pharyngeal tonsillar tissue. The tonsils generally reach their maximal size when the child is about 7 years of age and gradually atrophy. Cervical, axillary, and inguinal nodes are palpable in almost all infants and children. Occipital nodes may be palpable in about 5% of children under 12 years of age. Enlargement of postauricular, supraclavicular, epitrochlear, popliteal, mediastinal, and abdominal nodes is uncommon and suggests the presence of an associated pathologic process.

Lymph node enlargement results from one of two basic processes. The processes are proliferation of cells intrinsic to the lymph node and infiltration by extrinsic cells. Cells intrinsic to the lymph node that may undergo proliferation include lymphocytes, plasma cells, and histiocytes. This form of proliferation occurs in response to antigenic stimulation.

Infiltration of a lymph node involves invasion by malignant cells or by polymorphonuclear leukocytes in response to a local infection.

In attempting to determine the significance of lymphadenopathy, a number of facts should be ascertained that will facilitate reaching a diagnosis and instituting appropriate therapy.

The following questions should be answered:

1. Is the lymphadenopathy generalized (enlargement of more than two noncontiguous lymph node regions), or is it localized? Generalized lymphadenopathy is caused by generalized disease.
2. If the lymphadenopathy is localized, is it accompanied by signs of infection in the involved node? Is the node tender? Is the skin over the node warm or red?
3. If the lymphadenopathy is localized, is there evidence of infection in the drainage of the area of the lymph node or a history of recent antigenic introduction in the drainage area?
4. Which lymph nodes are involved in the process?

5. If the lymphadenopathy is generalized, what are the associated symptoms and signs? Of importance in the physical examination are the presence of hepatic and splenic enlargement, the size of the thyroid gland, and the presence of disease involving the heart, lungs, or joints. Is there any evidence of pallor or easy bruising?

GENERALIZED LYMPHADENOPATHY

Generalized lymphadenopathy does not usually present the same diagnostic dilemma to the physician as local lymphadenopathy. Generalized lymphadenopathy is usually associated with other abnormalities in the history, physical examination, or initial laboratory tests and thus enables the physician to reach a probable diagnosis.

The more common causes of generalized lymphadenopathy are listed below.

Infections must always be seriously considered in patients with generalized lymphadenopathy. Viral infections are probably the most common group of infections responsible for such a response. Viral infections associated with an exanthem such as rubella and rubeola should produce no diagnostic confusion. Infants and children with acquired cytomegalovirus infections or infectious mononucleosis may have nonspecific eruptions. The presence of more than 10% atypical lymphocytes in the peripheral blood smear should alert the physician to this diagnostic possibility.

With acute, overwhelming infections, the presence of fever, leukocytosis, signs of toxicity, and, perhaps, evidence of a focal lesion responsible for the dissemination process will generally alert the physician to the nature of the underlying disease.

Chronic infections with tuberculosis or syphilis may be causes of generalized lymph-

Causes of Generalized Lymphadenopathy

Infections
  Pyogenic infections
  Tuberculosis
  Syphilis
  Toxoplasmosis
  Brucellosis
  Histoplasmosis
  Malaria
  Typhoid fever
  Cytomegalovirus infection
  Infectious mononucleosis
  Exanthems (scarlet fever, rubella, rubeola)
  Infectious hepatitis
Collagen vascular diseases
  Lupus erythematosus
  Rheumatoid arthritis
Immunologic reactions
  Serum sickness
  Drug reactions
  Granulomatous diseases (sarcoid)
Drug-Induced
  Phenytoin
  Antithyroid medication
  Hydralazine
  Allopurinol
Storage diseases
  Gaucher's disease
  Niemann-Pick disease
Malignancies
  Leukemia
  Neuroblastoma (metastatic)
  Lymphomas
  Histiocytosis

adenopathy. This is a very unusual manifestation of these disorders in children.

In patients with rheumatoid arthritis or lupus erythematosus, the history is characterized by the presence of chronic, intermittent fever, evanescent rashes, and arthralgia and arthritis. Physical examination and laboratory test results may indicate the presence of disease involving the joints, kidney, lungs, liver, myocardium, and pericardium.

In patients with storage disorders that are associated with lymphadenopathy, the spleen and liver will also be enlarged. In young infants and children with these generalized disorders, evidence of cerebral involvement may dominate the clinical picture.

Although it is estimated that as many as 70% of pediatric patients with acute lymphoblastic leukemia will have generalized lymphadenopathy, this finding is rarely the initial manifestation of the disease. The clinical picture in these patients is dominated by a history of unexplained fever, general malaise, pallor, and easy bruising. With generalized lymphadenopathy, splenomegaly is invariably present.

The patient with histiocytosis frequently has associated skin involvement, a history of chronic otitis media, and evidence of disease involving the lungs, liver, and spleen.

REGIONAL LYMPHADENOPATHY

Regional lymphadenopathy, and most particularly lympadenopathy in the cervical area, produces the greatest diagnostic dilemma to the physician. The physician must decide if the lump is malignant and how long he can observe the patient before resorting to a biopsy or lymph node excision.

The area of involvement and the associated findings will facilitate a logical decision. For example, isolated supraclavicular lymph node involvement should always suggest the presence of malignancy. This is usually accompanied by signs of mediastinal disease and is generally a result of Hodgkin's disease or non-Hodgkin's lymphoma.

CERVICAL LYMPH NODE ENLARGEMENT

Isolated enlargement of the cervical nodes is generally the result of localized infection. The most common agents producing adenitis in this region are staphylococci and streptococci. Often a history of a recent upper respiratory infection will be elicited. The major causes of cervical adenopathy and their distinguishing characteristics are described in Table 79-1.

A systematic approach to patients with cervical adenitis is extremely important and a timetable that may ultimately lead to biopsy should be established.

When the cervical nodes are warm and tender and evidence of overlying infection is present in the overlying skin, diagnosis is relatively simple. These nodes should be aspirated for purposes of bacterial culture and smear for bacteriologic identification. In addition, a search should be made for a primary focus of infection in the scalp, mouth, pharynx, and sinuses. The submandibular nodes are most frequently enlarged in patients with infections in the ethmoid and maxillary sinuses. A history of cat scratch should also be elicited.

When the cervical node enlargement is nontender and not associated with signs of infection, other diagnostic procedures should accompany the initial evaluation. The following should be included: a complete blood count and smear to detect evidence of atypical lymphocytes, a heterophile test or a titer to detect the presence of Epstein-Barr virus antibodies, skin tests for both *Mycobacterium tuberculosis* and atypical mycobacteria, and a chest film.

If the cervical enlargement is accompanied by supraclavicular enlargement or if splenomegaly is present in the absence of evidence of a viral illness, recent immunization, or a drug allergy, an early lymph node biopsy should be obtained.

Table 79–1. Infectious Lymphadenopathy in Children and Adolescents: Differentiating Features in Ten Diseases of Different Etiologies

Etiology	Onset	Node Distribution	Fever–Toxicity	Hemogram	Diagnosis	Suppuration	Treatment
Streptococcus, group A	Abrupt, 2-3 days	Regional	Mild-marked	Leukocytosis	Aspiration and culture	Frequent	Penicillin, aspiration
Staphylococcus aureus	Abrupt, 2-3 days	Regional	Mod-marked	Leukocytosis	Aspiration and culture	Frequent	Keflex, dicloxacillin, aspiration, I&D
Cat-scratch disease	3-10 days	Regional	Mild-mod	Usually normal, min leukocytosis	Cat-scratch skin test, gram-negative bacteria skin/node	14%	Reassure, aspirate for pain
Mycobacterium tuberculosis	2-7 wk	Regional	Usually absent	Usually normal	PPDT>15mm	52%	INH, RMP, 1 yr Excision if no response
Nontuberculous mycobacterial disease	2-7 wk	Regional	Usually absent	Usually normal	PPD-T O-14 mm	74%	Excisional biopsy INH and RMP (rarely effective)
Infectious mononucleosis	1-2 wk	Gen ant and post cervical	Mild-mod	Lymphocytosis, atypical lymphs>15%	Monospot test, Epstein-Barr virus titers	No	Bed rest, symptomatic
Cytomegalovirus	1-2 wk	Gen ant and post cervical	Mild-mod	Lymphocytosis, atypical lymphs	Virus isolation, CF titer	No	Reassure, careful follow-up
Tularemia	1-7 days	Regional, 75% ulceroglandular	Mod	Leukocytosis	History and febrile agglutination	Frequent	Streptomycin IM for 6 d
Brucellosis	1-7 wk, several mo	Generalized	Mod-marked	Leukopenia, relative lymphocytosis	Blood culture, agglut. Brucella abortus	No	Tetracycline for 21 d
Toxoplasmosis	1-7 wk	Cervical ant and post generalized	Mild-marked	Lymphocytosis, atypical lymphs	IFA IgM> 1:1,000	No	Reassurance, if ill, pyrimethamine, SDZ

*Abbreviations used are: agglut, agglutination test; ant, anterior; CF, complement fixation; gen, generally; I & D, incision and drainage; IFA, indirect fluorescent antibody; IM, intramuscularly; lymphs, lymphocytes; INH, isoniazid; min, minimal; mod, moderate; post, posterior; SDZ, sulfadiazine; RMP, rifampin. (Margileth AM: Cervical adenitis. Pediatr Rev 7:13, 1985)

Guidelines for Diagnosis of Localized Noncervical Lymphadenopathy

Supraclavicular: Always consider mediastinal disease (tuberculosis, histoplasmosis, coccidiomycosis, sarcoidosis). Always consider lymphoma. In the absence of evidence of pulmonary infection, early node biopsy is indicated.

Axillary: Secondary to infections in the hand, arm, lateral chest wall or lateral portion of the breast. May be result of recently administered immunizations in the arm. Very common with BCG innoculations.

Epitrochlear: Secondary to infections on ulnar side of hand and forearm. Observed in tularemia when bite occurs on finger. Also observed in secondary syphilis.

Inguinal: Look for evidence of infection in the lower extremity, scrotum, and penis in the male, vulva and vagina in the female, the skin of the lower abdomen, perineum, gluteal region, or anal canal.

May be manifestation of lymphogranuloma venereum.

May represent metastatic disease from testicular tumors or bony tumors of the leg.

If all studies are not diagnostic, the patient can be treated safely for several weeks on the presumption that an undiagnosed, deep-seated bacterial infection is present in the node. Treatment should be with penicillin or a penicillin derivative in large doses. Careful measurements of the node should be performed. If at the end of 2 to 4 weeks of observation, the node has not changed in size or character or has grown painlessly larger, then node biopsy or excision should be performed.

It must be remembered that not all masses in the neck are of lymphoid origin. Palpable lumps in the neck may represent a cervical rib, thyroglossal cysts, branchial cleft cysts, cystic hygromas, goiters, and thyroid carcinomas.

BIBLIOGRAPHY

Knight PJ, Reiner CB: Superficial lumps in children: What, when and why? Pediatrics 72:147, 1983

Margileth AM: Cervical adenitis. Pediatr Rev 7:13, 1985

Part XIII: Oncology

80

Childhood Leukemia

The childhood leukemias represent about 35% of all childhood malignancies, with approximately 2500 new cases occurring each year in the United States. The leukemias can be classified as acute, chronic, and congenital. The terms *acute* and *chronic* originally referred to the relative duration of the illness prior to the death of the patient. *Acute leukemia* now connotes those diseases characterized by a predominance of immature hematopoietic or lymphoid precursors, while *chronic leukemia* refers to those conditions characterized by expansion of mature marrow elements. Congenital leukemia is a term reserved for the diagnosis of disease that appears during the first 4 weeks of life. It is estimated that 95% to 97% of all leukemia in the pediatric population is of the acute variety. Approximately 80% of the acute leukemia in children are lymphoblastic (ALL), 15% are myelogenous (AML), and the remainder are difficult to characterize and are classified as undifferentiated (AUL). The morphologic hallmark of acute leukemia is the blast form.

The disease may present either insidiously or abruptly. The abrupt form of presentation may be heralded by a serious hemorrhage, an acute infection, or an episode of respiratory distress. Typical presenting signs, symptoms, and physical and hematologic findings in patients with ALL are listed in Table 80-1.

Extramedullary leukemia may produce the initial symptoms and signs of the disease. Common extramedullary sites of disease include the central nervous system (CNS), the kidney, the testicle, bones, joints, and the gastrointestinal tract. One-half of patients with leukemia have evidence of cardiac involvement at autopsy, although only 5% of patients are symptomatic.

As depicted in Table 80-1, the initial laboratory findings may be quite variable. Although the triad of anemia, thrombocytopenia and abnormal white cell count and differential is the usual finding, approximately 10% of patients may have normal blood counts at the time of presentation, even when the bone marrow is found to be replaced with leukemic cells. Examination of smears of a bone marrow aspirate or biopsy is essential to the establishment of the diagnosis of leukemia. Normal bone marrow does not contain more than 5% blast forms, whereas leukemic marrow usually has at least 30% to 50% of the cells as blasts.

Table 80–1. Characteristics at the Time of Diagnosis of 137 Consecutive Children With Acute Lymphoblastic Leukemia (ALL)

Characteristic	No. of Patients
Signs and Symptom	
Lethargy/malaise	50
Fever/infection	43
Extremity/joint pain	31
Bleeding manifestations	24
Anorexia	17
Abdominal pain	9
CNS manifestations	3
Physical Findings	
Pallor	39
Hepatosplenomegaly	36
Ecchymoses/petechiae	24
Lymphadenopathy	12
Hematologic Findings	
Hematocrit (%)	
>35	9
30–34	7
21–29	41
<20	43
White Blood Count (mm³)	
<1000	3
1,000–5,000	25
5,100–25,000	45
25,000–100,000	19
>100,000	8
Platelet Count (mm³)	
>100,000	26
50,000–100,000	25
10,000–49,000	34
<10,000	15

The differential diagnosis of leukemia, particularly in those with a normal peripheral smear and blood counts, may include idiopathic thrombocytopenic purpura, neuroblastoma, juvenile rheumatoid arthritis, infectious mononucleosis, and infections that result in a leukemoid reaction or neutropenia. In patients who present with anemia, thrombocytopenia, and neutropenia, aplastic anemia must be excluded. Occasionally, patients with ALL may initially demonstrate bone marrow aplasia.

The basic principles of management of the child with acute leukemia include the following:

1. Prompt recognition and treatment of life-threatening complications at the time of initial diagnosis
2. Induction of complete remission using combination chemotherapy
3. "Consolidation" therapy after remission has been obtained
4. Continuous maintenance therapy with a combination of chemotherapeutic agents for a specific period of time

Treatment may produce metabolic emergencies such as hyperuricemia, hyperkalemia, and hyperphosphatemia with hypocalcemia. This metabolic emergency has been termed the acute tumor lysis syndrome and may be observed in the treatment of leukemia as well as other malignancies. Hyperammonemic coma may also complicate initial therapy. Other metabolic emergencies observed in leukemic patients include hyponatremia, hypokalemia, hypercalcemia, and lactic acidosis.

Hemorrhage as a consequence of thrombocytopenia and infection, particularly during periods of neutropenia, are always potential threats to life.

Prognosis has improved dramatically for children with ALL during the last two decades, and survival now approaches 70%. Table 80-2 lists factors that help to identify patients with good or poor prognosis.

CML represents about 2% to 5% of the childhood leukemias and can be classified into two distinct clinical syndromes: adult type CML (ACML), a disease virtually identical to that observed in adults, and juvenile CML, (JCML), a disease generally restricted to children. The distinquishing features of these two forms of chronic leukemia are listed in Table 80-3. For all practical purposes, the disease chronic lymphatic leukemia does not occur in the pediatric population

TABLE 80–2 Prognostic Groups As Defined By Children's Cancer Study Group

| | Prognostic Group | | |
Factor	*Good*	*Average*	*Poor*
WBC $\times$ 10^9/liter	<20	20–100	>100
Age, yrs	2–10	>10	<1
"Lymphoma" syndrome*	0	0–2	3 or more
Hgb. gm/dl	<10		>10
Liver, spleen, nodes	Not markedly enlarged		Markedly enlarged
Mediastinal mass	Absent	Absent	Present
CNS disease at Dx	Absent	Absent	Present
FAB morphology	L$_4$	L$_4$	L$_2$†
Ig classes decreased	0–1	0–3	0–3
% all patients	28.1	50.8	21.1
Continuous remission at 4 yrs (%)	92.1	55.0	45.7

*lymphoma syndrome = 3 or more features: Hgb>10 gm/dl, markedly enlarged liver, spleen, or nodes, and mediastinal mass.
†L$_2$+ = >25% L$_2$ lymphoblasts.
From Miller, D. R.: Childhood leukemias *In* Burchenal. J. H., and Oettgen. H. F. [eds.]: Cancer: Achievements, Challenges, and Prospects for the 1980's Vol. 2. New York. Grune & Stratton. 1981. (Reprinted by permission.)

Table 80–3. Clinical Characteristics of Adult Type Chronic Myelogenous Leukemia (ADML) and Juvenile Chronic Myelogenous Leukemia (JCML) in Childhood

Characteristics at Diagnosis	JCML	ACML
Age	Usually <4	Usually >4
Lymphadenopathy	Common	Unusual
Skin lesions	Common	Unusual
Bleeding	Common	Unusual
Bacterial infection	Common	Unusual
WBC > 100K	Unusual	Common
Hg <12	Common	Variable
Platelets	Usually decreased	Usually increased
Monocytosis	Common	Unusual
Circulating pronormoblasts	Common	Unusual
Hg F% increased	Common	Unusual
Philadelphia chromosome	Absent	>90%
Leukocyte alkaline phosphatase decreased	Variable	Common
Clinical course		
Median survival	1–2 years	4–5 years
Blastic phase	Unusual	Common

The presenting signs and symptoms in patients with ACML are a consequence of excessive accumulation of both mature and immature granulocytic cells. Anemia, pain, dysphagia, hypermetabolism, and massive splenomegaly may be present. The clinical course of ACML is quite variable. Reduction in leukemic cell load is usually accomplished by administration of busulfan or hydroxeurea. The need for treatment depends on the stage of the illness and the degree of symptomatology.

Patients with JCML may present with fever, persistent infections, organomegaly, skin rash, bleeding, and failure to thrive. Unlike ACML patients, patients with JCML usually do not respond to busulfan or hydroxyurea, and the mean survival for most treated or untreated patients is between 1 and 2 years. Bone marrow transplantation may offer the best chance for survival.

BIBLIOGRAPHY

Altman AJ, Schwartz AD: Malignant Diseases of Infancy, Childhood and Adolescence, 2nd ed. Philadelphia, WB Saunders, 1983

Brown AE: Management of the febrile, neutropenic patient with cancer: Therapeutic considerations. J Pediatr 106:1035, 1985

Grier HE: Chronic myeloproliferative disorders and myelodysplasia. In Nathan DG, Oski FA (eds): Hematology of Infancy and Childhood, 3rd ed, P 1064. Philadelphia WB Saunders, 1987

Murphy SB (ed): Acute lymphoblastic leukemia. Semin Oncol 12:79, 1985

Sallan SE, Weinstein HJ: Childhood acute leukemia. In Nathan DG, Oski FA (eds): Hematology of Infancy and Childhood, 3rd ed, P 1028. Philadelphia, WB Saunders, 1987

81

Wilms' Tumor

Wilms' tumor is an embryonal carcinoma arising in the kidney. It is the most common malignant neoplasm of the genitourinary tract in children and accounts for about 20% of all childhood solid tumors. The incidence is about 7.8 children per 1,000,000 per year in the United States, leading to approximately 500 new cases per year. The peak incidence occurs at 3 to 4 years of age, with 90% of all cases occurring in children under the age of 7.

Although the etiology of Wilms' tumor is unknown, about 15% of affected children will display other congenital anomalies that have been clearly associated with this tumor. About 1% of patients have aniridia, a condition with an incidence of about 1 in 50,000 in the general population. Another 2% to 3% of patients have hemihypertrophy, also a very rare condition in the general population. Children found to have either of these unusual anomalies deserve frequent evaluations to rule out the development of a Wilms' tumor. In addition, genitourinary anomalies (hypospadius, cryptorchidism, horseshoe kidney, polycystic kidney, or ureteral duplication) are found in 4% to 5% of patients, and musculo-skeletal disorders, such as clubfoot and hip dislocation, occur in about 3%.

Most children with Wilms' tumor present with an abdominal mass (80% to 90%), usually discovered by a parent while bathing or dressing the child. Other common presenting complaints include abdominal pain (30% to 40%), fever (23%), hematuria (21%), and hypertension (in one series, reported to occur in 63% of cases). It is important to remember that in about 5% of cases, the tumor will involve both kidneys.

The evaluation of any child with an abdominal mass should begin with a detailed history and physical examination, paying special attention to the associated anomalies noted above. Then, a thorough laboratory evaluation should be expeditiously undertaken, realizing that the differential diagnosis includes many distinct entities, including neuroblastoma, hydronephorsis, multicystic kidneys, splenomegaly, mesenteric cysts, duplication cysts, lymphoma, and rhabdomyosarcoma (see Chapter 38).

The initial laboratory evaluation should include a complete blood count, differential white blood cell count, platelet count, urinalysis, renal function tests, and liver function tests. Radiographic examinations must be undertaken to further delineate the structure and exact location of the mass, as well as to evaluate for metastatic disease and to document the patency of the inferior vena cava.

Plain films of the chest and abdomen should be obtained to evaluate for pulmonary metastases, the most common site for metastatic disease, and for the presence of calcifications within the mass, known to occur in 5% to 10% of Wilms' tumors. Intravenous pyelography should then be performed. Characteristic findings on IVP are distortion and displacement of the renal collecting system, although in about 10% of cases the affected kidney will not be visualized at all because of extensive disease. Renal ultrasonography and computed tomography may then be used to define the mass further, to study adjacent structures for metastatic disease, and to rule out involvement of the renal vein and inferior vena cava. Other studies, including urinary catecholamines (to rule out neuroblastoma), bone marrow aspirate and biopsy, skeletal surveys, bone scans, and CT scans of the chest and head may be used as specifically indicated in individual cases.

Several important prognostic factors have been identified for children with Wilms' tumor, including the following:

1. Tumor histology, divided into favorable versus unfavorable categories, with only 21% of those with favorable histology developing recurrent disease.
2. Lymph node involvement, with recurrences in 22% of those with negative lymph nodes versus 44% in those with positive nodes.
3. Patient age, with those less than 24 months of age having a better prognosis.
4. Tumor weight, with those weighing less than 250 g carrying a more favorable prognosis.

For the purpose of further classifying patients in terms of prognosis and the need for more aggressive therapy, the National Wilms' Tumor Study has established the following guidelines for staging Wilms' tumors:

Stage I—tumor is limited to the kidney and completely resected
Stage II—tumor extends beyond the kidney but is totally excised
Stage III—tumor extends beyond the kidney (within the abdomen) and is not completely excised, owing to infiltration of vital structures or the peritoneum
Stage IV—hematogenous metastases are present (*e.g.*, lung, liver, bone, and/or brain
Stage V—bilateral renal involvement

Advances in the treatment of Wilms' tumor have resulted in dramatic improvements in overall survival. Surgery, consisting of nephrectomy with complete excision of the tumor and exploration of the abdomen for extrarenal disease, remains the cornerstone of therapy. Most Wilms' tumors are radiosensitive, and radiation therapy is recommended for all tumors with extrarenal extension (stages II, III, and IV). Chemotherapy is also given to most children with Wilms' tumor, usually as a combination of vincristine and dactinomycin, although other agents such as adriamycin and cyclophosphamide may also be used.

Through careful study of various treatment combinations in patients whose disease had been well characterized (histology, stage, etc.), great strides have been made in the treatment of Wilms' tumor. Over 80% of patients can be expected to remain disease-free on a long-term basis, ranging from over 90% in those with stage I disease to about 50% in those with stage IV disease. Overall, children with Wilms' tumor have the best prognosis of any of the common childhood malignancies.

BIBLIOGRAPHY

Baum ES, Morgan ER: Wilms' tumor. Pediatr Ann 12:357, 1983

Cohen MD, Siddiqui A, Westman R et al: A rational approach to the radiographic evaluation of children with Wilms' tumor. Cancer 50:887, 1982

D'Angio GJ, Beckwith JB, Breslow NE et al: Wilms' tumor: An update. Cancer 45:1791, 1980

Green DM: The diagnosis and management of Wilms' tumor. Pediatr Clin North Am 32:735, 1985

82

Neuroblastoma

Neuroblastoma is the most common solid tumor in infants and young children. It occurs in approximately 9.6 white children and 7 black children per 1 million in the United States each year, making it the third most common childhood malignancy overall. At the time of diagnosis, 50% of patients will be under the age of 2, and over 75% will be under the age of 5. Arising from neural crest tissue, this tumor displays a remarkably high rate of early dissemination, with 70% of patients having metastatic involvement at the time of diagnosis.

The clinical manifestations of neuroblastoma may vary tremendously, depending both on the site of the primary tumor and the extent of metastatic disease. The primary tumor may be located in any area containing components of the sympathetic nervous system, with the 2 most common sites being the adrenal medulla and the sympathetic ganglia. About two-thirds of cases arise in the retroperitoneal region and present as an abdominal mass. These tumors also may cause urinary obstruction. Thoracic tumors may cause cough, dyspnea, or other signs of airway compression. Tumors arising from the cervical sympathetic ganglia may present as a neck mass or with Horner's syndrome (ptosis, myosis, anhydrosis, and exophthalmos).

The most common sites for metastic disease are the liver, skin, lymph nodes, bone and bone marrow. Thus, signs and symptoms may include hepatomegaly, lymphadenopathy, bone and joint pain, anemia, and skin nodules (especially in infants). Involvement of orbit is common in disseminated neuroblastoma and characteristically presents as proptosis with periorbital edema and ecchymosis. Constitutional symptoms, such as fever, anorexia, weight loss, and irritability, are also extremely common in patients with advanced disease.

Several less common manifestations of neuroblastoma deserve note because they are quite unique to this disease. Over 90% of neuroblastomas secrete catecholamines, and, although they are usually metabolized too rapidly to produce symptoms, some patients will present with hypertension or intractable diarrhea as a result of their effects. Another small group of patients will present with an opsoclonus–myoclonus syndrome, a neurologic disorder of unknown etiology that consists of an acute encephalopathy with opsoclonus, myoclonus, and truncal ataxia.

The initial evaluation of a child with suspected neuroblastoma should include quantitation of urinary catecholamines and delineation of the primary tumor. Elevated urinary catecholamines, most commonly vanillylmandelic acid (VMA) and homovanillic acid (HMA), are seen in over 90% of cases and may serve as useful markers subsequently in assessing both the response to therapy and possible tumor recurrence. The primary tumor and surrounding structures should be evaluated by appropriate radiographic studies. For abdominal tumors, a plain film will frequently reveal stippled calcifications within the tumor and an intravenous pyelogram (IVP) may show downward displacement of the kidney by an adrenal mass. Oblique views of the spine should be obtained in patients with primary disease in the chest to rule out widening of the intervertebral foramina due to intraspinal extension. Ultrasonographic examinations and computed tomography (CT) scans may be used, if necessary, to define the tumor more specifically.

Because of the extremely high incidence of tumor dissemination in these patients, all cases must undergo a thorough metastatic work-up. In addition to a history and physical examination, the evaluation should include a complete blood count, liver function tests, a skeletal survey, and a bone marrow aspiration in all patients. Other tests, such as bone scans, liver–spleen scans, CT scans, and myelograms may be used as clinically indicated.

The prognosis of neuroblastoma is related to the age of the child at diagnosis, to the site of origin of the tumor, and, most importantly, to the extent of disease at the time of diagnosis. Children who are under the age of 1 at the time of diagnosis have a survival rate of 74%, compared to 26% for those between 1 and 2 years of age and 12% for those over age 2. Tumors arising in the neck, posterior mediastinum, and pelvis carry a better prognosis than those arising in the abdomen, probably because of differences in dissemination at the time of diagnosis.

As with Wilms' tumor, a staging system for neuroblastoma has been established as follows:

Stage I: Tumor confined to structure of origin.

Stage II: Tumors extending in continuity beyond the structure of origin but not crossing the midline (may include ipsilateral lymph node involvement).

Stage III: Tumors extending in continuity across the midline (may include bilateral regional lymph node involvement).

Stage IV: Distant metastases present.

Stage IV-S: Patients under 1 year of age who would otherwise be stage I or II but who have remote spread of tumor to the liver, skin, and/or bone marrow, but not bone.

Patients with stage I, II, and IV-S disease carry a relatively favorable prognosis, with survival rates ranging from 63% to 85%. Children with stage III disease have a survival rate of 37% whereas those with stage IV involvement, unfortunately, representing over one-half of all cases, have a 2-year survival rate of only 5%.

Although neuroblastoma is generally considered to be a very aggressive tumor, another relatively unique feature of the disease is a high incidence of spontaneous remission, at times even in cases with widely disseminated disease. Overall, spontaneous remission appears to occur in about 7% of cases, most commonly in infants less than 6 months of age with stage I, II, or IV-S disease.

The treatment of neuroblastoma involves a combination of surgery, radiotherapy, and chemotherapy in most cases. Unfortunately, as opposed to many other childhood malignancies, little real progress has been made in this area in the past 20 years.

The surgical approach to neuroblastoma includes complete excision of the primary tumor whenever possible, sampling of lymph nodes for metastatic involvement, and, for abdominal tumors, a liver biopsy. In general, for patients with clearly unresectable tumors or widely disseminated disease, there is little evidence that surgery improves prognosis. Some experts, however, advocate aggressive debulking procedures, at times followed by a "second look" procedure after interval therapy has been given.

A variety of chemotherapeutic regimens have been used in patients with neuroblastoma and although many produce a good temporary response, the overall cure rate remains essentially unchanged. Commonly used drugs include cyclophosphamide, vincristine, adriamycin, *cis*-platinum, and epipodophyllotoxin (VM-26). These and other agents are being used in various combinations in ongoing clinical trials throughout the world.

Finally, although radiation therapy is also widely used in the treatment of neuroblastoma, its exact role remains unclear. Children with a localized primary tumor that was completely excised are generally cured by the surgical procedure alone and do not benefit from radiotherapy. In patients with stage III disease with gross residual tumor remaining after surgery, it may be of some benefit, particularly in reducing the tumor bulk. Its clearest roles are in the palliative care of patients with widespread disease and in the treatment of patients with spinal cord compression or obstructive phenomena.

Thus, neuroblastoma is a relatively common and rather unique tumor of infancy and early childhood. Although the prognosis is quite good for patients with localized disease, the majority of patients have metastases at the time of diagnosis and have a very poor prognosis. Intensive research efforts are ongoing in hopes of improving this situation, utilizing both conventional approaches and newer modalities such as immunotherapy and bone marrow transplantation.

BIBLIOGRAPHY

Evans AE: Staging and treatment of neuroblastoma. Cancer 45:1799, 1980

Hayes FA, Green AA: Neuroblastoma. Pediatr Ann 12:366, 1983

Lopez-Ibor B, Schwartz AD: Neuroblastoma. Pediatr Clin North Am 32:755, 1985

83

Brain Tumors

Brain tumors are the most common solid tumors in children and the second most common form of childhood malignancy overall. Their incidence for children under age 15 years is 2.4 per 100,000 per year, with approximately 1,200 new cases diagnosed in the United States each year. Although some variation exists between different tumor types, the peak age of incidence overall is between 5 and 10 years.

Approximately 60% of childhood brain tumors arise in the posterior fossa and are designated infratentorial. The most common of these are medulloblastomas, cerebellar astrocytomas, and brain stem gliomas (Table 83-1). Of supratentorial tumors in childhood, about 60% are located in the cerebral hemispheres, while the remainder arise in the midline, predominantly from the suprasellar, hypothalamic, and pineal regions.

Although the etiology of childhood brain tumors remains unknown, both hereditary and environmental factors are presumed important. Several hereditary conditions are clearly associated with intracranial tumors; most important, about 15% of children with neurofibromatosis develop brain tumors, and a smaller percentage of patients with both

Table 83–1 Incidence of Common Childhood Brain Tumors

Tumor Type	% of Cases
Infratentorial	
Medulloblastoma	20
Cerebellar astrocytoma	17
Brain stem glioma	9
Ependymoma	7
Supratentorial	
Cerebral hemisphere glioma	18
Craniopharyngioma	9
Optic nerve glioma	4
Meningioma	3
Pineal region tumors	3

tuberous sclerosis and von Hippel-Lindau disease are at a dramatically increased risk of developing an intracranial malignancy.

The presenting symptoms of brain tumors may vary widely, depending on their location, their rate of growth, their histology, and the age of the patient (Table 83-2). Tumors arising in the posterior fossa most commonly present with signs and symptoms of increased intracranial pressure, secondary to compression of the fourth ventricle with resultant hydrocephalus. These symptoms may include headache, characteristically occurring in the

495

Table 83–2 Common Presentations of Brain Tumors

Symptom	% of Cases
Increased intracranial pressure	85
Headache	70
Vomiting	75
Gait disturbance	40
Mental status changes	35
Visual symptoms	25
Hemiparesis	15
Seizures	10
Head tilt	10

morning upon awakening, vomiting, a 6th nerve (abducens) palsy, or a rapidly increasing head circumference. Further, since most infratentorial tumors involve the cerebellum, other signs may include gait disturbances, ataxia, impaired fine motor skills, nystagmus, and head tilt.

Supratentorial tumors less commonly produce hydrocephalus and are more likely to present with focal neurologic abnormalities, the nature of which vary depending on the location of the lesion. Frontal lobe tumors frequently present with mental status changes or hemiparesis, whereas temporal lobe involvement most commonly leads to focal seizures. Tumors arising from the pituitary gland, such as craniopharyngiomas, may present with endocrinologic abnormalities or with visual abnormalities secondary to involvement of the optic chiasm.

The differential diagnosis of brain tumors in children includes other mass lesions, such as subdural hematomas, infections of the central nervous system, congenital hydrocephalus, and other causes of neurologic dysfunction, such as toxic ingestions. After a careful history and physical examination, in nearly all cases, a computed tomography (CT) scan of the head with intravenous contrast should be the first step in the diagnostic evaluation. This should always be performed prior to a lumbar puncture if an intracranial mass or hydrocephalus is suspected. Other studies that may be useful in further delineating the tumor mass include angiography and magnetic resonance imaging. Pneumoencephalography, brain scans, and electroencephalograms (EEGs) rarely provide additional information but may prove useful in occasional patients.

The treatment of a child with an intracranial neoplasm requires a coordinated effort combining the skills of oncologists, neurologists, and neurosurgeons. The specific treatment plan will depend on the location of the tumor, the degree of infiltration into surrounding structures, the tumor histology, and the presence or absence of hydrocephalus. Surgical intervention is used to provide a biopsy to determine tumor histology, to relieve hydrocephalus (if present), and to attain maximum tumor removal. Radiation therapy is also used in a majority of patients, and chemotherapy is being used with increasing success in a variety of tumors. Corticosteroids are used to help control tumor edema.

SPECIFIC TUMOR TYPES

Medulloblastomas make up about 20% of all brain tumors in children. Their peak incidence occurs between the ages of 4 and 8 years, and they are more common in males than in females. They arise from the roof of the fourth ventricle, invade the cerebellar vermis, and commonly cause obstructive hydrocephalus. They are highly malignant tumors and tend to metastasize throughout the central nervous system. Complete surgical resection is generally not possible, and all patients receive postoperative staging (CT scan, myelogram, cerebrospinal fluid [CSF] studies, and bone marrow aspirate) and radiation therapy. The role of adjuvant chemotherapy is currently under study. Five-year survival rates of 40% to 55% have been reported in several series.

Cerebellar astrocytomas also comprise

about 20% of intracranial tumors in children. They affect males and females equally and show a mean age of onset of 6 to 7 years. They are usually slow growing, cystic, and tend to involve one cerebellar hemisphere without midline involvement. Hence, hydrocephalus is less common than with medulloblastomas and presenting complaints tend to include clumsiness and gait disturbances. Therapy and prognosis vary widely depending on the location, malignant grade, and histologic appearance of the tumor. Cystic, low-grade astrocytomas frequently can be excised completely, and they hold an excellent prognosis. Diffuse, high-grade astrocytomas, however, carry a much poorer prognosis even with significantly more adjuvant therapy.

Brain stem gliomas make up about 10% of childhood brain tumors and also most commonly present in the 3- to 8-year age-group. These tumors most frequently present with cranial nerve abnormalities (diplopia, dysarthria, facial weakness) or long tract signs secondary to compression of the corticospinal tract. They are generally very large by the time of presentation and hence are usually inoperable. Response to radiation is poor, and the role of chemotherapy is controversial. Overall, 5-year survival rates of 20% to 30% are reported for this devastating malignancy.

Ependymomas may arise from both supra- and infratentorial structures but most commonly arise from the floor of the fourth ventricle and thereby produce obstructive hydrocephalus. Complete surgical resection is rarely possible, and the potential for cure rests largely on the use of aggressive radiation therapy, frequently including the entire spinal axis. With such therapy, low-grade lesions carry a 5-year survival rate of 60% to 70%, while this figure drops to approximately 20% for high-grade lesions.

Although significant advances in the treatment of brain tumors have been made in recent years, owing both to improved surgical management and careful study of adjuvant radiotherapy and chemotherapy, the potential side effects of therapy are probably greater than for any other tumor. Surgical intervention may lead to significant disruption of normal brain tissue and radiation therapy to the central nervous system may produce devastating acute and chronic side effects. In addition, about 1.5% of children cured of a brain tumor will develop a second cancer. Hence, although we have good reason to be optimistic about the overall status of pediatric neuro-oncology, the outlook for all children, even those cured of their tumor, may be dampened by the side effects of therapy.

BIBLIOGRAPHY

Allen JC: Childhood brain tumors: Current status of clinical trials in newly diagnosed and recurrent disease. Pediatr. Clin North Am 32:633, 1985

Gjerris F: Clinical aspects and long-term prognosis of intracranial tumors in infancy and childhood. Dev Med Child Neurol 18:145, 1976

Walker RW, Allen JC: Pediatric brain tumors. Pediatr Ann 12:383, 1983

Yates A, Becker L, Sachs L: Brain tumors in childhood. Childs Brain 5:31, 1979

84

Malignant Bone Tumors

Bone tumors comprise slightly less than 5% of all childhood malignancies. Osteogenic sarcomas (osteosarcomas) are most common, accounting for about 60% of all cases, whereas Ewing's sarcomas account for another 30% of cases. The remaining 10% of childhood bone tumors are comprised of fibrosarcomas, chondrosarcomas, and non-Hodgkin's lymphomas of bone. Although the etiology of malignant bone tumors is unknown, there may in some cases be a relationship to growth, since both osteosarcomas and Ewing's sarcomas are seen most commonly in preteenage and teenage individuals during periods of rapid growth.

Most bone tumors present with localized pain at the site of the lesion, at times accompanied by overlying warmth and swelling. While there may also be varying degrees of soft tissue involvement, a palpable mass is usually not present initially. On occasion, bone tumors may present with symptoms due to metastatic disease, particularly involving the lungs.

The diagnosis is usually suggested by a lytic lesion on bone x-ray but must be confirmed histologically in all cases. Tissue for diagnosis may be obtained either by percutaneous nee-

dle biopsy or open biopsy. In addition to complete radiographic evaluation of the primary lesion, all patients with malignant bone tumors should undergo a chest x-ray and a chest computed tomography (CT) scan to rule out pulmonary metastases and a skeletal survey and/or bone scan to rule out other sites of bony involvement. Other evaluation should include a complete blood count, liver function studies elevated levels of alkaline phosphatase may be present), and a bone marrow examination in patients with Ewing's sarcoma or non-Hodgkin's lymphoma.

OSTEOSARCOMA

Over 60% of all cases of osteosarcoma occur in the second decade of life, with peak incidence coinciding with the adolescent growth spurt. Over 85% of cases occur before age 30. Osteosarcoma occurs most commonly in the metaphyseal ends of long bones; the distal femur is involved most frequently, followed by the proximal tibia and the proximal humerus. The tumor frequently extends from the intramedullary space through the cortex and into adjacent soft tissue structures.

Several different types of osteosarcomas have been described histopathologically. Tumors may be comprised primarily of spindle cells, giant cells, or small (round) cells. A fourth type, designated telangiectatic, contains vascular areas with pleomorphic cells. In all cases, the final diagnosis of osteosarcoma depends on the demonstration of osteoid material in the biopsy specimen.

The treatment of osteosarcoma has traditionally relied on amputation of the affected limb. Improvements in chemotherapy, however, have now made it possible to employ limb salvage procedures with increasing success. In these patients, en bloc resection of affected bone is employed, usually after intensive preoperative chemotherapy. Prostheses may then be implanted to maximize function.

The chemotherapeutic agents most commonly used for osteosarcomas are adriamycin and high-dose methotrexate with citrovorum factor rescue. Cyclophosphamide, bleomycin, dactinomycin, and *cis*-diamminedichloroplatinum are also used in some protocols. In most centers, chemotherapy is now included as a routine component of care, and it is of particular importance in patients with metastatic disease. Radiation therapy is of limited use for this tumor and is usually used only for palliative care.

Overall, although osteosarcomas remain devastating to the adolescents that they so frequently strike, actuarial disease-free survival rates have improved significantly in recent years, rising from 20% with amputation alone to 50% to 80% with surgery plus chemotherapy, at times even with limb-salvage procedures.

EWING'S SARCOMA

Like osteosarcoma, Ewing's sarcoma has a peak incidence between the ages of 10 and 20, although it is not as closely associated with the adolescent growth spurt. Over 75% of cases occur before the age of 20. Unlike osteosarcoma, this tumor rarely occurs in blacks.

Ewing's sarcoma most commonly arises in the femur but may also occur in flat bones such as the pelvis, the ribs, and the sternum. The typical radiographic picture is that of a lytic lesion with significant periosteal reaction. The presenting complaint is usually one of localized bone pain, often with associated swelling, tenderness, and warmth. Fever is not uncommon, and patients may present with anemia and leukocytosis as well. Occasionally, patients will present with symptoms of metastatic disease, most often involving the lungs.

Histologically, Ewing's sarcoma typically appears as a monotonous sheet of small, round cells with scanty cytoplasm. Areas of necrosis, calcification, and hemorrhage may also be identified. In about 10% of cases, a rosette-like pattern resembling metastatic neuroblastoma will be present.

The treatment of Ewing's sarcoma consists of both radiation therapy and chemotherapy in the majority of cases. While radiation therapy has traditionally been considered the most effective mode of treatment for the primary tumor, studies have now clearly demonstrated the benefits of adjuvant chemotherapy. The chemotherapeutic combinations most commonly employed include vincristine, actinomycin-D, cyclophosphamide, and adriamycin.

The role of surgical therapy remains relatively limited in this condition. However, because of the potentially severe side effects of the high-dose radiotherapy that is required, particularly retardation of limb growth, there is ongoing research studying the potential benefits of surgical extirpation. Current indications for surgery include cases in which the primary tumor is clearly resectable, especially for expendable bones such as a rib, and tumors arising from the phalanges, metacarpals, and metatarsals. In addition, many experts recommend amputation for Ewing's sarcoma of the extremities in children under the age of 8.

The prognosis for patients with Ewing's sarcoma varies both with the location of the primary tumor and the extent of disease. For those without soft tissue extension of the tumor and no metastatic disease, a 5-year survival rate as high as 87% has been reported. In contrast, however, in those with a primary tumor in the pelvis or with distant metastases, the prognosis is dismal, with survival rates of less than 20%.

BIBLIOGRAPHY

Jaffe N: Advances in the management of malignant bone tumors in children and adolescents. Pediatr Clin North Am 32:801, 1985

Rosen G: Management of malignant bone tumors in children and adolescents. Pediatr Clin North Am 23:183, 1976

Tebbi C, Freeman A: Osteogenic sarcoma. Pediatr Rev 6:55, 1984

85

Non-Hodgkin's Lymphoma

Non-Hodgkin's lymphomas (NHL) include a diverse group of malignant neoplasms of lymphoreticular cell origin. They bear little resemblance to Hodgkin's disease or to the adult variety of non-Hodgkin's lymphoma, but do, in fact, share many features with childhood acute lymphoblastic leukemia. Recent advances in the understanding and the treatment of NHL have produced a marked improvement in prognosis.

Lymphomas collectively rank third in frequency among the childhood malignancies, with NHL out-numbering Hodgkin's disease by a margin of 3 to 2. NHL rarely is seen under the age of 1 and affects primarily children between the ages of 5 and 15 years. It is much more common in males than in females with a ratio of 3 to 4:1.

Children with defects in host defense mechanisms are at particular risk for the development of NHL, in whom this malignancy is estimated to be between 100 and 10,000 times more common than in the general population. This high-risk group includes children with both congenital and acquired immunodeficiency diseases, including X-linked agammaglobulinemia, ataxia telangiectasia, Wiskott-Aldrich syndrome, and common variable hypogammaglobulinemia, as well as children receiving immunosuppressive therapy (*e.g.*, post-transplant).

The etiology of NHL remains an area of great interest. In addition to defects in immunoregulatory function, other postulated causes of NHL include viral infections, chromosomal aberrations, and environmental stress, such as benzene exposure. The role of viruses has received the most attention, particularly because of several animal models in which virus-induced lymphomas have been well characterized. In spite of intensive investigation, however, direct evidence for a viral etiology of NHL in man remains lacking, except possibly in the case of Burkitt's lymphoma in Africa, which has been closely associated with infection with Epstein-Barr virus.

NHLs include a diverse group of tumors that may arise from T cells, B cells, or non-T, non-B cells (null cells). Histopathologic classification systems have been established that are based on the cell type of origin as well as the degree of differentiation and the nodularity or diffuseness of the tumor. Nodular NHL is very rare in children, comprising only about 1% of cases. Approximately 40% to 50% are of T cell origin, an equal number are of B cell origin, and the remaining 5% to 10% are of null cell origin. Histologically, most undifferentiated tumors will be found to be of B cell origin, while the vast majority of lymphoblastic lymphomas are of T cell origin.

The clinical manifestations of NHL are equally diverse, depending primarily on the location of the primary tumor. Virtually any site of lymphoid tissue may be involved, including lymph nodes, Peyer's patches, the thymus, or extralymphatic sites (such as bone or skin). About one-third of patients present with lymphadenopathy, most commonly in the cervical, supraclavicular, and axillary areas. The node enlargement is usually painless and rapidly progressive; frequently, there will be associated mediastinal node involvement. Thirty percent to 40% of children with NHL will have their primary tumor in the abdomen, arising in the gastrointestinal (GI) tract, the mesentery, the ovaries, or retroperitoneal lymph nodes. These patients may present with an abdominal mass, distention, ascites, abdominal pain, vomiting, or, occasionally, with intussusception. Ten percent to 15% of patients will present with involvement of lymphoid tissues in Waldeyer's tonsillar ring, the nasopharynx, and the sinuses, while other less common primary sites include skin, bone, and the central nervous system.

The site of the primary tumor in NHL is frequently found to correlate with a specific histopathologic type and a characteristic clinical course. Tumors involving the mediastinum are usually lymphoblastic, of T cell origin, affect predominantly male adolescents, commonly involve the bone marrow, and often evolve to a picture indistinguishable from T cell leukemia. Tumors arising in the abdomen, however, are usually of B cell origin and undifferentiated histology, with a clinical course marked by local recurrence and, frequently, central nervous system (CNS)

involvement. Burkitt's lymphoma is an undifferentiated B cell malignancy that is particularly common in Africa, where it is the most common childhood tumor. In African children, it most commonly arises in the jaw or orbit and frequently involves the CNS, while in American children, it usually arises in the abdomen, rarely involves the CNS, and is associated with bone marrow involvement in about 60% of cases.

Although the initial presentation of NHL may be difficult to distinguish from many common childhood illnesses, the disease tends to progress rapidly, soon leaving little doubt as to its malignant nature. Hence, once the diagnosis of NHL is suspected, it is critical that a definitive diagnosis be established as efficiently as possible so that therapy may be instituted. Appropriate tissue samples must be obtained and studied not only for histopathology, but also for cell markers and cytogenetic analysis. Because of the heterogeneous nature of NHL, it is essential that all of these specialized studies be coordinated to make an accurate diagnosis.

Once the diagnosis of NHL has been established, an extensive evaluation must be undertaken to determine the extent of the disease. These staging studies must include a complete blood count, electrolytes, liver function tests, creatinine, urinalysis, bone marrow aspirate, lumbar puncture, bone survey (or bone scan), chest x-ray, and, frequently, computed tomography. It is also important to follow the serum lactate dehydrogenase, uric acid, calcium, and phosphorous, all of which may be abnormal in children with large tumors, especially once treatment is instituted. Other studies, such as ultrasonography, myelography, and intravenous pyelography should be utilized as clinically indicated.

Unfortunately, no single staging system for NHL has been uniformly accepted. Staging is difficult because, unlike many other childhood malignancies, the clinical course of

NHL may vary widely, depending on the site of the primary tumor and the cell type involved. The system most commonly used thus attempts to take into account both the extent of disease and the site of involvement.

Stage I: A single tumor (extranodal) or a single anatomic area (nodal), not including mediastinal or abdominal tumors.

Stage II: A single tumor (extranodal) with regional node involvement, or
Two or more nodal areas on the same side of the diaphragm, or
Two single extranodal tumors on the same side of the diaphragm, or
A primary GI tract tumor.

Stage III: Two single extranodal tumors on opposite sides of the diaphram, or
Two or more nodal areas above and below the diaphram, or
All primary intrathoracic tumors, or
All extensive primary intra-abdominal disease, or
All paraspinal or epidural tumors.

Stage IV: Any of the above with CNS or bone marrow involvement.

For Burkitt's lymphoma, an alternate system is generally employed. Stages A and B define tumors involving extra-abdominal sites only (A, one; B, two or more), stage C defines intra-abdominal tumors, and stage D includes intra-abdominal tumors with involvement of extra-abdominal sites. A fifth stage, designated AR, is added specifically to define stage C tumors that have been almost completely resected.

Advances in treatment of NHL over the last two decades have led to significant improvements in prognosis. For non-Burkitt's tumors, children with either stage I or stage II disease have a 2-year disease-free survival rate of over 80%, compared with 75% in stage III and 50% for stage IV. For Burkitt's lymphomas, survival rates for patients in stages A, B, or AR exceed 80%, while only about 40% of those in stages C and D survive.

Standard therapy for NHL includes multidrug chemotherapy and CNS prophylaxis using intrathecal medications. Realization that this malignancy resembles acute lymphoblastic leukemia has led to the successful use of several common antileukemic agents in NHL, including cyclophosphamide, vincristine, methotrexate, and prednisone. This approach, combined with routine CNS prophylaxis, underlies the great improvement in outcome that has occurred. While radiotherapy is also commonly employed, its exact role remains unclear, except in cases in which rapid reduction in tumor bulk is needed (*e.g.*, airway compromise). It should be stressed that in addition to specific therapy for the tumor, great care must be taken to prevent the potential metabolic complications that commonly occur in NHL, including hyperuricemia, uric acid nephropathy, hypercalcemia, and hyperkalemia. Because these tumors grow so rapidly, these complications (secondary to cell lysis) may be seen even before therapy is initiated. Vigorous hydration, allopurinol, and urinary alkalinization should therefore be employed routinely even before therapy is begun.

Thus, NHL defines a heterogeneous group of tumors that are characterized by lymphoreticular cell origin, rapid growth, dissemination, and, at times, evolution to an overt leukemic process. They present substantial biologic and therapeutic challenges, many of which are currently being met, as evidenced by the dramatic improvements in survival in recent years.

BIBLIOGRAPHY

Gardner RV, Graham-Pole J: Non Hodgkin's lymphoma. Pediatr Ann 12:322, 1983

Link MP: Non-Hodgkin's lymphoma in children. Pediatr Clin North Am 32:699, 1985

The Non-Hodgkin's Lymphoma Pathologic Classification Project. Cancer 49:2112, 1982

Wollner N, Exelby PR, Lieberman PH: Non-Hodgkin's lymphoma in children. Cancer 44:1990, 1979

Ziegler JL: Burkitt's lymphoma. N Engl J Med 305:735, 1981

86

Hodgkin's Disease

Hodgkin's disease accounts for about 40% of all childhood lymphomas. It occurs rarely in children under 2 years of age and has a peak incidence during the early to mid-teens. It affects boys more frequently than girls in children under the age of 12 but thereafter displays a nearly equal sex ratio.

Although the cause of Hodgkin's disease remains unknown, there has been a great deal of interest in recent years in a possible viral etiology. This interest is supported primarily by epidemiologic data, particularly reports of clustering of cases. In addition, the finding of high antibody titers to Epstein-Barr virus in many patients with Hodgkin's disease and the presence of Reed-Sternberg cells in occasional patients with infectious mononucleosis have heightened interest in this particular virus, although no direct relationship has been demonstrated. Other investigators argue that a genetic or environmental etiology may be more likely, although even fewer data exist to substantiate these claims.

Pathologically, the hallmark of Hodgkin's disease is the Reed-Sternberg cell. These are large, multinucleated cells with prominent nucleoli that are considered to be the malignant cell in Hodgkin's disease. Based on the ratio of Reed-Sternberg cells to lymphocytes and the degree of fibrosis of the tumor, four histopathologic types of Hodgkin's disease have been defined (the Rye classification): nodular sclerosis (50% of cases), mixed cellularity (25% of cases), lymphocyte predominance (20% of cases), and lymphocyte depletion (5% of cases). It is generally recognized that tumors of the lymphocyte depleted class are the most aggressive, leading to a strikingly less favorable prognosis than the other three types.

Over 90% of children with Hodgkin's disease present with painless adenopathy, most commonly in the cervical area. Up to one-half of patients will be found to have concomitant mediastinal or hilar adenopathy. Hodgkin's disease usually arises in a unifocal manner and extends along contiguous lymph node groups. Systemic symptoms, including fever, weight loss, anorexia, fatigue, and night sweats are usually not prominent but do occur in about 30% to 40% of cases.

A complete staging evaluation is critical in all patients with Hodgkin's disease for purposes of planning therapy and accurately assessing prognosis. As outlined in Table 86-1, this evaluation must include a complete

Table 86–1 Staging Evaluation in Hodgkin's Disease

History
Physical examination
Complete blood count
Erythrocyte sedimentation rate
Liver and renal function tests
Radiographic studies (chest x-ray, computed tomography [CT] scans)
Exploratory laparotomy (lymph node biopsies, liver biopsy, splenectomy)
Bone marrow aspirate and biopsy
Also consider: lymphangiography, skeletal survey, intravenous pyelography (IVP), bone scan, liver–spleen scan, gallium scan, serum copper level

history and physical examination, a complete blood count, liver function tests, renal function tests, radiographic studies (chest x-ray, abdominal and thoracic CT scans), bone marrow aspirate and biopsy, and exploratory laparotomy with splenectomy and biopsies of the liver and all lymph node groups below the diaphram. Lymphangiography, skeletal surveys, intravenous pyelography, bone scans, gallium scans, and liver spleen scans may be helpful in some cases. These studies serve both to determine the extent of disease at the time of diagnosis and to provide a baseline for future comparisons during and after therapy.

Using the data obtained in this extensive staging evaluation, all patients may be assigned to one of four stages under the Ann Arbor classification:

Stage I: Involvement of a single lymph node or single extralymphatic site.

Stage II: Involvement of two or more lymph node regions on the same side of the diaphragm.

Stage III: Involvement of lymph node regions on both sides of the diaphragm; may also include localized involvement of an extralymphatic site or the spleen.

Stage IV: Diffuse or disseminated involvement of one or more extralym-
phatic sites with or without associated lymph node enlargement (including all cases with liver involvement).

Each stage may be further subdivided into category A (*e.g.*, IIA), indicating no systemic symptoms, and B, indicating the presence of weight loss, fever, and/or night sweats. Overall, about 60% of children with Hodgkin's disease have stage I or II disease at the time of diagnosis, while about 25% have stage III disease and 15% have stage IV disease.

Standard therapy for pediatric Hodgkin's disease may include radiotherapy, chemotherapy, or both, depending on the stage of the disease and the location of the tumor. For children with stage I or II disease, primarily consisting of those patients with tumor confined above the diaphragm, radiotherapy generally is used alone with excellent results. For those with more extensive disease, combination therapy is most commonly used. Chemotherapy also is used with increasing success in the treatment of those patients experiencing relapse after receiving radiotherapy alone as the initial therapy. Agents in common use currently include adriamycin, vincristine, cyclophosphamide, procarbazine, bleomycin, and dacarbazine.

Most relapses in pediatric Hodgkin's disease occur within the first 2 years after diagnosis, and very few occur more than 4 years after the diagnosis. Hence, children should be evaluated at frequent intervals during this period of high risk of relapse. At least every 3 months, they should have a history taken, a physical examination, a chest x-ray, a complete blood count, a sedimentation rate, and serum chemistries, including determination of copper and ferritin levels. Any suspicion of relapse must be confirmed by a histologic diagnosis.

The treatment of Hodgkin's disease may result in both acute and chronic side effects. Myelosuppression may occur as a result of both chemotherapy and radiation therapy. Radiation pneumonitis and pericarditis may occur, and each of the chemotherapeutic agents has its own list of significant side effects. Splenectomized patients remain at significantly increased risk of overwhelming bacterial infection (particularly pneumococcal) for life. Hypothyroidism has been reported to occur in about two-thirds of patients undergoing mantle radiotherapy, and growth impairment may result from irradiation of vertebral bodies. Sterility is common in both males and females. Most importantly, it is clear that these children are at significantly increased risk of developing a secondary malignancy, most commonly acute myeloid leukemia.

In spite of the potential side effects of treatment, the overall outlook for children with Hodgkin's disease is very good. A 5-year disease-free survival rate of 75% to 80% can be expected for patients with disease in stages I to III, while for those with stage IV disease, survival rates ranging from 40% to 69% have been reported. Through careful patient classification and rigid clinical trials, we can be optimistic that these figures will improve in the future, while side effects of therapy are slowly reduced.

BIBLIOGRAPHY

Gilchrist GS, Evans RG: Contemporary issues in pediatric Hodgkin's disease. Pediatr Clin North Am 32:721, 1985

Lange B, Littman P: Management of Hodgkin's disease in children and adolescents. Cancer 51:1371, 1983

Proceedings of the symposium on contemporary issued in Hodgkin's disease: Biology, staging and treatment. Cancer Treat Rep 66:601, 1982

Tan CTC, Chan KW: Hodgkin's disease. Pediatr Ann 12:306, 1983

Part XIV: Neurology

87

Seizures

Seizures are extremely common in pediatrics, occurring in approximately 5% of all children. The majority of these occur in children under the age of 5, are associated with fever, and may be categorized as febrile seizures. Only a small proportion of children who have a seizure will actually develop epilepsy, a chronic condition characterized by recurrent seizures. Great strides have been made in recent years in the diagnosis and management of children with both febrile and afebrile seizures. This chapter will review the classification, evaluation, and management of childhood seizures.

FEBRILE SEIZURES

A febrile seizure has been defined by the National Institute of Health Consensus Development Conference as "a seizure, usually occurring between 3 months and 5 years of age, associated with fever but without evidence of intracranial infection or other defined cause." Febrile seizures occur in 3% to 4% of all children, with over one-half occurring between 9 and 20 months of age. A positive family history of febrile seizures will be obtained in up to 50% of cases.

Febrile seizures commonly occur early in the course of a febrile illness, during the initial rapid increase in body temperature. They most commonly consist of generalized tonic–clonic movements and rarely last more than 15 minutes. Thirty to 40% of children who have a single febrile seizure will have another, and of those, 50% will have a third. It must be emphasized that these recurrences do not constitute epilepsy.

Overall, the risk of developing epilepsy in children with febrile seizures is 2% to 3%, compared to a 0.5% risk in those without febrile seizures. Several risk factors have been identified for the development of epilepsy in children with febrile seizures. These include a family history of epilepsy, evidence of a neurologic abnormality prior to the onset of seizures, and an atypical febrile seizure (focal in nature, duration greater than 15 minutes, or recurrence within 24 hours). If two or more of these risk factors are present, the risk of epilepsy is 13%. Febrile seizures impart no increased risk of mental retardation, cerebral palsy, or other neurologic sequelae.

Every child who has had a febrile seizure should be carefully evaluated. Every effort should be made to determine the source of the fever by means of a thorough history and physical examination. While a lumbar puncture is not needed in all cases, it is the physician's responsibility to rule out meningitis as the cause of the fever (and seizure) in every case. This means that a lumbar puncture should be performed in any case in which meningitis cannot be ruled out on clinical grounds, particularly in those children under a year of age in whom the clinical detection of meningitis may be most difficult. In addition, one study identified five risk factors that helped to select those patients with febrile seizures and without meningitis: a physician visit within 48 hours before the seizure, the occurrence of seizures on arrival at the emergency room, a focal seizure, an abnormal findings upon neurologic examination, and suspicious findings on physical examination. A lumbar puncture should be performed if any one of these features is present.

Other routine laboratory evaluation is generally not indicated for children with uncomplicated febrile seizures. The use of an EEG remains somewhat controversial but, in general, is not predictive of either recurrence of febrile seizures or the development of epilepsy and hence is unwarranted. Other tests should be used only as needed for the evaluation of the fever's etiology. Routine analysis of serum electrolytes, calcium, or glucose is generally not indicated.

The management of febrile seizures is a difficult issue, not in terms of managing the acute seizure, but rather with regard to the prevention of future recurrences. For the child presenting in status epilepticus, management is essentially the same whether the child is febrile or afebrile. First, vital signs should be checked, an adequate airway should be ensured, and the patient should be positioned to minimize the risk of aspiration or physical injury. An intravenous catheter may then be placed while appropriate doses of medication are prepared. Necessary blood studies (if any)

may be obtained from this catheter. Then, if the seizures continue, intravenous diazepam (Valium) should be given at a dose of 0.2 to 0.3 mg/kg over a 2-minute period, with a maximum single dose of 10 mg. Equipment for artificial ventilation must be available, since diazepam is a potent respiratory depressant. A second dose may be given in 10 minutes, and if seizures still persist, phenytoin (Dilantin) or phenobarbital may be added to the regimen.

As noted, however, the more difficult question involves prophylaxis against future febrile seizures. Because these seizures tend to occur early in the course of a febrile illness, prophylactic use of antipyretics (acetaminophen) or anticonvulsants (phenobarbital) on an intermittent basis has not been successful. The basic question then becomes whether daily prophylactic anticonvulsant therapy is warranted to protect against the possible recurrence of febrile seizure. Although both phenobarbital and valproate sodium are effective when used in this manner, for most cases, the possible side effects of these medications make their use undesirable, especially considering that even though febrile seizures may be very frightening, they are not associated with neurologic sequelae. Thus, most experts consider chronic prophylactic therapy appropriate only for certain special cases, such as some children with atypical seizures, abnormal neurologic development, recurrent febrile seizures, or a family history of afebrile seizures.

AFEBRILE SEIZURES

Great efforts have been made in recent years to standardize the classification of seizures, using primarily electroencephalographic (EEG) data and the clinical characteristics of the seizure. These efforts have helped to provide data on the therapy, evaluation, and prognosis of the various seizure types seen in children. An outline of the classification system proposed in 1981 by the International League Against Epilepsy is seen in Table 87-1, dividing seizures into two main groups, those that are generalized in nature and those that are partial (localized) in nature.

GENERALIZED SEIZURES

Generalized seizures are characterized by bilateral involvement without local onset. Consciousness may be impaired, and this may even be the initial manifestation of the seizure. Motor involvement may be either major, as with tonic, clonic, or tonic–clonic seizures, or minor, as in absence seizures, myoclonic seizures, atonic seizures, or infantile spasms. EEG manifestations vary considerably with these different types of seizures, although all are characterized by bilateral involvement at seizure onset.

Tonic–clonic (grand mal) seizures are characterized by stiffness followed by rhythmic shaking. Tonic seizures have stiffness as their predominant manifestation, whereas clonic attacks have rhythmic shaking of the trunk and extremities without stiffening. Consciousness is lost, and the seizure is commonly followed by a period of drowsiness and, frequently, confusion. Incontinence is commonly noted, and transient focal neurologic deficits (Todd's paralysis) may occur.

Table 87–1 Seizure Classification

Generalized Seizures (Convulsive or Nonconvulsive)
  Absence
  Myoclonic
  Tonic/clonic/tonic–clonic
  Atonic
  Infantile spasms
Partial Seizures
  Simple partial (no impairment of consciousness)
  Complex partial (with impairment of consciousness)
  Partial seizures, which secondarily generalize

These seizures may occur at any age but have peak incidences between 2 months and 2 years of age and at puberty. Anticonvulsants commonly used are carbamazepine, phenytoin, phenobarbital, and valproate.

Absence (petit mal) seizures are typified by brief spells of unresponsiveness, usually lasting only 5 to 10 seconds. Motor manifestations are variable and may include complete cessation of movement, rhythmic movements of the eyes, or, less commonly, increased postural tone, myoclonus, deviation of the eyes, or autonomic changes. There may be many attacks per day, and the child may be accused of daydreaming or staring off into space. Absence seizures are most common in school-aged children and are rare under the age of 3 and over the age of 20. The EEG is characteristic with a spike and wave discharge at a rate of 3 per second. Ethosuximide is generally considered the drug of choice for these seizures, and the prognosis is very good for complete remission over time.

Myoclonic and atonic seizures are much less common seizure types but are noteworthy because of the management difficulties they present and their relatively poor prognosis. Myoclonic seizures are characterized by single or repetitive contractions of a group of muscles, while atonic (akinetic) seizures involve a sudden, momentary loss of postural tone. These seizures are often associated with a degenerative brain disease or other central nervous system (CNS) abnormality and may be exceedingly difficult to control.

Finally, infantile spasms deserve note, also primarily because of their poor prognosis. These seizures consist of sudden flexion of the head, accompanied by abduction and extension of the arms and flexion of the knees. They commonly occur in clusters and may number 20 or 30 in succession. They are associated with a characteristic EEG pattern termed hypsarrhythmia. Onset is typically noted between 3 and 9 months of age, at which time about two-thirds of patients will already be found to be developmentally delayed. Many of these patients will be found to have underlying CNS disease, including tuberous sclerosis, metabolic abnormalities, and damage secondary to anoxia or infections. Prompt treatment with adrenocorticotropic hormone (ACTH) or corticosteroids is recommended, although control may be difficult and side effects are common. Ultimately, the prognosis is quite poor, with only 10% to 20% of affected children attaining normal development and over one-half of cases going on to develop other seizure types later in childhood.

PARTIAL SEIZURES

In simple partial seizures, consciousness is maintained, and the symptoms produced by the seizure discharge depend on the specific area of the brain involved. Symptoms may be predominantly motor, sensory, autonomic, or psychic in nature. These seizures are more common in infancy than in childhood. They are often followed by rapid generalization of the seizure activity; in many of these cases, the focal component will not be recognized by the child or parent during the seizure but will instead be picked up by demonstration of a focal abnormality on the EEG or upon neurologic examination. Simple partial seizures are generally well controlled using carbamazepine, phenytoin, phenobarbital, or primidone.

Complex partial (psychomotor, temporal lobe) seizures commonly consist of purposeful but inappropriate motor acts, at times repetitive and lasting from minutes to hours. The patient often experiences an aura preceding the seizure and postictal depression following the episode. These seizures are less common in children than in adults. Carbamazepine is usually the drug of choice although phenytoin, phenobarbital, primidone, and valproate may all be effective in selected cases.

EVALUATION OF THE FIRST AFEBRILE SEIZURE

The first step in the evaluation of a child who has experienced a seizure is a complete history and physical examination. Details about the seizure episode should be carefully elicited, both to help confirm that the event was indeed a seizure and to begin to differentiate the various seizure types. Details about fever, focality, incontinence, loss of consciousness, postural changes, and postictal depression are all of critical importance. The physical examination must be very thorough, seeking any evidence of systemic disease as a cause of the fever (e.g., infection, metabolic illness) and any deficits in the neurologic or developmental examinations.

While no laboratory work-up should be considered absolutely routine, certain tests are useful and should be performed in most cases. These include determinations of serum glucose, electrolytes, and calcium, liver function tests, and blood counts. A lumbar puncture should be considered if there is any suspicion of CNS infection. An EEG should be performed on virtually all patients experiencing an afebrile seizure.

Although the EEG may be entirely normal unless a seizure occurs during the test, in other cases it may provide important diagnostic clues, such as the characteristic spike–wave pattern of absence seizures. Focal slowing on the EEG is an important finding because it may indicate the presence of a focal abnormality such as a tumor or focal encephalitis. Generalized slowing may be indicative of a more global problem such as metabolic encephalopathy.

Radiographic evaluation should be considered on a case-by-case basis. While skull x-rays are rarely useful, the computed tomography (CT) scan (and, possibly, nuclear magnetic resonance imaging) may be extremely helpful. A CT scan should not be considered routine but should be performed when there is focal slowing on the EEG, a focal deficit on neurologic examination, or continuing focal seizures. This is somewhat different from the approach in adults, in whom the likelihood of a tumor or vascular abnormality as a cause of the seizure is much higher.

TREATMENT DECISIONS

While drugs commonly used to treat the various seizure types were described previously, it is important to consider in more detail the indications for both the initiation and the discontinuation of anticonvulsant therapy.

It is clear that not all children who have experienced a first or even second seizure require anticonvulsant therapy. The decision to institute therapy must be made on an individual case basis and must take into account a variety of factors, including the age of the patient, the type of seizures experienced, and the risk of recurrence. Many studies have addressed the question of seizure recurrence in recent years, and these indicate that the risk of recurrence after a single generalized tonic–clonic seizure is relatively low, probably between 20% and 40%. Once a second seizure occurs, the risk of a third seizure is between 50% and 75%. The vast majority of recurrences occur within 1 year of the initial seizure.

With these numbers in mind, most experts do not recommend routine anticonvulsant use after a single tonic–clonic seizure but do strongly consider it for those children experiencing 2 or more seizures. The major advantage to treatment is a lesser risk of seizure recurrence (probably), while disadvantages lie primarily in the many side effects common to each of the anticonvulsant medications. Through careful monitoring, possible adverse effects can be minimized while efficacy is maximized. For children with absence and partial complex seizures, therapy should generally be initiated as early as possible because these seizures tend to recur much more frequently.

Finally, it has also been shown recently that, in many children, anticonvulsants can be successfully stopped without increasing the risk of seizure recurrence. In general, if a child has been seizure free for 2 years and has a normal EEG and neurologic examination, odds are very high (about 75%) that he will remain seizure free once anticonvulsants are stopped. Thus, parents can be reassured that, with most seizure types, the prognosis for their child is actually quite good, a far cry from the myths about epilepsy that remain quite prevalent.

BIBLIOGRAPHY

Delgado-Escueta A, Treiman D, Walsh G: The treatable epilepsies. N Engl J Med 308:1508, 1576, 1983

Gomez MR, Klass DW: Epilepsies of infancy and childhood. Ann Neurol 13:114, 1983

Joffe A, McCormick M, DeAngelis C: Which children with febrile seizures need lumbar puncture? Am J Dis Child 137:1153, 1983

NIH Consensus Development Conference on Febrile Seizures. Febrile seizures: Long-term management of children with fever-associated seizures. Pediatrics 66:1009, 1980

Shinnar S, Vining E, Mellits D et al: Discontinuing antiepileptic medication in children with epilepsy after two years without seizures. N Engl J Med 313:976, 1985

Vining E, Freeman JM: Management of nonfebrile seizures. Pediatr Rev 8:185, 1986

88

Neural Tube Defects

Open neural tube defects (NTD) afflict approximately 2000 live-born infants per year in the United States alone. Meningomyelocele, the least severe NTD, is the most common congenital malformation of the central nervous system (CNS). In recent years, clinicians and ethicists have disagreed profoundly about the early management of infants with meningomyelocele. Nonetheless, no one argues that even with prompt aggressive therapy and long-term multidisciplinary care, a survivor must often cope with substantial fixed motor and sensory losses, variable intellectual deficit, and/or learning disability, while at risk for progressive orthopedic deformities and a gamut of urologic complications. Potentially crippling, too, are the emotional, social, and economic stresses that accompany any chronic disability and that a neonatal onset can only exacerbate for both patient and family.

EMBRYOLOGY AND PATHOGENESIS

An understanding of the early embryogenesis of the CNS rationalizes the diverse phenotypes of the NTD. The CNS originates in the dorsal midline of the embryo as a plate of ecto-derm whose differentiation is induced by the notochord and adjacent mesoderm. This neural plate invaginates as its lateral margins fold toward the midline to form a neural groove. Midline fusion of these folds occurs first at the level of the lower medulla at 22 days' gestation and proceeds simultaneously in both rostral and caudal directions. Rostral closure of the neural tube at 24 days precedes caudal closure at the L1-L2 level by 2 days. At each level above this, normal development of the dura and axial skeleton (cranial vault and vertebrae) depends on a local interaction between mesoderm and a closed neural tube. The distal spinal cord (the conus medullaris and filum terminale) is modeled differently by internal canalization of solid neuroectoderm (4 to 7 weeks' gestation) and subsequent regression and differentiation that continues throughout gestation.

Although alternative explanations of the pathogenesis of NTD exist, available evidence supports a primary failure of neurulation (i.e., neural tube formation) with secondary maldevelopment of the overlying skeleton and soft tissues. This theory implies that the embryo suffers some critical insult at no later than 20 to 28 days' gestation.

516

Complete failure of neurulation (craniorachischisis totalis) prevents further normal development of the CNS; most affected fetuses are aborted. Rostral defects may be either complete or restricted, resulting in anencephaly or encephalocele, respectively. Similarly, disorders of neurulation caudal to the medulla cause a spectrum of malformation, ranging from total myeloschisis to meningomyeloceles of varying level and extent. Occult spinal dysraphic states originate as aberrations of caudal spinal cord development.

EPIDEMIOLOGY AND ETIOLOGY

The overwhelming majority of NTDs occur as a single malformation caused by a multifactorial inheritance, defined as the interaction of one or more mutant genes with some, usually unknown, environmental factor(s). A majority are associated with other congenital defects and arise secondary to single mutant genes (*e.g.,* autosomal-recessive Meckel-Gruber syndrome), chromosomal abnormalities (trisomies 13 and 18), teratogens, or as part of a syndrome or a complex anomalad (cloacal exstrophy).

Many factors influence the incidence of NTD. The incidence is higher in females, certain ethnic groups (particularly in United Kingdom natives of Celtic descent), and consanguineous marriages. A positive family history increases the risk of NTD in subsequent offspring at least 20-fold. Other findings implicate environmental, rather than genetic, factors in the etiology of NTD. These include the increased incidence in lower socioeconomic classes, the decreased incidence in Celtic people after transatlantic migration, and especially the marked general decline in the incidence of NTD over the last 50 years. Preliminary studies have reported that periconceptional vitamin supplementation may decrease the incidence of NTD in high-risk groups.

The risk of recurrence of an isolated NTD is influenced by family history, ethnic background and geographic locale. With one affected sibling, the risk to a subsequent sibling is 2% in the United States but 5% in the United Kingdom. Two affected siblings more than doubles these risks. The firstborn child of a mother with meningomyelocele has a 3% risk for an NTD. Meningomyelocele and anencephaly often are present in the same lineage. When an NTD occurs in association with other anomalies, the recurrence rate is higher and is determined by the mode of inheritance. Subsequent recurrence rate for the 5% of NTD associated with Meckel-Gruber syndrome is 25%.

ANENCEPHALY AND ENCEPHALOCELE

More than half of anencephalics are stillborn; the remainder die soon after birth. Pregnancies are complicated by increased rates of both pre- and postmaturity, as well as polyhydramnios. The diagnosis is obvious at delivery. Absence of the superior cranial vault gives these infants a characteristic frog-like facies. The cerebrum and hypothalamus are absent, and the upper brain stem and cerebellum are severely malformed. Perhaps half have associated open spinal defects. Notable abnormalities of the neurologic examination include slow stereotypic movements with decerebrate posturing and nonhabituation of primitive reflexes such as the Moro's reflex. Ninety percent of cases occur without a preceding positive family history. Anencephaly is a legitimate reason for a third trimester abortion.

An encephalocele is a herniation of brain tissue and/or meninges through a defect in the cranial vault. Seventy-five percent are located posteriorly, usually in the occipital midline; one-fourth present anteriorly as nasofrontal or nasopharyngeal masses. The size of a posterior encephalocele does not correlate with the severity of brain dysplasia. Outcome depends on the totality of CNS malformation. When indicated, surgery consists of resection and closure of the encephalocele and shunting of hydrocephalus as necessary. Nasopharyngeal encephaloceles generally present after infancy with nasal obstruction, epistaxis or recurrent meningitis. Encephalocele should be considered in the differential diagnosis of intranasal masses.

MENINGOMYELOCELE

Neonatal Evaluation

More than 80% of meningomyeloceles present in the lumbar, lumbosacral, and thoracolumbar areas. A small subset (10%) are meningoceles that involve the meninges but not the spinal cord; most are fully covered with skin and have an excellent prognosis. Defects affecting the spinal cord are, with rare exception, open. At delivery, these may be flush with the back or protrude in large, membranous sacs. All infants with meningomyelocele have vertebral and most have structural CNS abnormalities in addition to the open spinal cord defect. Of the latter, the most common are Arnold-Chiari malformation, hydrocephalus, occult (usually cervical) spinal cord lesions, and cerebral microgyria. Arnold-Chiari malformation includes variable degrees of downward displacement of the brainstem, cerebellar vermis, and fourth ventricle through the foramen magnum with elongation of the brain stem, and adjacent skull and cervical vertebral abnormalities. Hydrocephalus requiring a shunt results in at least 75% of the cases and may be either communicating or noncommunicating (secondary to aqueductal stenosis). Facial, pharyngeal, and laryngeal pareses are also associated with severe Arnold-Chiari malformation.

Most infants with meningomyelocele except those with severe hydrocephalus are born unsuspected after normal labor. Diagnosis at birth is straightforward in the case of open lesions; dermoid cysts, lipomas, hemangiomas, neurenteric cysts, nevi, and hamartomas must be considered in the differential of covered midline lesions. Rarely, meningoceles are occult, originating from the anterior sacral or lateral thoracic regions and present later as pelvic or posterior mediastinal masses.

Initial management of infants with meningomyelocele has two major aims: to prevent complications that may cause further irreversible damage and to define the neurologic level and identify any coexisting congenital anomalies. Parents are stricken to a variable extent by emotional turmoil and need appropriate understanding and support. A rapid multidisciplinary evaluation, although essential, cannot substitute for the early involvement of a committed pediatric generalist. The pediatrician must recognize the long-term implications of the diagnostic findings and then convey a realistic prognosis to the family. From the beginning, he must act as the child's advocate. Later, he will coordinate the multispecialty care effort and tailor therapy to the overall needs of the individual.

Immediate management always requires scrupulous care of the open lesion. Manual inspection is done only when necessary and with sterile technique. The defect should be dressed regularly with saline-soaked sterile gauze that is secured by a moisture-proof covering. This helps keep the lesion clean and minimizes further neural injury. Antibiotic therapy probably decreases the incidence of CNS infection and can be started except in the unusual case in which aggressive therapy is obviously not in the best interest of the child.

A deliberate physical examination will usually determine the neurologic level of the lesion with sufficient accuracy to afford a reasonable description of future functional activity. The lowest motor level of normal function is more reliably assessed and is more predictive than the sensory level. Key points of the physical examination include observation of voluntary movements and resting posture as well as careful inspection for muscle atrophy and joint deformity and dislocation. Determination of the sensory level is difficult in the neonate. There are often discrepancies between motor and sensory levels because the ventral spinal cord is often spared relative to its dorsal counterpart. Moreover, motor function may differ by up to two root levels between left and right sides. Occasionally, spinal injury may result from the delivery process or exposure to cold and reverses following stabilization and closure of the defect. In this case, initial examination usually will have revealed paradoxical paralysis of non-atrophied muscle groups.

Proceeding caudally from L1, muscle groups are innervated roughly in the following sequence: hip flexors > hip adductors > knee extensors > foot dorsiflexors > hip abductors > foot plantar flexors ≅ knee flexors ≅ hip extensors. The prognosis for ambulation and the likelihood of spinal and joint deformity change dramatically as normal function is attained in each successive muscle group. Lesions at L1-L2 or higher cause flaccid paralysis of the lower extremities that is complete except possibly for some hip flexion. Ambulation is futile, but mobility can be achieved with a wheelchair. Repair of bilateral hip dislocation is often contraindicated. Severe congenital and/or acquired scoliosis is common and may lead to future cardiopulmonary compromise without appropriate intervention. Lesions at S1 or below should always result in independent adult ambulation. Significant scoliosis is uncommon, but a variety of foot deformities may require orthopedic attention. Prognostication is more difficult for intermediate lesions (L3-L5). Some children with an L3 level ambulate with braces and crutches, only to become wheelchair dependent as adults. Infants with lower lumbar lesions should retain the ability to walk with aids into adulthood. Normal quadriceps function may be the single most important predictor of realistic adult ambulation. Full innervation of the hip adductors through L4 without balancing hip abductor function increases the chance of hip dislocation.

Parents also need a realistic appraisal of future intellectual capability. With early aggressive medical therapy cognitive abilities can be nearly normal. This assumes that massive hydrocephalus (cortical mantle less than 5 mm), overwhelming CNS infection, and other cerebral anomalies are absent at birth. The distribution of intelligence quotients (IQ's) of meningomyelocele patients in whom hydrocephalus is controlled and CNS infection avoided is slightly left-shifted compared to their siblings, but most have IQ's greater than 80. Regardless of IQ, visual motor integration skills are often delayed.

Identification and early treatment of hydrocephalus is critical for optimal outcome. The neurologic level correlates with the risk of hydrocephalus, higher-level lesions posing a greater risk. At birth, measurement of head circumference, palpation of sutures and fontanelles, and examination of the cranial nerves may suggest hydrocephalus and/or increased intracranial pressure. Transillumination of the skull will identify cortical mantle less than 1 cm in thickness. A normal head circumference does not rule out hydrocephalus. The evaluation of ventricular size should include ultrasonography or head CT scanning. Hydrocephalus may develop after birth, especially after operative closure of the defect. Serial measurement of head circumference and judicious repeat radiographic studies will identify these cases.

Urologic function must be assessed carefully throughout the neonatal period. Function often changes after birth or postoperatively. Voiding frequency and force of stream should be noted and residuals assessed by bladder palpation, Credé's maneuver, or catheterization. Laboratory studies should include serum blood urea nitrogen (BUN), creatinine, urine culture, and radiographic studies (intravenous pyelogram [IVP, voiding cystourethrogram [VCUG], radionuclide scans). Without proper management, infants with larger residuals and/or evidence of vesicoureteral reflux are at risk for renal infections and deterioration of renal function. Circumcision is contraindicated because the prepuce helps prevent chronic irritation. Twenty-five percent of males with meningomyelocele have cryptorchidism.

The birth of an infant with meningomyelocele confronts parents and physician with emotional, medical, and ethical dilemmas. The immediate question is always whether to pursue aggressive treatment. In the child with a very high defect, massive hydrocephalus and other significant congenital anomalies, surgical intervention would be heroic. Such a child is, however, uncommon. Many children even with high lesions have confounded expectations only to survive without surgical treatment and have thus incurred unacceptable morbidity. Withholding therapy on the basis of selection criteria derived from large population studies time and again has had disastrous consequences for individual patients.

On the other hand, aggressive therapy (e.g., surgical closure of the defect and treatment of hydrocephalus with ventriculoperitoneal shunts) has resulted in greater than 90% long-term survival at the same time that innovative urologic and orthopedic therapies and appropriate educational and emotional support have markedly improved the "quality of life" of survivors.

Parents need not be rushed into making a decision by the oft-cited 24- to 48- hour time limit. Recent evidence suggests that closure may be delayed as late as 1 week after birth without compromising CNS function. The extra time can be invaluable for parents to come to grips with their emotions, to grasp some of the medical implications and to participate more deliberately in the decision making process.

Childhood Care

In addition to providing routine pediatric care, the generalist must also coordinate the input of the neurosurgeon, orthopedist, urologist, physical therapist, and social worker. The special challenges of care are both medical and psychological: to guard the integrity of many organ systems and to foster independence and self-esteem.

Preservation of CNS function and intellectual potential is the foremost priority. Significant neurologic morbidity can result from shunt malfunction or infection. These complications present with nonspecific signs and symptoms (e.g., fever, headache, vomiting, lethargy, and irritability), and their differentiation from more common childhood illnesses can be difficult. The pediatrician must therefore react with a lower threshold to common complaints to ensure a timely evaluation. Seizure disorders develop in 25% of patients but usually respond well to standard anticonvulsants.

To the orthopedist falls the critical task of assisting the patient to achieve his maximum ambulatory potential. Early, he must be alert to progressive neurogenic deformities. These deformities are caused by an imbalance of muscle forces across a joint and can adversely affect future mobility. Casting procedures are only temporary until definitive surgery can be performed to restore the muscle balance. The use of a parapodium gives the infant an age-appropriate perspective on his environment and begins to promote his independence. Later, ambulation with braces, crutches, or other orthoses is possible for most patients. The orthopedist must also prevent significant kyphoscoliosis from developing.

The goals of the urologist are three: to preserve function, to prevent infection, and to facilitate continence appropriate for age. The initial radiographic assessment characterizes the degree of flaccidity or spasticity of the neurogenic bladder, describes renal parenchymal and ureteral anatomy, and identifies vesicoureteral reflux. Periodic follow-up through infancy monitors for developments requiring specific intervention. With flaccid neurogenic bladders, urologic goals are usually met with a combination of intermittent clean catheterization, antimicrobial prophylaxis and pharmacologic agents. Spastic bladders associated with high-grade reflux and hydronephrosis may require vesicoureteral reimplantations. By 6 years of age, urodynamic studies are possible in most children and allow more rational pharmacologic control of bladder and sphincter tone. These studies also help predict the effect on continence of surgical procedures such as artificial sphincter implantation and augmentation cystoplasty. Intelligent selection of these therapies has improved urinary continence in many patients. It is hoped that these newer management strategies will improve the long-term urologic outcome of patients with meningomyelocele, many of whom, in the past, would have died of complications of chronic renal failure.

Psychometric testing aids in the choice of an educational facility. Although most children perform well in a regular school setting, others have learning disabilities best addressed in special classes. Excellent medical care and sensitivity to the educational, emotional, and social needs of these children can help them achieve independent and productive lives.

PRENATAL DIAGNOSIS

Prenatal diagnosis is possible in greater than 90% of NTD. In high-risk pregnancies, the procedure of choice is amniocentesis for determination of amniotic fluid alpha-fetoprotein. This $alpha_1$-globulin is the predominant protein synthesized by the early fetal liver. Elevated amniotic fluid concentrations in NTD presumably occur secondary to transudation across neural membranes. Alpha-fetoprotein may be increased in cases of congenital nephrosis, omphalocele, upper gastrointestinal atresia, Turner's syndrome, sacrococcygeal teratoma, fetal distress, missed abortion, inaccurate dates, and maternal liver disease. Fetal blood contamination of amniotic fluid may also lead to a false-positive test result. False-negative results are the rule for closed NTD. Amniotic fluid concentration of this protein decreases with gestation; the optimum time of assay is between 14 and 16 weeks' gestation. A positive result should be followed by a detailed ultrasonographic examination. Mass screening for NTD has been performed in the United Kingdom using maternal serum alpha-fetoprotein levels but as yet is not routinely employed in the United States.

BIBLIOGRAPHY

American Academy of Pediatrics, Action Committee on Myelodysplasia, Section on Urology: Current approaches to evaluation and management of children with myelomeningocele. Pediatrics 63:663–667, 1979

Bahnson DH: Myelomeningocele and its problems. Pediatr Ann 11(6):528–540, 1982

Charney EB, Weller SC, Sutton LN et al: Management of the newborn with myelomeningocele: Time for a decision-making process. Pediatrics 75(1):58–64, 1985

Leonard CO: Counseling parents of a child with meningomyelocele. Pediatr Rev 4(10):317–321, 1983

McLaughlin JF, Shurtleff DB: Management of the newborn with myelodysplasia. Clin Pediatr 18(8):463–476, 1979

McLone DG, Czyzewski D. Raimondi AJ et al: Central nervous system infections as a limiting factor in the intelligence of children with myelomeningocele. Pediatrics 70(3):338–342, 1982

Myers GJ: Myelomeningocele: the medical aspects. Pediatr Clin North Am 31(1):165–175, 1984

Windham GC, Edmonds LD: Current trends in the incidence of neural tube defects. Pediatrics 70(3):333–337, 1982

89

Hydrocephalus

Hydrocephalus is a disorder characterized by an excessive volume of cerebrospinal fluid (CSF) in the ventricular system or in the subarachnoid space that is secondary either to anatomic or functional obstruction of CSF flow or, rarely, to overproduction of CSF. This definition excludes ventriculomegaly secondary to brain atrophy (hydrocephalus *ex vacuo*). Hydrocephalus is usually internal (involving the ventricular system) but may be external (involving primarily the subarachnoid spaces). External hydrocephalus may be associated with a genetic syndrome (*i.e.,* achondroplasia) or acquired following a central nervous system insult (*i.e.,* subdural hemorrhage). Most often it occurs in association with benign familial macrocephaly and has little clinical significance.

CSF MECHANICS

The highly vascularized choroid plexus, located in the lateral and third ventricles, produces the majority of CSF by active secretion of a hypertonic solution. Diffusion of water across the ependyma which lines the ventricles results in isosmolar CSF. In adults, the total CSF volume and the rate of CSF secretion are estimated to be 150 ml and 20 ml/hour, respectively. CSF mechanics in infants and children is similar to that of adults in that total CSF turnover takes place several times a day. Clearly, even a slight imbalance between CSF production and reabsorption may cause ventricular enlargement.

After secretion by the choroid plexus, CSF flow is mostly unidirectional. CSF passes from the lateral ventricles through the two lateral foramina of Munro into the midline third ventricle. From there, it courses caudally through the Sylvian aqueduct into a midline fourth ventricle, whence it exits *via* two lateral foramina of Luschka and the midline foramen of Magendie into dilated subarachnoid spaces known as cisterns to bathe the cerebellar and cerebral convexities. The cisternal system also connects the spinal (extracranial) and intracranial subarachnoid spaces. The fourth ventricle continues as the central canal of the spinal cord.

CSF reabsorption occurs primarily through projections of the arachnoid villi into the venous sinuses; a small amount is absorbed *via* the ventricular and spinal cord ependyma.

523

Internal hydrocephalus traditionally has been classified as noncommunicating or communicating. Noncommunicating hydrocephalus refers to an anatomical or mechanical obstruction to CSF flow within the ventricular system. This type of hydrocephalus may be congenital (*i.e.*, secondary to aqueductal stenosis with lateral and third ventricular dilatation and a normal-sized fourth ventricle) or acquired (*i.e.*, resulting from a posterior fossa tumor compressing the Sylvian aqueduct and/or the fourth ventricle). Communicating hydrocephalus is present when no obstructions hinder CSF flow into the cisternal system and the intracranial subarachnoid space; in this case, the entire ventricular system is dilated. Presumably, decreased CSF reabsorption functionally impedes CSF flow.

CONGENITAL HYDROCEPHALUS

Excluding hydrocephalus due to meningomyelocele, overt hydrocephalus at birth occurs at the approximate rate of 1 in 2000 pregnancies. The etiologies of congenital hydrocephalus in live-born infants who present for neurosurgical evaluation are listed in Table 89-1.

Aqueductal stenosis likely develops concurrently with the normal elongation of the mesencephalon at 15 to 17 weeks of gestation. In male infants, perhaps as many as 25% are due to X-linked inheritance. Clenched fingers and bilateral flexion deformities of the thumbs are diagnostic of X-linked inheritance in a newborn male with hydrocephalus. In the remaining male infants and in all female infants, the inheritance is multifactorial. The risk of recurrence with one affected female infant is 5%; with two affected infants, 10%. For X-linked hydrocephalus, the risk of recurrence in a subsequent male fetus is 50%. Natural history studies show that, while an occasional infant will have arrested hydro-

Table 89–1 Etiology of Congenital Hydrocephalus Overt at Birth

Aqueductal stenosis
    Males (75% multifactorial; 25% X-linked)
    Females (multifactorial)
Communicating hydrocephalus
Dandy-Walker malformation
Hydrocephalus associated with meningomyelocele
Autosomal chromosomal abnormality
    Trisomy 13
    Trisomy 18
    Translocation (13, 18)
Intrauterine infection (toxoplasmosis, cytomegalovirus, syphilis)
Congenital CNS tumor

cephalus, most infants die without treatment, and survivors incur severe retardation. Delivery by cesarean section and early neonatal shunt placement has improved survival and decreased morbidity.

Communicating hydrocephalus and the Dandy-Walker malformation likely arise from abnormalities in the formation of the subarachnoid spaces and in the perforation of the fourth ventricle at about 6 weeks' gestation. The Dandy-Walker anomaly includes congenital atresia of the foramina of the fourth ventricle with saccular dilatation of the fourth ventricle at the caudal end of the cerebellum. Other cerebral (*i.e.*, agenesis of the corpus callosum) abnormalities and polycystic kidneys may complicate this anomaly. Inheritance is probably autosomal recessive. Infants with the Dandy-Walker malformation frequently are dolichocephalic; that is, occipital enlargement increases the anterior-posterior dimension of the cranium but has little effect on the biparietal diameter. Posterior fossa involvement may cause nystagmus and paresis of the fourth to eleventh cranial nerves and, later, truncal ataxia. Seizures often present by a few months of age.

Outcome of infants with isolated communicating hydrocephalus is quite good with aggressive neurosurgical treatment; in a recent report of nine patients, mean IQ was 101. Follow-up of infants with the Dandy-Walker anomaly is less sanguine. Outcome hinges on the associated cerebral abnormalities.

Other causes of overt hydrocephalus at birth are less common and usually are associated with a dismal prognosis. Hydrocephalus in infants with an intrauterine viral, spirochetal, or protozoal infection results from an inflammatory fibrosis of the ventricular ependyma and/or the subarachnoid space with consequent obliteration of a ventricular channel or interference with CSF reabsorption. Some autosomal chromosomal disorders (trisomies 13 and 18) are associated with hydrocephalus. Very uncommonly, a congenital central nervous system tumor (i.e., teratoma) will obstruct ventricular flow.

Physical findings attributable to hydrocephalus are identical to those found in infants with meningomyelocele (see Chapter 88). It is notable that transillumination of infants with Dandy-Walker malformation may be misleading unless careful attention is given to the posterior fossa. Other physical findings may be helpful in establishing a specific diagnosis.

Infants with apparent hydrocephalus at birth should be thoroughly evaluated by cranial computed tomography (CT) scan. Hydrocephalus must be differentiated from other disorders such as hydranencephaly (complete absence of cerebral cortex), porencephaly (intracerebral cyst), and holoprosencephaly (grossly abnormal development of the prosencephalon). If hydrocephalus is confirmed, a careful search should be made for associated anomalies (agenesis of the corpus callosum, agenesis of the cerebellum, etc.). These additional abnormalities worsen the prognosis for survival and/or intellectual development. In infants with isolated hydrocephalus, aggressive neurosurgical treatment with ventriculoperitoneal shunt placement seems advisable.

The Fetus with Ventriculomegaly

Ultrasonographic diagnosis of fetal ventriculomegaly is now possible as early as 16 to 18 weeks of gestation. This diagnosis relies on measurements of the ratio of ventricular to hemispheric diameter. The top normal value of this ratio is 0.75 at 16 weeks but decreases to 0.40 by term. More important is documentation of progressive ventricular enlargement during gestation. In early fetal hydrocephalus, the anterior horns of the lateral ventricles are the first to dilate. Shortly thereafter, the posterior regions of the lateral ventricles enlarge. Late fetal hydrocephalus begins when the head circumference crosses percentiles. Again, abnormal cranial growth is apparent first in the frontal area. Late hydrocephalus may begin as early as 24 weeks or as late as 34 weeks.

The development of new surgical techniques has made it feasible to place ventriculo-amniotic shunts *in utero* in an attempt to treat fetal hydrocephalus. It was reasoned that treatment of selected fetuses might improve outcome relative to later postnatal surgery. It is fair to say, however, that the initial enthusiasm surrounding this procedure has been tempered by results that are thus far not too encouraging. A July 1986 progress report by the International Fetal Surgery Registry summarized results in 44 intrauterine shunt procedures. The procedure-related mortality rate was 10%. In addition, 22% of the fetuses had associated anomalies. In a subgroup of 32 fetuses with aqueductal stenosis, survival was increased (87.5%) compared to an untreated group of 20 fetuses (40%) gathered from three separate reports. However, only 37.5% (12 of 28) of the treated survivors were normal at follow-up versus 75% (6 of 8) of the untreated survivors. Certainly, a procedure that would only result in the survival of severely handicapped infants should be abandoned. Only prospective, controlled trials will determine if prenatal intervention is of benefit in any subgroup of fetuses with ventriculomegaly.

A diagnosis of fetal ventriculomegaly warrants a careful diagnostic evaluation to provide the most accurate prognostic and therapeutic counseling to the parents. Ultrasonography must search for neural tube defects (NTDs) and for other central nervous system abnormalities, as well as define the cortical mantle thickness. Despite a skilled examination, up to 25% of cases of spina bifida may not be apparent. Scrutiny should be directed to other organ systems, such as the kidneys and urinary tract, heart, limbs, and facial structures. Finally, the choroid plexus should be examined to exclude a papilloma. Amniocentesis allows determination of fetal chromosomes (banding should be performed to rule out translocation in addition to an obvious trisomy), sex (especially important if there is a previously affected male child), and alpha-fetoprotein level (see Chapter 88). Maternal serology may be helpful in identifying certain infectious causes of hydrocephalus. If a fetal chromosomal translocation is found, parental chromosomes should be studied to rule out the possibility of a balanced carrier.

If no poor prognostic signs are discovered, and the mother elects to continue the pregnancy, serial sonograms and assessment of fetal lung maturity help decide the best time for delivery. Rapidly progressive hydrocephalus with marked thinning of the cortical mantle may indicate the need for steroid therapy in an attempt to mature fetal lungs and allow elective delivery by cesarean section. Otherwise, it is better to wait at least until the fetal lungs are mature. In some cases, a nearly normal biparietal diameter (BPD) may make vaginal delivery possible. Cephalopelvic disproportion should always be addressed by cesarean section and not by a transvaginal cephalocentesis. Hopefully, delineation of the natural history of fetal ventriculomegaly (as distinct from neonatal hydrocephalus) will refine future obstetric management.

ACQUIRED HYDROCEPHALUS

Etiologies of acquired hydrocephalus are listed in Table 89-2.

Posthemorrhagic hydrocephalus in the premature infant is the most common cause of acquired hydrocephalus. Both obstruction to CSF flow and diminished CSF reabsorption may play a role in the pathogenesis. Hemorrhagic infarction and subsequent dissolution of periventricular cerebral tissue may also contribute to the "hydrocephalus". In these infants, ventricular dilatation is often present on ultrasound before head circumference growth is clearly abnormal or cranial sutures begin to widen. Symptoms of hydrocephalus relate to increased intracranial pressure. For instance, as the fontanelle becomes tenser, the neonate may develop bradycardia, hypertension, and apnea. Lethargy and vomiting are frequently present. Neurologic examination may reveal paresis of upward gaze (setting-sun sign) and serial decreases in lower extremity tone. Treatment is a complicated issue. Some infants are too tiny to undergo ventriculoperitoneal shunt placement; in others, residual ventricular blood and protein debris may result in early shunt failure. Most infants can be managed by some combination of diuretic therapy (*i.e.*, acetazolamide [Diamox] and

Table 89–2 Etiology of Acquired Hydrocephalus

Posthemorrhagic
Central nervous system infection
  Bacterial meningitis
  Tuberculous meningitis
Tumors (especially in the posterior fossa)
  Choroid plexus papilloma
  Astrocytoma
  Medulloblastoma
Arteriovenous malformation (*via* direct pressure)
Intraventricular or intracranial hemorrhage
  Systemic bleeding disorder
  Ruptured aneursym
  Arteriovenous malformation
  Trauma
Vitamin A intoxication

furosemide [Lasix]) to decrease CSF production, by serial lumbar punctures (if the hydrocephalus is communicating) or ventricular taps, or by temporary insertion of an external ventricular drain. In infants with progressive ventriculomegaly without other evidence of increased intracranial pressure, little consensus exists about optimal management.

In the older child, many signs and symptoms are referable to the underlying disease process. Signs and symptoms due to hydrocephalus *per se* depend on the rapidity of progression. Headaches are common but may vary in location, duration, and intensity. Early-morning headaches accompanied by nausea and vomiting are a classic sign of increased intracranial pressure. Personality changes may vary from irritability to indifference to somnolence. Alterations of vital signs may occur. Neurologic examination may reveal cranial nerve pareses, lower extremity spasticity, ataxia, and papilledema. Chronic hydrocephalus may affect growth, sexual maturation, and fluid and electrolyte balance secondary to hypothalamic dysfunction.

Diagnosis is easily confirmed by cranial CT scan. Therapy is directed at the underlying cause; hydrocephalus is treated by ventriculoperitoneal (VP) shunt placement. Serious postoperative complications of VP shunts include infection and shunt failure. Either complication can result in significant morbidity or mortality. Infections are likely to occur with organisms usually not considered to be pathogens *(Staphylococcus epidermidis)*.

BIBLIOGRAPHY

Alvarez LA, Maytal J, Shinnar S: Idiopathic external hydrocephalus: Natural history and relationship to benign familial macrocephaly. Pediatrics 77:901–907, 1986

Clewell WH, Johnson ML, Meier PR et al: A surgical approach to the treatment of fetal hydrocephalus. N Engl J Med 306:1320–1325, 1982

Habib Z: Genetics and genetic counselling in neonatal hydrocephalus. Obstet Gynecol Surv 36:529–534, 1981

McCullough DC, Balzer-Martin LA: Current prognosis in overt neonatal hydrocephalus. J Neurosurg 57:378–383, 1982

Manning FA, Harrison MR, Rodeck C et al: Catheter shunts for fetal hydronephrosis and hydrocephalus. N Engl J Med 315:336–340, 1986

Mealey J, Gilmor RL, Bubb MP: The prognosis of hydrocephalus overt at birth. J Neurosurg 39:348–355, 1973

Vintzileos AM, Ingardia CJ, Nochimson DJ: Congenital hydrocephalus: A review and protocol for perinatal management. Obstet Gynecol 62:539–549, 1983

Wapner RJ: Fetal surgery. In Nelson NM (ed): Current Therapy in Neonatal–Perinatal Medicine 1985–1986. Philadelphia, BC Decker, 1985

90

Cerebral Palsy

Cerebral palsy (CP) is defined as a "non-progressive disorder of motion and posture due to brain insult or injury occurring in the period of early brain growth (generally under 3 years of age)." Thus, the insult may have occurred prenatally, perinatally, or in early childhood.

CP occurs in 1 to 2/1000 live births. Currently, there are nearly one half million U.S. citizens with CP.

Most cases of CP are attributable to perinatal causes, such as anoxia, hypoxia, or cerebral hemorrhage. A few years ago, kernicterus was also a leading cause of CP, but with closer monitoring of serum bilirubin and aggressive therapy (phototherapy, exchange transfusion) of elevated serum bilirubin levels in neonates, the incidence of kernicterus has decreased markedly. Prenatal causes of CP include congenital defects in the architecture of the brain and infectious, toxic, nutritional, or physical insults to the fetus *in utero*. Postnatal causes of CP include head trauma, cerebral hemorrhage from any cause, infections such as encephalitis or meningitis, and encephalopathies due to toxic substances.

The terminology to classify the type of CP has lead to confusion in the past. Although there are various combinations and permutations, CP is either spastic (pyramidal tract insult) or extrapyramidal. Spasticity is associated with marked hyperreflexia, a positive Babinski's sign, contractures, and a clasp-knife hypertonicity (*i.e.*, a "give" or "catch" is noted when manipulating the limb). Extrapyramidal CP is associated with movement disorders (chorea, athetosis), mild hyperreflexia, a "lead-pipe" hypertonicity, and marked variability of the child's examination, depending on his emotions, posture, and sleep state. Hemiplegia involves two limbs on the same side. Double hemiplegia involved all four limbs, with the upper ones more involved than the lower ones. Quadriplegia involves all four limbs, with greater involvement of the lower ones. Diplegia involves all four limbs, with a *markedly* greater involvement of the lower limbs.

The CP-affected infant frequently comes to medical attention because the parents are concerned that the child is developmentally delayed (see Chapter 4 for normal developmental milestones). Other children come to attention during their acute insults (meningitis, head trauma, etc.) or are detected by their physicians at well-child visits. Parents may report that, during feeding, the infant thrusts his tongue, thereby making feeding extremely difficult, has a poor suck, gags, or arches himself. These problems are due to poor coordination of muscle groups. Parents may also report that the infant unilaterally fists and has a preference for one hand (hand preference normally appears in the second year of life). In the older infant and toddler, abnormal or clumsy crawling or walking is a common complaint.

When a child with any of the above complaints presents for evaluation, an entire physical examination is mandatory. Particular attention is paid to the child's overall development, muscle mass, skin lesions, and head size. There are also a number of maneuvers that the examiner should try with the child. These maneuvers are to detect resistance to joint movement/decreased range of motion (hypertonicity) and laxity of limb movement/increased range of motion (hypotonicity).

One maneuver involves taking the supine baby's hands and gently pulling the infant to a sitting position. Normal infants will flex their hips and knees and demonstrate good head control. A hypotonic infant will lack head control and will be quite lax. A hypertonic infant, on the other hand, will extend the hips and knees and come directly to a standing position rather than a sitting one.

Another maneuver is to place the infant in ventral suspension with the examiner supporting the infant under his axillae. Before 2 months, an infant in this position cannot maintain his head and neck in a horizontal plane with his trunk, but by 4 months of age, the infant will hyperextend his head and neck. If this hyperextension occurs much earlier than 4 months of age, the infant is hypertonic. If the infant in ventral suspension "scissors" his legs, there is increased tone in his hip adductors. The hypotonic infant in ventral suspension will extend, rather than flex, his elbows and knees.

Another maneuver is dorsiflexion of the ankle with the knee flexed. In the first 6 months, dorsiflexing the ankle will easily permit the dorsum of the foot to touch the shin. Limitation in or resistance to performing this maneuver in a young infant is characteristic of hypertonicity of the gastrocnemius muscles.

Finally, with the infant supine, if the legs can be abducted more than 160° with the knees flexed, there is hypotonicity of the hips. With the infant supine, if the elbow can be brought past the midline by pulling his hand across his chest, there is hypotonicity of the shoulders.

The persistence of two primitive reflexes that usually disappear by 4 to 6 months of age are useful screens for CP. An older infant who cannot break the obligatory extremity flexion during the asymmetric tonic neck posture is suspicious. Also suspicious is the persistence of the crossed extensor reflex. With the infant supine, the sole of one foot is roughly stimulated when the knee is extended. The other foot responds (in order) with flexion withdrawal, extension, abduction, and adduction. If this response persists after 4 months of age, CP is suggested.

Deep tendon reflexes are elicited to detect hyperresponsiveness or clonus (hypertonicity) or decreased responsiveness (hypotonicity). The infant should be relaxed during these assessments. The infant or child should be observed for involuntary movements, asymmetry of tone or movement, persistence of fisting, hand preference, and an inability to prop or balance oneself.

There are other maneuvers designed to identify the subtype of CP but these are beyond the scope of this section.

DIFFERENTIAL DIAGNOSES

CP is a static encephalopathy. Therefore, the first diagnostic task is to rule out a progressive encephalopathy. A primary or secondary progressive central nervous system (CNS) disorder should be considered if there is rapid and abnormal enlargement of the head (hydrocephalus, subdural effusion, tumor), organomegaly (storage diseases), retinopathy (neurodegenerative diseases), or a lack of or decreased deep tendon reflexes (myopathies, leukodystrophies, hypothyroidism). In addition, children with ambulation difficulties may have an orthopedic rather than a CNS abnormality.

The evaluation should be judicious, dictated by clinical findings and the history. If a progressive CNS lesion, such as hydrocephalus, is suspected, a cranial computed tomography (CT) scan is useful.

ASSOCIATED COMPLICATIONS

Children with CP frequently demonstrate cognitive deficits, vision and hearing problems, and orthopedic problems (*i.e.*, tightened/contracted muscles). Many children with CP have seizure disorders.

TREATMENT

There is no specific treatment of CP. The family must be supported emotionally both at the time of the initial diagnosis and throughout the child's life. The physician should offer this support. In addition, there are parent groups that are wonderful sources of peer support.

Children affected with CP usually benefit from the services of occupational, physical, and speech therapists. These professionals can teach parents methods to minimize contractures, to modify abnormal postures and tones, and to encourage speech. "Infant-stimulation" programs usually include the aforementioned therapists, a psychologist, a social worker, an orthopedist, and psychiatrist, and a vocational counselor. Children and parents are served in their homes and at a center where families can support each other. The exercises and techniques are tailored to the individual infant.

If severe, orthopedic abnormalities may require surgery, casting, or bracing, with the ultimate goal of independent ambulation.

Seizures are controlled with appropriate anticonvulsants. Muscle relaxants have also been used with mixed results.

BIBLIOGRAPHY

Molnar G: Cerebral palsy: Prognosis and how to judge it. Pediatr Ann 8:596–605, 1979
Nelson K, Ellenberg J: Neonatal signs as predictors of cerebral palsy. Pediatrics 64:225–232, 1979
Taft L: Cerebral palsy. Pediatr Rev 6:35–45, 1984
Vining E et al: Cerebral palsy. Am J Dis Child 130:643–649, 1976

91

Closed Head Trauma

Closed head trauma (CHT) is defined as a blow to the head or the acceleration of the head against another object. It is an extremely common complaint and accounts for many visits to pediatric health facilities.

CHT can be intentional, as in abuse or assault, or accidental. Young infants who are victims of abuse often sustain head trauma. However, young infants can also sustain head trauma when they are left unattended on beds or sofas and subsequently fall to the floor. Parents who leave their young infants unattended are either frankly neglectful or innocently ignorant of the fact that infants are so mobile.

Because they are so inquisitive about their environments and because their motor coordination is not fully developed, toddlers frequently sustain CHT. The episode may be as trivial as tripping over one's own feet and striking the head on a piece of furniture or as serious as falling down a flight of steps because of improper supervision or safety measures at the entrance to the stairs.

Older children are motorically active: they enjoy riding tricycles, bicycles, jumping rope, climbing, and swinging. All of these normal activities can lead to CHT because of inattention on the child's part, faulty equipment, or environmental conditions. CHT can also occur during childhood altercations between peers.

As the children grow older, motor-vehicle accidents and assault become the most common causes of CHT. Motor-vehicle accidents can be pedestrian (child is struck by an automobile), vehicular-operator (child's bicycle is struck by an automobile), or vehicular-passenger (unrestrained child in an automobile that is in an accident hits head on automobile's interior).

Historical information to be elicited includes a description of the injury and whether the child lost consciousness, seized, vomited, or was confused, somnolent, or irritable after the injury. If the child is verbal, he should be asked about the episode to determine how much of it he remembers. If the child is preverbal, the parent should be asked if the child's injury was immediately followed by crying. A history of previous CHT, previous injuries or "accidents," and previous or current abuse should be sought. Also important to elicit is whether the child has hemophilia, an abnormality of the bones, or a ventriculo-peritoneal (VP) or ventriculoatrial (VA) shunt in place.

The physical examination should be complete and include a neurologic assessment. The entire skull and especially the site of the injury should be palpated carefully for hematomas or a depressed skull fracture. Areas of ecchymosis on the face and skull, such as blood below the eyes (racoon's sign) and behind the ears (Battle's sign), should be noted. The ear canals should be checked for the presence of blood, and the tympanic membrane should be visualized to determine if there is a collection of blood behind it. The nose should be checked for blood or a clear nonmucoid discharge, which may represent leaking CSF. The eyes should be checked for hemorrhages in the sclerae, subconjunctivae, anterior chambers (hyphema), and retinae. The rest of the child's physical examination should include an assessment of other signs of trauma or abuse. The neurologic examination should be appropriate to the child's age but should include an assessment of the child's sensorium and motoric abilities.

Sometimes children with CHT present to medical care in a somnolent or agitated state. Young children with mild CHT frequently vomit after the event and become sleepy, especially if it is their nap time or bedtime. Depending on the circumstances of their injuries, other children are very frightened and nearly hysterical. For these reasons, such a child should be observed over several hours in the emergency room with repeated measurements of his vital signs and selected repetition of his physical examination until the examiner satisfies himself that the child's examination is stable or improving.

A skull film is not usually indicated unless (1) a depression is palpated in the skull, (2) a VP/VA shunt is in place, (3) the child's condition is questionable or deteriorating, (4) the child is a hemophiliac, (5) the child seized or experienced prolonged unconsciousness, or (6) bony facial areas have been injured. In some of these cases, it may be more prudent to obtain a computed tomography (CT) scan rather than a skull film.

Most pediatric cases of CHT are mild; the children are normal at evaluation. Frequently, even in mild CHT, children may vomit and become sleepy because of the time of day or the excitement of the event, but they, too, usually have normal findings on physical examination. Occasionally, children briefly lose consciousness after CHT. This is a concussion, and although a concussion victim may be amnesic for certain details of the injury, he usually has otherwise normal examination findings. Children with linear skull fractures also are usually normal on examination. However, if the linear fracture is in the area of the temporal artery, careful observation is necessary. The child with a depressed skull fracture may be symptomatic (depending on the site of the fracture and the depth of the depression) or entirely asymptomatic. Finally, the child with worsening neurologic signs (change in level of consciousness, respirations, blood pressure, pulse, seizures, paresis,. etc.) must be suspected of having subarachnoid or subdural bleeding.

Mild CHT requires no specific therapy except, perhaps, careful observation of the child over the next few days. Most linear skull fractures and concussions also require no specific therapy. Depressed skull fractures may require surgical elevation. Intracranial bleeding may require surgical evacuation of the blood.

BIBLIOGRAPHY

Billmire ME, Myers PA: Serious head trauma in infants—Accident or abuse? Pediatrics 75:340–342, 1985

Dershewitz R et al: Treatment of children with posttraumatic transient loss of consciousness. Pediatrics 72:602–607, 1983

Leonidas J et al: Mild head trauma in children—When is a roentgenogram necessary? Pediatrics 69:139–143, 1982

Rosman NP: Pediatric emergencies—Managing acute head trauma. Contemp Pediatr 3:24–46

Singer H, Freeman J: Head trauma for the pediatrician. Pediatrics 62:819–824, 1978

92

Headache

Headache is a very common presenting complaint in pediatrics. Most children with occasional headaches are never seen by physicians because they are treated at home. However, children with recurrent headaches (usually older children and adolescents) are frequently seen by health professionals. The parents of these patients may be concerned that headaches are the result of a brain tumor, which is, in fact, an uncommon cause of headaches.

The history should reveal as much information about the headaches as possible. Where is the headache located? Is the headache more likely to occur on certain days or certain times of the day? How frequently do headaches occur and how long do they last? What precipitates them, and what makes them better? Are the headaches accompanied by fever, neck pain, photophobia, nausea, vomiting, or auras? Has the headache ever awakened the child from sleep? Does the child have a history of allergies, head trauma, head surgery, or seizures? Does the child use medications or illicit drugs? Which ones? Does the child have difficulties with vision, hearing, or chewing? Is the child subjected to noxious physical environmental stimuli or the stress at home,

school, or socially? Is there a family history of headaches, especially migraines?

The physical examination should be complete. Particular attention should be paid to assessments of the eyes, ears, teeth, tempomandibular joints, sinuses, the skull (looking for areas of tenderness, asymmetry, bruits, etc.), and the neurologic examination.

DIFFERENTIAL DIAGNOSIS

Frontal headaches are common during viral illnesses, especially if accompanied by high fever. In an older child or adolescent with respiratory symptoms, frontal headaches, and pain on palpation of the area above the eyebrows might indicate frontal sinusitis. If the individual has pain on palpation of the maxillary sinus area, with or without periorbital edema, maxillary sinusitis might be present. Encephalitis and meningitis can also cause severe headache; in addition to headache and fever, meningitis is also accompanied by positive Kernig's and Brudzinski's signs. Encephalitis is frequently associated with changes in the sensorium.

Headaches accompanied by facial pain or

temporal headaches might indicate caries, dental abscesses, bruxism, or middle ear disease.

Headaches localized to the temples or to the neck muscles, without other physical signs, might be attributable to stress, especially if they occur at times of emotionally charged situations. Children with headaches might also be depressed; other psychosomatic symptoms are frequently present. Certain drugs, especially amphetamines, may cause headaches. Depending on the drug, other symptoms, such as changes in mood or appetite, are usually present.

Allergic children may develop headaches if they come in contact with the offending allergens. Noxious environmental stimuli, such as cigarette smoke and paint fumes, can also cause headaches in susceptible individuals.

The diagnosis of migraine headaches is based on classic presentation, although younger children do not always demonstrate it. Migraine is suggested by a paroxysmal, unilateral headache, preceded by an aura, nausea, or vomiting. A family history of migraine is frequently seen. Younger children may present with abdominal pain, vomiting, and ataxia without the "classic" headache.

Headaches may be caused by increased intracranial pressure, such as with intracranial bleeds, brain abscesses, pseudotumor cerebri, and brain tumors. The headache of a brain tumor is usually more severe in the morning. Vomiting may relieve the pain. Diplopia and changes in mental status, mood, and motor and sensory function develop later.

Although children with cerebral aneurysms may have chronic headaches, a ruptured aneurysm is associated with a severe headache, followed by confusion and loss of consciousness as the subarachnoid bleed proceeds.

Miscellaneous causes of headaches include severe anemia, seizures, hypertension, hypoglycemia, hyperventilation, hypoxia, hypercapnia, carbon monoxide poisoning, and head trauma.

TREATMENT

Treatment of the headache is directed toward its cause. Most uncomplicated headaches will respond to mild analgesics. This is especially true of headaches associated with fever. Headaches related to bacterial infections (sinusitis, meningitis, purulent otitis media, and dental abscesses) will improve when the infection is brought under control. When headaches are caused by stress or depression, the underlying psychological cause must be sought and addressed. Children whose headaches are precipitated by allergens or noxious environmental stimuli will improve when they are separated from these substances. An episode of migraine headaches cannot be treated once it is firmly established. However, the use of propranolol has been successful in preventing episodes or in abating an episode if taken prophylactically or very early in the episode's course. Mass lesions in the brain or intracranial bleeding are usually treated surgically.

BIBLIOGRAPHY

Barabas G: Management of headaches in childhood. Pediatr Ann 12:806–813, 1983
Prensky A: Differentiating and treating pediatric headaches. Contemp Pediatr 1:12–45, 1984
Shinnar S, D'Souza B: Migraine in children and adolescents. Pediatr Rev 3:257–262, 1982

93

The Hypotonic Infant

At the turn of the century, physicians recognized only two categories of hypotonia in infants. Werdnig and Hoffmann described infants who usually succumbed by early childhood to an inexorable progression of muscular weakness. In contrast, Oppenheim coined the term *myotonia congenita* to describe infants with stable hypotonia. Over time, the former diagnosis has been refined into one of the best characterized neuromuscular diseases, whereas an understanding of the workings of the neuromuscular unit has rendered the latter diagnosis obsolete. Today the differential diagnosis of hypotonia in infancy often requires a sophisticated battery of tests to assess the structure and function of the various components of the neuromuscular unit. It is likely that continued basic and clinical research will modify the current list of diagnoses.

EVALUATION OF HYPOTONIA

Hypotonia (floppiness) is defined as abnormally decreased tension in resting muscle. When evaluating infants, it is important to be familiar with the normal variation of tone with ges-

tational and postnatal age. During the third trimester, there is a strikingly ordered acquisition of flexor tone, which begins in the lower extremities and continues cranially. Truncal tone increases as well. These changes in tone also occur postnatally in healthy premature infants. Thus, the normal muscle tone of an infant born at 28 weeks's gestation, when examined 2 weeks after birth, is quite decreased in comparison to full-term infants; by 12 weeks of age, if all goes well, reexamination might reveal term-equivalent tone. If so, that would provide excellent reassurance for continued normal neurodevelopment.

Cerebral disturbances and disorders of the neuromuscular unit (the motor neuron, peripheral nerve, neuromuscular junction, and muscle) can produce hypotonia. Consequently, hypotonia is not an uncommon symptom in infancy. A systematic evaluation should include the family, prenatal, and postnatal history. On occasion, examination of the parents or other family members may give clues to or confirm a diagnosis. For example, a diagnosis of congenital myotonic dystrophy is supported by a history of polyhydramnios and the finding of the typical myopathic facies in a parent. The older infant should undergo detailed developmental testing.

Evaluation continues with a careful physical examination. The distribution of hypotonia must be noted (generalized versus focal, proximal versus distal, lower versus upper extremities), in addition to its severity (mild, moderate, marked). A "spastic catch" felt upon repeated flexion–extension of an extremity points to a cerebral etiology. Since hypotonia is not synonymous with weakness, assessment of strength is important. This may be difficult in an infant, but is best determined by observing spontaneous and elicited movements. Abnormal muscular activity also should be noted; for instance, fasciculations are the hallmark of diseases of the motor neuron. These may be most obvious in unusual locations; in Werdnig-Hoffmann disease, fasciculations of the tongue are characteristic. Determination of muscle bulk may provide valuable information in older children but might be misleading in the infant. Other key points of the neurologic examination include descriptions of deep tendon reflexes and the function of cranial and sensory nerves.

Laboratory evaluation is often necessary to establish a precise diagnosis. One or more of the following tests may be indicated: examination of cerebrospinal fluid (CSF) for protein and cell count, muscle enzyme (creatine phosphokinase [CPK], serum glutamic oxaloacetic transaminase [SGOT]) assay, electromyogram (EMG), nerve conduction velocity studies (NCV), and muscle biopsy for histologic, histochemical, electron microscopic, and biochemical studies.

Elevation of the CSF protein concentration usually indicates peripheral nerve disease; occasionally, a mild pleocytosis may also be observed, especially in the early stages. CPK can be elevated for many reasons other than muscle disorders (for instance, from an intramuscular injection); however, it is typically slightly increased in some diseases of the motor neuron and markedly elevated with certain myopathies. A normal level does not exclude muscle disease.

The EMG is an important clinical tool. It is useful for distinguishing disorders of the anterior horn cell, peripheral nerve, and muscle, as well as for demonstrating myotonia (failure of muscle relaxation) and myasthenia (muscle fatigability). The EMG measures the electrical potentials of muscle with a needle electrode and records them on an oscilloscope. Activity of a motor unit (a motor neuron and the muscle fibers it innervates) generates a potential that can be characterized in terms of its amplitude, duration, frequency, and shape. The amplitude and duration of a motor unit potential are a function of the number of muscle fibers innervated by the motor neuron. The number of individual potentials observed is a function of the number of motor units (*i.e.*, the number of intact anterior horn cells). A typical EMG records electrical activity both at rest and during muscular contraction. Any sustained electrical activity during muscle relaxation is abnormal. Abnormal potentials may be either fasciculations (high amplitude, long duration) or fibrillations (low amplitude, short duration). The former are seen in motor neuron disease and result from the reinnervation of denervated muscle fibers by outgrowths of adjacent axons belonging to diseased but still viable neurons. Fibrillations originate from denervated muscle fibers and may be present in disorders of the motor neuron and peripheral nerve. With contraction, the amplitude and duration of potentials are increased in motor neuron disease (reinnervation increases the number of muscle fibers per motor neuron), normal to decreased in peripheral nerve disease, and often strikingly decreased in muscle disease. Myotonia results in prolonged but gradually decreasing electrical activity following a single stimulus. Myasthenia is evidenced by diminution of the amplitude of the potentials with repetitive stimulation.

Nerve conduction velocity is decreased in peripheral nerve disorders, but results must be interpreted using age-dependent norms. Occasionally, open nerve biopsy is indicated. Muscle biopsy is best performed using an open technique under local anesthesia. In general, affected muscle should be sampled in acute disorders whereas more healthy muscle should be biopsied in subacute or chronic diseases. A large enough specimen must be taken on the biopsy to permit electron microscopic or biochemical studies should routine histologic and histochemical techniques prove insufficient. In general, muscle biopsy differentiates denervating disorders from intrinsic myopathies on the basis of grouped versus nongrouped atrophy. In addition, the biopsy may be the sole means of discriminating among many different myopathies.

REPRESENTATIVE DISEASES

Cerebral causes of hypotonia

As a group, cerebral disturbances are the most common cause of hypotonia in infancy. Table 93-1 lists the more prevalent etiologies. Several features help differentiate hypotonia secondary to a cerebral disturbance from other causes of hypotonia. Often there is additional evidence of cerebral dysfunction. Seizures are an especially specific indicator of a cerebral etiology and commonly occur after severe asphyxia or during metabolic derangements. Neurodevelopment may be delayed because of structural central nervous system abnormalities, asphyxial insult, hypothyroidism, chromosomal disorders (*i.e.*, trisomy 21) or other syndromes (*i.e.*, Prader-Willi). Neurodevelopmental history reveals a loss of milestones with degenerative nervous system

Table 93–1. Central Causes of Hypotonia

Hypoxic–ischemic encephalopathy
Intraventricular or parenchymal hemorrhage
Developmental defects
Metabolic
  Electrolyte disturbances (*i.e.*, hyponatremia)
  Hypoglycemia
  Hypocalcemia, hypomagnesemia
  Hyperbilirubinemia
  Drug toxicity (*i.e.*, maternal sedation)
  Inborn errors of metabolism
    Urea cycle enzyme deficiencies
    Disorders of organic acid metabolism
    Disorders of amino acid metabolism
Infection
  Sepsis
  Meningitis, encephalitis
Hypothyroidism
Trauma
Degenerative encephalopathies
  Gray matter (*i.e.*, Tay-Sachs disease)
  White matter (*i.e.*, adrenoleukodystrophy)
Spinal cord disorders
  Developmental defects
  Trauma

diseases. Secondly, the hypotonia due to a cerebral disturbance is usually generalized and not very severe; significant weakness is uncommon. Finally, deep tendon reflexes are preserved and may be hyperactive because of a lack of normal cerebral inhibitory input.

Spinal cord disorders

Trauma to the cord (for instance, during a difficult vaginal delivery) and structural abnormalities (meningomyelocele) are two important causes of focal hypotonia in the newborn.

Disorders of the lower motor neuron: Werdnig-Hoffmann disease

Werdnig-Hoffmann disease is the most common cause of severe hypotonia in the neonate. When it presents at or shortly after birth, this disorder is almost always fatal by the time the child is several years of age. Inheritance is autosomal recessive. A history of decreased fetal movement or the presence of contractures at birth indicate onset *in utero*. The clinical appearance of affected infants is arresting. Hypotonia and weakness are marked. In the most severe cases, the lower extremities assume a "frog-leg" posture and the upper extremities are held in abduction with shoulder rotation (the so-called "jug-handle" position). The thoracic respiratory muscles are always affected; the chest may be sunken or bell-shaped. The diaphragm is relatively spared. Involvement of pharyngeal muscle causes problems with swallowing and airway protection. In contrast, facial and sphincter muscles are unaffected. Pertinent findings on neurologic examination include lack of deep tendon reflexes and, possibly, fine muscle tremors. CSF, CPK and NCV are normal. EMG reveals fasciculations and fibrillations at rest, and increased amplitude and duration but a decreased number of motor unit potentials. Muscle biopsy confirms grouped atrophy.

The usual causes of death are progressive respiratory insufficiency and complications of aspiration.

Disorders of the peripheral nerve

As a group, these are very uncommonly recognized in infancy. A clearly abnormal sensory examination, together with decreased NCVs, points to this category.

Disorders of the neuromuscular junction: transient myasthenia gravis

Transient myasthenia gravis presents in approximately 15% of all infants born to mothers with myasthenia and may occur even if the mother is in clinical remission. Onset always occurs by 3 days after birth. The initial symptom is poor feeding due to decreased sucking ability. Generalized weakness is common, and hypotonia can be severe. Facial diplegia occurs in more than half of affected infants, but ptosis is relatively uncommon in the neonate. The disease may affect the respiratory muscles. Deep tendon reflexes are normal. The diagnosis is usually obvious given the maternal history, although, on occasion, a symptomatic infant provides the first indication of maternal disease. Symptomatic improvement to a test dose of neostigmine (0.1 mg/kg IM) is diagnostic. EMG is usually unnecessary, but will show a decremental response to prolonged nerve stimulation. Infants generally require a short course of anticholinesterase therapy. Prognosis is excellent with timely diagnosis.

Infant botulism is a relatively recently described cause of neuromuscular junction derived hypotonia. Onset may be insidious. Constipation is often a prominent symptom. Lack of pupillary responses helps differentiate this disorder from the myasthenias. In addition, EMG shows an incremental response. Presence of a high concentration of botulinum toxin in the stool is diagnostic.

Disorders of muscle: congenital myotonic dystrophy

Infants affected with this autosomal dominant disorder are always born to mothers with myotonic dystrophy; however, as with transient neonatal myasthenia, birth of the infant may lead to recognition of previously unsuspected disease in the mother. There is no correlation between the severity of disease in mother and infant. On the other hand, the severity of illness in a previous sibling influences the severity in subsequent offspring. If one sibling had severe congenital myotonic dystrophy, risk of severe disease in a subsequent pregnancy is approximately 30%; with a history of mild disease in a previous sibling, this risk falls to 5%.

Polyhydramnios is a universal historical feature in all infants with severe congenital disease. The cause of polyhydramnios relates to *in utero* swallowing dysfunction. The disease is apparent within hours to days after birth. Hypotonia may be pronounced; usually, it occurs in a generalized distribution but may, on occasion, be more marked proximally than distally. Facial diplegia and a characteristic tenting of the upper lip are hallmarks. Feeding problems result from pharyngeal dysfunction, and possibly from gastric dysmotility as well. Weakness may be present in respiratory muscles, including the diaphragm. Contractures, especially in the lower extremities, may be present with severe disease. Deep tendon reflexes may be absent, an atypical finding in most myopathies.

Mortality averages 50%. Among survivors, feeding and respiratory problems tend to improve gradually. Myotonia, usually difficult to detect in the neonate, later becomes conspicuous. On follow-up, almost all patients have some degree of mental retardation; the reason for this is unknown.

The EMG confirms myotonia. Muscle biopsy in the newborn period is not by itself diagnostic; usually, immaturity of muscle elements is noted.

BIBLIOGRAPHY

Brooke MH, Carroll JE, Ringel SP: Congenital hypotonia revisited. Muscle Nerve 2:84–100, 1979

Peterson H: Diagnosis of hypotonia in children: Types, differential diagnosis, and management. Pediatr Ann 5:30–38, 1976

Lewis DW, Berman PH: Progressive weakness in infancy and childhood. Pediatr Rev 8:200–208, 1987

Schmickel RD: Clinical Genetics Conference: Progress in understanding muscle disease. J Pediatr 109:1071–1073, 1986

Volpe JJ: Neurology of the Newborn, 2nd ed. Philadelphia, WB Saunders, 1987

Part XV: Rheumatology

94

Pain in the Extremities

Complaints of extremity pain are extremely common in pediatrics. In some cases, the etiology of the pain will be obvious based on the history and physical examination, frequently identifying minor trauma as the cause of the pain. In many other cases, however, particularly those involving chronic or recurrent pain, significant diagnostic challenges may be presented to the examining physician. This chapter will provide a framework for the evaluation of the child with limb pain, discussing the history, the physical examination, and the multiple diagnostic categories that must be considered.

The history should first focus on the character of the pain—its location, intensity, timing (e.g., onset, constant versus intermittent), and quality (dull, throbbing, sharp, stabbing, etc.). Factors that alleviate or aggravate the pain should be identified. Associated features such as swelling, stiffness, limping, weakness, and fatigue should be sought. Evidence of systemic disease must be pursued through a careful review of systems, asking about such symptoms as fever, weight loss, abdominal pain, and rash. Then, complete past medical, family, and social histories should be obtained in search of further diagnostic clues.

The physical examination should include not only an evaluation of the extremities, but also a thorough general examination, looking for any evidence of systemic disease that might be related to the pain. All four extremities and the spine should be examined carefully. Then, attention may be focused specifically on the area of pain, evaluating for erythema, warmth, swelling, tenderness, range of motion, muscle strength, muscle atrophy, and bilateral symmetry. If the lower extremities are involved, the gait should be observed carefully. Every effort should be made to identify the specific anatomic structures involved.

With the data obtained in the history and physical examination a differential diagnosis may be formulated. This must be done prior to laboratory evaluation so that unnecessary tests are not ordered; in fact, in most cases no laboratory tests will be required. The first step in this process is to decide which anatomic structures are most likely to be involved (i.e., bone, ligaments, muscles, tendons, cartilage, joint capsule, and/or bursa). Then, one must consider what the most likely etiology for the pain in that specific structure might be. The following etiologic categories should be considered:

543

Trauma. Trauma is the most common cause of extremity pain. Although the history will usually lead one to this diagnosis, this may not always be the case in infants and young children. The diagnosis of child abuse must always be considered, particularly if the history provided is inconsistent with the type or severity of the injury noted.

Infection. Bacterial infections of bones, joints, and soft tissues are serious problems that require prompt diagnosis and intervention (see Chapter 27). Clues to these diagnoses on the physical examination may include fever, a toxic appearance, swelling, erythema, extreme tenderness, and limited mobility. It is also important to remember that many other infectious diseases may have associated limb pain, as with myalgias in influenza and the reactive arthritis that may accompany *Salmonella*, *Shigella*, and *Yersinia* enteritis.

Inflammatory Disorders. The broad category of inflammatory disorders includes inflammatory conditions involving joints, synovium, muscles, and vascular structures. Examples include rheumatoid arthritis, systemic lupus erythematosus, dermatomyositis, polyarteritis nodosa, allergic reactions, and rheumatic fever. Each of these diseases is accompanied by characteristic physical and laboratory findings, frequently with evidence of multisystem involvement. The most common of these will be discussed in subsequent chapters.

Orthopedic Disorders. A wide variety of congenital and acquired conditions are included in the category of orthopedic disorders, the most common of which are chondromalacia patella, slipped femoral epiphysis, osteochondrosis of the femoral capital epephysis (Legg-Calvé-Perthes disease), and Osgood-Schlatter disease.

Neoplasia. Both benign and malignant tumors of bone, cartilage, muscle, nerve, and vascular structures may present with limb pain. It should also be noted that other malignant neoplasms, particularly acute leukemias and metastatic neuroblastoma, frequently present with bone and/or joint pain.

Hematologic Diseases. Although limb pain may occur in any severe anemia, the severe, recurrent pain seen in vaso-occlusive bone crises in sickle cell disease is the best example of a hematologic cause of extremity pain.

Idiopathic. Two important diagnoses fall into the idiopathic category. Transient (toxic) synovitis of the hip is a relatively common disorder primarily affecting children between the ages of 18 months and 12 years. Unilateral hip pain with limited range of motion are the classic features. It is a transient condition that is frequently associated with an intercurrent viral illness. The major difficulty is the differentiation of this condition from septic arthritis of the hip; making this distinction requires careful clinical and laboratory evaluation.

Growing pains are extremely common causes of extremity pain, occurring in about 15% of all children. These pains are recurrent, occur primarily at night, commonly involve the thighs, calves, and popliteal region, and principally affect children in the preschool-aged group. The pain may vary greatly in duration and intensity. The diagnosis is made based on a consistent history in a child who is otherwise well and who displays no significant physical findings.

Psychogenic. Some children and adolescents will have recurrent extremity pain that is apparently psychogenic in origin. It is important that this possibility be kept in mind and that family and social stresses be explored in the history.

This list is certainly not complete but should serve to organize one's approach to the child with extremity pain. Once a differential diagnosis has been formulated, specific laboratory tests may be used to help confirm the diagnosis, document the extent of injury, and plan a therapeutic regimen. Tests that might be used include x-ray studies, blood counts, sedimentation rates, and other specific tests (*e.g.,* bone scan, rheumatoid factor, antinuclear antigen, bone marrow aspirate), when clinically indicated. In the great majority of cases, a diagnosis may be reached with a minimum of laboratory investigation.

BIBLIOGRAPHY

McCarthy PL, Wasserman D, Spiezel SZ et al: Evaluation of arthritis and arthralgia in the pediatric patient. Clin Pediatr 19:184, 1980

Oster J, Nielson A: Growing pains. Acta Paediatr Scand 61:329, 1972

Passo MH: Aches and limb pain. Pediatr Clin North Am 29:209, 1982

Peterson HA: Leg aches. Pediatr Clin North Am 24:731, 1977

95

Juvenile Rheumatoid Arthritis

Juvenile rheumatoid arthritis (JRA) refers to a group of disorders characterized by chronic synovitis in childhood. There are estimated to be about 250,000 children in the United States with JRA. The cause of JRA is as yet unknown, although many theories have been proposed implicating infectious agents, immunologic abnormalities, and environmental stress. Several distinct subgroups of JRA have been defined that differ in terms of the pattern and severity of the arthritis, the degree of systemic (extra-articular) disease, and the age and sex ratios of affected patients.

Pathologically, affected joints are characterized by inflammation of the synovium, with hypertrophy, fibrinoid necrosis, and monocytic infiltration. Increased amounts of joint fluid are produced, commonly containing cell counts between 10,000 and 100,000 mm^3, consisting predominantly of polymorphonuclear leukocytes. Clinically, these affected joints are swollen, warm, painful, frequently limited in mobility, and, at times, erythematous. The inflammatory process is by definition chronic in nature, and over time there may be destruction of other joint structures. Prevention of permanent joint changes is a major goal of therapy.

In addition to joint involvement, it is important to remember that JRA may involve many other organ systems. As will be seen in the following discussion, common extra-articular manifestations of JRA include iridocyclitis, rash, fever, anemia, leukocytosis, lymphadenopathy, hepatosplenomegaly, and polyserositis.

As noted, several reasonably distinct subgroups of JRA have been defined by the American Rheumatism Association and others (Table 95-1). The major initial distinction is based on the number of joints involved: *pauciarticular* disease involves four or fewer joints, whereas *polyarticular* disease involves five or more joints. The following discussion will further define these subgroups, focusing

Table 95–1. Subgroups of JRA

Subgroup	% of patients
Systemic-Onset Disease	20
Polyarticular Disease	
Rheumatoid factor negative	25
Rheumatoid factor positive	10
Pauciarticular Disease	
Early childhood onset	25
Late childhood onset	15

on patterns of joint involvement, common extra-articular manifestations, and useful laboratory parameters.

SYSTEMIC-ONSET DISEASE

About 20% of children with JRA will present with an acute febrile illness, characterized by high intermittent fevers, an evanescent rash seen most commonly during temperature elevations, and multiple systemic manifestations, including lymphadenopathy, hepatosplenomegaly, anemia, leukocytosis, and polyserositis (pleuritis and pericarditis). Musculoskeletal complaints in systemic-onset JRA initially may consist only of arthralgias, myalgias, and transient arthritis. The systemic manifestations may go on for several months before resolving, to be followed in most patients by the development of some degree of chronic polyarthritis. Some patients will have more than one attack of systemic disease. Needless to say, making the diagnosis of JRA during this period of predominantly extra-articular disease may be most difficult, since signs and symptoms may mimic many viral illnesses and, at times, even malignancy.

This subgroup of JRA is seen slightly more commonly in males than in females. Both large and small joints may be affected, and about 25% of children will go on to develop severe, destructive arthritis. The disease may occur at any age, with a median age of onset of 5 years. Patients generally are seronegative for both antinuclear antibodies (ANA) and rheumatoid factors (RF).

POLYARTICULAR JRA

In polyarticular JRA, there is polyarticular arthritis without prominent systemic disease. About one-third of children with JRA fall into this category. Most experts agree that this subgroup may be further divided into two distinct subsets, based on the presence or absence of rheumatoid factor in the serum.

Seronegative (RF-negative) polyarticular JRA, accounting for about 25% of patients with JRA, may have its onset at any time during childhood. Females are predominantly affected. There is commonly a symmetrical polyarthritis involving both large and small joints. The ANA is positive in about 25% of patients. Systemic manifestations, most commonly fevers and mild anemia, may occur in some patients but are usually not a prominent feature. Although the arthritis is usually chronic and may produce significant distress for the child, fortunately, the response to therapy is generally quite good, and only 10% to 15% of patients will develop significant joint destruction.

Seropositive (RF-positive) polyarticular disease also predominantly affects females with a symmetrical polyarthritis of both small and large joints. Otherwise, however, this subset, accounting for about 10% of patients, is quite unique. In many ways, it is the childhood equivalent of classic adult rheumatoid arthritis, with severe destructive joint disease in a majority of patients in spite of therapy. Subcutaneous rheumatoid nodules commonly develop over pressure points (*e.g.*, elbow, heel, knuckles, extensor surfaces of fingers), and evidence of rheumatoid vasculitis occasionally may be seen. Onset is usually after the age of 8. In addition to high titers of rheumatoid factors, about 75% of patients will have a positive test for antinuclear antibodies, and a strong association with HLA-DR4 has recently been described.

PAUCIARTICULAR JRA

As noted, *pauciarticular* is the term used to describe disease involving four or fewer joints.

Occasional patients may have more than four affected joints but still be considered in this category based on other diagnostic criteria. Large joints are most commonly involved in an asymmetrical distribution. As with polyarticular JRA, it appears that there are at least two distinct subsets of patients with pauciarticular disease.

The first subset comprises about 25% of all children with JRA and is characterized by onset in early childhood, a high risk of iridocyclitis, a positive ANA in over 50% of patients, and a negative RF. Girls are predominantly affected, and most will develop disease before the age of 5. The knees, ankles, and elbows are most commonly involved, and very few patients go on to develop destructive joint changes. Although systemic complaints are overall unusual, about 50% of patients will develop iridocyclitis at some point. The eye disease may be insidious and display few symptoms until scarring has already occurred. Only through frequent slit lamp examinations will diagnosis be made early enough to prevent permanent damage. Consequently, most experts agree that a routine slit lamp examination should be performed by an ophthamologist four times a year for the first 10 years of the disease.

The second subset of pauciarticular JRA accounts for the final 15% of patients. It is characterized by later onset (generally, after age 8), male predominance, negative ANA and RF, a strong association with HLA-B27 (75% of patients), and predominant involvement of the joints of the lower extremities, including the hips. Many patients also will develop sacroiliac involvement, and some will have progression of the disease to the lumbar and thoracic spines, fulfilling criteria for the diagnosis of ankylosing spondylitis. Iridocyclitis may occur but is much less common than in early onset pauciarticular disease. Of note, a positive family history for ankylosing spondylitis, Reiter's syndrome, psoriasis, or inflammatory bowel disease is often found in these patients.

DIAGNOSIS

The diagnosis of JRA requires that three major criteria be fulfilled:

1. Onset during childhood.
2. Presence of arthritis on a chronic basis, generally considered to be greater than 6 weeks in duration (objective signs of synovitis, such as swelling, warmth, or erythema, must be present to fulfill this criterion).
3. Other conditions that may cause childhood arthritis must be excluded.

While these criteria may seem relatively straightforward, the diagnosis of JRA actually may be a most difficult task. The initial presentation may take a variety of forms and may not even include prominent joint disease, as in the subgroup with systemic onset. Even more important, the differential diagnosis of childhood arthritis is quite large, and before the diagnosis of JRA can be made the physician must rule out conditions such as acute rheumatic fever, septic arthritis, trauma, malignancy, the arthritis of inflammatory bowel disease, and numerous other rheumatic diseases, including systemic lupus erythematosus, psoriatic arthritis, and Reiter's syndrome. Distinguishing among these diseases requires a careful history and physical examination, searching specifically for features that might be associated with each diagnosis, and judicious use of the clinical laboratory.

Unfortunately, there are no specific laboratory tests for the diagnosis of JRA. The association of rheumatoid factors, antinuclear antibodies, and particular histocompatibility types with the various subgroups of JRA was described previously; while these are useful means of classifying patients, they are not specific and must be used with caution. Likewise, radiographs, blood counts, complement studies, sedimentation rates, and synovial fluid analyses are neither sensitive nor specific for the diagnosis of JRA, although they may be of tremendous help in excluding other conditions (*e.g.,* culture of synovial fluid to rule out septic arthritis).

THERAPY

The goals of therapy in JRA are to help the child to achieve as normal a life-style as possible, to prevent permanent joint (or eye) damage, and to minimize toxicity from the medications used. Successful achievement of these goals requires an understanding of the disease process and an ongoing assessment of the severity of joint involvement, the degree of joint destruction, the child's overall level of function, and the response to therapy, as well as an understanding of the impact that a chronic disease may have on a child and the family.

Anti-inflammatory agents, primarily salicylates, are the primary agents used to treat joint inflammation. Although it may take weeks to months to see their full effect, salicylates will adequately control the inflammatory process in the majority of cases, particularly in those patients in the seronegative polyarticular and pauciarticular subgroups. A number of other nonsteroidal anti-inflammatory drugs are available that appear to be comparable to salicylates in efficacy. For patients with severe disease that is unresponsive to these agents, usually among those with seropositive polyarthritis or systemic onset disease, therapy with gold salts, penicillamine, antimalarial agents, and, rarely, corticosteroids, may be added. Chronic iridocyclitis usually will be controlled using topical steroid therapy, although systemic steroids may at times be required.

In addition to pharmacologic therapy, management should include aggressive physical and occupational therapy to maximize musculoskeletal function. Orthopedic consultation may be required if joint deformity has been incurred. Psychological support should be provided throughout the illness, and children should be encouraged to lead as normal a life-style as possible. In most cases, there is reason to be optimistic because up to 80% of children with JRA will incur no serious disability as a result of the disease.

BIBLIOGRAPHY

Baum J: Treatment of juvenile arthritis. Hosp Pract September: 121, 1983

Brewer EJ, Bass J et al: Current proposed revision of JRA criteria. Arthritis Rheum 20:195, 1977

Brewer EJ, Gedalia A: The child with joint pain: An algorithmic approach. Contemp Pediatr 2:18, 1985

Cassidy JT: Treatment of children with juvenile rheumatoid arthritis. N Eng J Med, 314:1312, 1986

Schaller, JG: Juvenile rheumatoid arthritis. Pediatr Rev 2:163, 1980

96

Systemic Lupus Erythematosus

Systemic lupus erythematosus (SLE) is a systemic autoimmune disorder that may have its onset either in childhood or adulthood. The disease is characterized by the formation of a variety of autoantibodies, particularly to nuclear components, with multisystem damage due to the deposition of antigen–antibody complexes in tissues and in vessel walls. Although the etiology is as yet unknown, evidence suggests that the disease may be the result of a viral infection (or possibly other environmental stress) in a genetically predisposed host.

About one-third of cases of SLE present before the age of 20, most commonly during the teenage years. Presentation before the age of 5 is unusual. The overall prevalence of SLE in children is not well established, but it is estimated to be about one-tenth as common as juvenile rheumatoid arthritis. There is a marked female predominance at all ages, although the ratio of 9:1, as seen in teenagers and adults, falls to 3:1 or 4:1 in children under 12.

CLINICAL MANIFESTATIONS

Because the antigen–antibody complexes formed in SLE may be deposited in practically

any body tissue, the disease may present with a wide array of signs and symptoms. The American Rheumatism Association has developed criteria for the diagnosis of SLE, requiring that four of the 11 features listed in Table 96-1 be present, either serially or simultaneously, in order to make the diagnosis. As can be seen from this list, a high index of suspicion may be needed to make the diagnosis of SLE, particularly in its early stages, since many of the signs and symptoms may mimic those of other diseases.

In children, the most common presenting signs of SLE are fever, rash, arthritis, weight loss, and fatigue. The rash may take many forms, but in about half of patients, it will have a typical malar distribution, and photosensitivity will be described in about 40%. Other patients may have a characteristic discoid rash, appearing as erythematous raised lesions, frequently with keratotic scarring. The arthritis of SLE most commonly involves multiple peripheral joints and is generally nondestructive in nature.

Over time, up to 90% of children with SLE will develop renal involvement, characterized by proteinuria, hematuria, and the presence of casts in the urine. The majority of these patients will have a diffuse proliferative lesion

Table 96–1. Criteria for Diagnosis of SLE

Malar rash
Discoid rash
Photosensitivity
Oral ulcers
Arthritis
Serositis
   Pleuritis
   Pericarditis
Renal disorder
   Proteinuria
   Cellular casts
Neurologic disorder
   Seizures
   Psychosis
Hematologic disorder
   Hemolytic anemia
   Leukopenia
   Lymphopenia
   Thrombocytopenia
Immunologic disorder
   Positive LE preparation
   Anti-DNA (antibody to native DNA)
   Anti-Sm (antibody to Sm nuclear antigen)
   False-positive serologic test for syphilis
Antinuclear antibody

on renal biopsy. Renal function thus must be followed very carefully, with regular quantitations of protein excretion and creatinine clearance. In addition, hypertension will frequently accompany the renal disease of SLE, particularly in those patients on chronic steroid therapy.

Hematologic abnormalities are also extremely common in children with SLE, occurring in some form in the vast majority of patients. Leukopenia is seen in over half of cases, while a positive Coombs' test result and autoimmune thrombocytopenia may each occur in about one-third of cases. In addition, about one-fourth of patients will develop circulating anticoagulants with resultant clotting abnormalities.

Cardiopulmonary involvement may occur in up to 60% of all children with SLE. Pulmonary manifestations include pneumonitis and hemorrhage, serious complications that remain major causes of death in SLE patients. Cardiac abnormalities include pericarditis, myocarditis, and atherosclerotic heart disease as well as milder problems such as nonspecific heart murmurs and electrocardiographic (ECG) changes.

Central nervous sytem (CNS) involvement is also reported in over 50% of patients. Seizures, psychosis, strokes, and chorea are all possible manifestations. Other abnormalities, such as depression and anxiety, are frequently encountered and may be very difficult to differentiate from a functional disorder.

While these are the major clinical manifestations of SLE in children, other minor abnormalities are also extremely common. Lymphadenopathy, hepatosplenomegaly, and elevated liver function values are frequently present, indicating involvement of the reticuloendothelial system. Gastrointestinal manifestations include episodes of severe, intercurrent abdominal pain, most likely the result of vasculitis and/or serositis.

LABORATORY FINDINGS

In addition to the hematologic abnormalities described previously, children with SLE commonly manifest a variety of other laboratory abnormalities. All patients have circulating antinuclear antibodies, usually present in high titers and with specific patterns. Antibodies to native (double-stranded) DNA are highly specific for SLE and serve as useful markers of disease activity. Antibodies to the Sm antigen (a nuclear antigen separate from DNA) also are quite specific for SLE but are present only in a minority of patients. The LE preparation is positive in about 70% of patients but has largely been replaced by these more sensitive and specific tests.

A major mechanism of tissue injury in SLE occurs by means of complement activation secondary to immune complex deposition. Consequently, low levels of serum C3 and C4 are nearly always present in active lupus. These measures are useful diagnostically but are of even more value in monitoring disease activity. It is critical to remember, however, that certain inherited complement deficiencies may present with a lupus-like syndrome. Thus, a CH5O assay should also be performed (as a screening test for the absence of any complement components) in children with manifestations of SLE.

In addition to these highly specialized tests, other more basic tests, such as routine blood counts, urinalyses, and tests of renal function should be regularly performed. Patients with SLE are also particularly susceptible to a variety of infections, because of both the disease process and the immunosuppressive therapy used, and any evidence of infectious illness must be pursued with appropriate tests.

TREATMENT

The goals of therapy in SLE are to control inflammation, to suppress production of auto-antibodies, to promote normal growth and development, and to encourage as normal a life-style as possible, while at the same time making every effort to minimize toxic side effects from the medications used. Attaining these goals may be extremely difficult, and all children with SLE deserve referral to a specialist who has expertise in the diagnosis and management of this complex disease.

The first step in planning a therapeutic regimen is to determine the extent and severity of the disease, paying particular attention to possible renal involvement. As noted, antibody titers to DNA and serum complement levels are useful markers of disease activity. For patients with renal or other major organ involvement, corticosteroids are the mainstay of therapy. Although ideal dosage regimens have not been established, most experts recommend high initial doses to control active disease quickly, followed by a taper to the lowest possible dose. Patients must be monitored closely for flares in their disease, which will usually respond to a pulse of high-dose therapy. Unfortunately, the side effects of this chronic steroid therapy may be very serious, particularly in a growing child, making the disease seem even more difficult to manage in many cases.

Some patients with mild disease and no major organ involvement may be managed successfully with nonsteroidal anti-inflammatory agents such as aspirin or with antimalarials such as hydroxychloroquine. Conversely, a few patients will require immunosuppressive therapy (e.g., azothioprine, cyclophosphamide) because their disease remains under poor control on high-dose steroids or because steroid side effects have become unacceptably severe.

Hypertension is a common complication of SLE, and its control may require an aggressive medication regimen. Infections must be carefully and aggressively managed. Then, in addition to these pharmacologic modes of therapy, treatment of patients with SLE must include psychological support, as well as attention of diet and exercise, encouraging as much normal activity as possible.

PROGNOSIS

The prognosis for children with SLE has improved considerably over the last two decades. Once considered to be a rapidly fatal disorder in over half of all patients, current statistics show a 5-year survival rate of about 90% and a 10-year rate of 80%. Leading causes of death are renal failure, CNS disease, infection, and pulmonary lupus. Improved survival is most likely the result of a combination of factors, including earlier diagnosis, more careful monitoring, improved supportive care, and increased availability of dialysis and renal transplantation. Thus, while SLE should still be considered a severe, chronic, multisystem disorder, the prognosis is favorable in most patients.

BIBLIOGRAPHY

Rothfield N: Systemic lupus erythematosus. Pediatr Ann 11:397, 1982

Schaller J: Lupus in childhood. Clin Rheum Dis 8:219, 1982

Szer IS: The diagnosis and management of systemic lupus erythematosus in childhood. Pediatr Ann 15:596, 1986

Tan EM, Cohen AS, Fries JF et al: The 1982 revised criteria for the classification of systemic lupus erythematosus. Arthritis Rheum 25:1271, 1982

Appendix

Writing Orders

While entire books have been written on the subject of the medical record, very little attention has been devoted to the writing of medical orders. In fact, most physicians receive the sum total of their formal instruction in the art of order writing from an intern or resident during their first night on duty as a medical student. Although this system generally works, primarily because an intricate system of checks and balances is in place in most hospitals (*e.g.*, nursing, pharmacy), errors in medical orders remain frequent causes of mishaps in patient care. Such errors are, in fact, responsible for a substantial proportion of all malpractice suits against physicians.

The practice of writing orders is fairly simple as long as certain rules are followed. All orders should be clearly and explicitly stated. The importance of writing legibly cannot be emphasized strongly enough, particularly regarding medications and dosages. Each order should be dated, timed, and signed by the responsible physician. If an error is noted in an order, it should be crossed out with a single line and initialed by the physician. If an order must be canceled, this should be explicitly written as a separate order.

It is very helpful to establish a routine for writing admission orders. Although no particular format is critical, such a routine will help to ensure that no important measures are overlooked. An example of one commonly used scheme is as follows:

1. Admit to . . .
   - Specify ward and attending physician
2. Diagnosis
   - In this era of DRGs, the admitting diagnosis as stated on the order sheet is critically important. Be explicit! (*e.g.*, status asthmaticus versus asthma, diabetic ketoacidosis versus diabetes)
3. Condition
4. Allergies
5. Vital signs
   - Be specific; "per routine" is unacceptable
6. Activity
   - *e.g.*, Bed rest, bathroom privileges
7. Special nursing measures
   - *e.g.*, Daily weights, strict intake and output, respiratory isolation
8. Diet
9. Intravenous fluids

- Include fluid type, electrolyte content, and specific rate of administration
10. Medications
    - Be careful!
    - Write clearly and pay close attention to details like decimal points and units (*e.g.*, microgram versus milligram)
    - The route of administration (*e.g.*, IV, IM, PO, etc.) and the dosing interval must be clearly stated (*note:* tid does not necessarily equal q8 hours—decide what you really want the patient to receive)
    - For certain drugs, such as antibiotics and chemotherapeutic agents, the patient's weight and/or body surface area should be included on the order sheet along with the specific calculations used in arriving at a final doseage (*e.g.*, 200 mg/kg/day $\times$ 10 kg = 500 mg IV q6 hours)
    - PRN orders should be used judiciously with detailed indications for their use
11. Laboratory tests
    - Detail all tests and x-rays needed
12. NHO
    - These letters stand for "notify house officer" and may be used at your discretion; examples of commonly used NHO orders include:
        —NHO for temperature greater than 38°C—NHO for BP systolic greater than 140 mm Hg or BP diastolic greater than 90 mm Hg

This basic outline will generally stand up to even the toughest admission procedure. Specific components will be used to add to or change orders during the course of the hospital stay. Be careful to review standing orders on a daily basis. Finally, when an order is questioned by a nurse, pharmacist, therapist, or other physician, listen carefully because their checks and balances are critical to safe and effective patient management.

Index

Page numbers followed by *f* indicate figures; *t* following a page number indicates tabular material.